S0-BYI-723

Sterile Dosage Forms

Their Preparation and Clinical Application

Sterile Dosage Forms

Their Preparation and Clinical Application

Salvatore Turco, M.S., Pharm. D., F.A.S.H.P.

Professor of Pharmacy
Temple University School of Pharmacy
Philadelphia, Pennsylvania

4th Edition

Lea & Febiger

PHILADELPHIA · BALTIMORE · HONG KONG
LONDON · MUNICH · SYDNEY · TOKYO

A WAVERLY COMPANY
1994

Lea & Febiger
Box 3024
200 Chester Field Parkway
Malvern, Pennsylvania 19355-9725
U.S.A.
(215) 251-2230

Executive Editor — Michael Brown
Development Editor — Fran Klass
Project/Manuscript Editor — Jessica Howie Martin
Production Manager — Michael DeNardo

The use of portions of the text of The United States Pharmacopeia, Twenty-second Revision, official July 1, 1990, is by permission received from the Board of Trustees of The United States Pharmacopeial Convention, Inc. The said Convention is not responsible for any inaccuracy of quotation, or for any false or misleading implication that may arise by reason of the separation of excerpts from the original context.

Turco, Salvatore J.
    Sterile dosage forms: their preparation and clinical application
/ Salvatore Turco.—4th ed.
        p.   cm.
    Includes bibliographical references and index.
    ISBN 0-8121-1617-8
    1. Solutions (Pharmacy)—Sterilization. 2. Parenteral therapy.
I. Title.
    [DNLM: 1. Infusions, Parenteral. 2. Sterilization. 3. Dosage
Forms. 4. Drug Compounding. QV 778 T933s 1993]
RS201.S6T87 1994
615′.6—dc20
DNLM/DLC
for Library of Congress   93-24458
                                                                                CIP

First Edition, 1974
Second Edition, 1979
Third Edition, 1987

NOTE: Although the author(s) and the publisher have taken reasonable steps to ensure the accuracy of the drug information included in this text before publication, drug information may change without notice and readers are advised to consult the manufacturer's packaging inserts before prescribing medications.

Reprints of chapters may be purchased from Lea & Febiger in quantities of 100 or more. Contact Sally Grande in the Sales Department.

Copyright © 1994 by Lea & Febiger. Copyright under the International Copyright Union. All Rights Reserved. This book is protected by copyright. No part of it may be reproduced in any manner or by any means without written permission from the publisher.

PRINTED IN THE UNITED STATES OF AMERICA

Print number: 5 4 3 2 1

Preface

Since publication of the third edition of this book, interest in parenteral dosage forms has continued unabated. Over 320 million low-volume parenterals (LVPs) and over 100 million piggyback containers are used annually in the U.S. The proliferation of new parenteral antibiotics, chemotherapeutic agents, and other drugs has brought about widespread hospital use of parenterals.

Electronic mechanical equipment is now commonplace in hospitals. Its use and sophistication continue to increase. Newly designed electronic pumps have been developed for ambulatory use. Multi-electronic pumps have become available for multiple-drug infusion. Over 500,000 implantable infusion ports have been implanted into patients, and 100,000 new patients receive these implantable ports each year. New I.V. drug delivery systems have been introduced and are constantly evolving. Since the last edition, patient-controlled analgesia (PCA) is commonplace in medical centers. This technology allows the patient with pain to control the degree of analgesia. Although the National Coordinating Committee on Large Volume Parentrals (NCCLVPs) has been disbanded, (its work completed), many of its recommendations, such as I.V. admixture programs and I.V. teams, have been implemented. Particulate matter (PM) associated with parenteral products has been reduced, and the concepts associated with it are now well understood by manufacturers and clinicians. The use of parenteral nutrition (PN) has also increased.

PN in hospitals has been paralleled by home PN programs. Many patients, such as those with infectious and neoplastic diseases, administer PN to themselves at home. Growth in this area continues.

Centralized I.V. admixture programs are administered in more than 85% of all hospitals in the U.S. More stringent and complete guidelines for the preparation of parenterals by hospital pharmacists have been published. These guidelines, which will become recommendations in the near future, are a testament to the importance of parenteral preparation in the institutional setting. Packaging of parenterals has also undergone dramatic changes. Prefilled, premixed, prefrozen parenterals are now supplied, and newly designed plastic minibags (e.g., Add-Vantage) have been introduced. Premixed liquids (e.g., antibiotics, theophylline, heparin, lidocaine, dopamine) have become available. Multiple-dose containers (maxivials) have been developed to accommodate new methods of preparation of parenterals. Pharmaceutical manufacturers responded to the needs of pharmacists by addressing the packaging, labeling, and design needs required to facilitate patient care. The parenteral drug industry continues its efforts to meet higher standards of quality and to ensure the availability of sterile and particulate-free products.

A revolution in biotechnology of parenteral drugs has occurred. As of this writing, 14 bioengineered parenteral pharmaceuticals have been approved for clinical use, over 20 are awaiting final approval, and 120 are in phase III trials. Investigational new drugs (INDs) have been submitted for over 3200 products.

As we noted in the three previous editions, an information gap exists between those who manufacture sterile products and those who routinely prepare, dispense, and administer these products. We hope that this text will continue to narrow this gap by giving both groups a better understanding of what each must accomplish to achieve the best in patient care. Perhaps new insights into problem areas can be gained if those involved become better informed about the technology and requirements of others in the field. The answers to problems may exist in the application of knowledge we already possess. The pharmaceutical industry in the United States has become a 50-billion-dollar industry with multi-billion dollar companies that market billion-dollar drugs. And the growth continues unabated.

We acknowledge with sincere thanks the generous help received from our colleagues, Clyde Buchanan, Elaine P. Mackowiak, Murray M. Tuckerman, John D. Grabenstein, Faye Cosentino, and Stuart Feldman, and the pharmaceutical companies who supplied photographs for this text.

Philadelphia, PA   Salvatore J. Turco

Contributors

Gayle A. Brazeau
   Assistant Professor of Pharmaceutics
   University of Florida
   College of Pharmacy
   Gainesville, Florida

Clyde Buchanan, M.S.
   Director, Pharmaceutical Services
   Emory University Hospital
   Atlanta, Georgia

Faye Cosentino, R.N., B.S., C.R.N.I.
   Director of IV Therapy, *Retired*
   Laurence Hospital
   Bronxsville, New York

Stuart Feldman, Ph.D.
   Dean and Professor of Pharmaceutics
   University of Georgia
   College of Pharmacy
   Athens, Georgia

John D. Grabenstein, Ed.M., M.S., F.A.S.H.P.
   Major, United States Army Pharmacy Service
   Walter Reed Army Medical Center
   Washington, D.C.

Elaine D. Mackowiak, Ph.D.
   Professor of Pharmaceutical Chemistry
   Temple University
   School of Pharmacy
   Philadelphia, PA

Murray M. Tuckerman, Ph.D.
   Professor Emeritus of Pharmaceutical Chemistry
   Temple University
   School of Pharmacy
   Philadelphia, PA

Contents

CHAPTER

Introduction

Receiving medication by injection is an experience now common to all age groups. The advantages afforded by parenteral administration of drugs are well recognized by all medical practitioners. It is estimated that 40% of all drugs administered in hospitals are in the form of an injection. In some hospitals, the percentage of injectables is greater than 40%. Over 350 million units of large-volume parenteral solutions are used annually in U.S. hospitals. Market surveys indicate that over one billion disposable plastic syringes are used annually in American hospitals.

The sales of large-volume parenterals are approaching the one billion dollar mark. In 1976, infusion devices accounted for $185 million in sales. Such sales amounted to $585 million in 1982. By 1988, device sales were expected to account for over one billion dollars.[1] New innovations in drug therapy, systems, and packaging will force increased growth. Health care costs in the United States are approaching the one trillion dollar mark.

The term "parenteral" is applied to preparations administered by injection through one or more layers of skin tissue. The word is derived from the Greek words *para* and *enteron*, meaning outside of intestine, and is used for dosage forms administered by routes other than the oral route.

History of Parenteral Medication

The wide acceptance of parenteral drug therapy is the result of developments in many disciplines.[2-4] Early man's observation of insect bites and snake bites suggested to him that substances could be introduced into the body by puncture of the skin. Following the description of blood circulation in 1616 by William Harvey, English physician and physiologist, the possibility of intravenous injection of drugs gradually evolved. Harvey believed that death from the bite of a poisonous snake occurs because the poison is absorbed by the veins and circulated through the body. In 1665, Sir Christopher Wren

1

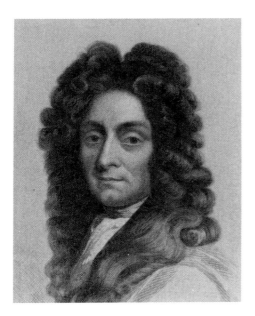

Figure 1–1. Christopher Wren (1632–1732), architect and astronomer, was the first person to inject medication into a dog's vein. (Courtesy of Free Library of Philadelphia and Wyeth-Ayerst Laboratories, Philadelphia, PA.)

(Fig. 1–1), professor of astronomy at Oxford and later to become a well-recognized architect, successfully put a dog to sleep by injecting opium into a vein of its hind leg by means of a quill attached to an animal bladder. The procedure was later performed in humans, using for injection opium, the so-called purging drugs, and water (Fig. 1–2). With crude apparatus, absence of pure drugs, and no knowledge of aseptic technique, the practice fell into disrepute. During the following two centuries, intravenous injections were primarily used in animal experimentation. With time, the observations gained from these experiences made a contribution to the concept of parenteral therapy.

Late in the eighteenth century, Edward Jenner used intradermal administration to perform his method of vaccination against smallpox. Various attempts at subcutaneous administration followed. In 1836, Lafarque, a French surgeon, punctured skin with a surgical lancet dipped in morphine to treat neuralgia. Francis Rynd, an Irish surgeon, dissolved morphine in creosote and introduced this solution under the skin in 1844. Sir Alexander Wood of Edinburgh used an instrument for injecting morphine through the skin and described it as "subcutaneous." The term "hypodermic" was coined by Charles Hunter, an English physician, who used an instrument similar to that employed by Wood. Hunter has been given the credit for recognizing subcutaneous injection as an effective route for the systemic absorption of a drug.[5,6] Charles-Gabriel Pravaz, a French surgeon, introduced a plunger-type syringe (Fig. 1–3) in 1853. In tracing the development of the hypodermic syringe, Van Itallie's study makes it evident that the present style of the syringe developed through the work of many men, no one man inventing the instrument (Fig. 1–4).[7] By 1860, subcutaneous therapy was practiced with the limited drugs available, but infections from the nonsterile devices and solutions were commonplace.

◆§(2)§◆
Delineatio Inſtrumenti Infuſorii,

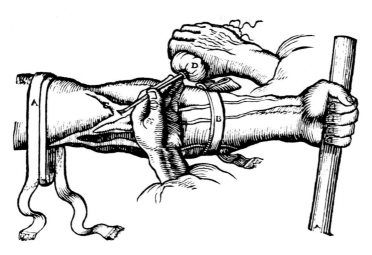

Figure 1–2. Intravenous injection into a man's arm, as illustrated in Latin treatise *Chirurgia Infusoria* by Johann Daniel Taylor (1634–1693). First ligature (A); second ligature (B); place for inserting instrument (C); and animal bladder holding liquid (D). (Courtesy of National Library of Medicine and Wyeth-Ayerst Laboratories, Philadelphia, PA.)

The observations of Pasteur and Lister pointing to the importance of aseptic technique did not immediately change the practical aspects of parenteral therapy. The materials used in fabricating the syringes did not lend themselves to satisfactory sterilization by heat, and the solutions frequently were heat labile. By 1880, it had become the practice of physicians to prepare their injections at time of use from tablet triturates. Uniform quantities of the drugs were molded into small tablets with sodium chloride or gelatin as the diluting material. The tablets were dissolved by warming them in water in a teaspoon prior to injection, then taking the solution up into the syringe. Although this practice resulted in uniform dosage and active solutions, no contribution was made toward the sterility of the injection.

By the 1890s, the medical literature was noting the importance of sterilizing both the syringe and the solutions. Progress had been made in the use of

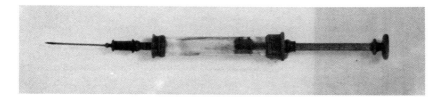

Figure 1–3. Metal (probably German silver) and glass syringe made in Philadelphia by Gemrig and Co. in 1857. The plunger's frictional surface is leather. (Courtesy of Mütter Museum and Wyeth-Ayerst Laboratories, Philadelphia, PA.)

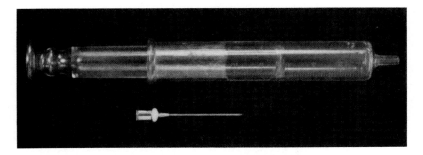

Figure 1–4. The Luer syringe was invented in 1896 in Paris by Karl Schneider of H. Wulfing Luer. (Courtesy of Mütter Museum and Wyeth-Ayerst Laboratories, Philadelphia, PA.)

bacteriologic filters, and improved methods were steadily being devised. These were the Chamberland and Berkefeld filters in the form of hollow cylinders of unglazed porcelain or of diatomaceous earth, and the Seitz, or asbestos pad, filter. Stanislaus Limousin, a French pharmacist, devised a container for storing sterile solutions and called it an "ampoule" (Fig. 1–5). The glass container had a long, tapering neck open at the end. After filling the tip of the glass, the neck was closed by sealing it with heat. The manufacture of parenteral solutions gradually passed from the hands of the individual pharmacist to pharmaceutical companies.

By the beginning of the twentieth century, the synthesis of arsphenamine by Ehrlich provided a material that dramatically demonstrated the effectiveness of parenteral therapy (Fig. 1–6). The era of chemotherapy was dawning.

Pyretic reactions continued to be associated with parenteral administration. The cause was attributed to several sources: the water used to make the solution, the chemicals themselves, and the devices used for administration. Florence Seibert in 1923 demonstrated that the source of the pyretic reactions was the water used to prepare the solutions.[8] Water not properly distilled and stored contained pyrogens, metabolic products of microorganisms. These sub-

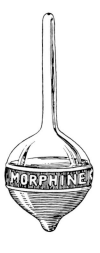

Figure 1–5. Stanislaus Limousin's design for the first ampul. Redrawn from original paper in Arch. Pharmacie, *1*, 145 (1886). (Courtesy of Wyeth-Ayerst Laboratories, Philadelphia, PA.)

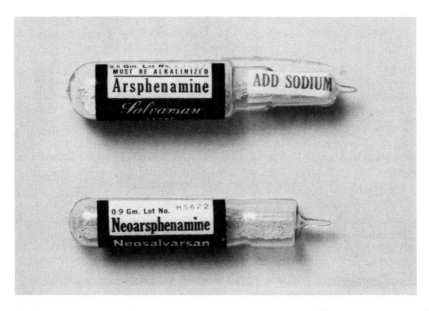

Figure 1–6. Ampul of arsphenamine and neoarsphenamine. Photographed from originals in the collection of Dr. Isadore Greenberg, Brooklyn College of Pharmacy (now Arnold and Marie Schwartz College of Pharmacy and Health Sciences), Long Island University. (Courtesy of Wyeth-Ayerst Laboratories, Philadelphia, PA.)

stances were responsible for the fever reactions that developed in those receiving parenteral injections. Care in using a pyrogen-free water as a solvent eliminated the fever response. Although the intravenous injection of glucose for nutritional purposes was first accomplished by Kausch in 1911,[9] it was not until a pyrogen-free water became available that dextrose was used extensively to make isotonic solutions and to provide calories. The deficiency of water and chloride in the patient suffering from Asiatic cholera was recognized by O'Shaughnessy during the cholera epidemics in England in 1832. The value of infusing water and salt solutions in cholera-stricken patients was demonstrated in the same year by Latta.[10,11] The practice died out until a suitable water vehicle was available to make the preparation of satisfactory infusion solutions possible.

Following the recognition of pyrogens, the first injectable solutions were made official in the *National Formulary V (N.F. V)* in 1926 under the name "Ampuls." At that time, there were six as compared to over 400 listed in the *United States Pharmacopeia U.S.P. XXII (U.S.P.)* and its supplements as injections. Sterile solutions were admitted to the U.S.P. XII in 1942 under the name "Injections." In addition, there are numerous sterile powders, sterile suspensions, and sterile ophthalmic solutions for which the compendium has established standards.

Development of Parenteral Packaging

In the development of parenteral therapy, changes continue to occur mainly in two directions: one in the packaging of parenteral preparations and the other in the methods by which they are administered. The single-dose glass ampul has changed little in basic design from that originally devised by Limousin. The next addition was the rubber closure for the glass vial. Because the closure can be pierced repeatedly, with the rubber resealing after the needle is withdrawn, the rubber-stoppered vial provides a container from which a number of doses of variable volume can be withdrawn and administered.

For certain drugs having fixed doses, the cartridge type of package has been devised. The cartridge generally consists of a glass tube, containing the sterile preparation, closed at both ends with rubber stoppers. The preparation is administered by placing the cartridge into a specially designed syringe to which a sterile needle is attached before administration. The empty cartridge is discarded. In some instances, the design of the cartridge holder permits it to be reused. To increase the convenience of administration of some products, the needle has been joined to the syringe at time of manufacture and designed as the package itself; the syringe contains the sterile preparation, and the sterility of the needle is maintained by a protective covering (see Chapters 12 and 14). After use, the syringe with needle attached can be discarded. It is in this form that parenteral packaging is currently developing.

Needle Sticks

It is estimated that more than 200,000 needle-stick injuries occur per year in the United States.[12] There is great concern about such injuries because of the risk of transmission of hepatitis B virus (HBV) and human immunodeficiency virus (HIV). It is estimated that 1 of every 14 hospitalized patients is an HIV carrier. Of hospital-related injuries to employees, 35% are caused by needle-stick/"sharps" punctures. Over a 12-month period in U.S. hospitals, approximately 18,000 hepatitis cases resulted from needle-stick accidents. One pilot study prevention program resulted in a 53% reduction in needle sticks.[13] Methods are being advocated to reduce needle-stick injuries, such as reduction of needle contact, providing a safe working environment, and disposable prefilled syringe cartridge disposal systems.

Jagger et al.[14] studied needle-stick injuries over a 10-month period in a university hospital and found that purchased disposable syringes had the lowest rate of needle sticks (6.9 for 100,000 syringes purchased).[3] Many of the injuries were the result of recapping. Millam[12] has reviewed some of the current devices available that may reduce needle-stick injuries.[1]

Listed below are some of these devices and their manufacturers:

    Safety-Lok Syringe—Becton Dickinson & Co.
    Monoject Safety Syringe with Safety Shield and Needle—Sherwood Medical
    Tubex Injection—Wyeth Ayerst
    Stick-Gard Safety Needle—International Medication System (IMS)
    Needle Point Guard—Needle Point Guard Inc.
    Protective IV Catheter—Johnson & Johnson
    Safe Stick—Phase Medical Inc.
    Intima—Deseret Medical & Becton Dickinson
    Needle-Lock Device—Baxter Healthcare Corp.
    Needle Less IV Access System—Baxter Healthcare Corp.
    Click Lock—ICU Medical Inc.

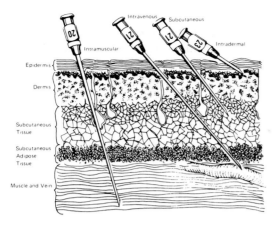

Figure 1–7. Routes of parenteral administration. Numbers on needles indicate size, or gauge, of needle based on outside diameter of needle shaft (see Chapter 14).

Development of Routes of Administration

The number of routes of administration also has increased, and new ones are being developed as the need for them arises. The routes currently used for parenteral therapy include intradermal, subcutaneous, intramuscular, intravenous, intra-arterial, and others (Fig. 1–7).

Intradermal (I.D.) Route

The drug is injected into the superficial layer of skin in intradermal administration, sometimes referred to as intracutaneous. Only small volumes of solution, in the order of 0.1 ml, can be administered by this route, and it is generally reserved for diagnostic tests and a limited number of vaccines. Absorption by this route is slow, resulting in a slow onset of drug action.

Subcutaneous (S.C.) Route

Injections of small volumes are given in the loose tissue beneath the skin, generally into the outer surface of the arm or thigh. Response to drugs administered by this route is more rapid than response to drugs administered intradermally. Subcutaneous administration is written on hospital pharmacy orders as "S.Q.," "Sub-Q," or "Hypo."

Intramuscular (I.M.) Route

Injection may be made into a muscle mass—intramuscular administration. A common site is the deltoid muscle in the upper arm, in which as much as 2 ml may be injected. Larger volumes, to a maximum of 5 ml, may be administered into the gluteal medial muscle of each buttock. Absorption by the intramuscular route is more rapid than it is by the subcutaneous route; it can be delayed or prolonged by administering the drug as a sterile suspension in either an aqueous or oily vehicle.

Intravenous (I.V.) Route

Large or small volumes of solutions can be administered into the veins for rapid effects. The results are predictable and potentially dangerous in that there is no retreat once the drug has been administered. Solutions of irritating drugs can be given by this route because of their rapid dilution with blood, or an intravenous fluid can be used as a diluent. This method of administration has *less* limitation as to volume, and the number and location of veins make for a readily accessible route.

Intra-Arterial Route

The intra-arterial route is infrequently used. Injection of a drug into an artery terminates in a target area, which may be an organ. The nature of the drug and the physiology of the circulatory system require intravenous injection, in which the drug becomes pooled and diluted throughout the blood system rather than going directly to an organ or tissue where the effects will be localized rather than generalized. The usual reason for using the intra-arterial route is to introduce radiopaque materials for diagnostic purposes, such as for arteriograms. Certain neoplastic drugs such as methotrexate are administered by this route. Arterial spasm and subsequent gangrene present problems that make the intra-arterial route hazardous.

Other Routes

Other, less commonly used routes include *intracardiac*, injection into a heart chamber; *intra-articular*, injection into a joint; *hypodermoclysis*, injection of a large volume of solution into subcutaneous tissue; *intraspinal*, injection into the spinal column; *intrasynovial*, injection into a joint fluid area, and *intrathecal*, injection into the spinal fluid. Parenteral drugs given by the intravenous or intraspinal route must be in solution. Parenteral emulsions, such as the nutritional fat emulsions, can be administered intravenously. Drugs administered by subcutaneous, intramuscular, or intradermal injection may be in the form of a solution, a suspension, or an emulsion.

Advantages of Parenteral Administration

The increasing use of parenteral administration is due partly to the number of advantages it offers:

1. An immediate physiologic response can be achieved if necessary, which can be of prime consideration in clinical conditions such as cardiac arrest, asthma, and shock.
2. Parenteral therapy is required for drugs that are not effective orally or that are destroyed by digestive secretions, such as insulin, other hormones, and antibiotics.
3. Drugs for uncooperative, nauseous, or unconscious patients must be administered by injection.
4. When desirable, parenteral therapy gives the physician control of the drug, since the patient must return for continued treatment. Also, in some cases, the patient cannot be relied upon to take oral medication.
5. Parenteral administration can result in local effects for drugs when desired, as in dentistry and anesthesiology.
6. In cases in which prolonged drug action is wanted, parenteral forms are available, including the long-acting steroids injected intra-articularly and the long-acting penicillins administered by deep intramuscular injection.

7. Parenteral therapy provides the means of correcting serious disturbances of fluid and electrolyte balances.
8. When food cannot be taken by mouth, or tube feeding, total nutritional requirements can be supplied by the parenteral route.[15]

Disadvantages of Parenteral Administration

Regardless of the parenteral route of administration, several disadvantages are inherent in parenteral procedures. The dosage forms must be administered by trained personnel, and require more time than those administered by other routes. Parenteral administration requires strict adherence to aseptic procedures, and some pain on injection is inevitable. Once a drug has been given parenterally, it becomes more difficult to reverse its physiologic effect. Finally, because of the manufacturing and packaging requirements, parenteral dosage forms are more expensive than are preparations given by other routes.

New life-saving techniques, such as cardiopulmonary resuscitation and parenteral nutrition (PN), along with life-saving antibiotics, have led to increased emphasis on parenteral therapy. The benefits derived from parenteral therapy have been overwhelmingly beneficial; however, advances in parenteral therapy have further complicated drug therapy. Complications have arisen from septicemia, fungal infections, intravenous admixture incompatibility, drug interactions, and the potential for needle sticks to cause hepatitis B or HIV infections.

Progress in the manufacture and packaging of sterile preparations will continue. The routes by which they can be administered may increase. However, their inherent requirements of sterility, freedom from particulate matter, freedom from pyrogens, and stability will remain the same. It is therefore essential that these requirements be appreciated not only by the manufacturer but also by all personnel who handle or administer sterile dosage forms. The requirements are relatively simple, but maintaining these requirements at all times remains an objective for all persons who prepare or administer sterile dosage forms.

References

1. Financial Analysts Federation, Health Care Seminar, Dec. 1, 1982. Franklin Plaza, Philadelphia, PA.
2. Griffenhagen, G.B.: The history of parenteral medication. Bull. Parenter. Drug. Assoc., *16*:12, (1962).
3. Miller, L.C.: A quarter century of success and failure in standardizing parenterals. Bull. Parenter. Drug. Assoc., *10*, 1 (1956).
4. Stormont, R.T.: The development and present status of parenteral drugs in medicine. Bull. Parenter. Drug. Assoc., *3*, 9 (1949).
5. Howard-Jones, N.: The origins of hypodermic medication. Sci. Am., *224*, 96 (1971).
6. Crellin, J.K.: Hypodermic medication—The rise and decline of a fashion. Pharm. Tech., *4*, 57 (June 1980).
7. Van Itallie, P.H.: The rugged beginnings of injection therapy. Pulse of Pharmacy, *19*, 3 (1965).
8. Seibert, F.B.: Fever-producing substances found in distilled water. Am. J. Physiol., *67*, 90 (1923).
9. Kausch, W.: Intravenous and subcutaneous nourishment with grape sugar. Dtsch. Med. Wochenschr., *37*, 8 (1911).

10. Kerr, D.N.S.: The history of intravenous therapy. J. Hosp. Pharm., *29*, 276 (1971).
11. Masson, A.H.B.: The early days of intravenous saline. Pharm. J., *217*, 571 (1976).
12. Milliam, D.: Avoiding needle-stick injuries. Nursing *90*, 61 (1990).
13. De Laune, S.: Risk reduction through testing, screening and infection control pre-cautions—with special emphasis on needle-stick injuries. Infect. Control Hosp. Epidemiol. 11 (suppl): 563 (1990).
14. Jagger, J., et al.: Rates of needle-stick injury caused by various devices in a uni-versity hospital. N. Engl. J. Med. *319*, 284 (1988).
15. Dudrick, S.J.: Rational intravenous therapy. Am. J. Hosp. Pharm., *28*, 82 (1971).

2

CHAPTER

Composition

When the term "sterile dosage form" is used, it refers to a product of a general group of pharmaceuticals having in common the characteristic of sterility, i.e., freedom from living microorganisms. Sterility is a required characteristic for these pharmaceuticals because of the method, site, or route of administration. Although many of the characteristics attributed to sterile pharmaceuticals, including the requirements for their handling and preparation, are also true for biologicals, differences exist because of the nature of the killed, attenuated, or live microorganisms used in preparing biological products. Unless otherwise stated, the following discussion concerns only sterile pharmaceuticals.

Types of Preparations

There are many ways to classify sterile dosage forms. Some classifications depend on the type of packaging involved, the products being referred to as single-dose units such as ampuls, prefilled disposable syringes or infusion solutions, and multiple-dose units as found in multiple-dose vials. For the purpose of writing regulations for their production and control, injectables are divided into two groups, small-volume parenterals (SVP) having a volume of less than 100 ml, and large-volume parenterals (LVP) having a volume of 100 ml or greater. Another approach is to indicate their clinical use as an irrigating solution, a dialysis solution, an allergenic extract, a diagnostic agent, or a sterile ophthalmic solution. The physical state of products has also served as the basis of differentiation among them, such as whether they are sterile solutions, sterile solids, sterile suspensions, or sterile emulsions. None of these classifications is complete. Therefore, the sterile dosage forms in general use are defined without regard to a given classification. In some instances, the definition given in the *U.S.P.* is included.

Injections

A drug in solution in a suitable vehicle, with or without added substances, intended for parenteral administration is designated an injection. An injection can be packaged as a single-dose unit or a multiple-dose unit; the volume can be as small as half a milliliter, such as Atropine Sulfate *Injection*, or as large as a liter, such as Dextrose *Injection*. The term can also be used for sterile emulsions.

Infusion Fluids

Intravenous infusion fluids constitute a group of single-dose injections characterized by their method of administration. They include preparations used for basic nutrition, such as Dextrose *Injection*; for the restoration of electrolyte balance, such as Ringer's *Injection* containing sodium, potassium, and calcium ions; for fluid replacement, a combination such as Dextrose and Sodium Chloride *Injection*; and for a number of special uses, such as total parenteral nutrition.

Radiopharmaceuticals

Radioactive chemicals used for organ function tests are frequently separated as a group of injections under the term "radiopharmaceuticals." They differ from other injections in that the drug is in a radioactive form; thus, different techniques are required in their preparation and handling.

Sterile Solids

Because some drugs do not have sufficient stability in solution to permit packaging them as injections, they are prepared as dry sterile solids to be placed in solution at time of use. If the sterile solids contain no buffers, diluents, or other added substances, they are labeled as the sterile drug, e.g., *Sterile* Sodium Nafcillin. If the dried sterile form of the drug also contains buffers, diluents, or other added substances, the preparation is labeled as the drug for injection, e.g., Amphotericin B *for Injection*. The difference in labeling indicates the presence or absence of added materials.

Sterile Suspensions

Drugs suspended in suitable parenteral vehicles are designated as sterile drug suspensions, e.g., *Sterile* Hydrocortisone Acetate *Suspension*. If the drug is in dry form and will give a suspension with the addition of a suitable parenteral vehicle, it is labeled as the sterile drug for suspension, e.g., *Sterile* Chloramphenicol *for Suspension*. Unlike injections, the two types of suspensions are never administered intravenously or injected into the spinal canal.

Ophthalmic Solutions, Suspensions, and Ointments

Drugs in solution or suspension administered by instillation in the eye are sterile preparations, although the term "sterile" is not generally included in their title, e.g., Sodium Sulfacetamide Ophthalmic Solution or Hydrocortisone Acetate Ophthalmic Suspension. They also differ from the preparations discussed previously in that they do not have the requirement of freedom from pyrogens because of the site of administration. In preparing ophthalmic ointments, the drug substances, either in solution or as micronized solids, are added to nonirritating ointment bases. The ointments are sterilized either by dry heat or by radiation; some are prepared as sterile preparations by the aseptic combination of sterile ingredients. They must be packaged in sealed containers and be free of objectionable particulate matter such as metal particles. Although they are sterile preparations, the term "sterile" is generally not included in the name, e.g., Hydrocortisone Acetate Ophthalmic Ointment or Gentamicin Sulfate Ophthalmic Ointment.

Solutions for Irrigation

Solutions used to bathe or flush open wounds or body cavities are defined as irrigating solutions and are used topically, never parenterally. Formerly, irrigating solutions were labeled using the same terminology as is used for injections. Sodium chloride solution that was to be used as an irrigating solution was labeled Sodium Chloride Injection, but it was packaged in a screw-cap bottle. Currently, the term "Sodium Chloride Irrigation" is used. The solution is packaged in screw-cap bottles. Irrigating solutions intended for single use should not be recapped and stored for subsequent use because of the great potential for contamination.[1]

Diagnostic Agents

Parenterally administered solutions for diagnostic purposes such as Evans Blue Injection, which is used in the determination of blood volume, also must meet the requirements of injections. A radiopharmaceutical injection administered parenterally for diagnostic purposes could also be included in this group.

Allergenic Extracts

Allergenic extracts are sterile concentrates of the allergens, or the substances responsible for unusual sensitivities in some persons, used for the diagnosis or treatment of allergenic reactions. Prior to use, the extracts are diluted to the desired concentration with aseptic technique and sterile diluting fluid. Because of the small dose, site of administration, and nature of the material, freedom from pyrogens is not a necessary specification for this dosage form.

Peritoneal Dialysis Solutions

The solutions used in the technique known as peritoneal dialysis act to decrease excess body waste, body fluids, serum electrolytes, and ingested toxic materials. They must meet the same requirements as injections for sterility, freedom from pyrogens, and freedom from particulate matter.

Pharmacy Bulk Packages

The manufactured bulk package is a sterile container for parenteral use that contains many single doses. These containers are intended for use in pharmacy admixture programs in which large numbers of doses are prepared. It is designed so that the rubber closure is penetrated only once, and is used in laminar flow hoods. Pharmacy bulk packages are exempt from the USP requirement that requires multipe-dose containers to have a volume no greater than 30 ml. They also have an exemption in that they are not required to have a bacteriostatic agent. Pharmacy bulk packages have special labeling and storage requirements.

Vehicles

The *U.S.P.* provides monographs with standards for a number of different types of water used for pharmaceutical purposes.[2] The ones pertaining to parenterals are discussed in the following sections.

Water for Injection (WFI)

The most widely used solvent for the preparation of parenteral dosage forms is Water for Injection. This type of water is specially prepared, collected, and stored in a manner ensuring that it can meet and maintain requirements for purity and freedom from pyrogens. It must be clear, colorless, and odorless, having a pH within the range of 5.0 to 7.0. Purity specifications limit the quantities of chloride, calcium, and sulfate ions; ammonia; carbon dioxide; heavy metals, oxidizable substances; and the total amount of dissolved solids present. The latter is not more than 10 parts per million (ppm) as determined by evaporating 100 ml Water for Injection to dryness and weighing the residue. Although this is the method recognized by the compendia, in practice the total dissolved solids are more often determined by measuring the conductivity of the water and expressing the solids content as parts per million sodium chloride. This has the disadvantage of measuring only the electrolytes present.

One of the most important characteristics of Water for Injection is freedom from pyrogens. Pyrogens are metabolic products of microbial growth and can occur wherever microorganisms are permitted to grow. Therefore, in obtaining pyrogen-free water, not only the equipment and feed water, but also the manner in which it is collected, are of importance. For large installations, the water is received in a closed stainless steel tank. For smaller systems, the water can be collected in sterile, pyrogen-free glass containers. In either case, Water for Injection must be used within 24 hours. To keep Water for Injection for a longer period, it must be stored under one of several conditions. It can be sterilized and protected against bacterial contamination during storage, in which instance it is labeled Sterile Water for Injection. Another means of maintaining it suitable for use is to store it at either 5° C or 80° C. The extremes of temperature prevent the occurrence of pyrogens by inhibiting the growth of microorganisms. For large installations in which Water for Injection has been received in closed stainless steel tanks, it is practical to keep the temperature of the tank and its contents at 80° C.[3] Smaller volumes can be stored at 5° C. If facilities for the proper storage of Water for Injection are not available and it is not to be sterilized, the water remaining at the end of the working day is discarded.

Water for Injection can be prepared either by distillation or by a recently developed process called reverse osmosis. In both cases, the quality of the feed water can influence the quality of the water produced. It is usually necessary to pretreat the feed water, either by filtration through a sand bed, charcoal, ion exchange resins, distillation, or by an initial passage through a reverse osmosis system to obtain a feed water of sufficient purity for the subsequent preparation of Water for Injection. Most systems for the preparation

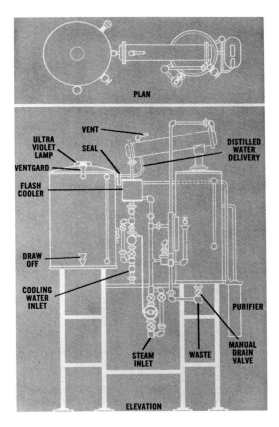

Figure 2–1. Water for Injection still and storage tank. (Courtesy of Barnstead and Still Sterilizer Co., Roxbury, MA.)

of Water for Injection include several of the processes mentioned, selected on the basis of the type of contaminants that must be eliminated from the feed water.

Distillation is a well-established process, and if the still is properly constructed and operated, water of the highest quality can be obtained (Fig. 2–1). The vapor generated by the still must be free of entrained water droplets possibly containing pyrogens and other contaminants from the feed water. Still designs frequently include devices to "scrub" the vapor to prevent water droplets from being carried over in the distillate. Stills are designed to operate at a given rate (gallons per hour); operation at a more rapid rate will result in carry-over of distillate from the evaporator. All parts of the still contacted by the vapor or distillate must be constructed from high quality materials, such as tin-coated metal, #304 or #316 stainless steel, or glass, to prevent metal contamination. The yield of pure water by distillation is approximately 10% of the total quantity of water used. Distillation is an expensive process because of the low yield, the energy requirements, and the resultant scaling problems.

Another accepted method for the preparation of Water for Injection is a process called reverse osmosis.[4,5] In the natural phenomenon of osmosis, the

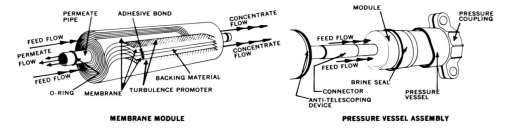

Figure 2–2. Spiral membrane module for water purification by reverse osmosis. (Reprinted with permission from Kunz, A.L.: Water purification and reverse osmosis. Bull. Parenter. Drug Assoc., *27*, 271 (1973).)

flow of water between two aqueous solutions of varying dissolved solid concentrations, separated by a semipermeable membrane, proceeds from the solution with the lower concentration into the solution with the higher concentration. Flow continues until the concentrations reach an equilibrium. The pressure head exerted by the second solution is called its osmotic pressure. In reverse osmosis, the direction of flow of the feed water passing through a semipermeable membrane can be reversed by applying pressure exceeding the osmotic pressure of the feed water. Owing to the characteristics of the semipermeable membrane, particulates and most dissolved solids are excluded, resulting in pure water passing through the membrane.

The semipermeable membranes used for reverse osmosis include the spiral-wound cellulose acetate membranes and the hollow fiber polyamide membranes. The cellulose acetate membrane takes the form of a thin film on a spongy backing material. The film is not completely intact, having openings reported to be in the range of 100 Å. Particulates, microorganisms, and dissolved organic compounds with molecular weights over 200 are rejected because of their molecular size. Thus, pyrogens are eliminated from the permeate. Dissolved electrolytes are rejected because of the repulsion of the ions from the surface of the membrane, higher valence ions being repelled a greater distance from the membrane. Rejection of small valence ions such as the chloride ions is not complete, and a small percentage of these ions passes through the membrane. These can be troublesome to eliminate. By pretreatment of the feed water and the use of a sufficient number of membrane passes, however, the chloride ion can be reduced to limits acceptable for Purified Water and Water for Injection.

For this application, the cellulose acetate membrane sheets are wrapped in a spiral configuration to form a coil and packaged within a metal cylinder. The feed water under pressure flows in one direction, and the permeate flows out through the center in another direction, as shown in Figure 2–2. The polyamide membrane material is spun into fine, hollow fibers with diameters in the range of 80 to 100 μ. The fibers are bundled, looped, and secured within a housing. The feed water under pressure passes through the fiber's walls, and the permeate is carried out through the open ends of the loop while the rejected water flows from the housing (Fig. 2–3).[6,7]

Water for Injection contains no added substances and is used for the preparation of parenteral solutions that are going to be sterilized after preparation. It is not used for the dilution of packaged parenteral products.

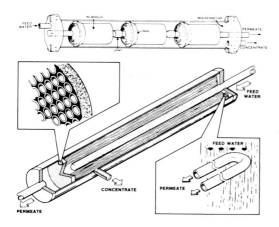

Figure 2–3. Hollow fiber module for water purification by reverse osmosis. (Reprinted with permission from Kunz, A.L.: Water purification and reverse osmosis. Bull. Parenter. Drug Assoc., 27, 273 (1973).)

Sterile Water for Injection (SWFI)

Sterile Water for Injection is Water for Injection sterilized and suitably packaged in single-dose containers not exceeding 1000-ml capacity. It contains no bacteriostatic agent. A higher total solids content is permitted in Sterile Water for Injection than in Water for Injection to allow for the material leached from the glass container during the sterilization process. When packaged in 30-ml or smaller containers, the limits are 40 ppm; 30-ml to 100-ml containers, 30 ppm; and larger than 100-ml, 20 ppm. This is the appropriate type of water for making parenteral solutions prepared under aseptic conditions and not sterilized by filtration or by autoclaving in the final container. For example, a dry powder, such as Sterile Sodium Phenobarbital, is placed in solution by aseptically adding Sterile Water for Injection, resulting in a sterile injection of sodium phenobarbital. Because it contains no antimicrobial agents, Sterile Water for Injection is packaged in single-dose containers not larger than 1 L capacity. It is labeled to indicate that it is not suitable for intravascular injection without its first having been made approximately isotonic by the addition of a suitable solute.

Bacteriostatic Water for Injection (BWFI)

Bacteriostatic Water for Injection is Sterile Water for Injection containing one or more suitable bacteriostatic agents. It is packaged in multiple-dose containers with no more than 30-ml capacity, and aliquots of the solution can be removed at various times owing to the presence of bacteriostatic agents that inhibit the growth of any accidentally introduced contaminant. When using this type of water, attention must be given to the compatibility of the bacteriostatic agents with the particular drug being placed in solution.

The most commonly used bacteriostatic agents are benzyl alcohol or a mixture of methyl- and propylparabens. When Bacteriostatic Water for Injection containing benzyl alcohol is used to solubilize Chloromycetin-Intramuscular, the material thickens slowly and makes it difficult to remove the antibiotic from the vial. The material is satisfactory if used within 2 hours. Another form of this drug, Chloromycetin Succinate, is compatible with solvents containing benzyl alcohol and may be used either intramuscularly or intravenously. Drugs such as thiopental sodium, atropine sulfate, phenobarbital sodium, sodium sulfadiazine, and sodium sulfathiazole are incompatible with Bacteriostatic Water for Injection containing the parabens. Erythromycin gluceptate must be reconstituted with preservative-free Sterile Water for Injection.

When reconstituting parenterals, the product brochure should be consulted and the recommended vehicle used. The pharmacist should not misconstrue this information and use a vehicle that is nearly similar, for example, interchanging Bacteriostatic Water for Injection with Sterile Water for Injection. In the former, the microbial preservative present may have an effect on the solubility and stability of the drug. Other injections occasionally used for the reconstitution of sterile solids include Sodium Chloride Injection and Bacteriostatic Sodium Chloride Injection. Again, the compatibility of the drug with the solvent must be recognized. The reconstitution of erythromycin lactobionate with Sodium Chloride Injection instead of with Sterile Water for Injection causes gel formation.

Also, because Bacteriostatic Water for Injection contains a bacteriostatic agent as an added substance, care must be exercised in administering volumes greater than 5 ml because each bacteriostatic agent has its own inherent toxicity. If volumes greater than 5 ml of the vehicle are required for reconstitution of a drug, the vehicle of choice is Sterile Water for Injection rather than Bacteriostatic Water for Injection. The various types of water are classified in Table 2–1.

Sterile Water for Inhalation

Sterile Water for Inhalation is water purified by distillation or by reverse osmosis, sterilized and packaged in single dose containers. It contains no antimicrobial agents except when used in humidifiers or similar devices that may become contaminated. The label indicates that sterile water for inhalation is not intended for parenteral administration.

Sterile Water for Irrigation

Sterile Water for Irrigation is water for injection that has been sterilized and packaged in single-dose containers. It contains no antimicrobial agents or other added substance. The USP permits the volume of the container to exceed a 1 liter capacity. This water is for general hospital use for irrigation and not intended for injection.

Other Common Solvents (USP)

Other common solvents include Sodium Chloride Injection, Bacteriostatic Sodium Chloride Injection, and Sodium Chloride Irrigation.

Oils for Injection

Because certain drugs, such as the steroids, some vitamins, and hormones, are not soluble in water to any extent but are soluble in oil, a number of vegetable oils are used as solvents, including soybean, peanut, cottonseed, corn, olive, sesame, and persic. The oils must be pure and meet official standards as to the quantities of free acids present. Oils of mineral origin, or hydrocarbons, cannot be used, since these materials are not metabolized by the body. Parenteral preparations in which oil is used as the solvent can only be administered intramuscularly. In order for an oil to be administered in-

TABLE 2–1. Comparison of Types of Water

Type	Preparation Method	Pyrogen-Free	Sterile	Packaging	Bacteriostatic Agent	Use
Purified Water U.S.P.	Distillation Ion exchange	No	No	Tight containers	No	Pharmaceutical solvent
Water for Injection U.S.P.	Distillation Reverse osmosis	Yes	No	1. Use within 24 hours or store below 5° C or over 80° C; or 2. sterilize; or 3. discard.	No	Manufacture of parenteral products that are going to be sterilized.
Sterile Water for Injection U.S.P.*†	Distillation Reverse osmosis	Yes	Yes	Single-dose containers	No	Same as Water for Injection above; as sterile solvent for sterile solids, for dilution of sterile solutions provided aseptic technique is used. Same as sterile solvent
Bacteriostatic Water for Injection U.S.P.‡§	Distillation Reverse osmosis	Yes	Yes	Multiple-dose and single-dose containers	Yes	Same as sterile solvent
Sterile Water Irrigation*	Distillation Reverse osmosis	Yes	Yes	One liter or larger; wide mouth; does not need to meet particulate matter requirements for LVP, to be labeled "For irrigation only" and "Not for injection."	No	Irrigating solution
Sterile Water for Inhalation	Distillation Reverse osmosis	Yes	Yes	Single-dose containers	Yes No	Humidifiers Inhalation

*No added substances including bacteriostatic agents.
†Not suitable for intravascular injection without having been made isotonic.
‡Consider compatibility between bacteriostatic agent and drug.
§Benzyl alcohol or combination of paraben esters commonly used.

travenously, it must first be emulsified to give a stable emulsion as found in Intralipid (KabiVitrum Laboratories, Inc.). In this injection, soybean oil is emulsified in Water for Injection, using egg yolk phospholipids as the emulsifying agent and glycerin as a stabilizer. Clinically, it can be administered intravenously to provide a source of calories.

Added Substances for Parenterals

In the formulation of parenteral preparations, it is common practice to consider the inclusion of a group of ingredients, known as added substances, to increase the usefulness and stability of solutions. Consideration of a chemical as an additive depends on its value in one of the following categories: (1) to maintain the drug's solubility; (2) to maintain the solution's physical and chemical stability; (3) to maintain the sterility of the solution when a multiple-dose package is used; or (4) to ease parenteral administration by reducing pain on injection or tissue irritation. A survey of added substances found in parenteral products used in the United States revealed a limited number of compounds being used.[8] The reluctance to introduce new materials is based on the necessity of lengthy and costly safety testing.

In preparing parenteral solutions, the objective is to provide at time of use a sterile solution or suspension of the labeled drug in the potency stated that is safe to use if the directions for administration are followed. The philosophy involved in selecting additives embraces the following principles. Every parenteral product represents an individual pharmaceutical system with its own characteristics and requirements. These requirements may change as the concentration of the drug changes, as the packaging components are modified, or as one method of administration is given preference over another. Thus, for added substances in general, the value of the discussion is somewhat limited. Because of the methods of administration, more stringent limitations are placed on additives for parenterals than on those for any other dosage form. The additives chosen are limited in both number and quantities. They are selected with the knowledge that they are not going to interfere with the therapeutic efficacy of the drug and are harmless in the amounts administered. Colorants are never added to parenteral formulations.

Although the commonly used additives are considered nontoxic in the quantities used, modification of dosage requirements or method of administration by the user (neither intended by the manufacturer) can invalidate this assumption. This was indicated in the use of glucagon for the treatment of myocardial failure. Glucagon (Lilly) is a crystalline polypeptide hormone usually used in counteracting severe hypoglycemic reactions in diabetic patients. It is packaged as a lyophilized powder in 10-mg quantities. The diluting fluid (10 ml) contains glycerin, 1.6%; phenol, 0.2%; and sodium hydroxide or hydrochloric acid for adjustment of pH. In cardiotherapy, 100-mg doses have been administered. If the lyophilized powder is reconstituted with diluting fluid prior to its addition to a larger volume of an intravenous fluid, doses of 100 mg result in the administration of 200 mg phenol, which may be toxic.[9,10] Likewise, the fact that cardiac arrhythmias were observed after the administration of 100 mg dexamethasone has suggested the possibility that the arrhythmias may have been due to the preservatives, methyl- and propylparaben. In addition to the 100 mg dexamethasone present as the phosphate ester, the injection contained creatinine, 200 mg; sodium citrate, 50 mg; sodium hydroxide to adjust the pH; sodium bisulfite, 25 mg; methylparaben, 27.5 mg; and propylparaben, 5 mg.[11]

Another reported example concerns the unexpected toxic symptoms observed after administration of a certain peritoneal dialysis fluid.[12] The dialysis solution contained dextrose, 7%; sodium chloride, 0.62%; sodium lactate, 0.39%; calcium chloride, 0.026%; magnesium chloride, 0.015%; and sodium bisulfite, 0.05%. Sodium bisulfite is used extensively in concentrations as high as 0.31% (equivalent to 0.2% sulfur dioxide) as an antioxidant to prevent discoloration of parenterals, but rarely are these fluids administered in volumes comparable to those used in peritoneal dialysis, perhaps as high as 10 to 40 L/day. Subsequent toxicity studies on rabbits revealed that rapid absorption of sodium bisulfite from the peritoneum does occur, and the ability of the organism to remove the bisulfite by oxidation or urinary excretion is lost when the levels in blood are increased. Thus, it was concluded that the administration of 500 mg sodium bisulfite per liter is dangerous and that it should not be used. These examples demonstrate dramatically that the presence of added substance in injections must be considered when unusual doses are given or when the method of administration is modified.

Maintenance of Solubility

To maintain the drug in solution, it is sometimes necessary to include an additional solubilizing agent, either a miscible cosolvent or a chemical solubilizer. Among the solvents frequently used are polyethylene glycols 300 and 400, propylene glycol, glycerin, and ethyl alcohol.[13] Barbiturates, antihistamines, and cardiac glycosides are examples of drugs requiring these solvents. In addition to their aid in solubilization, the presence of organic solvents can retard the hydrolysis of numerous drugs. Occasionally, the hospital pharmacist is called on to prepare extemporaneously a parenteral solution containing a drug that is not soluble in Sterile Water for Injection. Preparing these solutions with water-miscible organic solvents not generally used, or using known vehicles in amounts larger than are normally used, can be dangerous practices.

When organic solvents are used for parenteral administration, it is necessary to have toxicity specifications for the solvent as a raw material included. A case has been reported of a marketed drug that produced nephrotic symptoms. Investigation revealed that the probable cause was neither the drug nor the pure solvent but the impurities in the solvent produced by aging. The instability of the solvent (polyethylene glycol 300) produced toxic decomposition products.[14]

In addition to organic solvents, other chemicals have been used to maintain the solubility of drugs. In developing a satisfactory parenteral form of the steroid hydrocortisone phosphate (as the monosodium salt), a fine trace precipitate believed to be the free hydrocortisone alcohol was formed. The difficulty was overcome by solubilizing the alcohol with creatinine, N-methyl creatinine, or niacinamide.[15] Niacinamide also was used to solubilize riboflavin before the availability of the highly soluble riboflavin phosphate.[16]

Other examples of solubilizers in parenteral solutions include sodium benzoate to solubilize caffeine in Caffeine Sodium Benzoate Injection and the excess of ethylene diamine in Aminophyllin Injection to maintain the solubility of theophylline. Again, we emphasize the necessity of knowing the toxicity of any additive selected to solve a solubilization problem.

To a limited extent, nonionic surfactants, such as the polysorbates (Tweens, Atlas Chemical Company) and polyoxyethylated derivatives (Emulpor El-620, GAF Corporation), have been used to solubilize drugs, especially the oil-soluble vitamins, for intramuscular administration. When present in solution with other additives, however, surfactants can present problems in chemical or physical incompatibilities. The binding and inactivation of a number of preservatives by polysorbate 80 have been reported.[17]

Maintenance of Stability

Once present in solution, a drug may be subject to both oxidative and hydrolytic changes. To prevent degradation of drug by oxidation, antioxidants may be present, either alone or in combination with chelating agents. Inert gases used both during processing and in packaging can also be helpful.

Antioxidants are easily oxidized and have lower oxidation potentials than do the drugs they are meant to protect. The most commonly used antioxidants are the sodium or potassium salts of the metasulfite, and sulfite ions.[18,19] The choice of the salt depends on the pH of the system to be stabilized, metabisulfite being used at low pH values, bisulfite for intermediate pH values, and sulfite for higher pH ranges. In most instances, sulfur dioxide is the active component, and the quantity used is not more than that equivalent to 0.2% sulfur dioxide. Other agents include acetone metabisulfite, ascorbic acid, thioglycerol, and cysteine hydrochloride.

Because most oxidative degradation processes of pharmaceuticals are autooxidative in nature, involving chain reactions that require only small amounts of oxygen to initiate the process, reduction of oxygen concentration alone may not be sufficient to eliminate completely the possiblility of degradation. Frequently, chelating agents are effective in enhancing the activity of antioxidants. By forming complexes with trace amounts of heavy metals, the catalytic activity of the metals in the oxidation process is eliminated. The most commonly used agent is the sodium salt of ethylene-diamine tetraacetic acid, although similar claims have been made for certain of the dicarboxylic acids, such as tartaric acid and citric acid. Synergistic action is claimed for various combinations of antioxidants and chelating agents. Numerous examples of parenteral solutions that employ combinations are to be found in the patent literature.

Another common procedure to stabilize a solution containing oxygen-sensitive materials is to use vehicles that have been flushed with an inert gas, such as nitrogen or carbon dioxide, and the maintenance of the solution under a blanket of inert gas during processing. Further protection is given the solution in the final package by subdividing it into the containers under an inert gas. For example, Sodium Bicarbonate Injection is prepared and packaged in an atmosphere of carbon dioxide, and sterile solutions of the phenothiazine derivatives are filled under a nitrogen atmosphere.

Further enhancement of the drug's stability in solution may require the addition of a buffer system. When a buffer is required, attention must be given to buffer capacity, buffer range, and the effect of the buffer on the stability and activity of the product.

Maintenance of Sterility

Suitable substances to prevent the growth of microorganisms accidentally introduced into multiple-dose containers during use constitute another important group of additives. It should be realized that there is no universal agent satisfactory for all preparations, nor is a given concentration of a particular antimicrobial agent satisfactory for all preparations. Each product must be considered as to its own requirements. Minor formulation changes, e.g., changing the concentration of the drug, can result in an unsatisfactory preservative system. In a survey of antimicrobial preservatives currently being used, Akers noted the limited number of acceptable agents, the toxicity and stability problems encountered, and the difficulties in proper evaluation of preservative activity.[20]

As parenteral solutions become more complex in composition, and as packaging materials become more sophisticated, these conditions can substantially influence the effectiveness of the traditionally employed antimicrobial preservatives. Because of the potential toxicity of antimicrobial agents, care must be taken in selecting the agent and its concentration. This is particularly important in preparations that are given parenterally in volumes larger than 5 ml. The *U.S.P.* gives maximum limits for certain preservatives. For cationic, surface-active compounds, such as benzethonium chloride, benzalkonium chloride, Myristyl-gamma-picolinium Chloride, and mercury-containing compounds, such as phenylmercuric nitrate and Sodium Ethyl Mercurithiosalicylate, the limit is 0.01%. For phenol, cresol, and chlorobutanol, the limit is 0.5%. No maximum limits are suggested for the parabens and benzyl alcohol. Methyl- and propylparabens are frequently used in the combination of 0.18% for the methyl ester and 0.02% for the propyl. Benzyl alcohol is commonly used at 0.9% concentration; when its local anesthetic action is also desired to reduce pain on intramuscular injection, the concentration may be as high as 1.5%.

Although reports on antimicrobial agents are numerous in the literature, it is difficult to evaluate conflicting claims as to preservative activities and stability. There have been many reports of the interaction of commonly used preservatives with macromolecular materials, the pH dependence of some preservatives for effective activity, the chemical instability of the preservative itself, the interaction of the preservative with the active component of the solution, and the interaction of the preservative with the packaging components. The complete disappearance of a preservative from a parenteral solution is not an infrequent occurrence. It is usually due to the absorption of the antimicrobial agent by the rubber closure. In addition, there must be an awareness of the stability of the preservative to the sterilization process.

To determine the effectiveness of an antimicrobial system for parenterals, an inoculum containing a known number of organisms (*Candida albicans, Aspergillus niger, Escherichia coli, Pseudomonas aeruginosa,* and *Staphylococcus aureus*) is added to the preparation. The preparations are incubated at 32° C, and the microbial preservative system is considered adequate if there is no significant increase in the number of organisms. The adoption of this test has helped the formulator to evaluate the comparative activity of preservatives in his particular formulation.

In the clinical environment, there is a lack of agreement as to how many times or how long multidose vials will remain sterile after the initial entry. A number of factors make unanimity difficult, such as technique used, environment, storage conditions, the drug, preservatives used in the vial, and the number of entries made into the container.

One study illustrated the weakness of the bacteriostats methyl- and propylparabens, in concentrations of 0.05% and 0.005% respectively, in sodium chloride injection 0.9% and sterile water for injection when compared to other agents.[21]

The recommended guidelines from literature reviews range from 7 days to 3 months. With proper storage, handling, and labeling, 30-day dating after initial entry seems prudent.[22]

Ease of Administration

Whenever possible, it is the practice to make parenteral solutions isotonic with the body fluids. Although some may question the value of adjusting the tonicity of solutions when the volume to be administered is small, attention to this fact does not detract from the therapeutic efficacy of the preparation. Historically, this has been done by making the colligative properties of the parenteral solution comparable to those of the body fluids. Solutions made iso-osmotic with the body fluids may not be isotonic with respect to the erythrocytes.[23] With new products, it is necessary to do in vitro hemolysis studies; additives present in parenteral solutions can contribute to the overall hemolytic characteristics of the solution. When solutions are hypotonic, either sodium chloride or dextrose is added to increase the osmotic pressure of the solutions. When the desired concentration of the drug in solution is hypertonic, the manufacturer has no choice but to prepare a hypertonic solution. By changing the route of administration or by slowing the rate of injection, the clinician can alleviate, to some extent, the discomfort resulting from administration of the solution. A solution that is irritating by the intramuscular route may be less irritating when given intravenously at a slow rate, because of its rapid dilution with blood in the vein. The hypertonic parenteral nutrient solutions are administered via the subclavian vein leading directly to the heart, where the solutions are diluted rapidly.

Other additives sometimes present to improve the ease of administration include benzyl alcohol and other local anesthetics. With Keflin, tetracylcine, and Coly-Mycin Injectable, 1% injections of Xylocaine or procaine are frequently used as the diluent to reduce pain on intramuscular injection. Small quantities of hydrocortisone and heparin are sometimes added to amphotericin B to reduce vein irritation. Epinephrine hydrochloride at a concentration of 1:100,000 is frequently used with local anesthetics or other drugs to serve as a vasoconstrictor, prolonging the local effect of the drug.

Added Substances for Sterile Suspensions

When formulating sterile aqueous suspensions, there is the added problem of adequately dispersing the insoluble drug, usually in the particle size range of 10 μm, in the vehicle. Uniform distribution of the drug is required to ensure an adequate dose at the concentration per unit volume indicated on the label. Improper formulation can result in caking of the insoluble material at the bottom of the container, making it difficult to disperse, to take up in a syringe, and thus to administer. To avoid caking, the additives in sterile suspensions include flocculating agents such as benzyl alcohol or phenyl-ethanol.[24] The presence of a suspending agent such as sodium carboxy-methylcellulose or hydroxyethylcellulose increases the viscosity and acts as a colloidal protectant for the suspended solid. Wetting agents such as polysorbate 80, Pluronic F-68 (Wyandotte Chemical), or sorbitan trioleate also help to keep the solid material in suspension. Additives similar to those found in injections are used as antimicrobial preservatives and to adjust the vehicle for isotonicity.

Added Substances for Ophthalmic Solutions

The administration of ophthalmic solutions by instillation is considered topical rather than parenteral. Therefore, in the formulation of ophthalmic solutions, it is not unusual to use a different group of added substances, including buffers, antimicrobial preservatives, chemicals to adjust tonicity, and thickening agents. Some physicians prefer ophthalmic solutions packaged in single-dose containers without any additives, owing to the incidence of hypersensitivity to this group of chemicals.

Lacrimal fluid has a pH of about 7.4 and has some buffering capacity. For ophthalmic solutions of certain drugs, such as the alkaloidal salts, in which the therapeutic efficacy depends on the availability of the alkaloidal base, the solution is buffered near the pH of the tear fluid, yet sufficiently low to keep the alkaloidal material in solution until after instillation. Phosphate or acetate buffers are usually used. For local anesthetic solutions in which the activity is not pH-dependent, the solutions usually are not buffered.

Normal tear fluid has a tonicity value comparable to 0.9% sodium chloride solution. Solutions instilled in the eye should exert an osmotic pressure comparable to that of the tear fluid so that these solutions are not irritating to the mucosal membranes of the eye. This characteristic assumes a greater importance in eyewashes, in which a relatively large volume of solution is used, than in eye drops, in which the eye can rapidly adjust to the difference in osmotic pressure.

When ophthalmic solutions are packaged in multiple-dose containers, they must include an antimicrobial agent to prevent the growth of any microbial contaminant accidentally introduced into the package during use. Among the commonly used preservative compounds are benzalkonium chloride, 0.01% to 0.001%; chlorobutanol, 0.5%; phenylmercuric nitrate, 0.002% to 0.001%; methylparaben, 0.1% to 0.03%, in combination with propylparaben, 0.01%. Ethylenediaminetetraacetic acid (EDTA), 0.1% to 0.01%, has been used in combination with benzalkonium chloride to enhance the latter's activity against *Pseudomonas aeruginosa*. Other agents which have been used include benzyl alcohol, chlorhexidine diacetate, phenylethanol, and polymyxin B sulfate.[25] As mentioned in the discussion on injections, each ophthalmic solution must be recognized as an individual system, and what is adequate for one formula may not be satisfactory for another. The compatibility of the drug and the additive must be considered; the effectiveness of a preservative system can be evaluated with the same microbiologic test that is used for evaluating the preservative systems for parenterals. Ophthalmic solutions for surgical procedures are packaged as single-dose units and do not contain preservatives.

Frequently, the viscosity of the ophthalmic solution is increased by the addition of a suitable, water-dispersible polymer, such as methylcellulose, hydroxypropylcellulose, or polyvinyl alcohol. In a study using subject acceptance as the criterion of choice, hydroxyethylcellulose was found to be the preferred polymer.[26] The increased viscosity aids in holding the solution in contact with the mucosal tissue, thus increasing the effectiveness of the drug present in solution.

The added substances and their concentrations in sterile dosage forms are listed on the label. Insight into the physical and chemical natures of the drug in solution can be gained by careful study of the ingredients found there. Such insight is frequently useful in determining the physical compatibility of sterile dosage forms with other agents.

References

1. Kaczmarek, E.R., Sula, J.A., and Hutchinson, R.A.: Sterility of partially used irrigation solutions. Am. J. Hosp. Pharm., 39:1534, (1982).
2. United States Pharmacopeia XXII, U.S. Pharmacopeial Convention, Inc., Rockville, MD, 1990, p. 1456.
3. Giorgio, R.J.: Considerations in the design of hot circulating Water for Injection systems. Pharm. Tech., 2, 19 (Dec., 1978).
4. Kunz, A.: Water purification and reverse osmosis. Bull. Parenter. Drug Assoc., 27, 266, (1973).
5. Frith, C.F., Dawson, F.W., and Sampson, R.L.: Water for Injection USP XIX by reverse osmosis. Bull. Parenter. Drug Assoc., 30, 118, (1976).
6. Juberg, D.L., Pauli, W.A., and Artiss, D.H.: Application of reverse osmosis for the generation of Water for Injection. Bull. Parenter. Drug Assoc., 31, 70 (1977).
7. Jacobs, P.: Use of reverse osmosis for the production of parenterals in the hospital pharmacy. Pharm. Weekblad., 116, 342, (1981).
8. Wang, Y.J., and Kowal, R.R.: Review of excipients and pH's for parenteral products used in the United States. J. Parenter. Drug Assoc. 34, 452 (1980).
9. Cronk, J.D.: Correspondence: Phenol with glucagon in cardiotherapy. N. Engl. J. Med., 284, 219 (1971).
10. Spodick, D.H., Byrne, M.J., and Pigott, V.M.: Correspondence: Phenol in glucagon diluent. N. Engl. J. Med., 284, 500 (1971).
11. Schmidt, G.B., Meier, M.A., and Sadove, M.A.: Sudden appearance cardiac arrhythmias after dexamethasone. JAMA, 221, 1404 (1972).
12. Halaby, S.F., and Mattocks, A.M.: Absorption of sodium bisulfite from peritoneal dialysis solutions. J. Pharm. Sci. 54, 51 (1965).
13. Spiegel, A.J., and Noseworthy, M.M.: Use of nonaqueous solvents in parenteral products. J. Pharm. Sci., 52, 917 (1963).
14. Kessenich, W.H.: The solutions for the problems we share. Bull. Parenter. Drug Assoc., 14, 11 (1960).
15. Charnicki, W.F., and King, R.E.: U.S. Patent 2,970,944 (Feb. 7, 1961).
16. Stecher, P.: U.S. Patent 2,480,517 (August 30, 1949).
17. Bahal, C.K., and Kostenbauder, H.B.: Interaction of preservatives with macromolecules. J. Pharm. Sci., 53, 1027 (1964).
18. Lachman, L.: Antioxidants and chelating agents as stabilizers in liquid dosage forms. Drug Cosmetic Industr., 102, 36, 43 (1968).

19. Akers, M.J.: Preformulation screening of antioxidant efficiency in parenteral products. J. Parenter. Drug Assoc., *33*, 346 (1979).

20. Akers, M.J.: Considerations in selecting antimicrobial preservative agents for parenteral product development. Pharm. Tech., *8*, 36 (May, 1984).

21. Plott, R.T., et al.: Iatrogenic contamination of Multidose Vials in simulated use. Arch. Dermatol. *126*, 1441 (1990).

22. Moi, S., et al.: Time limit on multidose vials after initial entry. Hosp. Pharm. *26*, 805 (1991).

23. Ansel, H.C.: Intravenous solutions and the erythrocyte. Am. J. Hosp. Pharm., *21*, 25 (1964).

24. Portnoff, J.B., Cohen, E.M., and Henley, M.W.: Development of parenteral and sterile ophthalmic suspensions. Bull. Parenter. Drug Assoc., *31*, 136 (1977).

25. Eriksen, S.P.: Preservation of ophthalmic, nasal, and otic products. Drug Cosmetic Industr., *107*, 36 (1970).

26. Dudinski, O., Finnin, B.C., and Reed, B.L.: Acceptability of thickened eye drops to human subjects. Curr. Therap. Res., *33*, 322 (1983).

Characteristics

Sterility and freedom from particulate matter are common characteristics of all sterile dosage forms. The forms administered parenterally are also pyrogen-free. For drug products, stability becomes an additional consideration because the objective of the manufacturer is to provide at time of use a sterile solid, solution, or suspension of the drug, in the potency stated on the label, that is safe to use if the directions for administration are followed.

Sterility

All dosage forms administered parenterally, ophthalmic solutions, and any medical device used in conjunction with the administration of such agents must be sterile, i.e., free from all living microorganisms. The freedom from microorganisms is ensured initially by subjecting the product to a valid sterilization process, then packaging the product in a form that ensures the retention of this characteristic. The term "sterile" is an absolute one and should never be used or considered in a relative manner. One should never refer to a product as partially or almost sterile.

It is also expected that in subsequent handling of the product for administration, the aseptic technique of the manipulator will ensure the continued exclusion of living microorganisms. Proper aseptic techniques for the preparation and administration of sterile dosage forms are discussed in later sections.

Freedom from Particulate Matter

Particulate matter refers to the mobile, undissolved substances unintentionally present in parenteral products. The presence of particulate matter in parenteral solutions has been a concern since the conception of this route of administration. Although the parenteral route can provide a lifesaving, convenient, necessary, and effective method of administration, some believe that extraneous, unintended foreign matter constitutes one of its hazards.[1]

The composition of unwanted particulate matter is varied. In some instances, the composition is common to many sources, whereas in others it is individual to a specific source. Extraneous materials found in parenterals include cellulose and cotton fibers; glass, rubber, metal, and plastic particles; undissolved chemicals; rust; diatoms; and dandruff. The theoretic possibilities include any environmental material to which the product is exposed.

Biologic Significance

Clarity, or the absence of visible particulate matter, has always been considered a requirement for parenteral products. Initially, this requirement was based on the psychologic effect that a solution with visible material might have on the patient receiving the injection, as well as on the conclusions that might be drawn concerning the company that markets injectables with visible material floating in the solutions. When glass ampuls became popular as packaging materials, concern was noted about the probability of glass particles showering into the solution when the ampul is opened. Animal studies, which consisted of intravenously injecting suspensions of ground glass into rabbits, did not reveal any harmful effects on the animals, which continued to gain weight and thrive.[2] Therefore, until recently, concern for particulate matter in solutions was largely based on the psychologic effects on the user.

In 1964, the work of two Australian pathologists showed the development of emboli in lungs of rabbits that had received large volumes of parenteral solutions intravenously.[3,4] These results stimulated renewed interest in the significance of particulate matter. Although the evidence accumulated to this time is circumstantial, measures have been taken by the industry and by those who use the products to eliminate particulate matter from solutions. It is possible that particulate matter in intravenous solutions can be harmful, especially to geriatric patients, who may receive large volumes of infusion fluids, and to hospitalized patients, who are recumbent and have sluggish pulmonary circulation. In addition, the patients may be under concomitant therapy with corticosteroid and other drugs, which may modify tissue response, so that a localized granulomatous process could become diffuse throughout the lung.

Although the biologic effects of particulate matter may be vague at the present time, the quality control ramifications are clear. Particulate matter is undesirable, and constant efforts must be made to eliminate its sources and occurrence.

The *U.S.P.* has established particulate standards regarding the number and dimensions of particles in large-volume parenterals, and in small-volume parenterals where the monographs require it.[5]

Sources

Particulate matter can be contributed to a parenteral product from many sources and activities: (1) the solution itself and the chemicals comprising it; (2) the manufacturing process and its variables, such as the environment, equipment, and personnel; (3) the packaging components in which the product is contained; (4) the sets and devices used in administering the product;

and (5) the manipulations involved in the preparation of the product for administration as well as the environment in which it is prepared.[6,7]

During the manufacture and packaging of the solution, the environment, personnel, and filling equipment can contribute to particulate matter. The environment and equipment are more easily monitored than are the personnel. Identification of particulate matter can be helpful in locating the sources and eliminating them. Particles 50 μm or larger can be detected by visual inspection. For smaller particles, special instrumental techniques must be used. All the techniques require scrupulously clean equipment and environment for satisfactory performance, although the procedures are based on different physical principles. The membrane, or microscopic, method consists of passing a solution through a membrane filter, followed by microscopic examination of the particles retained on the membrane. While on the membrane, the particles can be sized, counted, and possibly identified.[8,9] By photographing the membrane, a permanent record of a sample can be obtained; however, the method is tedious and difficult when done manually. Automatic image analysis systems (πMC System, Millipore; Omnicon Pattern Analysis, Bausch and Lomb) have been proposed for the rapid measurement and counting of particles obtained by the membrane method.[10]

In the U.S.P., the microscopic membrane method is used to determine the number of particles in large-volume parenterals. For small-volume parenterals, the method calls for the use of an electronic liquid-borne particle counting system, utilizing a light-obscuration sensor such as the HIAC/Royco Counter. The British Pharmacopoeia (B.P.) uses the Coulter Counter (Coulter Electronics), which detects and measures particles by a change in electrical resistance. Hopkins and Young found that both the Coulter Counter and the HIAC/Royco Counter give results comparable to the microscopic method provided reasonable precautions are taken to eliminate air bubbles and clean techniques are followed.[11]

Packaging components, such as the glass or plastic container or the rubber closure, can generate particulate matter if they are not washed and handled properly. The administration device, whether it be a syringe or the infusion tubing for intravenous fluid, can also generate particulate matter.

During storage, the solution can generate particulate matter, owing to chemical reactions among components of the solution, reaction of the chemical components with the packaging materials, or degradation of the solution itself.

Regardless of the care used by the manufacturer in eliminating particulate matter, the sterile product must be handled in its administration, and this constitutes another potential source for particulate contamination. When administering the product, the manipulator opens the ampul or pierces the rubber closure of the vial. The source of foreign material now becomes the glass from breaking of the ampul or the rubber particles generated by the coring process, the needle and syringe, and the human and environmental factors associated with aseptic technique. At time of administration, the sources are primarily environmental, that is, improper aseptic technique and improper methods of administration.

Control and detection of particulate matter have long been of concern to the industry. Originally, a clarity test was devised by the manufacturer whereby the contents of each container were swirled and viewed against a light and a dark background under a light of given intensity. Particles of lint, rubber, and other debris float or settle to the bottom of the container. Air bubbles can be differentiated by the fact that they rise to the surface and dissipate. Normal human vision, however, can detect particles only in the range of 50 μm under these conditions, or perhaps 25 μm for reflective particles such as glass. Inspectors grow fatigued, and visual acuity depends on factors such as the degree of attentiveness, emotional stress, and personal comfort. Thus, levels of discrimination vary greatly from inspector to inspector. This procedure, formerly recognized as an official standard method, is still used, but is no longer an official method because, in a court case, it was ruled that the test is an arbitrary one and therefore cannot serve as a standard.

Attempts have been made to automate the process.[12] One method is to view the containers under magnification while they are spun mechanically. Another approach has been to detect particles in movement electronically, automatically rejecting the containers having particles larger than 5 μm in diameter.

Standards have been established in the *U.S.P.* to limit particulate matter occurring in large volume injections intended for administration by intravenous infusion. The microscopic membrane procedure is followed. The large-volume parenteral injection meets the standard if it contains not more than 50 particles per milliliter that are equal to or larger than 10 μm (50,000 per liter), and not more than 5 particles per milliliter that are equal to or larger than 25 μm in linear dimension (5000 per liter).

The *U.S.P.* proposes that a small volume injection, i.e., one having a volume of less than 100 ml, will meet the requirements if it contains not more than 10,000 particles per container that are equal to or greater than 10 μm in effective spherical diameter and/or 1000 particles per container equal to or greater than 25 μm in effective spherical diameter. As previously indicated, the counting is done using an electronic liquid-borne particle counter with a light-obscuration sensor.

Freedom from Pyrogens

Early in the practice of parenteral administration of drugs, pyretic reactions were observed frequently. These reactions were malaise, headache, and increased fever. Terms such as "salt fever," "serum fever," "protein fever," and "salvarsan fever" were commonly used to denote the reactions. The causes for these effects, as the names indicate, were attributed to several sources: impurities found in the glass of the syringe or package container, the chemical itself, the pH of the solution, the rubber tubing used in administering the solution, and even the temperature of the solution. It was not until the classic observations of Florence Seibert in 1923 that the substances responsible for these untoward reactions from the injection of parenteral drugs were recognized as bacterial in origin, and that the organisms primarily occurred in the water used as the solvent. By carefully distilling the water before use and storing it properly, Seibert demonstrated that these fever-producing materials (bacterial endotoxins) could be eliminated.

The term "pyrogen" had originated earlier in reference to a fever-producing substance obtained from spoiled meat; it is derived from the Greek words meaning "production of fire." Later, pyrogen was used to designate any fever-producing agent.

Definition

Pyrogens, or bacterial endotoxins, are defined as metabolic products of living microorganisms, or the dead microorganisms themselves, causing a specific pyretic response upon injection. They occur whenever microorganisms are allowed to grow. Regardless of their microbial source, they appear to have similar properties. Chemically, they are considered to be lipopolysaccharides, soluble in water but insoluble in organic solvents.[13] They can be filterable macromolecular solids with molecular weights reported to be as low as 15,000 or as high as 4 million. Because they are soluble in water, neither sterilization with moist heat under pressure nor filtration through sterilizing filters eliminates pyrogens, although these processes eliminate the living microorganisms. Pyrogens produced by gram-negative microorganisms are the most potent. Dry pyrogen extracts appear to be stable over long periods; even pyrogenic aqueous solutions lose little of their activity over years.

Pharmacologic Effects

The effects of the administration of pyrogens vary not only with microbial source of the pyrogen but also with the species of the animal receiving the injection. The rabbit is among the species most sensitive to pyrogens, and for this reason had been used traditionally as the test animal in the official test for the detection of pyrogens.

Other variables in the response to pyrogens are the route of administration and the volume of solution administered. Pyrogens assume a greater importance in the intravenous administration of drugs than in the subcutaneous or intramuscular administration. This is a result not only of the route of administration but also of the fact that larger volumes are given intravenously than by other routes.

In man, the pyrogenic reaction is manifested by fever and chills. Following injection, there is a latent period of 45 to 90 minutes, than a rapid rise in body temperature, followed by chills, headache, and malaise. The chills last 10 to 20 minutes, reaching a peak in the second or third hour. Usually, the effects can be controlled by the administration of an antipyretic drug, but a rise in temperature in selectively ill patients could conceivably have severe consequences on the course of an illness. Also, a pyrogenic reaction to a product indicates poor technique and handling on the part of the manufacturer or manipulator during the product's preparation or administration. Thus, it is a reaction that all manufacturers seek to avoid because it is an indictment against their product and company name.

Occurrence

When pyrogens do occur in parenteral products, they come from one of three sources: the water used as the solvent; the containers with which the solution has come into contact during its preparation, packaging, storage, or administration; or the chemicals used in the preparation of the solution.

The most common source of pyrogens is the water used to make the solution. Although water itself is a poor culture medium, contamination can occur by airborne or dust-borne microorganisms. As discussed previously, this is why the only water used in the preparation of parenteral products is Water for Injection. If distillation is used to prepare Water for Injection, the still must be properly designed and operated. Because pyrogens are nonvolatile, they are removed from the feed water by distillation. The pyrogen-free distillate is collected in pyrogen-free and sterile containers. If the containers are not pyrogen-free, the pyrogens on the container are dissolved in the water, thus making it pyrogenic. If the container is not sterile, microorganisms are able to grow and produce pyrogens, resulting in a pyrogenic solvent. Water for Injection, when collected in pyrogen-free and sterile containers, must be used within 24 hours for the preparation of parenteral products that are going to be sterilized within this period. If Water for Injection is to be kept for a longer period, it can be stored in pyrogen-free, sterile containers at either 5° C or 80° C (temperatures at which microorganisms will not grow) to eliminate the possibility of pyrogens. An alternative is to sterilize Water for Injection, thereby maintaining sterility until time of use. After sterilization, it is labeled "Sterile Water for Injection" and as such has no restrictions as to when it may be used, provided that it is packaged properly.

In pharmaceutical plants provided with a distribution system for Water for Injection, the pipe lines circulating the solvent are subject to the same requirements as when the solvent is collected in glass bottles. Materials of construction must be chosen so as not to alter the chemical quality of the water. In the piping, cracks and crevices must be avoided to reduce the accumulation of material or bacteria. To accomplish this, the system should be constructed of welded stainless steel. Usually, the Water for Injection remaining from daily production is discarded rather than stored at the end of the day.

Pyrogens can be eliminated from metal and glass containers by dry heat. When this is not practical, owing to the size of the containers or the nonavailability of proper dry heat equipment, pyrogens can be eliminated by rinsing the containers well with pyrogen-free Water for Injection; the pyrogens, being water-soluble, are removed by repeated rinsings.

The same requirement must also be applied to the filling equipment, the containers and components used in packaging the product, and the devices used in administering the parenteral injection, whether the latter be a syringe or an administration set for an infusion solution. Again, when it is not practical to eliminate pyrogens with dry heat, the equipment must be thoroughly washed with Water for Injection. Wet equipment, when allowed to dry over a period of time under ordinary room conditions, can be a source of pyrogen contamination.

The chemicals used in the preparation of parenteral products can be the source of pyrogens, although they are not the most common source. Chemicals from natural sources or those prepared by fermentation processes, including dextrose, fructose, sodium citrate, phosphate salts, amino acids, and heparin, can become pyrogenic if contaminating microorganisms are allowed to flourish at some point in the processing of the chemicals and are not removed by subsequent treatment to isolate the chemicals. When a chemical is found to be pyrogenic, it is best to use another lot of the chemical, or another source for the chemical. As a specification, freedom from pyrogens is not commonly listed for chemicals. An exception has been ampul-grade ascorbic acid, which indicates that the chemical has been tested and found free from pyrogens. This specification is one that usually must be determined by the manufacturer using the chemical.

Elimination of Pyrogens

Being organic compounds, pyrogens can be destroyed with high heat by oxidation, or "burning up." Satisfactorily high temperatures are 250° C for 30 to 45 minutes or 180° C for 3 to 4 hours. Although this method is effective for pyrogens contaminating glassware and metal containers, it is not practical for solutions. Pyrogens in solutions are eliminated chemically by oxidation with peroxides, acids, and alkalis, but these agents also destroy the drugs and other chemicals in solution. Absorption of pyrogens in solution by asbestos and charcoal has also been reported to be effective, but the drugs and other chemicals in solution are also partially or completely removed. Having relatively high molecular weights compared to those of the drugs in solutions, synthetic filter media may offer the means of selectively removing pyrogens from solution.[14] At present, however, these media do not offer a practical approach for eliminating pyrogens from a contaminated parenteral solution. The best approach, from a practical point of view, is to prevent them from occurring by making certain that the parenteral solutions are made with pyrogen-free chemicals, Water for Injection, and pyrogen-free equipment and are packaged in pyrogen-free containers.

Pyrogen Test

To substantiate the fact that parenteral solutions, as well as devices for their administration, are free of harmful quantities of pyrogenic contaminants, samples taken from each production batch are subjected to a pyrogen test for pyrogens. The traditional test is a biologic one employing the rabbit as the test animal, because the rabbit is highly sensitive to pyrogens (Fig. 3–1). Samples of the parenteral solution are injected into the ear veins of three rabbits to determine whether the samples cause an increase in body temperatures. The test is a limiting one, i.e., it allows for the presence of pyrogens but physiologically limits the quantity. Temperatures above prescribed limits indicate the presence of pyrogenic material. To test devices, the devices are washed with Sterile Water for Injection and the washings are injected into the rabbits' ear veins. The rabbit test used today is essentially the same as that developed by Seibert in the 1920s and has been recognized throughout the world as the official method. It has all the disadvantages of a biologic method, namely, variability of response and difficulty in controlling all the influencing factors. The procedure for performing the pyrogen test is described in the *U.S.P.*. Most hospital pharmacies send samples to commercial laboratories for pyrogen testing. The official test is not satisfactory for testing some parenteral agents because of their pharmacologic effect on the rabbits. Some drugs may be inherently pyrogenic, whereas others, such as morphine and its derivatives, appear to mask the pyrogenic effect.

An alternate approach for detecting pyrogen contamination is the bacterial endotoxins test using the reagent, limulus amebocyte lysate. Originally developed as a rapid in vitro test for radiopharmaceuticals, the test has been further developed and has gained recognition, by both the *U.S.P.* and the

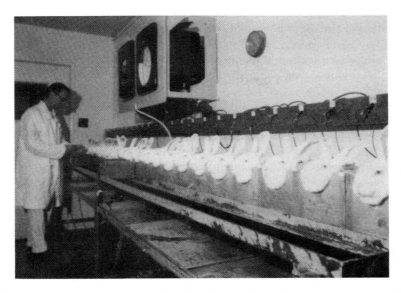

Figure 3–1. Pyrogen test using rabbits. (Courtesy of Scientific Associates, Inc., St. Louis, MO).

Food and Drug Administration as being suitable for injections and medical devices.[14] The amebocytes, or circulating blood cells, of the horseshoe crab *(Limulus polyphemus)* contain a protein that clots in the presence of bacterial endotoxins (pyrogens). Prepared as a lyophilized powder, the amebocyte lysate has been shown to be a sensitive reagent for the detection of pyrogens in parenteral solutions. When present in solution with pyrogens, the lysate causes gelation of the solution that can be visually observed within 60 minutes. The advantages of the test's simplicity, sensitivity, and reproducibility have been recognized. Comparison testing of endotoxin solutions by both the limulus lysate test and the *U.S.P.* pyrogen test has confirmed that the former test is the more sensitive and reliable.[15]

Implications of Pyrogens in Clinical Practice

Freedom from pyrogens is a characteristic required of all parenteral products and the devices used for their administration. Because of rigorous adherence by pharmaceutical manufacturers to good manufacturing practices and control procedures, pyrogenic reactions from commercial preparations are relatively rare. Cases of pyrogenic contamination have been reported for Antihemophilic Factor, Mannitol Injection, Methicillin, and Normal Serum Albumin.[16,17] Clinically, it is difficult to ascertain the extent and consequences of pyrogenic incidences and responses. Physicians frequently fail to associate an increase in temperature with a pyrogen-contaminated product, but such cases have been reported.[18] The decline in frequency of these incidents is the result of better industrial technology as well as the increased use of disposable administration sets and other equipment.

Stability

In developing a sterile dosage form, prime consideration is given to the stability of the drug. Drugs in solution tend to be less stable than drugs in dry form. For parenteral administration, a solution or suspension is required, and factors regarding drug stabilization are carefully considered. The selection of added substances aids in the maintenance of physical and chemical stability. For solutions, physical stability usually refers to the physical appearance of the product on storage. The formation of precipitates or color usually indicates instability. Drug degradation is not necessarily indicated by visual changes; a subpotent solution can remain clear and colorless. It is the responsibility of the manufacturer to ensure the stability of the prduct by proper formulation and packaging.[19,20] Packaging components assume an important role in determining product stability. Not only must they be inert with respect to their own physical and chemical characteristics, but they must in no way modify or react with the chemicals present in the solution. For light-sensitive drugs, packaging requirements include containers of amber glass or light-resistant cartons to protect the solutions from changes caused by light.[21] If special storage conditions are required, these should be clearly printed on the label.

It is the responsibility of the manufacturer to ensure that a given batch of a parenteral product is stable by periodically conducting assays on samples retained by the quality control group. Once the package is opened, however, and its contents are added to another solution or are repackaged in another container, stability can no longer be ensured and depends on a large number of variables.

When the stability of a drug in solution cannot be maintained over a reasonable period of time, the solution may be lyophilized. Lyophilization is the process of rapidly freezing and drying the frozen sterile solution of drug under high vacuum. The water present passes from the solid state to the vapor state without passing through the liquid phase. Drying leaves a sterile residue containing the drug and other additives; the dried material can be restored to solution at time of use by adding the proper sterile diluent. A lyophilization chamber is depicted in Figure 3–2.

When formulating a drug solution for lyophilization, a chemical or diluent, such as mannitol, is added to the solution to give a structure, or matrix, to the dried residue. The solution of the drug is prepared, sterilized by filtration, and aseptically subdivided into the final sterile containers. Trays of containers are placed in the lyophilization chamber. After lyophilization, a "plug" of residue equivalent to the original volume of the solution remains in the container. The containers are aseptically removed and closed. The term "lyophilize" means "love to dissolve," and the rapidity with which the solid returns to solution indicates the reason for the name of the process. Many parenteral dosage forms have been made commercially possible by means of this process, and its technology is rapidly developing. The process and its application to pharmaceuticals have been reviewed.[22]

Another drying method used commercially to prepare sterile powders for reconstitution is spray-drying. This method is being used for a number of antibiotic powders. Under carefully controlled aseptic conditions, a sterile solution of the antibiotic is sprayed into the top of a cone-shaped chamber through

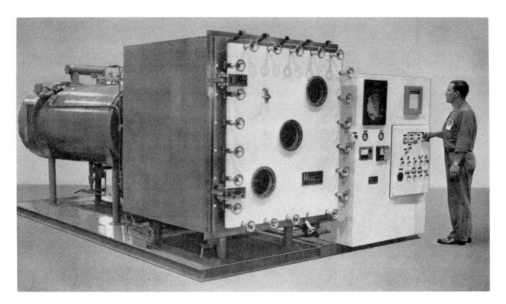

Figure 3–2. Lyophilization chamber. (Courtesy of Hull Corporation, Hatboro, PA.)

which warm air is circulating. The atomized droplets dry rapidly as they fall through the warm air. The spray-dried particles are homogeneous, uniform in size, and nearly spherical in shape; the latter characteristic gives the powder good flowing characteristics. After collection, the bulk sterile powder is subdivided into sterile containers.

When preparing parenterals and other sterile dosage forms commercially or extemporaneously, or when using them clinically, the characteristics of sterility, freedom from particulate matter, freedom from pyrogens, and stability must be recognized and given proper attention.

References

1. Lockhart, J.D.: Medical Significance of Particulate Matter in Large Volume Parenterals. FDA Symposium of Safety of Large Volume Solutions. Washington, DC, July 28–29, 1966, p. 23.
2. Brewer, J.H., and Dunning, J.H.F.: An *in vitro* and *in vivo* study of glass particles in ampules. J. Am. Pharm. Assoc., Sci. Ed., *36*, 289 (1947).
3. Garvan, J.M., and Gunner, B.W.: Intravenous fluids: A solution containing particles should not be used. Med. J. Austral., *2*, 140 (1963).
4. Garvan, J.M., and Gunner, B.W.: The harmful effects of particles in intravenous fluids. Med. J. Austral., *2*, 1 (1963).
5. The United States Pharmacopeia, XXII Revision, Easton, PA, Mack Publishing Co., 1990, p. 1471.
6. Davis, N.N., Turco, S., and Sively, E.: Particulate matter in I.V. infusion fluids. Bull. Parenter. Drug Assoc., *24*, 257 (1970).
7. Turco, S., and Davis, N.: Clinical significance of particulate matter: A review of the literature. Hosp. Pharm., *8*, 137 (1973).
8. Trasen, B.: Membrane filtration technique in analysis for particulate matter. Bull. Parenter. Drug Assoc., *22*, 1 (1968).
9. McCrone, W.C., Draftz, R.G., and Delly, J.G.: The Particle Atlas. Ann Arbor, MI, Ann Arbor Science Publishers, 1970.

10. Levy, J.D., McCarthy, C.J., and Stevens, R.E.: Application of image analysis for rapid determination of particles in parenteral solutions. Bull. Parenteral Drug Assoc., *31*, 299 (1977).
11. Hopkins, G.H., and Young, R.W.: Correlation of microscopic counts with instrumental particle counts. Bull. Parenter. Drug Assoc., *28*, 15 (1974).
12. Louer, R.C., Jr., Russoman, J.A., and Rasanen, P.R.: Detection of particulate matter in parenteral solutions by image projection: A concept and its feasibility. Bull. Parenteral. Drug Assoc., *25*, 54 (1971).
13. Good, C.M., and Lane, H.E., Jr.: The biochemistry of pyrogens. Bull. Parenter. Drug Assoc., *31*, 116 (1977).
14. Parenteral Drug Association: Depyrogenation. Technical Report No. 7, 1985.
15. Food and Drug Administration: Draft Guideline for Validation of the Limulus Amebocyte Lysate Test as an End-Product Test for Human and Animal Parenteral Drugs, Biological Products, and Medical Devices. Rockville, MD, 1983.
16. Ann. Drug Recalls, J. Am. Pharm. Assoc., *10*, 577 (1973).
17. Ann. APhA Newsletter, Oct. 9, 1976.
18. Spengler, R.F., Melvin, V.B., Lietman, P.S., and Greenough, W.B.: Febrile reactions after methicillin. Lancet, Feb. 2, 1974.
19. Lin, S.: Stability testing program for parenteral products. Bull. Parenter. Drug. Assoc., *24*, 83 (1970).
20. Lin, S.: Comparison of accelerated stability data with shelf-life studies. Bull. Parenter. Drug Assoc., *34*, 269 (1969).
21. Lin, S., and Lachman, L.: Photochemical considerations of parenteral products. Bull. Parenter. Drug Assoc., 23:149 (1969).
22. Williams, N.A., and Polli, G.P.: The lyophilization of pharmaceuticals: A literature review. J. Parenteral. Sci. Tech., *38*, 48 (1984).

4

CHAPTER

Large-Scale Preparation

Whether sterile products are prepared on an industrial scale or made extemporaneously by the hospital pharmacist, the raw materials used, the procedures involved, the packaging, and the care taken determine whether the final products will have the required characteristics previously described. Quality must be built into the products from the beginning; it cannot be imparted after the products have been made. Although the extemporaneous preparation of one or two units of sterile products by the hospital pharmacist may appear to be simpler than the preparation of tens of thousands of units by a large group of personnel in an industrial setting, in essence there is a great similarity in factors that must be considered. The main differences are found only in the steps taken, owing to the large quantity of materials used and the number of personnel involved in industrial operations. In the following discussion, the preparation of a large number of units of sterile products is described. In Chapter 5, the conditions necessary in the extemporaneous preparation of a few units are described, and the similarities between the two operations are noted.

Environmental Control

If sterile products are to be free from particulate matter, they must be prepared, sterilized, and packaged in an environment free of particulate matter. In the overall processing, certain steps have more critical requirements than others. In Figure 4–1, note that critical steps include the preparation of the filling area, the procedures of washing and sterilizing the packaging components, and the preparation of the personnel who fill or subdivide the product into its final package.

The filling area, or room in which the solution is subdivided into its final package, is critical, because at this point, the solution is exposed to both the environment and the personnel involved. Thus, this area must be maintained

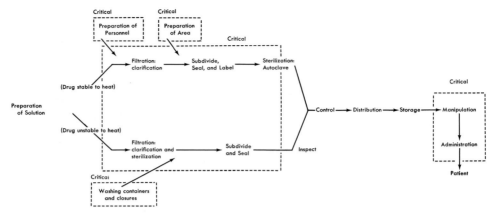

Figure 4–1. Flow sheet for the preparation of sterile products.

as free as possible from particulate matter, such as dust, lint, and fibers. The air supplying these areas can be passed through high efficiency particulate air (HEPA) filters capable of removing particles of 0.3 μm or greater with an efficiency of 99.97%. Microbial contaminants present in air are usually found on dust and other particulate matter and are also hereby removed. Thus, the filtered air coming into this critical area is free of both particulate and microbial contamination. The air is supplied under positive pressure, i.e., the air in the critical area, having a higher pressure than air in the adjoining areas, flows outward when doors are opened. This prevents particulate contamination from sweeping into the critical filling area.

The critical filling area is constructed from materials that can easily be cleaned and disinfected. The walls can be stainless steel or regular wall material covered with an epoxy resin paint. Likewise, the work surfaces and floor are smooth and free of cracks and crevices. The entire facility may be irradiated with ultraviolet lamps to ensure the disinfection of all surfaces exposed to the rays and to maintain sterility once personnel have entered the room. Personnel must be protected from ultraviolet irradiation while they are working in this area.

Laminar Air Control

From his work in the space technology program in the early 1960s, Dr. Willis Whitfield developed the concept of laminar air flow while trying to improve on conventional clean rooms.[1] He noticed that filtered air forced through wall or ceiling ducts creates swirls in the airstream that can trap particles and microorganisms in a room. His concept of laminar air flow is a bank of filtered air that moves through a work area in a parallel configuration and at sufficient speed to sweep contamination with it and create a minimum of turbulence (Fig. 4–2). Laminar flow is defined in federal regulations as "air flow in which the entire body of air within a confined space moves with uniform velocity along parallel lines with a minimum of eddies." The velocity of the air for effective laminar air flow is usually stated as 90 ± 20 feet per minute throughout the undisturbed room area.

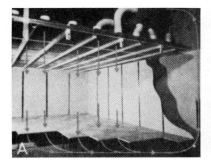 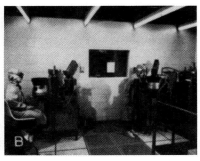

Figure 4–2. *A,* Vertical laminar air flow in production facility. Air turbulence is minimized and environmental control can be achieved. *B,* Prefiltered air is forced through a high efficiency particulate air (HEPA) filter and flows downward over filling equipment, continually bathing the area with clean air. (Courtesy of Wyeth Laboratories, Philadelphia, PA.)

The concept of laminar air flow has been applied in the parenteral drug industry in a number of ways. Some companies, when building new facilities, have constructed laminar air flow rooms for their critical operations. In these rooms, an entire wall consists of HEPA filters through which the air is forced. The most critical operations are placed closest to the laminar air flow wall, and the less critical are placed farther away. Laminar air flow units have been placed above filling machines, with the vertical laminar air flow washing all particulate material from the area where the open containers receive the solutions. Constructed in the form of hoods, laminar air flow equipment is used extensively for sterility testing and for aseptic manipulations in hospitals; the latter application is discussed in the next chapter.

By federal standards, clean rooms have been classified into three groups: Class 100, Class 10,000, and Class 100,000.[2] This classification is based on the particle count. The maximum allowance of particles permissible is 0.5 μm and larger or 5.0 μm and larger. The limits are expressed as follows:

  Class 100—Particle count not to exceed a total of 100 particles per cubic foot of a size 0.5 μm and larger.

  Class 10,000—Particle count not to exceed a total of 10,000 particles per cubic foot of a size 5.0 μm and larger, or 65 particles per cubic foot of a size 5.0 μm and larger.

  Class 100,000—Particle count not to exceed a total of 100,000 particles per cubic foot of a size 05 μm and larger, or 700 particles per cubic foot of a size 5.0 μm and larger.

All clean room facilities must be monitored to ensure that they are receiving proper maintenance.[3,4] The rooms are monitored for both viable and other particulates to confirm adherence to established standards. The microbial content of the ambient air can be determined by settle plates (fallout plates) or mechanical air-sampling devices such as the Anderson sampler and the Reynier slit air sampler. Settle plates consist of open Petri dishes containing sterile nutrient agar, which are exposed to the air for a prescribed length of time. After the plates are incubated at a specified temperature and for a specified period of time, a count is made of the number of colonies on each plate. The disadvantages of the technique are that only the larger particles settle rapidly and that the volume of air tested is not known. These drawbacks are avoided when the mechanical air-sampling devices are used. Air is drawn through these instruments at a specified rate over a Petri dish containing sterile nutrient medium. After incubation, the counts can be expressed as the number of colonies per cubic foot of sampled air. Surface swabs subjected to the same procedures are used to determine microbial contamination of floors and flat surfaces.

Nonviable particulates are counted by electronic devices such as the Royco particle counter. Standards are established, and deviation from these standards for both viable particles and other particulates can be readily detected. Cleaning procedures and schedules are of utmost importance in maintaining the low levels of particulate contamination required for the satisfactory manufacture of sterile products.

Likewise, HEPA filters, whether they are located in hoods, walls, or ceiling, must be routinely checked for the presence of cracks and the maintenance of proper velocity (see "Environmental Control" in Chap. 5). Manufacturers of laminar flow equipment, as well as private laboratories, offer maintenance contracts for the continued safe operation of the equipment.

Personnel

The greatest source of particulate matter and possible microbial contamination in the preparation of sterile products, and the most difficult to monitor, is the personnel involved. When working in this critical area, personnel are garbed in jumpsuits, including hood and gloves. Their shoes are covered with disposable boots. The uniforms are most satisfactory when made from monofilament fabrics, such as Dacron or Ty-Vek, which do not shed lint or fibers. By nature, the personnel should be conscientious and reliable. The best standard operating procedures fail when they are not followed. Motivation of personnel is accomplished by giving them a thorough understanding of the importance of their tasks, and such motivation becomes critical to the operation. These personnel include not only the persons involved in the filling operation but also those given responsibility in other areas, such as maintenance. Failure to do their jobs adequately can result in the failure of the production lot, or worse, the passing through control of a lot of material that fails in one or more of the requirements for sterility, freedom from particulate matter, or freedom from pyrogens.

Packaging Components

Materials used for packaging and administering parenterals include components made of glass, rubber, stainless steel, and plastic. Regardless of its composition or form, the packaging material constitutes a likely source for stability problems, particulate matter, and pyrogens.[5] Since the initial use of glass for sterile products early in this century, much progress has been made in glass technology, and many problems rising from its use as a packaging material have been solved.

Glass

The degree of resistance of the product to glass varies with the type of product to be packaged in the container. The chemical attack rate of aqueous solutions on glass is high but varies with the pH and the constituents of the aqueous solution. On the other hand, solutions of a hydrophobic nature, such as oils, organic solvents, or dry sterile solids, show little chemical attack on the glass. Aqueous solutions containing heat-stable drugs frequently are terminally sterilized in the final glass container, and the heat of the sterilization process accelerates the chemical attack on the glass. The chemical attack by parenteral products on glass is caused primarily by released alkali, which can cause deleterious effects on the parenteral solution following changes in pH, composition, color, and stability.

Glass is made by fusing amorphous silicon dioxide (sand) with metallic oxides at high temperatures.[6] The characteristics of the resultant glass depend on the nature and quantities of the alkaline earth and metal oxides. Glass prepared from silica, in combination with a relatively high amount of boron oxide and small amount of the alkaline earth oxides, is a borosilicate glass with high chemical stability, low coefficient of thermal expansion, and high resistance to heat shock. Glass containing no boron oxide and high quantities of the alkaline earth oxide is a "soft" glass having poor chemical and heat resistance. The latter glass is more easily worked (i.e., molded), and therefore is lower in cost. Amber glass used for products sensitive to light contains manganese oxide, which gives the glass its color.

For parenteral products, the compendia have classified glass based on its resistance to water attack and its release of alkali. The *U.S.P.* classification is as follows: Type 1—highly resistant borosilicate glass; Type II—treated soda-lime glass; and Type III—soda-lime glass. Type II glass is essentially soda-lime glass that, after being molded into the desired form, is treated with acidic gas under controlled humidity and elevated temperatures to neutralize the alkali present on the surface of the glass; the alkali forms sodium sulfate, which is subsequently removed in washing the containers. The sterilization of glass packaging components is also influenced by the type of glass. Glass components molded from Type I glass may be sterilized before or after filling with solution, whereas Type II glass *should* be sterilized by dry heat before filling; Type III glass *must* be sterilized by dry heat before filling.

Initially, glass packaging components for new products are made from Type I glass to eliminate as many container problems as possible. As experience and stability data are collected for a product, the manufacturer may find it possible to use a less expensive glass, such as Type II or Type III. Products having a pH greater than 7.0, or one that may become alkaline before the expiration date, should not be packaged in Type II or Type III glass containers. Type II glass containers may be used for solutions having pH values less than 7.0. Both Types II and III are suitable for oils and sterile powders.

One source of precipitate observed in solutions packaged in glass results from the reaction of components of the solution with the alkali leached from the glass, or the leaching of metallic ions, which act as catalysts for other reactions. Solutions containing phosphates, citrates, or tartrates are subject to flake formation, owing to reaction with materials from the glass. Precipitates

TABLE 4–1. Composition of Rubber Packaging Components

Component	Composition
Rubber	Natural, neoprene, or butyl
Vulcanizing agent	Sulfur
Accelerator	Guanidines, sulfide compounds
Activator	Zinc oxide, stearic acid
Fillers	Carbon black, kaolin, barium sulfate
Plasticizer	Dibutyl phthalate, stearic acid
Antioxidants	Aromatic amines

were observed when commercially prepared solutions of dextrose 5% in water are combined with solutions containing 40 mEq potassium chloride.[7] The precipitate was shown by analysis to be silica and alumina. It is highly probable that the silica was material leached from the glass container.

Another example of the leaching of solids from glass is the total solids requirements for Sterile Water for Injection. Whereas Water for Injection has a limit of 10 ppm, Sterile Water for Injection is permitted higher limits depending on container size: 40 ppm for containers up to and including 30-ml size, 30 ppm for containers 30- to 100-ml size, and 20 ppm for larger sizes. A greater limit is permitted for Sterile Water for Injection because of the leaching of material from the glass during sterilization. The requirement decreases as the volume increases because the ratio of the volume to the wetted inner surfaces decreases.

Rubber

To provide closures for multiple-dose vials, intravenous fluid bottles, plugs for disposable syringes, and bulbs for ophthalmic pipettes, rubber is the material of choice. Its elasticity, ability to reseal after puncture, and adaptability to many shapes make it unique. One must remember, however, that the composition of any single piece of rubber represents the combination of many ingredients to give it the characteristics required. To understand some of the problems arising from the use of rubber for packaging components, it is necessary to understand the variety of materials in the final composition of the package (Table 4–1).

The rubber compound is the basic ingredient, and this polymer is vulcanized in the presence of sulfur with heat. The vulcanization reduces plasticity and improves the resistance of the rubber to changes in temperature. To increase the rate of vulcanization, compounds such as guanidine derivatives are present as accelerators; these in turn are activated with materials such as zinc oxide and stearic acid. The tensile strength, hardness, and permeability are influenced by materials such as carbon black and barium sulfate; these materials are called fillers. Plasticizing agents and antioxidants are added to reduce the effect of oxygen on the rubber compound. The rubber and the additives are mixed, then subjected to heat and pressure during the molding process for the given rubber packaging components. Thus, the rubber piece that serves as a closure for a parenteral vial or a plug in a disposable syringe is a complex material.

Several problems originate from the rubber closure. It the closure is incompatible with the solution, the solution can become discolored, turbid, and degraded. Surface-active agents in the solution can extract chemicals from the closures; the extractives in turn can catalyze or react with ingredients in the solution, causing physical or chemical instability. There may be loss of the preservative or other added materials in the solution, owing to their absorption into the closure. For moisture-sensitive sterile solids, the closure may permit the transfer of moisture, causing the degradation of the drug. For every product, the compatibility of the rubber closure with the sterile solution, suspension, or powder must be determined and the best closure selected. Once a given rubber closure has been selected for a parenteral product, the rubber manufacturer has the responsibility to maintain consistently all characteristics of the closure. To do this, tests such as ash, specific gravity, ultraviolet, and infrared spectrophotometric analysis of solvent extract are used.[8,9]

One of the most frequently encountered problems associated with rubber closures is that of coring.[10] Coring is the generation of rubber particles cut from the closures when needles or medical devices are inserted; the particles are known as "cores" (see "Techniques of Parenteral Administration" in Chap. 6). Cores are deposited in the solution or remain in the cannula. It is believed that the cores are cut from the lower surface of the closure when the heel of the needle enters the rubber. Although coring is primarily attributed to the design of the needle, the composition of the rubber used for the closure also can influence the degree of coring. The tendency of a rubber closure to core sometimes represents a compromise in composition to obtain a rubber closure with good stability.

Coring is observed at time of use of the product. Unduly large gauge needles increase the chance of coring. Some precautions may be taken to minimize it. A minimum gauge needle should be inserted with the bevel side up at an angle less than 45 degrees. After penetration of the closure, but before entrance into the container, the needle should be in the vertical position. Rubber closures on products that require refrigeration or freezing become more prone to coring. Delaying the reconstitution of the product until after the closure has warmed to room temperature alleviates the coring tendency. Similar care must be exercised when inserting plastic spikes into large-volume intravenous fluids. The prepared or reconstituted product should be examined for cores. The presence of cores indicates that the product should be discarded, or in some instances, it may be necessary to remove the cores by filtration to salvage the product.

Plastic

The plastic used in preparing packaging material is also complex.[10] The primary constituent is the plastic polymer, usually polyethylene or polypropylene. The polymers differ in their characteristics. Polyethylene exhibits low water absorption, high resistance to most solvents, and low resistance to heat. For this reason, polyethylene items cannot be sterilized by autoclaving. On the other hand, polypropylene shows high resistance to most solvents and can be autoclaved. In addition to the plastic polymer, other chemicals are added to modify the physical characteristics of the material, e.g., plasticizers to improve flexibility; stabilizers to protect the plastic from light and discoloration;

accelerators to increase the rate of polymerization of the resin; antioxidants to retard oxidation; fillers to modify physical properties such as strength; colorants; and lubricants in the case of molded pieces. The composition of the plastic and of the solution determines the degree of reactivity between the additives of the plastic and the components of the solution. Substances can be leached from the plastic into the solution, and ingredients from the solution can be absorbed by the plastic. The plastic may be permeable to moisture, permitting loss of volume and modification of concentration of the solution. The degree to which these problems occur depends on whether the plastic device or container, such as a disposable plastic syringe, is for short-term, one-time use, or whether the device is to be used as a package in which a solution is to be stored over a long period.

Preparation of Packaging Components

Before being used to package sterile products, glass and rubber components are washed and sterilized. Improper handling of packaging materials in the preparation stage is one of the greatest sources of contamination by particulate matter. Glass containers received in cardboard and chipboard boxes contain dust generated by these packaging materials. This dust and other particulates are difficult to eliminate, and frequently, the empty glass containers are vacuumed before washing. Another approach to reducing troublesome particulates has been the use of "shrink wrapping." Groups of empty glass containers are wrapped tightly together with plastic film before shipment, thus eliminating the contact of the glass with the cardboard cartons. The glass containers are passed through a number of cycles in automatic washing equipment. The cycles vary depending on the type of equipment, but usually consist of rinsing the container alternately with cold water and then with steam. The expansion and contraction of the glass break down films and allow steam to penetrate and clean the surface. This "shock treatment" promotes the removal of all particulate material. The washing consists of the following steps: (1) outside, rinse with filtered water; (2) inside, rinse with steam; (3) outside, rinse with filtered water; (4) inside, rinse with steam; (5) outside, rinse with filtered water; (6) inside, rinse with steam; (7) inside, rinse with steam. Rough treatment of glassware in the washing equipment or during handling can generate glass particulate matter, which subsequently contaminates the filled containers. After washing, the glass containers are placed in stainless steel boxes and are rendered pyrogen-free and sterile by means of dry heat. The handling area for the wet containers is maintained under vertical laminar air flow to prevent the particulates in the environment from contaminating the clean wet containers (Fig. 4–3). After heating, the containers are moved to a sterile area and allowed to cool.

Washing procedures for glass containers have been made more effective for removing particulate matter by including a fluoride treatment in the wash cycle. The containers are washed with either dilute hydrofluoric acid or ammonium bifluoride solutions. The glasses are allowed to remain in contact with the fluoride solution for approximately 30 seconds before the solution is rinsed away. This treatment removes a thin surface layer of the glass with its ad-

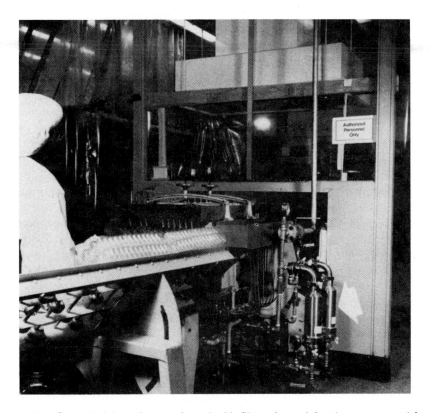

Figure 4–3. Cozzoli vial washer equipped with filters (arrow) for the water used for the two final rinses. The washed vials pass from the machine into a laminar air flow area. (Courtesy of Pall Trinity Micro Corporation, Cortland, NY.)

herent particulate matter. When this procedure is used, the safety of personnel must be a consideration.

As a method of sterilization, dry heat is not as efficient as moist heat, and therefore higher temperatures and longer exposure times are required. Dry heat sterilization is effective for oxidizing, or "burning up," and sterilizing chemicals and oils, provided temperatures below their decomposition temperatures are used. Many variables must be considered in using dry heat sterilization, including size of the oven, size of the load, arrangement of the load, and nature of the material being sterilized. Ovens usually have circulating forced-air heat. Glass containers are usually heated at 180° C or higher for 4 hours. This period would be in addition to the time necessary for the contents to reach 180° C and would vary considerably with the factors mentioned previously.

In preparing rubber components such as closures and plugs, the objective is to eliminate surface dirt, rubber particles, and water-soluble extractives, and to render the closures sterile. The danger is that, if they are handled roughly, particles will be generated by the rubbing surfaces of the rubber pieces; this can be a source of particulate matter found later in the filled container. Methods of preparation vary in the industry, but usually they consist of gently agitating the closures in a mild detergent, thoroughly rinsing the detergent away, autoclaving the closures immersed in Water for Injection several times, autoclaving the wet closures in a suitable sealed package, and drying at low heat. Autoclaving involves the use of moist heat under pressure. Autoclaving the closures in Water for Injection allows extraction of the water-soluble constituents before the closure is placed on a filled container and autoclaved. If this step were not performed, any water-soluble extractives present would pass into the parenteral solution.

Plastic containers are usually washed with filtered air to remove particulate material, then are suitably wrapped and sterilized with ethylene oxide. One of the great advantages of ethylene oxide sterilization of plastics is that the gas, owing to its ability to diffuse and penetrate, sterilizes the plastic materials after they have been assembled and placed in their final packaged form. Chemically, ethylene oxide is a cyclic ether, a liquid to 10° C; above this temperature, it is a gas. It is miscible with water and common organic solvents. On the skin, it acts as a vesicant, and on inhalation, it has the toxicity of ammonia gas. It forms an explosive mixture with air and therefore is usually used in combination with carbon dioxide (10% ethylene oxide and 90% carbon dioxide) or fluorinated hydrocarbons (12% ethylene oxide and 88% fluorinated hydrocarbons). For some industrial applications, 100% ethylene oxide is used.

As in dry heat sterilization, many variables have to be considered when using ethylene oxide as a sterilant. The material to be sterilized is wrapped and placed in a chamber, which is subsequently heated to 130° F to increase the effectiveness of the ethylene oxide. The relative humidity of the chamber and the moisture content of the material are important factors in determining the efficacy of the method. Under ideal conditions, a relative humidity of 30 to 50% is desirable. Sufficient ethylene oxide is introduced into the evacuated chamber to reach a concentration of 450 mg per liter. An exposure time of 4 hours or longer is used, depending on the material, type of packaging, and size of the chamber. After the sterilization cycle is completed, the material is placed in quarantine for 5 days to 2 weeks to allow the residual ethylene oxide to vaporize. The time required for the residual amount of ethylene oxide to dissipate depends on the nature of the material, the method of packaging, and the conditions under which the material was sterilized.[11]

Another concern in the use of ethylene oxide is the presence of reaction products; ethylene oxide can react with water to form ethylene glycol, with chloride ion to form 2-chloroethanol, and with sulfhydryl groups to form 2-mercaptoethanol. When present in sufficient concentration on the sterilized item, these reaction products can cause untoward and toxic reactions. As a sterilization process, ethylene oxide must be adapted to the material and conditions involved. Recommendations can be considered only in general terms.

Preparation of Product

Equipment used for the preparation of sterile products should be clean, sterile, and free of pyrogens. If the size of the mixing containers precludes the elimination of pyrogens with dry heat, they should be thoroughly rinsed with Water for Injection prior to use. The purest chemical grades of the added substances should be selected. Following its formulation in a clean but not necessarily sterile area, the solution is ready to be taken into the sterile filling

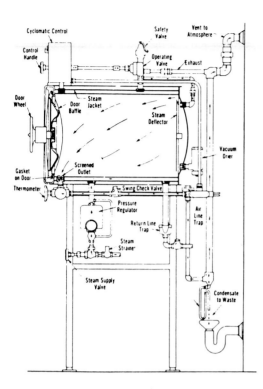

Figure 4–4. Schematic drawing of parts of an autoclave. (Courtesy of American Sterilizer Company, Erie, PA.)

areas. In some manufacturing facilities, the mixing tanks are taken into the filling areas; in other facilities, the solution is pumped through the lines installed through the walls. Because the solution is not sterile at this point, it should be packaged and sterilized within 24 hours. If this is not possible, the bulk solution must be sterilized and stored as a sterile solution.

Clarification and Sterilization

Subsequent handling depends on whether the drug in solution is heat-stable or heat-labile. Heat-stable solutions are clarified (passed through a suitable filtration medium to remove particulate matter), subdivided into the final containers, sealed, and subjected to terminal sterilization by autoclaving (Figs. 4–4 and 4–5). Heat-labile solutions are passed through a suitable filtration medium for both clarification and sterilization, and then subdivided into the final sterile containers and sealed (see Fig. 4–1).

In general, filtration media can be divided into two broad groups, depth filters and screen filters. Depth filters have been made from asbestos, fritted glass, and unglazed porcelain. They trap particles in tortuous channels, thereby clarifying the solution. All the media are available in a large number of pore sizes, the finest being suitable for removing microorganisms with subsequent sterilization of the solution. These media represent an older group of filters. As a group, they have a number of disadvantages and have been replaced by the screen-type filters for clarification and sterilization of parenteral solutions.

Screen or membrane filters are made from cellulose esters, microfilaments, polycarbonate, synthetic polymers, silver, or stainless steel in the form of films 1 to 200 μm thick. The films have a meshwork of millions of microcapillary

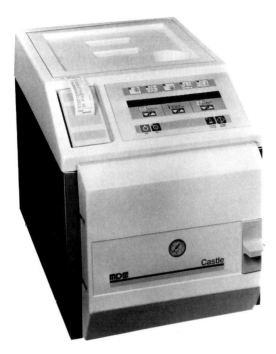

Figure 4–5. Tabletop autoclave designed to sterilize heat and moisture-stable materials. (Courtesy of Castle Company, Rochester, NY.)

pores of uniform size. Membrane filters are available in a number of pore sizes, ranging from 8 to 0.22 μm. Membranes having pore sizes 0.45 μm and smaller are considered to be sterilizing filters, i.e., capable of removing microorganisms as well as other particulate material. Because the pore volume of a membrane filter represents approximately 70 to 85% of the total filter volume, relatively high flow rates are obtained compared to those obtained with the depth filters. Membranes are used either as single sheets of varying diameters supported within stainless steel holders or as fluted columns packaged within plastic cartridges.

In addition to the main clarifying and/or sterilizing filtration steps, filters may be placed at other sites in the filling line. The sterile, clarified solution may be filtered again as it leaves the bulk tank or immediately before it passes through the filling needle into the final container. Clarifying filters are placed on line after the main clarifying and/or sterilizing filtration to remove particulate matter generated by the filling lines and the equipment regulating the filling volume.

Vertical laminar air flow units are frequently placed directly above the filling machine to prevent particulate matter in the environment from falling into the open container while it is being filled. An excess volume of solution is placed in all parenteral containers so that the labeled volume of solution can be withdrawn from the container; a 10% excess is used for a 1 ml container and 2% for a 100-ml container. The *U.S.P.* provides a guide listing the recommended excess volume for a container of a given size. Slightly larger allowances are made for viscous solutions. Checking for proper volume fill is an in-process control as well as a control for the finished package.

When the solution is subdivided into glass vials or bottles the containers are sealed with rubber closures and aluminum caps. The aluminum caps crimped

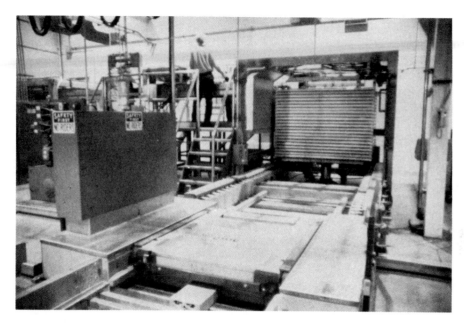

Figure 4–6. Sterilization of LVP bag equipment. (Courtesy of Abbott Laboratories, North Chicago, IL.)

onto the containers over the rubber closures hold the closures securely and protect the surface of the closure prior to use. The center tab or perforated center can be removed and the exposed area of the closure disinfected prior to injecting the needle to withdraw the solution. To close ampules, the stems are sealed by fusion of the glass, either by tip-sealing or by pull-sealing. In tip-sealing, the ampule is rotated while the tip of its stem is held in a hot flame, usually obtained by burning a mixture of natural gas and oxygen. The tip closes by fusion of the glass, forming a "bead." In pull-sealing, the ampule is rotated in a hot flame directed at a point midway down its stem. When the glass softens, the top is pulled off and the glass fuses at the breaking point. The pull-sealing method results in fewer leaking ampules and is preferred in large scale operations where it is an automatic process.

When the aqueous parenteral product is heat stable, the sealed final container can be sterilized by autoclaving. This type of processing is known as terminal sterilization, sterilization of the aqueous solution after it has been packaged. The sterilization of LVP bag equipment by autoclaving is shown in Figure 4–6.

Autoclaving is the most widely used and most reliable sterilization method available. Steam normally has a temperature of 100° C, but its heat content can be increased by placing the steam under pressure. At sea level and under 15 pounds of pressure, the temperature of steam rises to 121° C. Pressure plays no role in the sterilization process other than to increase the temperature of steam. When the steam contacts a cooler object, it imparts its heat to the object until the latter reaches 121° C. The mechanism of action of steam is the coagulation of protein, which thus disrupts the vital processes of the organism. Once the entire object or the total contents of a container reach

121° C, sterilization requires only 10 minutes. The time required for the autoclave and the contents to reach the sterilization temperature is referred to as the "lag time." The lag time is subject to a number of variables, and these variables in turn determine the length of the sterilization cycle.

Variables that must be considered in determining the lag time include the size of the autoclave, the nature of the material in the load, and the manner in which the material is arranged in the autoclave. The larger the autoclave, the longer the time required to heat it to 121° C. The nature of the material, e.g., whether cloth or metal, influences the rate at which heat penetrates the load. Consider two ampules, one 5 ml and the other 50 ml, both containing Water for Injection. The time required for the contents of the 50-ml ampule to reach 121° C will be longer than that for the 5-ml ampule. Once the contents of the two ampules reach 121° C, the sterilization time will be the same. Loading the autoclave chamber is important, inasmuch as it determines how easily steam will have access to the load. For example, tightly packed bed linen requires a long sterilization cycle in an autoclave because of the time required for the steam to penetrate to the center of the material.

Because of the importance of knowing when conditions of sterilization have been achieved, it is common practice to include sterilization indicators in the load. A number of types of sterilization indicators are available. They may indicate by either physical or chemical changes the temperatures attained, or they may be biologic indicators based on the ability of the available heat to destroy heat-resistant bacterial spores. Regardless of type, it is important that indicators be distributed throughout the load to demonstrate that proper heating conditions have been reached.

The simplest sterilization indicators consist of chemicals that undergo change in color when subjected to temperatures of 121° C. These chemicals may be present on tape used to wrap packages for the autoclave, or they may be impregnated on cardboard and placed strategically throughout the load. Chemicals melting at 121° C and contained in glass capsules can be used. The change of the material from a crystalline form to a melted form indicates that the sterilization temperature has been reached.

The most reliable and precise sterilization indicators are thermocouples (electrical thermometers) inserted in various parts of the autoclave load. The temperature at each site is recorded continuously on a time chart located outside the autoclave. The time chart provides a permanent record of the conditions under which the autoclave load was sterilized.

Currently, the use of biologic indicators is being recommended. Biologic indicators are spores of heat-resistant organisms, such as *Bacillus stearothermophilus*, held in suspension in ampules or impregnated on paper. The ampules or spore strips are placed strategically throughout the load, and following sterilization, the indicators are placed in a sterile nutrient medium and incubated. If conditions of sterilization have been reached, the spores will not grow. When growth occurs, it is an indication that conditions of sterilization were not attained. Sterilization indicators are an important aspect of control. Their proper use and interpretation help to prevent the release of nonsterile products. Biologic indicators are available not only for steam sterilization, but also for dry heat and ethylene oxide sterilization procedures.

TABLE 4–2. *U.S.P. XXII* Official Tests for Parenteral Products*

Title	Page in USP XXII
Injections	1470
Clarity test	1470
Definition	1470
Vehicles	1470
Added substances	1471
Containers	1471
Volume in containers (overfill)	1471
Labeling	1471
Packaging and storage	1472
Particulate matter	1596
Sterilization	1706
Methods	1706
Biological indicators	1625
Sterility testing	1483
Antimicrobial Agents—Effectiveness	1478
Bacterial Endotoxins Test	1493
Pyrogen Test	1515
Container Specifications	1570
Light transmission	1570
Chemical resistance (glass)	1571
Biological test (plastic)	1572
Physiochemical test (plastic)	1497
Permeation	1570

*Individual monographs specify assay, pH, identification test, and other requirements.

Control

When tens of thousands of units are prepared on an industrial scale, control measures appear to be more complex and greater in scope than those exercised by the hospital pharmacist who prepares one or two units extemporaneously. In both instances, however, control measures are taken to assure that each unit will provide at time of use a sterile preparation of the labeled drug in the potency stated that is free of particulate matter and pyrogens and that is safe to use if the directions for administration are followed. Controls used by the industry to ensure that the product meets their claim include chemical assays for the drug substance and antimicrobial preservative, when one is present; pH specification; freezing point depression value; sterility test; pyrogen test; clarity test; and, in some instances, safety testing (Table 4–2).

Sealed ampuls are routinely tested for proper sealing through the leaker test. In this test, the ampuls are immersed in a dye solution (methylene blue), and a vacuum is applied. When cracks or other openings caused by an incomplete seal are present in any of the ampuls, a vacuum forms within the leaking ampul. Then, when the outside vacuum is released, the vacuum within the leaking ampul draws the dye solution into the ampul. The ampuls with the colored contents can then be easily identified as "leakers" and removed. It has also been suggested that vial closure systems be subjected to integrity testing to demonstrate that sterility will be maintained during the lifetime of

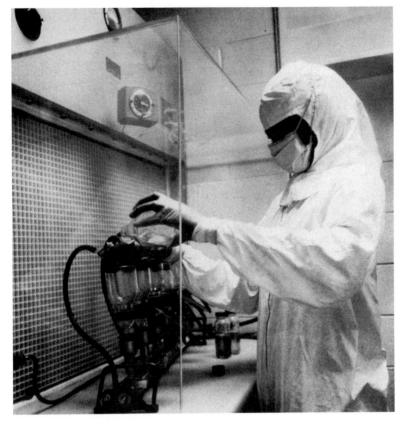

Figure 4–7. Sterility test using the membrane filtration method. (Courtesy of Elkins-Sinn, Inc., Cherry Hill, NJ.)

the product. Both physical and microbiologic methods have been proposed for determining vial-closure integrity.[12]

Chemical assay of the preparation ensures that the product initially contains the labeled amount of drug substance and serves as the basis for future stability testing. The presence of the antimicrobial preservative in the proper concentration is also determined initially and can be rechecked at later dates for its stability with time in the formulation. Agreement of the solution's pH and freezing point depression values serves as a qualitative indication that the quantities of additives stated in the formula have been used.

Each batch of a parenteral product is subjected to a sterility test to meet the requirements of the compendium. In terminal sterilization, each autoclave load is considered to be a batch. In a cold sterilization process, the units filled during a normal 8-hour working day are considered to be a batch. The number of samples removed for sterility testing depends not only on the sterilization method, but also on the procedure to be used for sterility testing.

There are two official methods of sterility testing—the direct transfer of the samples to sterile culture media and the membrane filtration procedure. In the first method, aliquots of the samples are transferred aseptically into each of two sterile culture media, fluid thioglycollate medium and soybean casein

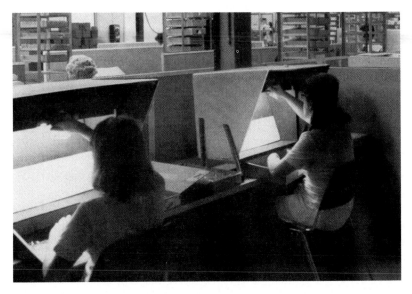

Figure 4–8. Visual inspection of parenteral containers for clarity or absence of particulate matter. (Courtesy of Elkins-Sinn, Inc., Cherry Hill, NJ.)

digest. The inoculated fluid thioglycollate medium samples are incubated at 32° C, and the soybean casein digest samples at 22° C for 14 days. Negative and positive controls are prepared, along with the samples. For the product to pass the sterility test, none of the tubes with either medium can show turbidity or signs of growth (except the positive control) at the end of the incubation period.

In cases in which the parenteral product contains a bacteriostatic agent or the drug substance present in the product possesses inherent bacteriostatic activity, the membrane filtration procedure is followed (Fig. 4–7). In this method, the entire contents of the samples are filtered through a sterile membrane filter having a porosity of 0.45 μm, thereby isolating any microbial contaminants present on the membrane. The membrane is washed with a sterile diluting fluid to remove all traces of the bacteriostatic agent. The membrane is then aseptically removed and divided into two segments. One part is placed into 100 ml of sterile fluid thioglycollate medium, and the other is placed into 100 ml sterile soybean casein digest. The former is incubated with a positive and negative control at 32° C for 7 days, and the latter with controls at 22° C for 7 days. The product passes the sterility test if no turbidity or signs of growth appear at the end of the incubation period. The exact procedures for sterility testing are found in *U.S.P. XXII*.[13]

Samples of the production batch are tested in rabbits for the presence of pyrogens (see "Pyrogen Test" in Chap. 3). Certain drug substances, owing to their physiologic activity, make pyrogen testing in rabbits difficult; administration of a normal human dose to rabbits can be toxic and can result in death of the rabbits. In some cases, the limulus lysate test is applicable.

All units in a production batch are checked individually for clarity, i.e., for the absence of particulate matter. The contents of the container are swirled before a well-lighted white and black background, and those containers with particulate matter are rejected (Fig. 4–8).

With many products, an acute LD_{50} toxicity test (safety test) in the mouse is performed to assure that the total packaged product has no greater inherent toxicity than did previous batches. Changes in the toxicity of preparations can come from many sources, including the raw materials used, the packaging components, and errors made during the compounding of the solution.

Labeling

After satisfactory completion of the control tests, the material is labeled. By law, the labels of parenteral products must indicate the vehicle used, if other than Water for Injection; the drug; and all additives, with the percentage of each present. If the product is for veterinary use, it must be so stated; if it is intended for irrigation, the label must indicate that it is not intended for injection. Expiration dating is required for all products.

References

1. Whitfield, W.J.: Microbiological studies of laminar flow rooms. Bull. Parenter. Drug Assoc., *21*, 37 (1967).
2. Federal Standards No. 209a: Clean Room and Work Station Requirements, Controlled Environment. Washington, DC, General Services Administration, 1967.
3. Kladko, M.: Fundamentals of clean rooms. Pharm. Tech., *6*, 72 (May) (1982).
4. Frieben, W.R.: Control of the aseptic processing environment. Am. J. Hosp. Pharm., *40*, 1928 (1983).
5. Nedich, R.L.: Selection of container and closure systems for injectable products. Am. J. Hosp. Pharm., *40*, 1924 (1983).
6. Adams, P.B.: Surface properties of glass containers for parenteral solutions. Bull. Parenter. Drug. Assoc., *31*, 213 (1977).
7. Kramer, W.: Precipitates found in admixtures of potassium chloride and dextrose 5% in water. Am. J. Hosp. Pharm., *27*, 548 (1970).
8. Wood, R.T.: Validation of elastomeric closures for parenteral use. J. Parenter. Drug Assoc., *34*, 286 (1980).
9. Hopkins, G.H.: Improved procedures for selection of rubber closures. Pharm. Tech., *2*, 34 (June) (1978).
10. Hopkins, G.H.: Factors Influencing the Coring of Rubber Closures. Technical Report No. 9. Phoenixville, PA, The West Company, 1958.
11. Handlos, V.: Hazards of ethylene oxide sterilization. Arch. Pharm. Sci. Ed., *7*, 147 (1979).
12. Frieben, W.R.: Integrity testing of vial closure systems used for parenteral products. J. Parenter. Sci. Technol., *36*, 112 (1982).
13. The United States Pharmacopeia, XXI Revision, Easton, PA, Mack Publishing Co., 1990, p. 1483.

CHAPTER

5

Extemporaneous Preparation

Parenteral Manufacturing in Hospitals

The hospital pharmacy literature of the 1950s and 1960s dealt considerably with parenteral manufacturing. Hospital pharmacies were acquiring additional personnel, space, and equipment to meet their needs. Many hospitals were manufacturing intravenous solutions, irrigating solutions, and other small-volume parenterals. In many cases, quality control was lacking. Several factors shifted the trend of parenteral manufacturing from hospitals to industry.

The responsiveness of industry to the hospitals' needs ensured superior-quality products at reasonable cost. The parenteral drug industry filled the gap in product line, and many pharmacists soon realized it was to their advantage to purchase all available products rather than to manufacture them.

Studies first published in 1962 shocked the hospital world by disclosing that one medication error was committed for every six or seven doses of drugs administered. These early studies showed that deficiencies existed in drug distribution and that the pharmacist was not involved in assuming the responsibility for safe and effective drug therapy in hospitals. These deficiencies, together with increasing sophistication in hospitals and increased complexity of drug usage, made greater demands on the pharmacy department.

At present, it is necessary in some institutions to prepare extemporaneous injectables that are not available commercially. The extent of extemporaneous parenteral preparation in hospitals depends on whether the pharmacy departments have the trained individuals and proper equipment to provide this service.

Parenteral preparation in a hospital includes intravenous admixtures, syringe prefilling, and parenteral compounding. The latter includes bulk compounding and extemporaneous preparation of injectables. Preparations included in bulk compounding are intravenous fluids (being manufactured in only a few hospitals), irrigating solutions, and solutions for peritoneal dialysis. In large

TABLE 5–1.   Parenteral Drugs Manufactured in Hospitals

Number of hospitals surveyed	82
Number of respondents	41
Number of manufacturing any product	3
Different drug entities manufactured	68
Reason stated for manufacturing:	
Not commercially available	56
Cost (less expensive)	12

From Turco, S.J.: Hosp. Pharm., 8, 103 (1973).

teaching hospitals with research facilities and qualified personnel, radiopharmaceuticals are prepared. The preparation of ophthalmic solutions is limited to those not commercially available; the preparation of allergens is almost nonexistent, and only a few hospitals manufacture injections, which are commercially available. The results of a recent survey are shown in Table 5–1.

Most hospitals, in addition to lacking space, have additional disadvantages that make them undesirable for good manufacturing areas. Unauthorized personnel have easy access to the area, and physical disadvantages include overhead pipes, exposed drains, and general poor condition of the physical plant. The quality control practiced by the hospital manufacturing department has been questioned by many because of its lack of space and of adequate facilities; lack of personnel; lack of good control procedures; and lack of work volume necessary for the staff to become proficient.

A few hospitals maintain a manufacturing department when there is a wide discrepancy between the cost of commercially available products and that of hospital preparation. The manufacturing area does provide facilities for research on new formulations, which are frequently required, and also provides a useful area for the training of students, pharmacists, residents, and others. The paramount reason for a manufacturing area is to prepare drugs that are commercially unavailable. Some drugs are commercially unavailable because of lack of demand, and others present stability problems for the manufacturer.

The greatest need for parenteral manufacturing exists in the area of extemporaneous compounding. Medical students, residents, interns, and staff physicians frequently request new drug items reported in the literature. Removal of this component of service would restrict the physician in the use of new therapies and even some old ones.

Environmental Control

First consideration is given to the environment in which the parenteral products are to be prepared. The hospital's lack of specially constructed facilities can be overcome with a laminar air flow hood for the critical parts of the operation.[1–3] Under normal circumstances, air is in a turbulent state and contains thousands of suspended particles per cubic foot. Some of the suspended particles carry microorganisms. With changing air currents, the particles that settle out on surfaces and objects can readily be recycled into the environment. A laminar air flow hood filters the ambient air, thus removing the particles and microorganisms, and places the air in a directional move-

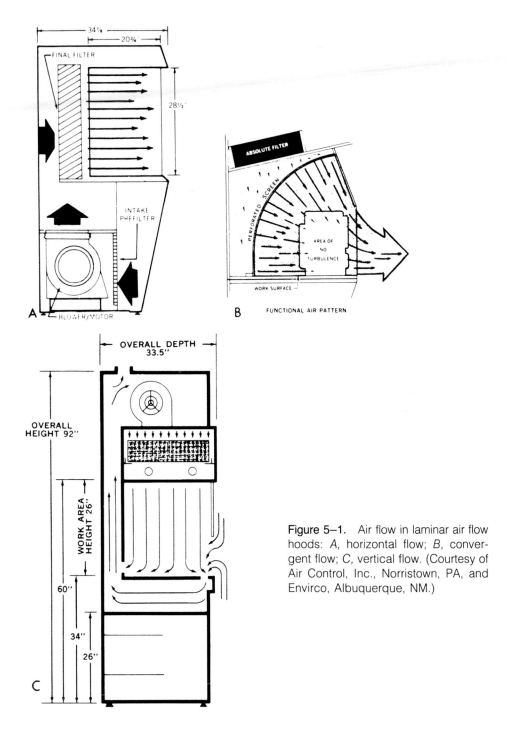

Figure 5–1. Air flow in laminar air flow hoods: *A,* horizontal flow; *B,* convergent flow; *C,* vertical flow. (Courtesy of Air Control, Inc., Norristown, PA, and Envirco, Albuquerque, NM.)

ment at a velocity that produces an area free of particles and microorganisms. The directional flow pattern of a laminar air flow hood can be horizontal, vertical or a combination of both, called "convergent" (Fig. 5–1). For the extemporaneous preparation or manipulation of sterile dosage forms, any of the patterns is satisfactory. In some applications, one type of flow is preferred; for example, when the work involves infectious material or a noxious chemical, a closed vertical air flow hood is required to protect personnel and environment.

The greatest disadvantage of laminar air flow is the false sense of security it may give the operator. The use of laminar air flow requires the same precautions and aseptic techniques that would be followed without its presence. The operator must appreciate that laminar air flow does not remove microbial contaminants from surfaces; it is not a sterilization process. Therefore, the significance of the microbial load present on materials placed in the hood should be recognized. Another danger in using laminar air flow is the failure to maintain the hood's operating efficiency, which would reduce its value.

The laminar air flow station is preferably located in an area where it will not be subjected to strong drafts of air from outside sources or to excessive activity in front of the hood. Minor disadvantages encountered in its operation are the heat generated by the motor and the noise produced in a small area. The laminar air flow hood is operated at least 15 minutes prior to use to allow the hood to purge itself of particulate matter. Before use, the grill protecting the high efficiency particulate air (HEPA) or absolute filter may be vacuumed, and the top surface of the work area may be cleaned with a suitable disinfectant.

In a typical horizontal laminar air flow hood, air from the room is taken in at the lower front through a coarse prefilter, usually composed of spun glass (Fig. 5–2). The air is blown into the distribution plenum and through the HEPA filter to maintain a velocity of 230 ± 90 cm/min. The filter consists of banks of filter medium, a fiberglass composition or similar fibrous material, separated by corrugated kraft paper or aluminum pleats (Fig. 5–3). The separators on both sides of the filters act as baffles to direct the air in a laminar flow, i.e., a uniform parallel flow. The filter removes 99.97% of all particles 0.3 μm or larger, thus removing inert solid material as well as airborne microorganisms. The size of these particles can be appreciated when the sizes of other material particles are compared with them: ground talc, 0.5 to 60 μm; bacteria, 0.3 to 30 μm; viruses, 0.003 to 0.05 μm; pollens, 10 to 100 μm; tobacco smoke, 0.01 to 1 μm; and human hair, 30 to 200 μm. The construction of the filter and the air velocity, not readily perceptible to one standing in front of the hood, provide a body of air that sweeps the workbench clean and maintains this state of cleanliness (Fig. 5–4). This directional air flow prevents the formation of eddies of air and maintains the integrity of the internal environment. The outward air pressure also prevents nonsterile room air from entering the hood area.

Some laminar flow hoods are equipped with easily read static pressure gauges that indicate when pressure builds up behind the filter owing to the clogging of the filter. This pressure buildup indicates that the HEPA filter needs changing. The filter in a laminar air flow hood should be replaced when the velocity of air across the work surface area falls below 22 m/min. Under normal conditions, and if the prefilters are changed at monthly intervals, the filters may last for a year or longer.

Proper installation of the HEPA filter is important. To determine whether the filter is properly installed and functioning, the manufacturer or certifier

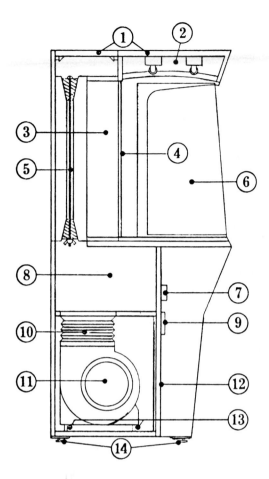

Figure 5–2. Typical horizontal laminar air flow hood: overhead access panels (1); cabinet lights and diffuser (2); HEPA filter (3); egg-crate outflow grid (4); sliding wedge lock (5); transparent end panels (6); filter-life gauge (7); pressure chamber (8); power and light switches (9); flexible collar (10); multi-air blower (11); prefilter and inflow grill (12); shock mounts (13); levelers and height adjustment (14). (Courtesy of Abbott Laboratories, North Chicago, IL.)

passes dioctyl phthalate (DOP) smoke into the intake of the hood. Dioctyl phthalate forms an invisible smoke with an average particle size of 0.3 μm. A leak in the filter or improper installation of the hood is indicated if the smoke passes through the filter and is detected by a smoke photometer.

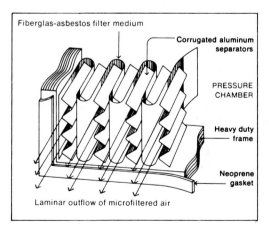

Figure 5–3. Construction of high-efficiency particulate air (HEPA) filter. (Courtesy of Abbott Laboratories, North Chicago, IL.)

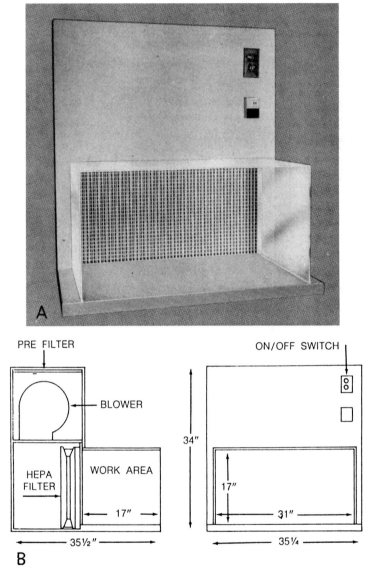

Figure 5–4. Laminar air flow station, bench: illustration (*A*) and diagram (*B*). A console model is also available. (Courtesy of Travenol Laboratories, Inc., Deerfield, IL.)

Laminar hood installations should be checked every six months for leaks and proper operation.[4] When testing equipment is not available within the organization, private laboratories can be hired to inspect laminar air flow hoods routinely. A simple means to determine whether the velocity of air is satisfactory is with an anemometer (Fig. 5–5). When properly maintained, a laminar air flow hood can provide the hospital pharmacist with an environment suitable for preparing or handling sterile preparations.

When working in the hood, the operator should wear sterile gloves and guard against sneezing or coughing. A direct open path between the critical

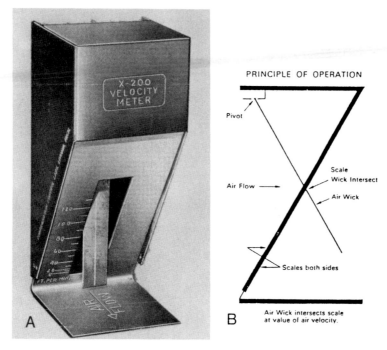

Figure 5–5. Anemometer for determining velocity of air in a laminar air flow hood; illustration (A) and diagram (B). (Courtesy of Contamination Control Laboratories, Livonia, MI.)

work area and the filter should be maintained; no equipment should be placed in front of or near the critical work area. Dead spaces form in back of objects, as indicated in Figure 5–6. Working too near the front edge of the bench can also create air turbulences, which can pull air from the room or around the personnel into the hood. To observe air patterns in a hood, small amounts of smoke can be released in the hood. The area of turbulent air behind an object can be seen, and in this turbulent area, which extends three to six times the width of the object, the smoke moves in a circular pattern. Avis has summarized the classification of biologic safety cabinets (Table 5–2).

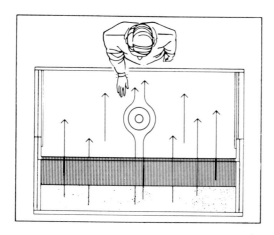

Figure 5–6. Dead spaces can form behind objects placed in stream of laminar air flow. (Courtesy of Abbott Laboratories, North Chicago, IL.)

TABLE 5-2. Classification of Biologic Safety Cabinets*

Classification of Class II Cabinets	Recirculated Air (%)	Exhausted Air (%)	Inflow Air Velocity (ft/min)	Source of Exhaust Airflow	Exhaust Requirements	Ducts and Plenums
Type A	70	30	75	From plenum common with supply to work area	Exhausted into the buffer room or vented to the outside through a HEPA filter	Contaminated ones are under positive pressure
Type B_1 (Formerly Type 2)	30	70	100	Directly from rear of work area	Exhausted to the outside through a HEPA filter	Contaminated ones are under negative pressure
Type B2	0	100	100	Directly from work area	Exhausted to the outside through a HEPA filter	Contaminated ones are under negative pressure
Type B3	70	30	100	From plenum common with supply to work area	Exhausted to the outside through a HEPA filter or into the buffer room	Contaminated ones are under negative pressure

*Summarized from Standard No. 49 of the National Sanitation Foundation. Cf. reference 4.
Reprinted from Avis, K. E.: Appropriate laminar-flow cabinets for pharmaceutical applications. Pharm. Technol. (November), 1987.

Personnel

Individuals selected to work with the hospital pharmacist in the extemporaneous preparation of sterile products should have good personal health habits and be capable of developing well-organized work routines. They should be cognizant of the importance of careful planning and the observance of details as well as of the importance of their task regardless of the routine aspects of the operations. Emphasis should be placed on their understanding of the end use of the products they help to prepare. Training should be provided to ensure their appreciation for the reasoning behind the precautions and care taken in following the required procedures.

Aseptic technique becomes a way of thinking, an attitude, toward the maintenance of sterility. For the inexperienced manipulator, aseptic procedures are tedious, but coordination develops with experience, and the aseptic techniques involved in preparing and handling sterile preparations become natural to the operator. The quality of the sterile products prepared is directly related to the manipulative skills of the hospital pharmacist and those working with him.

Packaging Components

All packaging components of the final container for the sterile product must be sterile, free of particulate matter, and free of pyrogens. After the components have been wrapped in a manner that ensures maintenance of sterility and protection from particulate matter prior to their use for packaging, the suitable sterilization process must be selected. Regardless of the method of sterilization, packaging components should be washed and sterilized as the need for them arises. In general, they should not be prepared and stored for long periods of time, i.e., for more than 2 weeks. Longer periods may be satisfactory, but the hospital pharmacist should prove to his own satisfaction that under his operating procedures this is the case.

Glass Components

As described in Chapter 4, glass can vary considerably in its resistance to attack by water and chemicals. Because there is not time for extensive stability studies in a hospital, only glass packaging components made from Type I glass should be used. Ordinarily, glass causes problems of physical and chemical stability; the use of Type I glass diminishes these problems.

Glass packaging components can be sterilized either by dry heat or by autoclaving. When sterilized by dry heat, the components are rinsed well with distilled water or Water for Injection* and are placed in covered stainless steel boxes. If boxes are not available, the containers may be placed in glass beakers and covered with aluminum foil, which will also protect the containers until time of use. If only a small number of units are required, they can be wrapped together in aluminum foil.

---

*Pyrogen-free water is called "Water for Injection." In facilities where a bulk supply of Water for Injection is not maintained. Sterile Water for Injection (SWFI), available commercially in liter containers can be used.

When a hot air oven is not available, the glass components are rinsed well with Water for Injection, wrapped in a material suitable for autoclaving, such as kraft paper or muslin, and autoclaved. The sterile packages can be dried after autoclaving by allowing them to remain in the warm autoclave with the door open, or they can be air dried. The wrapping materials and the handling methods during washing and sterilization procedures can generate particulate matter that will later be discernible in the product. When facilities are not available for preparation of containers, empty sterile, pyrogen-free vials with closure can be purchased commercially.

Rubber Components

In preparing rubber components, it is important not only to render them sterile and pyrogen-free but also to remove particles adhering to them from the manufacturing process and to extract from them any water-soluble material that could eventually find its way into the preparation. Surface debris and dirt are removed by washing the rubber pieces in a mild detergent solution, such as sodium pyrophosphate, with agitation. The rubber components are rinsed repeatedly with Water for Injection to remove traces of the detergent and pyrogens. To remove the water-extractable materials, the washed components are immersed in Water for Injection and autoclaved for 20 minutes. The autoclaving step is repeated once. The washed components are dried and stored in suitable, covered containers.

Before use, the required number of rubber components are immersed in Water for Injection, rinsed well to remove particulate matter and pyrogens, and drained. They are wrapped in paper and autoclaved for 20 minutes to render them sterile. Some operators prefer to immerse them in Water for Injection for autoclaving and to remove them with sterile forceps or with a sterile-gloved hand because they are used in the packaging of the sterile preparation.

Plastic Components

Plastic components are washed with filtered air to remove particulate material and wrapped in either plastic, such as a polyethylene bag, or paper prior to sterilization with ethylene oxide. A sterilization indicator for ethylene oxide is placed in one of the packaging components to assure the operator that the sterilant has penetrated both the wrapping material and the component. Ethylene oxide penetrates polymeric materials at varying rates, depending on the thickness and composition of the material.

When an ethylene oxide sterilizing chamber is available, the material is sterilized according to the manufacturer's directions. Usually, the cycle consists of a 30-minute humidification period, heating the contents of the chamber to 130° F, and exposing the material to an atmosphere of ethylene oxide at the concentration of 450 mg/L for 4 hours. After the removal of the sterilant with vacuum, the material is stored under room conditions for 48 hours or longer to allow the residual ethylene oxide to dissipate.

When an ethylene oxide chamber is not available, the so-called bag method has been used for small quantities of material (Bard ETO, C.R. Bard, Inc.). The wrapped plastic material is placed in a polyethylene bag with an ampul containing a liquid mixture of ethylene oxide and Freon. The end of the bag is closed by twisting and secured with a wire. While holding the ampul in the closed bag, the top is broken, and the ethylene oxide-Freon mixture is released. The mixture vaporizes under room conditions, and the bag fills with the sterilant vapor. The bag is placed in a stainless steel can, and the can is closed and inverted. After 24 hours, the contents are removed from the can and plastic bag. The sterile plastic components are quarantined for 48 hours or longer to remove the residual ethylene oxide.

Because ethylene oxide and its reaction products such as ethylene glycol and 2-chlorethanol are irritating to the skin and mucous membranes, gas-sterilized materials must be aerated to allow residual amounts of these toxic substances to dissipate.[5] This precludes their immediate use after sterilization. The time required for the elimination of these residual substances varies with the nature of the material, the overwrap used, temperature, air flow, and other environmental conditions.[6] Paper and cloth overwraps allow more rapid elimination than do plastic coverings. Cases of reactions to ethylene oxide-sterilized materials have been reported, including injury following the use of an anesthetic mask that had been in contact with a patient's face, respiratory tract irritation after use of ethylene oxide-sterilized equipment, and contact dermatitis.[7-9] In the past, some commercial products were recalled, owing to the ethylene oxide residues found after the products had been distributed.

Injections

For preparation of bulk solutions, it is not necessary to use the laminar air flow hood. Containers such as beakers or stainless steel cans and other pieces of apparatus should be rinsed well with Water for Injection if the equipment is not sterile and pyrogen-free when stored. It is good practice to restrict use of the equipment to the manufacture of sterile preparations. After use, they can be covered, rendered sterile and pyrogen-free by dry heat, and stored. When no hot air oven is available, an alternate method is to wash them with Water for Injection, rinse them well, cover, and autoclave. After drying, they can be stored. With either of these methods, the equipment is maintained pyrogen-free and ready for use.

Bulk solution is prepared following the appropriate formula and adjusting the pH when required, prior to making the solution up to final volume with Water for Injection. For small volumes, it is convenient to use volumetric flasks for greater accuracy. At this point, the solution is pyrogen-free because the containers, the solvent, and, it is hoped, the chemicals are pyrogen-free. Particulate matter from the chemicals, personnel, and environment is present. The bulk solution is not sterile, because it has not yet been subjected to sterilization. After preparation, the solution must be sterilized and packaged within 24 hours.

Selection of the sterilization method to be used (autoclaving or filtration through a microbiologic filter medium) depends on whether the injection is heat stable or heat labile. A heat-stable injection may be sterilized after it has been placed in the final container; a heat-labile bulk solution is sterilized by filtration through a suitable sterile filtration medium, then divided aseptically as a sterile solution into sterile containers. When there is a question regarding the heat stability of the injection, filtration is the process to use.

When the solution is to be autoclaved in its final container, it is still necessary to filter the solution to remove any particulate matter before filling. In this instance, the filtration procedure would be designated as a clarification step.

Several media can be used for clarification and sterilization, including the cellulose ester membrane and filters prepared from unglazed porcelain, fritted glass, and diatomaceous earth. Asbestos formerly was used, but it is no longer considered suitable for parenterals because it is questionable whether a solution can be filtered through asbestos without contaminating the filtrate with fine invisible asbestos fibers.

Screen or membrane filters are made from cellulose esters, synthetic polymers, microfilaments, polycarbonates, silver, or stainless steel. Owing to their advantages, availability, and ease of handling, cellulose ester membranes are rapidly becoming the most widely used medium for the clarification and sterilization of parenteral solutions regardless of the volumes involved (Gelman Instrument Company; Johns-Manville; Millipore Corporation; Nucleopore; Pall Corporation; Selas Corporation). These filters are thin films, 1 to 200 μm thick, available in diameter sizes from 13 to 293 mm. The membranes are inert to most aqueous solutions, but may be attacked by a number of organic solvents. In the latter instance, solvent-resistant membranes made from other polymers are available (Fluoropore, Millipore Corporation; Teflon, Johns-Manville).

The membrane films consist of a meshwork of millions of microcapillary pores of uniform size ranging from 8 μm to 0.22 μm. The membrane having 0.22 μm pores is considered to be the sterilizing filter capable of removing microorganisms. Because the pore volume of a membrane filter represents approximately 70 to 85% of the total filter volume, relatively high flow rates are obtained. Their high surface retention can result in clogging, and when large volumes or highly particulate-contaminated solutions are filtered, prefilter pads (depth filters) should be used. The prefilter traps the greater portion of the larger foreign particulates, allowing the smaller pores to trap the microorganisms. Other characteristics include (1) minimal absorption of fluid, (2) low retention of fluid, (3) chemical and biologic inertness, (4) stability when dry to temperatures as high as 125° C, (5) no shedding of filter material, and (6) disposability. The membranes are fragile to handle, but when supported, they withstand pressure differentials as high as 10,000 psi. Pyrogens and viruses are not removed by membrane filters.

The integrity and proper placement of a membrane filter in a holder can be checked by determining the bubble point (Fig. 5–7) or performing the forward flow test.[10,11] Depending on its porosity, each size membrane has a characteristic bubble point. The bubble point is the pressure required to push a gas through a liquid-saturated filter. Until the bubble point of the filter in question is reached, the gas will not displace the liquid in the matrix. The forward flow test measures the number of pores above the critical diameter for a given porosity and ensures proper sealing within the filter housing. These tests may be used as in-process quality control procedures, being performed both before and after filtration to ensure the integrity of the membrane.

Filtration for Clarification and Sterilization

Regardless of the volume of solution to be filtered, there is a suitable unit to hold a membrane filter of the desired porosity. For small volumes, less

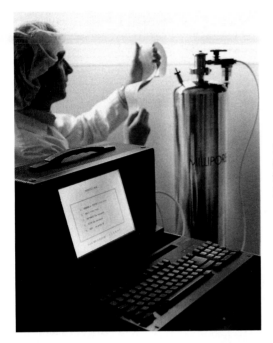

Figure 5–7. Bubble test apparatus to ensure the integrity of a membrane filter. (Courtesy of Millipore Corporation, Bedford, MA.)

than 100 ml, a stainless steel or plastic unit containing the sterilizing membrane and fitted on a Luer-Lok syringe can be used (Fig. 5–8).[12] Sterile plastic filter holders (Swinnex; Millex) complete with membranes are available commercially as disposable units. The plastic filter holder (Swinnex) from which the used membrane can be removed is reusable. The filter holder is molded from polypropylene plastic and withstands autoclaving. The membrane can be replaced, and the entire unit can be suitably wrapped and autoclaved. The stainless steel holders are handled in a similar manner (Fig. 5–9).

For volumes of 100 to 1000 ml, glass or stainless steel filter units holding the membranes can be autoclaved and used with sterile receiving flasks and negative pressure (vacuum). Larger volumes should be filtered with positive pressure, i.e., compressed gas forcing the solution through the filter rather than a vacuum pulling it through (Figs. 5–10 and 5–11). This involves the use of a pressure tank, stainless steel filter holder, and receiving container. As the volume of the solution increases, filter membranes of larger diameters can be selected to increase the flow rate.

The filtration or clarification operation is carried out in the laminar air flow hood to eliminate contamination from the environment and the personnel. For large volumes, not usually encountered in extemporaneous filling, it is desirable to have a completely closed filtration collection system. For small volumes that can be prepared within the confines of the laminar air flow hood, this is not required.

Subdivision of Solution

In subdividing a solution into its final container, a syringe, a Cornwall syringe, or a pipetting device designed to deliver a measured volume repeatedly

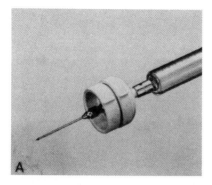

Figure 5–8. *A,* Swinnex disposable filter unit, *B,* Schematic diagram of the Swinnex disposable filter unit. (Courtesy of Millipore Corporation, Bedford, MA.)

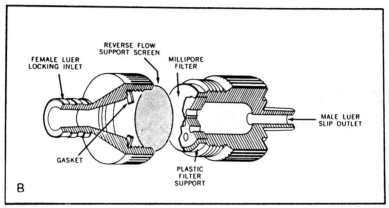

may be used (Fig. 5–12). An excess of solution is placed in each container to allow withdrawal of the volume stated on the label. The device used for subdividing is washed well with Water for Injection and autoclaved before use.

Usually, it is most convenient for the hospital pharmacist to package the

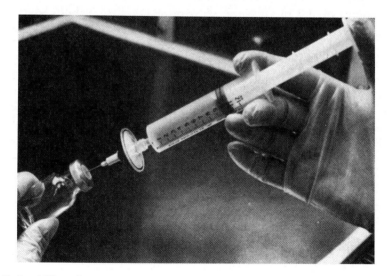

Figure 5–9.   Millex disposable filter unit in use. (Courtesy of Millipore Corporation, Bedford, MA.)

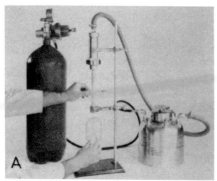
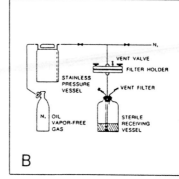

Figure 5–10. *A*, Sterilization of large volume by membrane filtration with pressure vessel and stainless steel holder for the membrane. *B*, Schematic diagram of sterilization by membrane filtration. (Courtesy of Millipore Corporation, Bedford, MA.)

solution in rubber-stoppered vials or glass syringes. When the solution is incompatible with rubber, however, it may be necessary to use ampuls. Glass ampuls are sealed by fusing the tip of the stem by either tip-sealing or pull-sealing. In pull-sealing, the tip of the stem is held loosely with a pair of forceps, and the ampul is rotated while the center of the stem is placed in a hot flame. When the glass softens, the top is pulled off, and the glass fuses at the breaking point. In tip-sealing, the ampul is rotated mechanically with its tip in a hot flame. If the tip remains in the flame for too long, the glass forms a bubble, owing to the expansion of the air in it, and a poor seal results. Portable ampul tip-sealers are available (Cozzoli Machine Co.). Usually, a

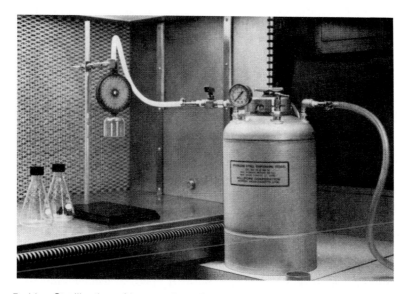

Figure 5–11. Sterilization of large volume by membrane filtration with a pressure vessel. The filter illustrated (Twin 90, Millipore) is presterilized, disposable plastic unit containing two 90-mm diameter filters, pore size 0.22 μm. (Courtesy of Millipore Corporation, Bedford, MA.)

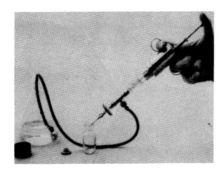

Figure 5–12. A Cornwall syringe with a Millex unit attached offers a convenient way to fill a series of vials while removing particles and microorganisms. (Courtesy of Millipore Corporation, Bedford, MA.)

combination of natural gas and oxygen is burned to obtain sufficient heat for melting the glass.

Leaking ampuls are detected by immersing the sealed ampuls in a vacuum jar containing a dye solution. A vacuum is pulled on the chamber and released after a brief period. In the process, leaking ampuls lose their solutions, thus creating a vacuum within them. When the chamber vacuum is released, the vacuum created in leaking ampuls draws the dye solution into the ampuls so that they can be detected. Undetected leakers can result in contaminated injections.

The material to be used in the subdivision is arranged in the laminar air flow hood in a manner that promotes the orderly filling of the solution. The equipment is positioned so that the empty containers, the filling operation itself, and the filled but unsealed containers are not obstructed in any way from the laminar air flow. After the containers are sealed, they may be removed from the hood.

Solutions that are to be terminally sterilized in the final container are removed to the autoclave; solutions sterilized by filtration and subdivided are ready for control.

Practical Problem

Because a particular solution is not available from any commercial source, a physician asks pharmacy services to supply it. The solution contains ingredient A, 100 mg/ml; ingredient B, 25 mg/ml; ingredient C, 50 mg/ml; and ingredient D, 3 μg/ml. The sterile solution is to be packaged in 10-ml vials for addition to liter bottles of dextrose or sodium chloride injection for intravenous feeding.

Day before Preparation

1. One hundred 10-ml vials are washed, packed in inverted position in covered containers, and placed in a hot air oven for at least 4 hours at 180° C to render them sterile and pyrogen-free.
2. A cellulose membrane having a porosity of 0.22 μm (47 mm diameter) is placed in a clean stainless steel filter holder. The locking ring of the filter holder is tightened loosely. Both ends of the filter holder are wrapped with kraft paper, and the entire unit is wrapped in nylon or autoclaving paper and sterilized in the autoclave for 20 to 30 minutes.

3. The Tygon or rubber tubing to be used in conjunction with the sterilization setup is washed well with Water for Injection, wrapped, and autoclaved for 20 minutes.
4. The glass container into which the solution will be filtered is washed, covered, and placed in the hot air oven for 4 hours at 180° C to render it sterile and pyrogen-free.
5. The Cornwall syringe or other pipetting unit to be used in subdividing the sterile solution into sterile vials is assembled, adjusted to deliver a volume of 10.3 ml, washed well with Water for Injection, wrapped, and autoclaved for 20 minutes.

Day of Preparation

1. The laminar air flow hood is wiped down with disinfectant solution, and the blower is turned on.
2. One hundred rubber closures are rinsed well with Water for Injection, immersed in Water for Injection in a covered container, autoclaved for 20 minutes, and removed to laminar air flow hood.
3. The following materials are arranged in the hood:
   Wrapped sterile membrane filter and holder
   Tygon tubing for pressure tank
   Sterile receiving flask
   Sterile Cornwall syringe adjusted to deliver 10.3 ml
   Covered container with sterile-pyrogen-free vials
   Sterile cylindrical graduate, 25 ml, to check the delivery of the Cornwall syringe
   Sterile covered beaker to act as waste container
   Two pairs of sterile gloves and a pair of sterile forceps, if desired, for application of rubber closures
4. Preparation of the solution

   Formula:

mg/ml	Ingredient	g/L
100	A	100.00
25	B	25.00
50	C	50.00
0.003	D	0.003
qs	Water for Injection qs	1000.0 ml

   Procedure:
   Warm 750 ml of Water for Injection to 80° C. Add and dissolve ingredient B by stirring. After solution cools to room temperature, add and dissolve ingredients A and C.
   Dissolve 10.0 mg of crystalline ingredient D in 10 ml of Water for Injection. Add an aliquot of 3 ml to the solution containing the other ingredients, and make up to a volume of 1000 ml with Water for Injection.
5. Sterilization of the solution
   Rinse a stainless steel pressure tank with Water for Injection, drain, and add the prepared solution.

TABLE 5–3.   Temperatures and Times of Exposure for Dry Heat Sterilization

Temperature		Time of Exposure
(°C)	(°F)	(minutes)
170	340	60
160	320	120
150	300	150
140	285	180

        Remove the wrapping from the membrane filter holder while it is in the hood, and assemble the setup. Tighten the locking ring of the filter holder, and connect holder to the pressure tank with the sterile Tygon tubing.

        Using an inert gas, such as compressed nitrogen, apply pressure to the tank, and force the solution through the sterilizing membrane into the sterile receiving container.

6. Subdivision of the solution

        Put on the sterile gloves, open the wrapped Cornwall syringe, and place the sinker of the syringe in the sterile solution. Check the delivery volume of the syringe; if satisfactory, fill the sterile vials. With sterile forceps, apply sterile rubber closures to the vials as they are filled. (This should be done by the second operator.) After the entire batch is filled, apply aluminum seals, and seal with a hand crimper.

7. Testing

Sterile Solids

Occasionally, the hospital pharmacist may receive a request for a chemical or drug substance to be made available as a sterile powder. When the sterile solid is not available commercially, the pharmacist has difficulty meeting the request because of his limited means for sterilization. In the industry, drug substances such as antibiotics are isolated from sterile solutions with aseptic processing. The sterile bulk material is then subdivided aseptically into the final containers. Steroids crystallized from sterile solutions under controlled conditions and with aseptic handling are isolated as sterile bulk powders.

Another approach for preparing sterile solids is lyophilization. Aqueous solutions of the drug substance are sterilized by filtration through a suitable microbiologic filter, and the sterile filtrate is lyophilized under aseptic conditions to give a sterile solid. Water-insoluble drugs such as the steroids can be placed in an organic solvent such as dioxane (peroxide-free), sterilized by filtration, and lyophilized. Facilities for those operations are not available to the hospital pharmacist. Usually, a hot air oven is the only means at his disposal for sterilizing dry solids.

Dry heat sterilization can be used for a limited number of dry solids. The materials must be stable to relatively high temperatures and long periods of heating. Sterilization is a function of time versus temperature; the relationships suggested in sterilization texts are given in Table 5–3. The time of exposure indicates the period after the entire quantity of material has reached the temperature shown.

The temperature selected for dry heat sterilization depends on the heat stability of the chemical. The temperature must be below the decomposition point of the chemical. The "lag" time, or period required for the entire quantity of the material to reach the selected temperature, depends on the ability of heat to penetrate the material, the quantity involved, and the manner in which it is placed in the hot air oven. For example, dry heat penetrates a chemical more quickly if it is exposed as a layer $1/2$ inch thick than if the same quantity is placed in a layer 1 inch thick. The only means of determining when the material has reached the sterilization temperature at which the oven is set is to have a thermometer or thermocouple in the center of the material. Different chemicals, or the same material in different quantities, must be considered as individual cases, each with its own requirement. Following sterilization, samples should be aseptically removed from the bulk powder and tested for sterility.

Practical Problem

A request is received for 100 g of sterile barium sulfate. Because it is inorganic, barium sulfate is stable at high temperatures, decomposing above 1600° C. The temperature-time ratio of 170° C can be used. One hundred grams of barium sulfate are placed in each of two 500-ml beakers and covered with aluminum foil. They are placed side by side in the center of the hot air oven, and a thermometer is inserted in the center of the material in the second beaker. When the temperature reaches 170° C as indicated by the thermometer, the 1-hour sterilization period begins. Following sterilization, samples of the powder are tested for sterility. Two containers of the same size with the same quantity of the same material are placed in the same general location in the oven; the one containing the thermometer serves as a control while the second one remains covered. We assume that if the powder in the control beaker is satisfactory, the powder in the second beaker is also satisfactory.

Sterile Suspensions

Sterile suspensions are prepared by the aseptic combination of the sterile solid having particles of the desired size with the sterile vehicle. Aqueous vehicles can be sterilized either by autoclaving or by microbiologic filtration. Autoclaving of suspensions is not recommended, because it is doubtful whether a contaminated solid can be sterilized throughout by moist heat. In addition, heating the suspension results in increased solubility of the suspended solid in the vehicle. Upon cooling, the solid recrystallizes from the vehicle as particles of varying dimensions. Oily vehicles cannot be sterilized by autoclaving because of their nonaqueous nature; they are usually sterilized with dry heat or filtration.

Quality Control

The best guarantee that a product will conform to what is stated on its label is strict adherence by conscientious personnel to good manufacturing procedures. Regardless of the quantity of control testing, quality cannot be tested into a product. Quality is there because of the ingredients used, the procedures followed, and the personnel involved in its preparation. These aspects assume a greater importance in extemporaneous preparation of sterile products because of the limited time available for testing prior to their use. The nature of the clinical environment places necessary demands on the pharmacist because economic and time considerations make it impractical, and in many instances impossible, to do extensive testing. Control tests for a single, extemporaneously prepared injection become impractical and prohibitive in cost to the patient. This does not preclude good judgment and good procedures, however. Proved test procedures must be established and periodically evaluated. Performing a number of these tests at regular intervals provides a means of monitoring or evaluating procedures, environment, and personnel. Therefore, in instances in which control testing is waived, it is done so on the basis that performance of stated procedures in the past produced satisfactory qualities and repetition of the same procedures will again produce the desired qualities.

As stated previously, the three characteristics required of all sterile products are sterility, freedom from pyrogens, and freedom from particulate matter. To perform a sterility test, a randomly selected sample of the product is aseptically added to a sterile nutrient medium; the inoculated medium is incubated under optimum conditions for microbial growth.[13] The premise is that microbial contaminants present in the product will grow under these conditions. For some types of products, the membrane filtration method for sterility testing is more convenient to use than other methods. In this procedure, the sample contents are filtered through a sterile membrane. If microbial contaminants are present, they will be collected on the membrane. With aseptic technique, the membrane is divided into two parts, and each part is placed in a different culture medium for incubation. The procedure is especially applicable when the drug substance itself possesses bacteriostatic properties, when the preparation contains a bacteriostatic agent, or when the product is an oil. The appearance of turbidity in the culture medium indicates microbial contamination.

The details of the official methods for sterility testing are found in the *U.S.P.*[14] Sterility testing for small production batches of 20 to 200 units requires that 10% of the production batch be sampled. For batches of less than 20 units, a minimum of 2 samples is tested. The procedures followed differ, depending on the nature of the materials, the sterilization process, and whether sterilization indicators are used. The microbiologic departments in most hospitals are equipped to do sterility testing.

It is the exceptional hospital that is equipped to test products for pyrogens. The cost of sending preparations to private laboratories for testing, as well as the time involved, may be prohibitive. This does not preclude, however, either the routine pyrogen testing of Water for Injection, if used by the pharmacy in the preparation of sterile products, or the random selection of products for pyrogen testing. Satisfactory production and storage of Water for Injection, along with its proper handling, play a major role in eliminating pyrogen problems from extemporaneously prepared products. When a given product is pre-

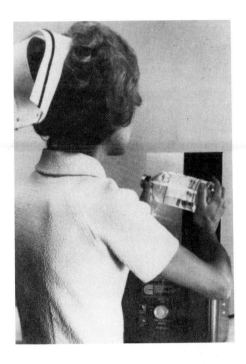

Figure 5–13. Inspection of intravenous fluid for particulate matter prior to administration. (Courtesy of Contamination Control Laboratories, Livonia, MI.)

pared on a large scale and stored for future use, utilization of the pyrogen test as a control procedure is in order.

The inspection of the finished sterile package for the presence of particulate matter can be easily done on a routine basis. Not only is it good practice to observe the contents for clarity at time of preparation, but also it should be part of the routine prior to the administration of a parenteral product. The clarity test consists of swirling the contents of the container and viewing them against a well-illuminated light and dark background (Fig. 5–13). When particles are detected, the unit is rejected.

In the limited number of instances in which a given product is prepared on a large scale and stored for future use, it is advantageous to determine the potency of the preparation by chemical or microbiologic assay. This serves as a basis on which to assess or evaluate questions arising as to its activity and sterility. The hospital's clinical laboratory can be helpful in assisting with control procedures.

When possible, it is advantageous to both the pharmacist and the patient to use commercially prepared sterile products. When the desirable dosage form is not available, the hospital pharmacist is able to prepare a satisfactory product provided he understands its requirements and the relatively simple procedure for meeting them.

In addition to preparing a suitable product, it is part of the pharmacist's responsibility to ensure that the individual requesting the product has the authority to make the request and is knowledgeable in the use of the drug. Proper dosage and route of administration should be ascertained before manufacture. If time or cost factors prohibit adequate testing, the physician should be made aware of this fact. In all instances, commercially available products should be sought first. Although the limited availability of facilities, equipment, and control methods can be considered to be disadvantages, the hospital pharmacist has the advantage of being personally involved with the product throughout the entire period of its preparation. New draft guidelines have been proposed by the American Society of Hospital Pharmacists.[15] These guidelines describe quality assurance procedures for pharmacy-prepared sterile products.

References

1. Brier, K.L., Latiolais, C.J., Schneider, P.J., et al.: Effect of laminar air flow and clean room dress on contamination rates of intravenous admixtures. Am. J. Hosp. Pharm., *38*:1144 (1981).
2. Frieben, W.R.: Control of the aseptic processing environment. Am. J. Hosp. Pharm., *38*, 1928 (1983).
3. National Coordinating Committee on Large Volume Parenterals: Recommended methods for compounding intravenous admixtures in hospitals. Am. J. Hosp. Pharm., *32*, 261 (1975).
4. Bryan, D., and Marback, R.C.: Laminar air flow certification. Am. J. Hosp. Pharm., *41*, 1343 (1984).
5. Guess, W.L.: Residual ethylene oxide and reaction products in polymers. Bull. Parenter. Drug Assoc., *24*, 68 (1970).
6. Handlos, V.: The hazards of ethylene oxide sterilization. Arch. Pharm. Chemie. Sci. Ed., *7*, 147 (1979).
7. Ethylene oxide hazards. Clin-Alert, Louisville, KY, Science Editor, Inc. June 30, 1969.
8. Ethylene oxide sterilization. Clin-Alert, Louisville, KY, Science Editor, Inc. December 30, 1969.
9. Hanifin, J.M.: Ethylene oxide dermatitis. JAMA, *217*, 2 (1971).
10. Pall, D.B.: Quality control of absolute bacteria removing filters. Bull. Parenter. Drug Assoc., *58*, 1301 (1969).
11. Reti, A.R.: An assessment of test criteria in evaluating the performance and integrity of sterilizing filters. Bull. Parenter. Drug Assoc., *31*, 187 (1979).
12. Low Volume Sterilizing Filtration. Application Report AR-11. Millipore Corporation, Bedford, MA, 1969.
13. Bowman, F.W.: The sterility testing of pharmaceuticals. J. Pharm. Sci., *58*, 1301 (1969).
14. The United States Pharmacopeia, XXII Revision. Easton, PA, Mack Publishing Co., 1990, p. 1483.
15. Draft Guidelines on Quality Assurance for Pharmacy-prepared Sterile Products. Am. J. Hosp. Pharm. *49*, 407 (1992).

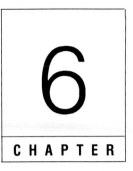

CHAPTER

Handling and Administration

Faye Cosentino

The Patient

For members of all health care professions, the well-being of the patient is the primary goal at all levels of treatment and care, including the administration of parenteral medications.

Persons who become patients continue to differ from one another as much as they did before becoming patients. Health care personnel have tended to expect a stereotyped reaction from patients: They are to be cooperative at all times and not question or suggest changes in procedures and routines. They are to believe that everything is being done for their own good. Most important, they are not to complain. Behavior not in line with that expected of a good patient is likely to be considered uncooperative. Failure to recognize the patient as an individual can endanger his well-being and deter the members of the health care professions from their primary roles.

When ill, an individual assumes a different role from the one he had when in good health. In the process of adapting himself to the role of the patient, an individual's behavior changes in an attempt to adjust to something new. Some people adjust to new circumstances with a greater facility than others. The seriousness of an illness from a medical viewpoint may not necessarily be a useful indicator in predicting a person's attitude and reaction to his illness. Some patients whose illnesses may be considered minor in terms of

Some material in this chapter has been retained from Chapter 6 of the previous edition, authored by Robert E. Young.

complete recovery view their states with great alarm and concern. Other patients experiencing serious illnesses may show little emotional reaction or concern.

It cannot be assumed that a patient's fears and anxieties can and will be eliminated. Health care personnel can take many avenues that may ease the emotional and physiologic distress of a patient. Health care personnel can offer a unique service to patients when available knowledge is used to promote therapeutic relationships.

Emotional Reactions to Illness

Fear, anxiety, and stress are emotional reactions to illness. Physiologic responses to emotion are well organized, and even when emotion is strong, the body responds harmoniously. What may be disorganized is the behavior resulting from an emotional experience. A person experiencing extreme fear may be so consumed by emotion that his behavior becomes erratic; thus, he is less effective in eliminating the cause of his fear. Among fears common to patients are the fear of the unknown and the fear of needles.

Expectation of harm or unpleasantness characterizes fear. The body normally reacts by attempting to avoid or withdraw from threat. Fear places the body in a state of readiness for action to avoid or to escape harm. Health care personnel who take the time to discuss procedures and to explain the reasons for their use prior to their implementation can do much to alleviate patients' fears resulting from misconceptions and fear of the unknown.

Anxiety is an uneasiness of mind caused by apprehension of danger or misfortune. It is most often a persistent generalized fear of the unknown associated with some future event. The predominant characteristic is the lack of awareness as to its cause. Anxiety is vaguely organized in the mind of the patient, who feels helpless and uncertain concerning the appropriate action to take. Anxiety is difficult to handle because the person lacks insight as to its cause and feels defeated, and the physiologic symptoms expressed are fatigue, insomnia, diarrhea, urgency to void, nausea, anorexia, and excessive perspiration. At times, the patient may think that his heart stands still.

Stress occurs most frequently when situations necessitate an increased and often prolonged effort to adapt, or adjust. Any factor that disturbs the physical, psychologic, or physiologic equilibrium of the body may be stressful. The body strives to eliminate the factor causing the stress. Stress is a highly individualized experience, in much the same manner as is the threshold of pain; some patients appear to tolerate more stress than others. The important aspect is how the patient perceives and meets the situation causing the stress. It is a rare patient who does not experience it.

In general, patients expect health care personnel to orient them to the hospital environment. Nearly everyone is afraid of the unknown. To be left alone in a hospital room without explanations, consideration, or orientation can be a frightening experience. Health care personnel who help the patient feel that he is not just another person aid in developing the desirable climate in which to care for him. This helps greatly in alleviating fears, anxieties, and stresses.

Psychologic Aspects of Drug Therapy

Concern only for the pharmacodynamic effects of drugs on the patient leaves much to be desired in health care personnel. The hospital environment potentiates the symbolic meaning and psychologic effects that can result from the administration of drugs. Because the patient and health care personnel are in close communication in the hospital, the attitude of the latter toward the psychologic effects of drugs plays a great role in the care of the patient. Drug therapy can influence the behavior, sense of well-being, and emotional state of the patient in addition to its physiologic action. Psychologic responses to medications can mimic pharmacologic reactions, such as adverse reactions, including allergic reactions.

Drugs hold symbolic meanings for patients. The foremost one is help. Effectiveness can be accelerated if the health care personnel instill in the patient's mind the idea of the benefits to be derived from the therapy. The psychologic practice of reinforcement does much to prolong the effectiveness of the drug administered. It is an accepted fact that the effectiveness of certain drugs on the body occurs only in the presence of an appropriate mental state. The patient's belief and faith confer positive benefits.

The second drug symbol is related to its inherent activity or power. The patient can become dependent on the drug's action to meet more successfully the stresses with which he is confronted. Herein lies the way to addiction produced by a sense of well-being. The emotional need is often subconscious, but the drug provides the patient with strength and a temporary sense of security. When a patient's needs cannot be met independently, his incapacity to face reality can be overcome by his dependency on specific drugs, such as narcotics, amphetamines, and alcohol.

When the patient is unable to face the reality of a cure granted by a specified drug, he considers it a danger. He may resist taking the drug, refuse to have the prescription refilled, or even throw it away. This unhealthy phenomenon usually occurs when the patient cannot face reality and uses his illness to meet a dependency his emotional state requires. He fears the loss of this dependency by its pharmacologic correction and a return to emotional stability.

Drug therapy can produce a feeling of ambivalency. The conscious wish for a return to health may be in conflict with the subconscious gratification of his needs which are dependent on his illness. When this conflict occurs, some symptoms may be relieved, whereas others may be grossly magnified.

Drug fantasies can best be alleviated by an honest explanation of the action expected of a drug. Fantasies are often exhibited by the patient's feeling that the drug is too weak or too strong and by his taking it upon himself to correct the dosage according to his desired needs. Some fantasies are based on fear, as implied by the terms used to designate the drugs, e.g., "radioactive drugs," "sedatives," and "antidepressants." It is important to determine what the patient knows and believes about drugs before administration so that drug fantasies are minimized.

Patients who believe that they are allergic to a certain drug, for real or imagined reasons, are likely to react with fear or panic when use of the drug is contemplated. Rejection of a patient's claim of allergy without evidence can result in dire consequences. A patient's reaction to the side effects of a particular drug may be reduced if the patient has been prepared in advance for their occurrence. The route of administration may cause an adverse reaction to the drug. The patient's attitude can change a drug's effectiveness both psychologically and physiologically.

Drugs may interfere with judgment, mood, sense of values, motor ability, and coordination. Particular care must be exercised in the administration of certain drugs because of the side reactions they cause. For example, antihistamines can cause drowsiness, depression, and a decrease in alertness.

Medications tend to be more effective when the patient believes in his capacity to get well and has a strong desire to regain his health. Such therapy also helps him to believe that the health care personnel are sincerely interested in his health. The patient's past and present conditioning to drugs, illnesses, hospitals, and health care personnel, as well as his health goals, help to determine his reactions to drugs. Health care personnel must exercise great caution and must remember that one of the most important deterrents to successful drug therapy occurs when the patient and the health care team have divergent goals.

Personnel Administering Parenteral Drugs

Legally, the only person in the health care team who may prescribe drugs for a patient is a physician, or in some instances, a dentist. Once the medication order has been written, the personnel administering drugs can include the nurse (registered, graduate, student, licensed practical), the pharmacist, the pharmacy technician, and intravenous therapists. Medications are prescribed by physicians, but other members of the health care team administer them. This discussion mainly concerns the latter group.

Personnel administering medication must help the patient to accept it and must sometimes reinforce the patient's confidence in the physician who prescribed it. The administration of medication is meaningful to the patient. If it is administered later than usual, if it is diluted more or less than the previous dose, if it is given in a different manner, if it is not producing results as he thinks it should, the patient may become disturbed.

Thoughtful consideration of the patient's comfort influences his acceptance of the medication. The personnel administering the medication should assist the patient in assuming a comfortable position, one compatible with his condition and the route of administration. Giving the patient a brief explanation of what is to be done and what is expected of him is also helpful.

If permitted by the institution, a brief explanation should be given as to the purpose of the medication and any effects that might be frightening. For example, because he has had an operation, an epileptic patient accustomed to taking his anticonvulsant agent orally every 4 to 6 hours is suddenly given the drug intramuscularly without any explanation. The patient will be upset because of his fear that without his medication he may have a grand mal seizure. The patient who is taking phenazopyridine hydrochloride should be informed that his urine will be orange-red because of the medication. If the drug depresses the central nervous system appreciably, the necessary limitations of activity should be explained and emphasized.

If the medication is to be administered by means of a needle, the injection can be a frightening experience regardless of the patient's age. The memory of a previous unpleasant experience or of comments made by a friend may cause him to dread any form of administration with a needle.

To administer the drugs intelligently, it is helpful for personnel to understand the patient's disease process and diagnosis. Knowledge of the physician's plan of therapy is likewise essential. The person giving the medication should know the local and systemic actions of the drug as well as its toxic manifestations and side reactions.

Specific components of a drug order written by a physician should be present before the drug is administered: (1) the name of the patient, (2) the date and time at which the order was written, (3) the generic name of the therapeutic agent, (4) the concentration and dosage of the drug, (5) the time and frequency of administration, (6) the route of administration, and (7) the physician's signature and registration number, if required.

Personnel must take precautions to make certain that the person receiving the medication is the one scheduled to receive it, and that the drug being administered is the one prescribed. The medication record must be compared with the patient's identification bracelet. If there is no identification bracelet, the drug should not be administered. In most hospitals, it is the responsibility of the head nurse to see that every patient has an identification bracelet.

The preferred route of administration is the one that permits the maximum therapeutic response and, at the same time, is the easiest on the patient. Clinical response can alter drug therapy. For this reason, drugs are withheld before certain laboratory tests or for some clinical indications. Morphine sulfate is withheld if the respirations are 12 or less per minute, and oral drugs are withheld if the swallowing reflex is absent of if persistent nausea and vomiting are present. Knowledge of these clinical signs can be used as a guide to consult with the physician for further orders.

Techniques of Parenteral Administration

When administering drugs by injection, care must be taken to prevent infection. Both the administration devices and the drug preparation must be sterile and free of pyrogens and foreign material. Of equal importance is strict adherence to a good hand-washing procedure before compounding or administering an injection. The basic procedure for hand-washing consists of using a good emulsifying agent, producing sufficient friction by rubbing to remove bacteria from the hands, then rinsing thoroughly.

Parenteral products should be examined before and after admixture. Hanging intravenous solutions are inspected periodically for the formation of precipitates or for changes in color. Prior to use, the presence of particulate matter can be detected by viewing the contents against a dark and a light background. This inspection can show particles of approximately 50 μm (the optical limitation of the human eye). Gross microbial growth caused by cracked containers is usually seen in clumps of floating or stringy material. Microbial contamination is not always visible, however. Particles of lint, rubber, and other debris float or settle to the bottom of the container; air bubbles can be differentiated because they rise to the top and dissipate.

Frequently, the compounder is required to open an ampul or vial to reconstitute the product. The source of foreign material now includes the glass

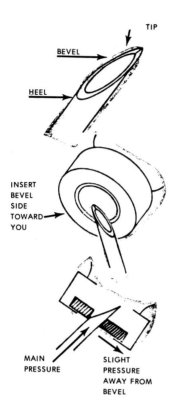

TIP

BEVEL

HEEL

INSERT
BEVEL
SIDE
TOWARD
YOU

MAIN
PRESSURE

SLIGHT
PRESSURE
AWAY FROM
BEVEL

Figure 6–1.   Proper method of inserting needle into rubber stopper to prevent coring.

from breaking the ampul, rubber generated by the coring process, the needle
and syringe, and the human and environmental factors.

Coring, i.e., the cutting of a piece of rubber from the closure by the needle,
occurs in varying degrees in parenteral products. The manufacturer's primary
concern is stability of the product. The rubber formation he chooses may compromise its coring ability. Products that require refrigeration or freezing become more prone to coring. In some instances, it is wise to delay reconstitution until the closure has risen to room temperature. The use of extra-large
gauge needles to penetrate rubber closures increases the chance of coring;
therefore, minimum-gauge needles are recommended. The rubber closure
should be penetrated with a minimum-gauge needle, with the beveled edge
up at an angle less than 45°, and the needle should be elevated to a vertical
position just before its entrance into the vial (Fig. 6–1). The alcohol swab
used to disinfect the closure can contribute lint fibers and alcohol to the product. One should avoid penetrating the closure before evaporation of the excess
alcohol.

Ampuls can cause a considerable amount of glass generation during breakage. Glass becomes more obvious when paint from the color-banded type of
ampul also falls into the product. The withdrawal of glass can be minimized
by holding the ampul in an upright position, slightly tilted, when inserting
the needle, and avoiding the outer surface of the neck of the ampule. The
needle should not be lowered to the base of the ampul, but held slightly
above, to avoid drawing glass particles into the syringe. The use of a 5-μm
filter needle prevents admixture contamination with large-size particulate mat-

ter. Strict aseptic techniques must be used during compounding to prevent bacterial contamination of the admixture.

When administering drugs intravenously, personnel should be aware of the recommended dosage range, required dilutions, recommended flow rate, desired effects of the drug, and the side effects. The predictable side effects may include dry mouth, accelerated pulse, and drowsiness. Unpredictable effects may include hypersusceptibility, idiosyncrasies, or allergic hypersensitivities to the drug. The administrator should recognize possible toxic manifestations of the drug and be aware of any dangers involved in administration, such as adverse reactions resulting from an incorrect rate of infusion.

If any of the following untoward reactions are experienced by the patient, the drug should be discontinued immediately, the vein kept open, and the physician notified: shock, chest pain, difficult breathing, cyanosis, excessive sweating, unusual change in pulse rate and rhythm, unusual drowsiness or loss of consciousness, vomiting, or convulsions.

When possible, the entire procedure should be carefully explained to the patient prior to venipuncture, to avoid misunderstandings, to allay apprehension, and to obtain the patient's consent. Critically ill patients are particularly prone to exaggerated fears, which trigger vasovagal reactions from the autonomic nervous system. The reactions may be manifested by syncope but can readily be alleviated if the therapist appears confident and uses all possible resources to reassure the patient. If the patient is ignored, vasoconstriction can readily occur. Peripheral collapse severely limits the availability of sites for venipuncture. If several attempts are necessary to institute therapy, the procedure becomes extremely traumatic to the patient and may undermine the course of therapy. Only skilled personnel should be permitted to administer parenteral therapy to apparently difficult patients.

In several ill cardiac patients, therapy may not only be difficult, but may pose a real physiologic threat to the patient. Fear incites stimulation of the adrenal medulla, and vasopressor production is stimulated. Hormones are secreted into the system, causing a chain reaction of sodium and chloride retention, causing cellular retention; loss of cellular potassium, causing intravascular water retention; increased vascular system load, causing pulmonary edema. For these reasons, the patient must be considered carefully before venipuncture.

Personnel administering parenteral fluids should have a thorough knowledge of the components of intravenous administration devices. These include basic intravenous sets, pediatric sets, secondary sets, volume control units, specialty sets, blood and blood component sets, filters, cannulae, and electronic pumps and controllers.

The individual starting the infusion is often preoccupied with the disease state of the patient and other responsibilities. The stress placed on the practitioner by the emergency, often involving immediate demands for livesaving parenteral drugs, leads to a tendency to minimize concern about contamination. In the event of cardiac arrest, anaphylactic shock, or any other life-threatening situation in which time is of the utmost importance, adherence to strict aseptic techniques may not be possible. If sterility has been compromised, the entire intravenous system, including the cannula, should be replaced as soon as the patient has been stabilized.

Three acceptable skin disinfectants for an intravenous preparation are (1) 1% or 2% tincture of iodine followed by complete removal with 70% alcohol, (2) a 30-second cleansing with povidone iodine without removal, and (3) a full 60-second vigorous scrub with 70% alcohol. An area approximately 2 inches in diameter is cleansed in a centrifugal manner, starting at the proposed insertion site and working outward in a circular motion.

Intramuscular Technique

Technique	Comments
1. Gently tap the selected site of injection with the fingers several times.	Stimulation of the peripheral nerves helps to minimize the initial reaction when the needle is inserted.
2. Cleanse the area thoroughly with a centrifugal motion.	Pathogens present on the skin can be forced into the tissues by the needle.
3. With the thumb and the first two fingers, press the tissue down firmly in the direction of the thigh.	Compression of the subcutaneous tissue helps to ensure that the needle will enter the muscle. Moving the tissue downward will help to disperse the solution and seal the needle track when the tissue is permitted to return to normal position.
4. Hold the syringe in a horizontal position until ready to inject.	The pull of gravity may alter the position of the plunger of the syringe, causing a loss of drug.
5. When ready to inject, quickly thrust the needle into the tissue at a 90-degree angle.	Quick injection minimizes pain. Thrust helps to insert the needle.
6. As soon as the needle is in place, slowly pull back on the plunger to determine whether the needle is in a blood vessel. If blood is noted, pull the needle back slightly and test again.	Muscle tissue is vascular. Drugs injected into the blood stream are absorbed immediately; in intramuscular administration a slower rate is desired. In addition, unintended injection into a blood vessel may cause damage.
7. If no blood enters the syringe, inject the solution.	This indicates proper location of needle in muscle, not in a blood vessel.
8. Remove the needle quickly.	Slow removal of the needle pulls and traumatizes the tissues and may cause discomfort.
9. Rub the area.	Rubbing aids in distribution and absorption of the solution.

Direct Intravenous Injection With Small Vein Needle (SVN)

Technique	Comments
1. Connect syringe with medication to needle adapter.	Be sure to flush tubing and needle.
2. Place patient on back in semi-Fowler's position with arms below heart level.	Supine position permits access to both arms. Blood flow is increased when arms are below heart.
3. Apply tourniquet 4 to 6 in. proximal to intended entry site.	Tourniquet increases venous distention. Vein becomes more visible and easier to palpate, and cannula placement is facilitated.
4. Have patient open and close fists. Observe and palpate a suitable vein.	Muscle contraction increases venous flow toward venipuncture site. Palpation is required to affirm a soft "bouncing" vein, and ensures that the vessel is not an aberrant artery.
5. Release tourniquet.	Release of tourniquet at this time prevents prolonged hemostasis.

6. Perform skin prep.

Proper cleansing removes bacteria.

7. Reapply tourniquet. With thumb of one hand, retract on vein and soft tissue downward about 2 in. distal to venipuncture site.

Tourniquet and downward retraction on vein promote vein stabilization and prevent vein from rolling.

8. Hold needle by wings, almost parallel with arm, directly in line with vein.

Wings provide needle stability. Parallel angle lessens risk of piercing posterior wall of vein.

9. Enter skin and vein with one quick step.

A one-step entry assures adequate vein placement for a short SVN. A blood return is noted when vein is entered.

10. Carefully thread needle into vein.

Full needle insertion is required to ensure secure vein entry.

11. Remove tourniquet.

Removal of tourniquet at this time alleviates hemostasis and vein occlusion.

12. Gently withdraw small amount of blood.

Withdrawal of blood reaffirms secure vein entry.

13. Slowly inject medication. At frequent intervals, withdraw on plunger to obtain blood return.

Inject drug at manufacturer's recommended rate. Frequent testing for blood return assures secure vein cannulation. Monitor patient for any signs of adverse reactions. If any occur, stop injection immediately.

14. Remove needle with one smooth, quick step.

Quick removal of needle prevents traumatization of venous wall and impedes hematoma formation.

15. Apply pressure at site of venipuncture.

Pressure prevents hematoma formation.

Intermittent Intravenous Techniques

Heparin Lock or Intermittent Catheter (INT) In Situ

Technique	Comments
1. Connect needle no larger than 22 gauge and no longer that 1 in. to syringe with medication or I.V. tubing. Flush I.V. tubing and needle with admixture or drug.	A short, small-gauge needle prevents leaving a large hole in the cap and prevents puncture of catheter or tubing. All air must be flushed from the system to prevent air embolism.
2. Cleanse port end of cap with antiseptic swab.	Cleansing port end removes bacteria from injection site.
3. If drug or admixture is incompatible with heparin, device must be flushed with normal saline before and after drug administration.	Flushing with normal saline removes heparin from device prior to drug administration and prevents contact with heparin after administration.
4. Insert needle into center of injection cap. Hold cap with one hand while inserting needle with other. Tape connection if prolonged use is intended.	Holding injection cap with hand stabilizes device and prevents mechanical irritation at site. Do not force insertion if obstruction is felt; instead, realign needle angle. Taping connection prevents needle dislodgement.
5. Withdraw syringe plunger or squeeze tubing to obtain blood return.	Patency of vein is ascertained, and infiltration is prevented.
6. Inject drug/admixture at recommended rate.	Administering medication at rate recommended by manufacturer decreases risk of untoward reactions.
7. Hold device firmly, and withdraw needle.	Holding device firmly while withdrawing needle prevents accidental device dislodgement.

8. Flush device with heparin solution.

Heparin flush prevents cannula occlusion. Be sure to re-prep injection site prior to flush, and stabilize device during needle entry and withdrawal.

Catheter With Obturator in Situ

Technique	Comments
1. Prepare syringe with medication or flushed I.V. tubing.	All air must be removed from syringe or tubing to prevent air embolism.
2. Place sterile 2 × 2 in. sponge under cannula hub.	Sterile field is provided to perform connection, and risk of touch contamination is reduced.
3. Remove and discard obturator from cannula in situ.	Obturator must not be reused.
4. Connect syringe with medication/I.V. tubing adapter into cannula hub.	The sterile sponge can be used to perform the connection to reduce risk of touch contamination.
5. If using I.V. tubing and system, which are to remain in place, secure connection with tape.	Risk of disconnection is prevented.
6. Withdraw plunger or squeeze tubing to obtain blood return.	Patency of vein is checked, and infiltration is prevented.
7. Inject medication or admixture at recommended rate.	Administering medication at rate recommended by manufacturer decreases risk of untoward reactions.
8. Remove syringe/I.V. tubing.	Cannula is held firmly to prevent accidental cannula dislodgement.
9. Insert new sterile obturator.	Obturator should be firmly locked in place.

Established Intravenous Infusion

Technique	Comments
1. Connect needle no larger than 22 gauge and no longer than 1 in. to syringe with medication.	A short, small-gauge needle prevents leaving a large hole in the cap and prevents puncture of catheter or tubing.
2. Flush needle with drug solution.	All air must be flushed out of needle to prevent an air embolism.
3. Cleanse rubber flashbulb or injection port with antiseptic swab.	Cleansing removes bacteria from injection site.
4. Insert needle into one of the small circles on the flashbulb or into Y-site injection port.	Some sets contain small circles on flashbulb. If circles are present, needle must be placed inside any circle. If circles are not present, any part of flashbulb may be used. Some sets do not contain a flashbulb, but have a Y-site injection port.
5. Open infusion clamp, and allow infusion to run for a few seconds.	Free flow affirms patent cannula. If free flow is not possible, I.V. must be restarted before medication is given.
6. Regulate drip to a moderate rate.	If the medication is incompatible with the I.V. admixture, the tubing must be flushed with normal saline before and after drug administration. If the medication and I.V. mixture are compatible, allowing the I.V. to run dilutes the drug, causing less vein irritation and affirms a patent line throughout the drug administration.

7. Inject medication at recommended rate.	Administering medication at rate recommended by manufacturer decreases risk of untoward reactions.
8. Stabilize flashbulb or Y site while withdrawing needle.	Accidental cannula dislodgement or tubing disconnection is prevented.
9. Allow solution to flush vein, then regulate to prescribed rate.	Flushing vein after drug administration dilutes drug in vein and decreases risk of chemical phlebitis.

Piggyback Method With Established Intravenous Infusion

Technique	Comments
1. Be sure that the primary tubing contains a back checkvalve.	The back checkvalve is needed to shut off primary flow automatically while piggyback line runs. The primary flow resumes automatically when the piggyback flow stops.
2. Lower primary container on hanger.	This increases pressure of piggyback flow that is needed to shut off back checkvalve.
3. Cleanse Y-site injection port directly below back checkvalve with antiseptic swab.	Cleansing removes bacteria from injection site.
4. Close flow clamp on piggyback tubing, and connect to piggyback container. Hang container on I.V. pole.	
5. Insert needle of piggyback tubing into center of Y site. Tape connection.	Tubing comes with needle permanently attached.
6. Lower piggyback container, open flow clamp, and allow fluid from primary container to fill tubing and half of drip chamber. Close flow clamp.	Filling tubing, while connected to primary line, prevents air contamination with drug in piggyback container. This is especially important when handling antibiotics and cancer chemotherapeutic agents.
7. Hang piggyback container on I.V. pole, open clamp all the way. Use the clamp on primary tubing to regulate drip rate to manufacturer's recommended rate of administration.	Pressure from the piggyback fluid pushes against the back checkvalve and stops the fluid from the primary line. The flow clamp on the piggyback tubing should be all the way open to allow for full pressure. All regulation of drip rate must be done by the primary tubing clamp.
8. When the piggyback container is empty, the primary line starts to run. Regulate primary line to desired drip rate.	When the fluid in the piggyback system is released, the back checkvalve releases and allows the primary line to run automatically.
9. If there is air in the piggyback tubing, refill with fluid from primary line. Close piggyback flow clamp.	Flush air from tubing in same manner as first tubing flush. To administer next dose of drug, change containers and repeat procedure.

Connecting Secondary Line With Established Intravenous Infusion

Technique	Comments
1. Connect secondary container, tubing, and 20-gauge, 1-in. needle. Flush tubing and needle.	A 20-gauge needle prevents needle from bending. A 1-in. needle prevents piercing of primary I.V. tubing. Flushing the system prevents air blockage or air embolism.
2. Reaffirm that I.V. site and primary line are without complications.	The primary line must be functioning properly for the secondary line to run.
3. Cleanse the flashbulb or injection port with an antiseptic swab.	Cleansing removes bacteria from injection site.

Technique	Comments
4. Insert needle into a circle of the flashbulb or into the Y-site injection port.	Some sets contain small circles on flashbulb. If circles are present, needle must be placed inside any circle. If circles are not present, any part of flashbulb may be used. Some sets do not contain a flashbulb, but have a Y-site injection port.
5. Securely tape connection.	Taping prevents to-and-fro motion, which increases risk of contamination and prevents needle dislodgement.
6. If intermittent administration is desired, close flow clamp of unwanted container, and regulate flow of desired container.	This method of administration allows intermittent dosage of either solution or continuous flow of both solutions.
7. If simultaneous administration of both solutions is desired, regulate each flow clamp to its desired flow rate.	When both admixtures are run at one time, they must be compatible.
8. If one container runs dry, lowering that container allows the fluid from the other container to fill the tubing and displace the air.	Air in either tubing will cause air blockage, or if infused, a possible air embolism.

Connecting Volume Control Set With Established Intravenous Infusion

Technique	Comments
1. Prepare volume control set with fluid container, according to manufacturer's instructions.	Some membrane volume control sets require special steps to fill drip chamber. Fill burette with approximately 15 ml of fluid. Then perform OSCAR: (O) open flow clamp, (S) squeeze drip chamber, (C) close flow clamp, (A) and (R) release drip chamber. Other sets fill the same as a standard I.V. tubing.
2. Attach a 20-gauge, 1-in. needle. Flush tubing and needle.	A 20-gauge needle prevents needle bending. A 1-in. needle prevents piercing primary I.V. tubing. Flushing the system prevents air blockage or air embolism.
3. Reaffirm that I.V. site and primary line are without complications.	The primary line must be functioning properly for the volume control set to run.
4. Insert needle into a circle of the flashbulb or into the Y-site injection port.	Some sets contain small circles on flashbulb. If circles are present, needle must be placed inside any circle. If circles are not present, any part of flashbulb may be used. Some sets do not contain a flashbulb, but have a Y-site injection port.
5. Securely tape connection.	To-and-fro motion, which increases risk of contamination, is prevented. Needle dislodgement is prevented.
6. Fill burette chamber with desired amount of fluid.	
7. If set is to be used for administration of drug, cleanse injection site on top of burette with an antiseptic swab.	Because these sets have a high risk of contamination, owing to repeated injections, it is not recommended that they be used for intermittent medication administration, except in the neonate or newborn, where fluid overload is a serious problem. Cleansing the injection site removes bacterial contamination.
8. Inject completely dissolved medication into the injection port on top of the burette.	All medication must be completely dissolved before it is added to any further solution.
9. Rotate burette.	Rotation of burette ensures proper mixing of medication and solution.

10. If primary admixture and burette medication are incompatible shut off primary solution. If fluid overload is a concern, shut off primary solution.

The primary solution and burette medication may run at the same time by regulating each clamp individually. If incompatibility is present, they must not run at the same time.

11. Infuse the burette medication at the recommended rate.

All medications should be administered at the rate recommended by the manufacturer to lessen the risks of untoward reactions.

12. When the burette chamber is emptied, the flow stops running, and air will not fill the tubing. Close clamp.

The valve in the burette shuts automatically when the burette chamber is empty of fluid. To reestablish flow, fill chamber with desired amount of fluid.

Continuous Intravenous Technique With Over-the-Needle Catheter (ONC)

Technique	Comments
1. Prepare I.V. container and tubing. Flush system.	Air must be flushed from the tubing to prevent air blockage or infusion of air with possible embolism. All equipment must be assembled prior to start of venipuncture.
2. Place patient on back in semi-Fowler's position with arms below heart level.	Supine position permits access to both arms. Blood flow is increased when arms are below heart.
3. Apply tourniquet 4 to 6 in. proximal to intended entry site.	Tourniquet increases venous distention. Vein becomes more visible and easier to palpate, and cannula placement is facilitated.
4. Have patient open and close fists. Observe and palpate a suitable vein.	Muscle contraction increases venous flow toward venipuncture site. Palpation is required to affirm a soft "bouncing" vein and assures that the vessel is not an aberrant artery.
5. Release tourniquet.	Release of tourniquet at this time prevents prolonged hemostasis.
6. Perform skin prep.	Proper cleansing removes bacteria.
7. Reapply tourniquet. With thumb of one hand, retract vein and soft tissue downward about 2 in. distal to venipuncture site.	Tourniquet and downward retraction on vein promote vein stabilization and prevent vein from rolling.
8. Hold cannula by the stylet hub at a 45-degree angle in line with vein.	Holding cannula by stylet hub prevents touch contamination of catheter hub and prevents turning of catheter, which would result in breaking of the catheter-stylet seal. A 45-degree angle prevents skin drag upon entry.
9. Quickly insert cannula through skin, along side of vein. Do not pierce vein with skin entry.	A two-step entry, skin first and vein second, permits access into veins that cannot be entered with one step.
10. Lower cannula at an angle almost parallel with the skin.	Lowering cannula in this way permits vein entry without piercing posterior vein wall.
11. Maintaining skin traction, quickly enter vein for approximately $1/2$ in.	Vein entry must be approximately $1/2$ in. to ensure entry of both stylet and catheter.
12. Blood return through the stylet assures vein entry. Hold stylet firmly with one hand while threading the catheter off the stylet with the other hand. Thread catheter into vein.	Holding the stylet firmly and sliding catheter into vein assures that stylet will not puncture catheter. If obstruction is felt, do not force catheter; remove entire unit, and start over at another site. *Never rethread stylet back into catheter*, as it can cause a catheter embolism.
13. Remove tourniquet.	Hemostasis and vein occlusion are alleviated. Hematoma formation at entry site is prevented.

14. Place sterile 2 × 2 in. sponge under catheter hub. Remove and discard stylet. Connect I.V. tubing. Stabilize cannula with tape.

Sterile field is provided for catheter-tubing connection. Cannula stabilization prevents mechanical irritation.

15. Open flow clamp, and allow fluid to run.

Adequate flow rate reaffirms proper vein placement.

16. Apply sterile dressing.

Sterility of site is ensured.

17. Secure dressing with tape. Apply second strip of tape to looped I.V. tubing.

Any tubing stress is not relayed to venipuncture site.

18. Document dressing with date, time, type, gauge and length of cannula, and your initials.

Such information is necessary to maintain system and to ensure full cannula removal.

Intermittent Intravenous Therapy

Intermittent intravenous therapy may be administered secondary to a primary-keep-vein-open (KVO) line, by intermittent catheter (INT) or heparin lock, or by a catheter with an obturator. The primary tubing of the KVO line contains a back checkvalve. When the primary container is lowered on a hanger, fluid pressure from the higher secondary solution shuts the back checkvalve off and prevents the primary line from running. When the secondary container is empty, lack of pressure releases the valve, and the primary solution starts running automatically. Patency of the intermittent catheter and heparin lock is maintained, between usages, with a low-dose heparin flush. A catheter with obturator consists of two separate parts. To use this device, the obturator is removed, and the catheter hub is connected directly to the intravenous tubing or syringe. After each use, a new sterile obturator is securely locked in place.

The advantages of a primary KVO system for intermittent drug administration are as follows. (1) It allows for the least number of entries into the system to administer medications; thus, it has the least risk of touch contamination. (2) It requires the least amount of nursing time to administer the medication. (3) Because it requires no flushes or tubing replacements, it is the least costly method.

Disadvantages of a primary KVO system include the following. (1) It requires continuous administration of intravenous fluid between doses of drugs, which may be harmful to patients on strict limitations of fluid intake. (2) It requires the patient to be continuously connected to the infusion.

The main advantage of an intermittent catheter (INT), a heparin lock, or a small vein needle (SVN) is that they allow patients freedom from infusions between drug administrations. Whether a patient will receive less total fluid than with a KVO system depends upon the procedure used to administer the drug. Disadvantages of this method of administration include the following. (1) If the tubing is flushed after each dose to ensure full drug delivery to the patient, and if the patient is receiving two or more drugs daily, the total fluid volume may be more than with the KVO system. If the tubing is not flushed, and an inline filter is used, as much as 20% of the drug may be discarded with the tubing. If incompatibility of drugs with heparin is a concern, the device requires a normal saline flush before and after drug administration. Each time a drug is given, the injection cap must be punctured; thus, a total of four punctures could be involved. Each puncture increases the risk of touch contamination. To ensure sterility, new equipment should be used for each drug delivery; thus, this method can be very costly.

The catheter with obturator has the same advantages and disadvantages as the INT or heparin lock except that it requires no heparin. Heparin incompatibility is therefore not a problem.

Transfusion Therapy

Transfusion therapy is used to replace blood volume, to replace oxygen carrying capacity, and to replace coagulation factors. Transfusions may be given with whole blood, packed red cells, frozen cells, washed cells, fresh frozen plasma, cryoprecipitates, platelet concentrates, and 5% or 25% human serum albumin.

The majority of blood components require ABO and Rh antigen-antibody compatibility testing prior to administration.

All patients receiving blood or blood components must be identified by hospital identification bands, and if possible, by stating their name before starting the transfusion. This policy minimizes the risk of the patient receiving the wrong blood, which would result in a fatal reaction.

Whole blood and red-cell components must be given through an administration set containing a blood filter. Non-red-cell components may be given through a special component administration set. A blood warmer may be required for massive, rapid transfusions and for patients with cold agglutinins. The venipuncture procedure is the same as for an infusion. A large-gauge cannula may be required for rapid administration of packed red cells. When the transfusion is completed, the blood set must be replaced with a fresh infusion set if intravenous fluids are to follow the transfusion.

Possible immediate transfusion reactions include hemolysis, fever, allergy, circulatory overload, hypothermia, and citrate toxicity, Possible delayed reactions include hepatitis, syphilis, malaria, and AIDS. All reactions must be treated according to hospital policy. The treatment varies according to the type and severity of the reaction. It may be necessary to stop the transfusion, or slowing of the drip rate and administration of antihistamines may be appropriate. The blood bank must be notified of any reaction, so that appropriate investigation may be instituted and future reactions avoided.

Initiating and Maintaining an Intravenous System

In an effort to reduce infections related to intravenous systems, the Centers for Disease Control (CDC) have published guidelines for the insertion of the cannula and maintenance of the system. The National Intravenous Therapy Association (NITA) has published standards of care to minimize all I.V.-related complications. Examples of these recommendations are:

1. Strict aseptic techniques should be followed during cannula insertion, during admixture, and during any manipulations of the system.
2. If hair removal is necessary, it should be cut with scissors and not shaved because shaving causes skin microabrasions, which can increase the risk of infection.

3. The insertion site must be prepped with an acceptable disinfectant prior to cannula insertion.
4. The cannula should be securely anchored to prevent to-and-fro motion, to lessen the risk of mechanical irritation.
5. The puncture site should be covered with a sterile dressing. Unsterile tape should not touch the site.
6. The system should be maintained as a closed unit as much as possible. Injection ports should be disinfected immediately prior to use.
7. All peripheral I.V. cannulae should be changed every 48 to 72 hours.
8. All I.V. solution containers should be used or discarded after 24 hours.
9. All I.V. tubing and component parts should be changed every 24 to 48 hours, preferably at time of container change.
10. All insertion sites should be checked every 8 hours. The site should be palpated through an intact dressing. If any tenderness, redness, or edema is noted, the dressing should be removed and the site carefuly examined.
11. The site should be changed immediately at the first sign of any complication.

Complications of Intravenous Therapy

Local complications occur frequently, but are usually not of a serious nature. Systemic complications must be recognized and treated immediately, as they are always life-threatening.

Local Complications

Hematoma occurs when blood escapes from the vein into the surrounding tissue. The patient usually complains of tenderness at the site. Treatment consists of extremity elevation with cold compresses for the first 24 hours, followed by warm compresses. Hematoma formation can be prevented by venipuncture expertise, utilizing a two-step entry method, and upon cannula removal, application of pressure until all bleeding has stopped.

Infiltration occurs when intravenous fluid or drugs are injected into the surrounding tissue. This complication may result from an unsuccessful venipuncture, or the vein may have been pierced by the cannula or broken after a successful entry. Edema is usually visible, and the skin may be cold to touch. If the infiltration is large, the patient may complain of pain. To check for an infiltration while the intravenous system is running, place a tourniquet above the site tightly enough to stop venous flow. If the infusion continues to drip, an infiltration is occurring. Treatment consists of relocation of the infusion site, elevation of the extremity, and application of warm compresses. Intravenous sites should be checked frequently for signs of infiltration to minimize the amount of fluid or drug infused into the tissue. Because small vein needles easily cause infiltration, they should not be used for administration of vesicant drugs. Secure cannula placement with adequate stabilization helps prevent this complication.

Phlebitis is an inflammation of the vein. Symptoms include pain, heat, redness, and swelling. The infusion must be relocated, the extremity elevated, and warm wet compresses applied. To prevent phlebitis from recurring, underlying causes should be investigated, and if possible, altered. Causes may include traumatic vein entry, large-gauge cannula, mechanical irritation from unstabilized cannula, leaving cannula in site for too long a time period, and administration of drugs known to cause phlebitis, with the possibility of further dilution and/or filtration.

Site infection may be present without systemic complications. A purulent discharge may be noted. Local redness and pain are usually present. The intravenous site and all equipment must be changed immediately to prevent septicemia. The cannula tip and any drainage are cultured to verify infection. Warm wet compresses are applied. Prevention is best achieved through adherence to strict aseptic techniques during venipuncture and all intravenous system manipulations.

Systemic Complications

Septicemia related to intravenous administration of drugs is a systemic infection that is usually suspected if fever occurs without any other found cause. Symptoms include fever, chills, headache, and general malaise. The entire intravenous system must be changed immediately. All equipment, including container, tubing, and cannula tip, must be cultured. The symptoms frequently subside after cannula and equipment change. Antibiotic therapy may be necessary. Prevention of septicemia related to intravenous administration of drugs requires adherence to strict aseptic techniques during admixture, venipuncture, and all manipulations of the intravenous system.

Circulatory overload results from giving too much fluid too fast. Signs and symptoms include engorged neck veins, increased blood pressure, elevated central venous pressure (CVP), rapid respirations, and shortness of breath. The infusion should be changed to a KVO rate, the head of the bed should be elevated, and the patient should be made warm with extra blankets, if necessary, to increase the peripheral blood volume so that some of the fluid load is taken off the central system. The physician must be notified immediately because diuretics, morphine, and oxygen are usually required. Prevention of circulatory overload includes keeping an accurate intake and output record, with prompt attention given to insufficient output for intake, maintaining accurate infusion flow rates, and in elderly patients, maintaining semi-Fowler's position and keeping the extremities warm.

Speed shock occurs when a foreign substance is injected so rapidly that toxic plasma levels are reached in the blood, heart, and brain. Symptoms include syncope, shock and cardiac arrest. Treatment varies according to the specific drug involved and the degree of shock present. Prevention is possible by always giving drugs at the rate recommended by the manufacturer. This may require the use of electronic control devices for the administration of potent drugs.

Air embolism is a potential complication of every infusion; however, it is most frequently seen with central catheters and malfunctioning pumps. Symptoms occur suddenly and include chest pain, cyanosis, decreased blood pressure, weak rapid pulse, rise in CVP, and loss of consciousness. To treat air embolism, one immediately places the patient on the left side in Trendelenburg's position. This allows the air to be trapped in the right atrium. The physician must be notified immediately, as prompt removal of the air may be necessary to save the patient's life. Prevention includes having the patient perform Valsalva's maneuver using catheter insertion and tubing changes, or whenever the needle or catheter is opened to air. The use of Luer-Lok, air-eliminating filters has been shown to prevent this complication. All pumps must be checked before usage to ensure that the air detection system is working.

Catheter embolism occurs when a catheter is served within the vein. Usually the patient has no symptoms. If the severance occurs during peripheral insertion, placement of a tourniquet at the joint above the insertion, tight enough to stop venous flow, may trap the embolism peripherally and allow surgical removal. All catheters should be radiopaque to allow for radiologic location. The surgical removal of a central catheter embolism depends on its location and the condition of the patient. To prevent this complication, when inserting an over-the-needle catheter (ONC), the stylet must never be rethreaded back into the catheter. When inserting an inside-the-needle catheter (INC), the catheter must never be withdrawn back through the needle. If a central catheter has a needle remaining in place, the tip must always be secured within the needle protective cover.

Pulmonary embolism occurs when a blood clot occludes the pulmonary vascular system. Symptoms include those of respiratory, circulatory, and cardiac distress. Treatment consists of aggressive anticoagulation therapy. Prevention includes the use of adequate blood filtration during transfusions, filtration of intravenous admixtures for large particulate matter, prevention of thrombophlebitis, and avoidance of the lower extremities for infusion therapy.

Summary

When administering parenteral drugs, personnel must know the patient— his fears, idiosyncrasies, allergies, and disease—and the physician's plan of treatment. Personnel must be knowledgeable about the drugs being used— the physiologic effects, possible adverse reactions, and antidotal treatment. They must use strict aseptic techniques and know the various routes of administration, and the equipment required and reaction time expected for each specific route. The well-being of the patient can best be served when all of this information is put to use.

General References

American Association of Blood Banks (AABB): Safe Transfusion. Washington, DC (1981).
Center for Disease Control (CDC): Guidelines for the Prevention and Control of Nosocomial Infections. Atlanta (1983).
National Intravenous Therapy Association (NITA): Intravenous Nursing Standards of Practice. NITA Journal, 5, 1, 19 (1982).
Plumer, A.L.: Principles and Practice of Intravenous Therapy. 3rd Ed. Boston, Little, Brown and Co., (1982).

7

CHAPTER

Biopharmaceutic Factors Influencing Drug Availability

Stuart Feldman and Gayle A. Brazeau

For a pharmacologically active drug to be therapeutically effective, it must reach the site of its activity in the body in sufficient amounts and at a sufficient rate that the desired pharmacologic effect takes place. In other words, the drug molecule must be available to the site of action. Several factors can influence the therapeutic response to a given drug. The physicochemical properties of the drug and its dosage form and the biologic characteristics of the patient play a role in the clinical response to a given drug. The study of the relationship between the physical and chemical properties of the drug and its dosage form and the biologic effects observed following the administration of the drug in the dosage form is termed "biopharmaceutics."

The *biologic availability*, or *bioavailability*, of a pharmaceutic dosage form expresses the relationship between the efficiency of absorption from a test preparation and that from a standard preparation. For example, the availability of a drug from an intramuscular or subcutaneous dosage form may be compared with that of an equivalent dose of the drug administered intravenously. Another definition of bioavailability, which is useful in describing drug availability from parenteral dosage forms, is that availability represents the amount of intact drug that reaches the systemic circulation.

The therapeutic response to a given drug can be controlled in many ways. The techniques can be utilized to alter the onset and duration of clinical activity, and include (1) selection of the route of administration, (2) choice of the dosage regimen, (3) choice of the specific drug analog, (4) use of other drugs in the therapeutic regimen, and (5) selection and preparation of the

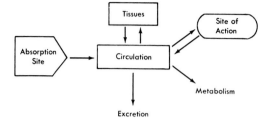

Figure 7–1. Pharmacokinetic scheme for the absorption, distribution, metabolism, and elimination of a drug from a parenteral dosage form.

formulation, including both active and nonactive ingredients. All these factors can influence the time course of a drug in the body, which in turn may alter the clinical effectiveness of the medicinal agent. Figure 7–1 represents an overall pharmacokinetic scheme for the parenteral administration of drugs and the resulting absorption, distribution, metabolism, and elimination of the active drug molecule.

The routes of administration used in parenteral drug therapy are quite numerous. In many instances, the choice of a route of administration is governed by the desire to obtain rapid-onset drug activity and to achieve high levels of drug at the site of action. Sometimes the drug is delivered directly to the site of action. The administration of drugs by intrathecal, intracisternal, intracardiac, intradermal, or intravenous injection exemplifies this approach. Parenteral routes of administration that require an absorption step before the drug can gain access to the systemic circulation and the site of action are the intramuscular, subcutaneous, and implantation routes.

Physicochemical Influences on Bioavailability

Dissolution Rate

The process by which a drug in a solid form goes into solution is termed "dissolution." When a drug is administered in solid form, whether orally in the form of tablets, capsules, or suspensions, or parenterally in the form of an intramuscular suspension or pellet, the rate of absorption of the drug across the biologic membrane is frequently found to be controlled by the slowest step in the sequence:

$$\text{Solid Drug} \xrightarrow{\text{Dissolution}} \text{Drug Solution} \xrightarrow{\text{Absorption}} \text{Absorbed Drug}$$

In many instances, the slowest step in the sequence is the dissolution of drug in the fluids at the absorption site. In this instance, any factor influencing the rate of solution of this drug also influences the absorption of the drug across the biologic membrane.

The rate at which a drug is absorbed can have an important influence on the concentration of the drug in the blood. The importance of this influence can be appreciated by examination of Figure 7–2, depicting the blood levels of a hypothetic drug suspension after intramuscular injection of three different dosage forms. If it is assumed that a certain concentration of drug in the blood is needed for a pharmacologic effect, it is easy to see how, in dissolution rate-

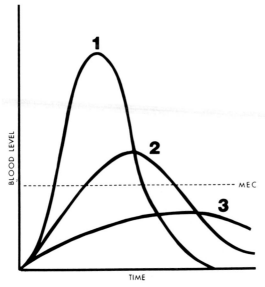

Figure 7–2. Hypothetic blood level versus time curves following the absorption of a drug from three different dosage forms administered by intramuscular injection. The dashed line represents the minimum effective concentration (MEC).

limited absorption, the dissolution rate can affect the absorption rate of the drug. Formulation 1 in Figure 7–2 dissolves rapidly, and the blood concentration of drug rises rapidly with time. In a relatively short time, the drug achieves the minimum effective concentration (MEC) necessary for therapeutic activity. Formulation 2 has a lower dissolution rate than has formulation 1, and a longer time is needed before therapeutic levels of drug are achieved. It is also important to note that the concentration of drugs in the therapeutic range does not extend over a long interval. The dissolution rate and the absorption rate of formulation 3 are so slow that therapeutic levels of drug in the blood are never achieved.

Several factors can influence the dissolution rate of drugs in pharmaceutic dosage forms. The factors and their effect on dissolution rate are easily recognized if one applies a simple equation that has been used to predict the rate at which a drug goes into solution. The equation, first derived by Noyes and Whitney,[1] is as follows:

$$\text{Dissolution} = K \cdot D \cdot S \, (C_s - C) \qquad\qquad \text{Eq. 1}$$

where C is the concentration of drugs in solution at time t, C_s is the equilibrium solubility of the solute at the experimental temperature, S is the surface area of solid drug, D is the diffusion coefficient of the drug, and K is a constant. Inspection of Equation 1 yields several important observations. The relationship of D, S, and C_s to the dissolution rate is a direct proportion, meaning that changes, whether increases or decreases, in these terms directly increase or decrease the dissolution rate. For example, decreasing the particle size of the solid in the dosage form increases the total surface area of the drug present in the dosage form. The increased surface area results in an increased dissolution rate. An excellent example of this effect can be seen in the work of Buckwalter and Dickison, who studied the effect of particle size on the absorption of procaine penicillin G suspensions by the intramuscular

TABLE 7–1. Penicillin Serum Concentration in Rabbits One Hour After Intramuscular Injection of Aqueous Suspensions of Procaine Penicillin G

Particle Size (μm)	Average Blood Level (units/ml)
150–250	1.37
105–150	1.24
58–105	1.54
35–38	1.64
<35	2.40
1–2	2.14

Data from Buckwalter and Dickison[2]

route.[2] They found that the most rapid absorption occurred from procaine penicillin G suspensions containing the smallest crystals. The average blood levels of procaine penicillin G one hour after intramuscular injection as a function of particle size are summarized in Table 7–1.

It is also possible to utilize the effect of particle size on drug dissolution to obtain a release of the active drug over a longer period. Increasing the particle size of the drug in suspension results in decreased surface area, lower dissolution rates, and a lower rate of absorption of the drug from the site of injection. An example of the influence of particle size on pharmacologic activity has been reported by Schlichtkrull from an investigation of insulin absorption.[3] The crystal size of insulin is an important consideration in determining the onset and duration of insulin activity in man. A long-acting insulin (Ultralente) showed a slow decline in blood sugar levels and an extended depression of the blood sugar level for longer than 10 hours after administration to rabbits when the particle size was 50 μm, but showed a steep fall in blood sugar for 4 hours after administration and then a rapid rise to almost normal levels when a suspension of small crystals (5 μm), was administered.

By altering the solubility of the drug, C_s, the dissolution rate can be either increased or decreased. Several factors can alter the solubility of a drug. Polymorphism, the existence of a substance in more than one crystalline form, is responsible for a number of clinically significant differences in drug activity. In general, there is only one stable crystalline form of a drug. Other polymorphic forms are less stable and usually have greater solubility. The greater solubility results in a faster dissolution rate and, therefore, more rapid absorption of the drug. This has been found to be the case with novobiocin[4] and chloramphenicol,[5] which can exist in either the stable crystalline form or the amorphous form. In both instances, only the amorphous form exhibits biologic activity.

The influence of polymorphism on the absorption of drugs from parenteral dosage forms is further elucidated by the subcutaneous implantation of two forms of methylprednisolone into rats.[6] The average absorption rate from the more soluble polymorphic form II was about 1.7 times the absorption rate of drug in the stable form I. In vitro studies show that the dissolution rate of form II is about 1.4 times faster than that of form I.[7]

Another method of altering the solubility of drugs that are either weak acids or weak bases is by modification of the pH in the solution surrounding each

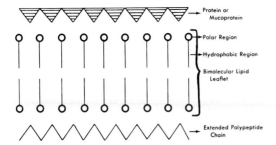

Figure 7–3. Bimolecular leaflet model of cell membrane structure.

solid particle. If the solubility of drugs can be appreciably increased in this "diffusion layer," an increased dissolution of the solid can be obtained. The pH of this diffusion layer is not necessarily the same as the pH of the body fluids such as blood, lymph, or serum. The pH of the diffusion layer in subcutaneous measurements in rats was found to range from a low of 3.57 to a high of 9.00, depending on the drug used, whereas the pH of the rat blood was between 7.3 and 7.4.[6] Although the pH effect on drug solubility and absorption may not always be critical with parenteral formulations, the pH of the diffusion layer may have an extremely important influence on drug solubility and dissolution rate with other routes of administration, especially oral administration of drugs.

Also of importance when considering the effect of dissolution rate on drug absorption is the viscosity of the parenteral solution or suspension. The viscosity of the solution or fluid in which a drug dissolves can affect the dissolution rate by altering the diffusion coefficient of the drug. At higher viscosities, the diffusion coefficient of the drug is reduced, resulting in a decrease in dissolution rate. In mice, it has been found that the use of 35% vol/vol aqueous glycerin as the solvent decreased the acute toxicities of subcutaneously administered isoniazid and streptomycin sulfate compared with the acute toxicities of the aqueous solutions of these drugs.[8,9] These results are presumably due to the increased viscosity and lower diffusion coefficients of the drugs in the aqueous glycerin systems.

Partition Coefficient and Lipid Solubility

Before an active drug molecule can reach the general circulation and become distributed throughout the body, it must first cross some biologic membrane. The properties of this membrane often can play an important role in the therapeutic activity of the drug. Biologic membranes are highly complex structures that are primarily composed of lipids and proteins. In general, the membrane structure is one in which a lipid layer is sandwiched between protein layers. The lipid layer is the backbone of the membrane and is made up of complex lipid molecules such as phospholipids and cholesterol. The molecules are arranged so that the lipid portion, or nonpolar end, of each molecule is directed inward, and the polar portion faces toward the outer surface. The layers of protein give strength to the membrane. Figure 7–3 is a simplified diagram of a cell membrane.

The lipid properties of biologic membranes are important in the absorption of drugs. For example, from the composition of the membrane, it is reasonable to assume that a cell presents a lipophilic barrier to materials outside the membrane. When one remembers that a complex membrane is made up of a number of cells, it becomes evident that all the membranes of the body can be considered similar lipophilic barriers to drugs that must cross them to reach the site of action. Drugs having the proper lipophilic characteristics are able to penetrate the biologic membranes in much the same way as a drug molecule partitions across an oil-water interface. This phenomenon has been shown to be the case, as most drug molecules penetrate cell membranes in relation to the lipid solubility of the drug. Passage of drugs across the membrane of the oral cavity, through the gastrointestinal epithelium, through the skin, and into the bile, central nervous system, tissue cells, and kidney has been found to be related to the lipid solubility of the drug molecule in question. Even with the intravenous administration of drugs, where absorption into the body is not a problem, distribution of the drug to the site of action and to other tissues in the body depends greatly on the lipid-solubility characteristics of the drug.

Another aspect to be considered when discussing the relationship of lipid solubility to drug absorption concerns the drug molecules that are either weakly acidic or weakly basic. These molecules can exist in either the un-ionized or the ionized state, and the degree of ionization depends on the dissociation constant (K_a) of the drug and the pH of the environment. This property of these drug molecules can greatly affect the passage of drugs across biologic membranes. The greater lipid solubility belongs to the un-ionized form of the drug molecule, and therefore, the un-ionized molecule can penetrate most membrane barriers more readily than can the ionized form of the drug.

The Henderson-Hasselbalch equation for the ionization of a weak acid, HA, can be derived from the following equations.

The ionization of a weak acid is given by:

$$HA + H_2O = H_3O^+ + A^- \qquad \text{Eq. 2}$$

The dissociation constant, K_a, can be calculated from:

$$K_a = \frac{(H_3O^+)(A^-)}{(HA)} \qquad \text{Eq. 3}$$

The Henderson-Hasselbalch equation for the weakly acidic drug is obtained by taking the logarithm of both sides of Equation 3 and multiplying by minus one, resulting in the equation:

$$pH = pK_a + \log \frac{(A^-)}{(HA)} \qquad \text{Eq. 4}$$

By repeating the same steps for a weakly basic drug, the following equation can be obtained:

$$pH = pK_a + \log \frac{(B)}{(BH^+)} \qquad \text{Eq. 5}$$

where B is the weak base and BH^+ is its acid conjugate. For acidic drugs at pH values below their pK_a, the drug molecule would exist predominantly in the un-ionized form, the form best suited for passage of the drug across the biologic membranes. In alkaline pH, where the drug is largely in the ionized, lipid-insoluble form, the rate of membrane penetration would be relatively low, and access to the site of biologic activity would be reduced.

The interrelationship of dissociation constant and lipid solubility, the pH at the absorption site, and the absorption characteristics of various drugs across biologic membranes is known as the *pH-partition* theory.[10]

Interaction Between the Drug and the Dosage Form

In many instances, the so-called inert ingredients in a pharmaceutic dosage form can affect the availability of the active drug from the complete product. The major reason for decreased availability of the active drug in the presence of these adjuvants is an interaction, or complexation, between the components of the dosage form. The binding of a drug to some inactive, nonabsorbable substance results in a drug complex that is also nonabsorbable. The following scheme should help to illustrate the problem:

$$\begin{array}{ccc} \text{Active} & + \text{Inert Binding} \rightleftharpoons & \text{Drug} \\ \text{Drug} & \text{Agent} & \text{Complex} \\ \downarrow & & \\ \text{Absorbed} & & \\ \text{Drug} & & \end{array}$$

The drug complex cannot be absorbed across the biologic membrane; thus, the rate of drug absorption is reduced. If the complex is easily dissociable, then the bioavailability is not reduced. If a water-insoluble complex is formed, however, there is a good possibility that the total amount of drug absorbed from the dosage form will be reduced.

The work of Brigham and Nielson illustrates the effect of complexation on drug absorption.[11] These workers found that the acute subcutaneous toxicities of streptomycin and dihydrostreptomycin sulfates in mice were reduced when small amounts of calcium pantothenate were added to the aqueous media. The chronic toxicities of the preparations were identical. The interaction between the streptomycin and calcium pantothenate resulted in a more slowly absorbed antibiotic, and therefore, in lower acute toxicity. Because the antibiotic eventually may have been completely absorbed from the dosage form, the long-term toxicities were identical.

There has been some evidence that formation of a drug complex with greater lipid-solubility characteristics than the drug alone results in more rapid absorption of the active drug molecule. For example, complexation of prednisolone with dialkylpropionamides results in greater absorption of the steroid across the rat's small intestine.[12] The usefulness of this approach for parenteral formulations has yet to be evaluated.

The possible effects that can occur from the addition of either supposedly inert, nonactive ingredients or other active constituents to the dosage form should be pointed out by the pharmacist to the patient. The pharmacist should be absolutely certain that the addition of these adjuvants will in no way alter the therapeutic activity of the medicinal agent.

The interaction between a drug molecule and an adjuvant resulting in the formation of a more slowly absorbed complex can be used to prolong the activity of parenteral dosage forms.

Physiologic Factors Influencing Drug Absorption

Several factors inherent to the biologic system can influence the absorption of drugs from parenteral dosage forms. The following section discusses these factors and their influence on the absorption process.

One of the most important influences on drug absorption is the route by which the drug is administered. Intravenous injection results in immediate and total access of the active drug molecules to the body. Other routes of administration, such as intramuscular or subcutaneous routes, require an absorption step before a drug can gain access to the body and therefore reach the site of its intended activity. Thus, any factors that influence this absorption step also influence the rate at which active drug enters the body. Besides the physicochemical properties of the drug molecule, the physiologic factors such as blood flow from the injection site can be important in determining drug activity.

It has been found that, after subcutaneous injection, the active drug is absorbed by diffusion of the drug into the capillary network at the absorption site.[13] The greater the blood flow in the capillary network to and from the absorption site, the greater is the absorption rate of the drug. Therefore, any factor that influences the flow of blood at the absorption site also influences the rate of absorption. For example, epinephrine has been shown to reduce the subcutaneous absorption of a number of drugs. The mechanism of the absorption-delaying effect of epinephrine is the constricting action of the drug on the vascular bed in the zone of absorption which reduces blood flow through the absorbing area and decreases absorption. Enhanced absorption of drugs has been noted in the presence of hyaluronidase.[13] Presumably, the effect is caused by the spread of the injected drug solution over a larger area of connective tissue, exposing the drug to a larger absorption surface.

Administration by the oral route can influence the parenteral absorption of certain drugs. For example, in experiments on rabbits, Schou showed that the subcutaneous absorption of sulfacetamide was markedly increased following the systemic administration of cortisone.[14]

Other influences on blood flow in capillaries at the absorption site may also effect drug absorption. For example, increased muscular activity, resulting in increased blood flow to the muscles, may result in an increase in absorption rate of drugs from the site of an intramuscular injection. Boger and co-workers found that the level of body activity influenced the duration of effective penicillin blood level after intramuscular administration of procaine penicillin G suspended in oil to patients with lobar pneumonia and to ambulatory control patients.[15] In the group of 10 patients with pneumonia, the mean duration of penicillin plasma concentrations above 0.039 unit/ml was 33 hours. In the 9 ambulatory patients, the mean was 12 hours.

Dosage Form Considerations

Intravenous Injection Formulations

The injection of drugs by the intravenous route provides the drug with direct access to the systemic circulation. The concentration of drug in the blood after a rapid intravenous injection reaches a maximum within 4 minutes, the time required for mixing the drug solution with the blood. The duration of therapeutic effect after an intravenous injection is determined by the initial dose and by the distribution, metabolism, and excretion parameters associated with the therapeutic agent. For most drugs, the overall elimination process is first-order, and the biologic half-life is independent of the initial dose. This means that in a given time a certain fraction of drug in the blood disappears regardless of the initial concentration. This would indicate that the intravenous formulation is not a useful method to achieve sustained blood levels for drugs with short biologic half-lives. In these instances, constant blood levels can be achieved by continuous intravenous drip. Other possibilities for prolonging drug blood levels include the use of complexation, protein binding, and microencapsulation. These methods require more investigation, however, before they can be used routinely.

Intramuscular and Subcutaneous Injection Dosage Forms

The injection of intramuscular and subcutaneous dosage forms results in lower but more sustained blood levels of drugs than do intravenous dosage forms. As discussed in a previous section, intramuscular and subcutaneous injections require an absorption step before the drug reaches the circulation. Several different types of intramuscular or subcutaneous dosage forms, however, can show different biopharmaceutic and therapeutic properties. Among the dosage forms available are (1) aqueous solutions, (2) aqueous suspensions, (3) oleaginous solutions, and (4) oleaginous suspensions. Each of the dosage forms presents different characteristics, from the administration of the drug in its formulation to the appearance of the active agent in the circulation.

Aqueous Solutions. Parenteral formulations of water-soluble drugs in aqueous solution, in most instances, provide the most rapid absorption rates when administered by the intramuscular or subcutaneous routes. In these dosage forms, only two steps are required for absorption: the drug must be transported from the bulk solution at the injection site to the biologic membrane, and the drug must penetrate this barrier so that it can reach the systemic circulation. The factors influencing drug absorption from this type of dosage form are the viscosity of the fluid at the site of injection, the concentration of the drug in the dosage form, and the degree of activity of the patient.

Aqueous Suspensions. Aqueous suspensions of drugs present another step in the critical processes leading to absorption. This step, the dissolution process, has been discussed previously and can profoundly influence both the rate of release of the drug from the dosage form and the total time required for the drug to be released from the dosage form. Alteration in the solubility of the drug in the parenteral formulation, in the particle size of the suspended solid, and in the amount of drug present may affect the variables and the effects they may have on the release of drug from suspension dosage forms in which dissolution is the rate-determining step.

TABLE 7–2. Effect of Formulation Variables on Release of Drug from Dissolution Rate-Limited Suspension Dosage Forms

Formulation Variables			Effect on Release	
Solubility in Water	Particle Size	Total Amount of Drug in Dose	Rate	Duration of Absorption
Constant	Constant	Increase	Increase	Unchanged
Decrease	Constant	Decrease	Decrease	Unchanged
Constant	Decrease	Constant	Increase	Decrease
Constant	Increase	Constant	Decrease	Increase
Increase	Constant	Constant	Increase	Decrease
Decrease	Constant	Constant	Decrease	Increase

Adapted from Simonelli, A.P., and Dresback, D.S.: Principles of formulation, parenteral dosage forms. In Perspective in Clinical Pharmacy. Edited by G. Francke and A.K. Whitney. Cincinnati, OH, Drug Intelligence and Clinical Pharmacy; 1972, p. 399.

Oleaginous Solutions. A dosage form of a drug dissolved in an oleaginous vehicle is useful when a water-insoluble drug is involved. Many of the problems associated with aqueous suspension dosage forms, such as control of particle size, chemical instability in water, and changes in drug crystal form, can be avoided by the use of an oleaginous vehicle. Many factors that influence the release characteristics of drugs from aqueous solutions apply equally to the oleaginous solutions, including viscosity of the injection fluid. An additional step in the process involves the transport of the drug across the oil-biologic fluid interface. This step is usually quite rapid, however, and is usually not the rate-limiting step.

Oleaginous Suspensions. The factors influencing the absorption of drugs from aqueous suspension and oleaginous solution dosage forms apply to the oleaginous suspension. For cases in which the dissolution of the drug in the oil phase is the rate-determining step, Table 7–2 provides useful information as to the effects of formulation variables on the drug release patterns.

Drug Absorption and Bioavailability From Intramuscular Injection

Intramuscular administration of drugs is a widely utilized parenteral route of drug delivery. Exact doses of drugs can be administered by this route, but the rate of drug absorption may vary widely. Many of the factors discussed in the previous sections can influence the rate of drug absorption from the intramuscular injection site.

Recent studies have indicated that the site of injection is an important influence on drug absorption rate.[16–18] Cohen and associates examined lidocaine levels in plasma after injection of the drug into the deltoid muscle (arm), lateral thigh, or buttocks.[16] Sixty-nine patients with proved or suspected myocardial infarction were administered 200 mg of lidocaine intramuscularly. Higher lidocaine plasma levels were obtained after injection into the deltoid muscle than after injection into the lateral thigh. Both of these injection sites gave higher lidocaine plasma concentrations than injection into the buttocks. The

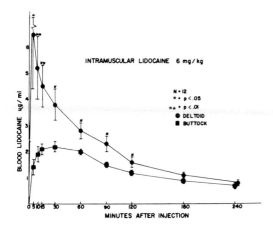

Figure 7–4. Blood lidocaine levels following high-dose (6 mg/kg) I.M. 10% lidocaine injection into the deltoid and gluteal muscles. Note the rapid development of high therapeutic levels following intradeltoid administration. (From Zener et al.[17])

low plasma levels of lidocaine after injection into the buttocks were attributed to the high affinity of fatty tissue for lidocaine and the generally low vascularity of this area. Similar results for lidocaine injected intramuscularly into the deltoid muscle and buttock were reported by Zener and co-workers.[17] These workers found that intradeltoid injection produced higher blood lidocaine levels and more rapid development of peak blood levels than did injection into the buttocks. They also raised the possibility of the effect of exercise on absorption from the intramuscular site. Because the patients were hospitalized and in bed, there was minimal exercise of the buttock (gluteal) muscles, whereas movement of the deltoid muscles was less restricted. The blood levels of lidocaine following injection of 6 mg/kg into the two sites are illustrated in Figure 7–4. Significantly higher blood lidocaine levels were attained from deltoid injection than from gluteal injection.

Studies with cephradine, a cephalosporin antibiotic, reveal sex differences in the intramuscular absorption of drugs.[18] Six male and six female volunteers each received a single intramuscular injection of cephradine once weekly for three consecutive weeks. The drug was injected into the gluteus maximus, vastus lateralis, or deltoid muscle. Cephradine serum concentrations were similar in males irrespective of the site of injection. Serum levels of the cephalosporin in females were similar to those of males when the drug was injected in the deltoid or vastus lateralis sites. Much lower levels were found in females, however, after injection into the gluteus maximus muscle. These comparative data are presented in Table 7–3 and raise some interesting possibilities of the influence of sex differences on the intramuscular absorption of drugs.

TABLE 7–3. Peak Cephradine Concentrations (µg/ml) in Plasma after Intramuscular Injections* at Different Sites of Male and Female Volunteers

Injection Site	Males	Females
Gluteus maximus	11.1	4.3
Deltoid muscle	11.7	10.2
Vastus lateralis	9.8	9.4

*Injected dose = 475 mg.
Data from Vukovich et al.[18]

Intramuscular injection of benzodiazepines is a common route of administration in cases in which rapid sedation is indicated. The justification for this route is that the onset of effect is rapid and therefore desirable; however, there have been reports that chlordiazepoxide, when given in large doses by the intramuscular route, may be slowly effective or ineffective. In studies performed in healthy volunteers, oral doses of 50 mg were more rapidly absorbed than equivalent doses administered intramuscularly.[19] The average concentration of chlordiazepoxide in blood after intramuscular administration was 52% lower than the concentration achieved after oral administration. A similar occurrence has been reported for diazepam.[20,21]

Many drugs with limited aqueous solubility are often formulated in solution for parenteral administration through the use of pH and alteration and organic cosolvents. The most commonly used solvents include propylene glycol, ethanol, and the low molecular weight polyethylene glycols.[22] If adequate quantities of the organic cosolvents are not utilized in the formulation, dilution by fluids at the site of injection could lead to precipitation at the injection site. This precipitation could result in severe vascular irritation or other tissue injury at the injection site, and could in turn significantly alter the bioavailability of the drug. Studies with phenytoin, the antiepileptic drug, have illustrated this occurrence.[23–25] Phenytoin is a rather insoluble drug (solubility: 14 μg/ml at pH 7). The preparation available for parenteral administration is a propylene glycol and alcohol aqueous solution adjusted to pH 12. When the drug is administered intramuscularly, the decrease in pH results in conversion of the sodium salt to the free acid and the precipitation of phenytoin in interstitial water at the injection site. These crystals have a low rate of dissolution, and therefore, the drug is absorbed at a low rate from the injection site. Studies have shown that absorption from a single intramuscular dose occurs over a 4- to 5-day period.[26] Wilder and associates presented evidence to show that after resumption of oral administration following the intramuscular injection of phenytoin, there was a gradual rise in phenytoin plasma levels, which could lead to adverse neurologic effects.[25]

Although the absorption of phenytoin from the intramuscular injection site is variable and painful, owing to the high pH of the injection and the propylene glycol solvent, this route may be of some value for sustaining established therapeutic plasma levels when the patient is unable to take the drug orally. A method has been prepared for shifting from oral to intramuscular phenytoin administration in patients requiring parenteral therapy for as long as two weeks.[25]

Serum creatine phosphokinase (CPK or creatine kinase-CK) increases after the intramuscular injection of commonly utilized formulations and/or drugs. Classes of drugs that have been associated with increases in serum CPK levels include cephalosporin antibiotics, benzodiazepines, phenothiazines, and local anesthetics. Besides the active drugs, these parenteral formulations are composed of a wide variety of excipients (viz., antimicrobial preservatives, solubilizers, wetting agents, emulsifiers, tonicity modifiers, suspending agents, lubricants antioxidants, chelating agents, or oleaginous vehicles,[27] and it has been suggested that skeletal muscle damage may be at least partly caused by the excipients within the formulation.[28] Investigators have demonstrated a good correlation between the release of CK and tissue injury at the site of injec-

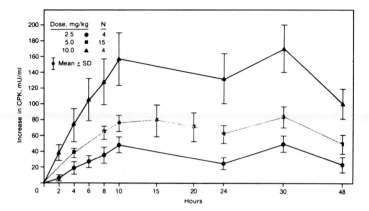

Figure 7–5. Time course of CPK activity increase in 5 subjects after intramuscularly given pralidoxime chloride. Concentration of pralidoxime chloride was 300 mg/ml, and volume was proportional to dose. (From Nora, Smith, and Cameron.[29])

tion,[29–31] as well as a correlation between those formulations known to be painful upon injection and muscle injury at the injection site.[29,32–35] It has been suggested that CPK release can be caused by either factors related to the physicochemical properties of the formulation and injection (e.g., dose and volume of the injection, osmolarity, speed of injection) or a direct chemotoxic effect on the muscle fibers (e.g., a direct effect on cell membrane permeability or a disruption in cellular homeostatic processes). The relationship between muscle injury at the site of injection and bioavailability (both rate and extent) is unclear; however, one study in rabbits reported that the degree of skeletal muscle damage caused by the organic cosolvents (namely, propylene glycol and polyethylene glycol) did not seem to affect the bioavailability of a diazepam tracer dose.[36]

Similar studies have shown that a substitution or replacement of propylene glycol by polyethylene glycol in the formulation of a diazepam injectable does not affect bioavailability relative to the commercial formulation, but may reduce pain or the presence of adverse reactions.[37,38]

Sidell and co-workers examined the influence of dose of drug, volume of injected solution, and osmolarity of the injection of pralidoxime chloride and sodium chloride on CPK activity.[39] An increase in CPK activity in blood was found to be directly related to the concentration and osmolarity of the injected solution when the volume was kept constant, and directly related to the volume when the concentration or osmolarity was kept constant. Figure 7–5 illustrates that the time course of CPK actively increases after intramuscular administration of pralidoxime chloride in varying volumes and doses. The findings suggest that diluent may make a significant contribution to the increase in CPK observed after intramuscular administration of drugs. This is of importance in patients with suspected acute myocardial infarction, when the convenience of intramuscular drug administration must be weighed against the diagnostic importance of serum CPK.

Recent work by Cockshott and co-workers suggests that the majority of injections intended to be intramuscular may actually be delivered into fat.[40] In these studies, it was found that less than 5% of the women and less than 15% of the men received an intramuscular injection in the gluteal muscles when a 3.5-cm needle was used for the injection. Thus, it appears that the majority of "intramuscular" injections may have been intralipomatous. These findings raise a number of important questions concerning the efficacy of intramuscular versus intralipomatous injections. The differences between the effects of introducing drugs into fat or muscle have not been well studied, but some findings suggest that there may be important changes. The data of Cohen,[16] Zener,[17] and Vukovich[18] discussed previously may result, in part, from injection of the drug into the fat rather than the muscle of the buttock. Absorption of a drug from fat may occur at a lower rate than from muscle tissue. A more superficial injection, however, may avoid some of the recognized complications of an intramuscular injection. An injection into fat lowers the possibility of the drug being injected into a vein or arteriole and may result in a lower degree of tissue damage. In addition, there may be a lower likelihood of nerve palsies or bacterial infections. The issue of whether an intramuscular or an intralipomatous injection is therapeutically better needs to be resolved by further research. Some have suggested that disposition of a drug into muscle is desirable, and a needle should be chosen whose length is appropriate for the site of injection and for the patient's deposits of fat.[40]

Drug Absorption From Subcutaneous Injection

Absorption from the subcutaneous route of administration is influenced by the same factors that determine the rate of absorption from intramuscular sites. The vascularity in the regions of subcutaneous injection is poorer than that of muscle tissue and may lead to slower absorption. It may be possible to increase the absorption rate by application of heat to increase flow to the injection site. Absorption can be slowed by adding a vasoconstrictor to the injection solution, such as is done with local anesthetics. This serves to prolong the effects of the local anesthetic agent.

The absorption of drugs following subcutaneous injection can be through either the capillaries or the lymphatic system associated with the site of injection. Supersaxo and co-workers showed a linear relationship between the molecular weight of water-soluble compounds and the proportion of the dose absorbed lymphatically.[41]

Insulin is the drug most commonly administered by the subcutaneous route. The duration of action of insulin is mainly controlled by its crystallinity. Nora and associates, in a series of studies in diabetic children, found that with either subcutaneous or intramuscular injection, the absorption rate of insulin is about 50% faster after injection into the arm than after injection into the thigh.[42] This could potentially lead to differences in control of the disease.

In studies to examine the potential hemodynamic influences of 200 mg of lidocaine administered subcutaneously into the antecubital fossa as a local anesthetic *prior* to *cardiac catheterization*, Schwartz and co-workers found mean peak levels of lidocaine of 0.28 to 0.49 μg/ml.[43] These low levels would produce no alteration in hemodynamic function and tend to indicate poor absorption of lidocaine from this subcutaneous site.

Biopharmaceutics of Intrathecal Injections

In some circumstances, drugs must be administered directly into cerebrospinal fluid (CSF) to achieve effective concentrations. The intrathecal route of administration is associated with a high incidence of side effects, some of which may be attributable to formulation components.

Injection of drugs intrathecally is accomplished by way of the lumbar spinal cord, basal cisterns, or lateral ventricles. Factors such as solution volume and specific gravity, as well as the patient's position, have been reported to influence drug distribution within the central nervous system.

Formulation considerations for intrathecal injections have been reviewed in a recent article.[44] Vehicle, solution pH and osmolarity, preservatives added, physical state of the drug, addition of detergents and protein, all may have an influence on the patient's tolerance to the injected formulation. Further studies are necessary to examine the factors surrounding the injection of drugs intrathecally and the formulation considerations necessary to minimize toxicity.

Parenteral Administration of Peptides and Proteins

The use of parenteral administration is increasing with the advent of new peptide and protein products. The low bioavailability of therapeutic peptides following oral administration combined with the difficulties and liabilities associated with intravenous injections has lead to an increased interest in drug administration by the subcutaneous and intramuscular route. New therapeutic peptides that have been administered either subcutaneously or intramuscularly include human chorionic gonadotropin (hCG), recombinant erythropoietin (r-epo), tissue type plasminogen activator (t-PA), atrial natriuretic factor (ANF), and adenosine deaminase (AD).[45-50] Subcutaneous or intramuscular administration may provide a means to prolong systemic half-life and/or therapeutic activity. Factors that have been shown to affect the rate and extent of absorption include the site of injection, the use of absorption enhancers, and chemical modifications of the protein.[47,48,51] Modifying proteins through the covalent binding of polyethylene glycol provides a means to reduce immunogenicity at the injection site which could, in turn, improve drug availability.[50]

Parenteral Drug Delivery Systems

Liposomal encapsulation of drugs, both conventional and new therapeutic peptides, intended for parenteral administration, may provide a means to achieve systemic sustained release or provide targeted drug delivery while reducing immunogenicity and systemic or local adverse reactions. Long-circulating liposomes have been shown to have the potential to prolong the biologic activity of a therapeutic peptide.[52] Compared to the absorption of solutions, the intramuscular absorption of liposomally encapsulated drugs is reduced, with the rate of drug release from the site of injection a function of the liposome composition and size.[53,54] The encapsulation of compounds into liposomal formulations may provide a means to target specifically to the lymphatic system because lymphatic uptake seems to play a major role in intramuscular absorption.[54,55] Other delivery systems that have been shown to prolong drug release from injection sites or increase the circulating half-life include biodegradable microcapsules or microparticles, multiple water emulsions, and the chemical modification of peptides through the covalent addition of polyethylene glycol.[56–58]

This chapter was designed to give the reader an appreciation of the physical, chemical, and biologic factors that can influence the absorption, availability, and therefore, the activity achieved. These processes are involved with the distribution, metabolism, and elimination of the therapeutically active drug, and it is difficult for the pharmacist to influence these processes. He can, however, control the design and preparation of the parenteral dosage form. It is in this capacity that the pharmacist can play a major role in drug therapy. An understanding of the principles of biopharmaceutics enables him to advise the physician better in the selection of parenteral dosage forms.

References

1. Noyes, A.A., and Whitney, W.R.: The rate of solution of solid substances in their own solutions. J. Am. Chem. Soc., *19*, 930 (1897).
2. Buckwalter, F.H., and Dickison, H.L.: The effect of vehicle and particle size on the absorption, by the intramuscular route, of procaine penicillin G suspension. J. Am. Pharm. Assoc., Sci. Ed., *47*, 661 (1958).
3. Schlichtkrull, J.: Insulin Crystals, Copenhagen, Ejnar Munksgaard Publisher, 1958.
4. Mullins, J.D., and Macek, T.J.: Some pharmaceutical properties of novobiocin. J. Am. Pharm. Assoc., Sci. Ed., *49*, 245 (1960).
5. Almirante, L., DeCarneri, I., and Coppi, G.: Relation between the therapeutic activity and the crystalline and amorphous state of chloramphenicol stearate. Farmaco (Prat)., *15*, 471, (1960).
6. Ballard, B.E., and Nelson, E.: Physicochemical properties of drugs that control absorption rate after subcutaneous implantation. J. Pharmacol. Exp. Ther., *135*, 120 (1972).
7. Hamlin, W.E., Nelson, E., Ballard, B.E., and Wanger, J.G.: Loss of sensitivity in distinguishing real differences in dissolution rates due to increasing intensity of agitation. J. Pharm. Sci., *51*, 432 (1962).
8. Prescott, B., Kauffman, G., and James, W.G.: Means of increasing the tolerated dose of streptomycin in mice. Antibiot. Chemother., *8*, 27 (1958).
9. Prescott, B., Kauffman, G., and James, W.G.: Further studies on effect of glycerine on toxicity of isoniazid-streptomycin mixtures in mice. Antibiot. Chemother., *8*, 225 (1958).
10. Gibaldi, M.: Biopharmaceutics and Clinical Pharmacokinetics. 2nd Ed. Philadelphia, Lea & Febiger, 1977, p. 27.
11. Brigham, R.S., and Nielson, J.K.: The effect of calcium pantothenate on the acute and chronic toxicity of streptomycin and dihydrostreptomycin in mice. Antibiot. Chemother., *8*, 122 (1958).
12. Hayton, W.L., and Levy, G.: Effect of complex formation on drug absorption. XII. Enhancement of intestinal absorption of prednisone and prednisolone by dialkypropionamides in rats. J. Pharm. Sci., *61*, 362 (1972).
13. Schou, J.: Absorption of drugs from subcutaneous connective tissue. Pharmacol. Rev., *13*, 441 (1966).
14. Schou, J.: The influence of cortisone on the subcutaneous absorption of drugs. Acta Pharmacol. Toxicol. (Kbh), *14*, 251 (1958).
15. Boger, W.P., Oritt, J.E., Israel, H.L., and Flippin, H.F.: Procaine penicillin G in oil. I.: Plasma concentration; preliminary observations on its use in pneumonia. Am. J. Med. Sci., *215*, 250 (1948).

16. Cohen, L.S., Rosenthal, J.E., Horner, D.W., et al.: Plasma levels of lidocaine after intramuscular administration. Am. J. Cardiol., 29, 520 (1948).

17. Zener, J.C., Kerber, R.E., Spivack, A.P., and Harrison, D.C.: Blood lidocaine levels and kinetics following high-dose intramuscular administration. Circulation, 47, 984 (1973).

18. Vukovich, R.A., Brannick, L.J., Sugarman, A.A., and Neiss, E.S.: Sex differences in the intramuscular absorption and bioavailability of cephradine. Clin. Pharmacol. Ther., 18, 215 (1975).

19. Greenblatt, D.J., Shader, R.I., and Koch-Weser, J.: Slow absorption of intramuscular chlordiazepoxide. N. Engl. J. Med., 291, 1116 (1974).

20. McCaughey, W., and Dundee, J.W.: Comparison of the sedative effects of diazepam given by the oral and intramuscular routes. Br. J. Anaesth., 44, 901 (1972).

21. Root, B., and Loveland, J.P.: Pediatric premedication with diazepam or hydroxyzine: Oral versus intramuscular route. Anesth. Analg., 52, 717 (1973).

22. Yalkowsky, S.H., and Rubino, J.T.: Solubilization by organic cosolvents I: Organic cosolvents in propylene glycol-water mixtures. J. Pharm. Sci., 74, 416 (1985).

23. Wilensky, A.J., and Lowden, J.A.: Inadequate serum levels after intramuscular administration of diphenylhydantoin. Neurology, 23, 318 (1973).

24. Serrano, E.E., Roye, D.B., Hammer, R.H., and Wilder, B.J.: Plasma diphenylhydantoin values after oral and intramuscular administration of diphenylhydantoin. Neurology, 23, 311 (1973).

25. Wilder, B.J., Serrano, E.E., Ramsey, E., and Buchanan, R.A.: A method for shifting from oral to intramuscular diphenylhydantoin administration. Clin. Pharmacol. Ther., 16, 507 (1974).

26. Kostenbauder, H.B., Rapp, R.P., McGovern, J.P., et al.: Bioavailability and single dose pharmacokinetics of intramuscular phenytoin. Clin. Pharmacol. Ther., 18, 449 (1975).

27. Wang, Y.J., and Kowal, R.R.: Review of excipients and pH's for parenteral products used in the United States. J. Parenter. Drug Assoc., 34, 452 (1980).

28. Vukovich, R.A.: The effect of multiple intramuscular placebo injections on injection site tolerance and serum creatine phosphokinase activity. Curr. Therap. Res., 18, 706 (1975).

29. Steiness, E., Rasmussen, F., Svendsen, O., and Nielsen, P.: A comparative study of serum creatine phosphokinase (CPK) activity in rabbits, pigs, and humans after intramuscular injection of local damaging compounds. Acta Pharmacol. Toxicol., 42, 357 (1978).

30. Surber, C., and Sucker, H.: Tissue tolerance of intramuscular injectables and plasma enzyme activities in rats. Pharm. Res., 4, 490 (1987).

31. Williams, P.D., et al.: An in vitro model for assessing muscle irritation due to parenteral antibiotics. Fund. Appl. Toxicol., 6, 10 (1987).

32. Grim, M., Rerabkova, L., and Carlson, B.M.: A test for muscle lesions and their regeneration following intramuscular drug application. Toxicol. Pathol., 16, 432 (1988).

33. Steiness E., Svendsen, O., Rasmussen, F.: Plasma digoxin after parenteral administration. Local reaction after intramuscular injection. Clin. Pharmacol. Therap., 16, 430 (1974).

34. Kronborg, I., Hunt, D., and Goble, A.J.: Elevation of serum creatine kinase levels after intramuscular injections of lignocaine. Med. J. Aust., 1, 635 (1975).

35. Wilensky, A.J., and Lowden, J.A.: Inadequate serum levels after intramuscular injection of diphenylhydantoin. Neurology, 23, 318 (1973).

36. Brazeau, G.A., and Fung, H.-L.: Effect of organic cosolvent-induced skeletal muscle damage on the bioavailability of intramuscular [^{14}C]diazepam. J. Pharm. Sci., 79, 773 (1990).

37. Korttila, K., Sothman, A., and Andersson, P.: Polyethylene glycol as a solvent for diazepam: Bioavailability and clinical effects after intramuscular administration, comparison of oral, intramuscular, and rectal administration, and precipitation from intravenous solutions. Acta Pharmacol. Toxicol., 39, 104 (1976).

38. Shah, A.K., Simons, K.J., and Briggs, C.J.: Physical, chemical, and bioavailability studies of parenteral diazepam formulations containing propylene glycol and polyethylene glycol. Drug. Dev. Indust. Pharm., 17, 1635 (1991).

39. Sidell, F.R., Culver, D.L., and Kaminskis, A.: Serum creatine phosphokinase activity after intramuscular injection: The effect of dose, concentration, and volume. JAMA, *229*, 1894 (1974).

40. Cockshott, W.P., Thompson, G.T., Howlett, L.J., and Seeley, E.T.: Intramuscular or intralipomatous injections? N. Engl. J. Med., *307*, 356 (1982).

41. Supersaxo, A., Hein, W.R., and Steffen, H.: Effect of molecular weight on the lymphatic absorption of water-soluble compounds following subcutaneous administration. Pharm. Res., *7*, 167 (1990).

42. Nora, J.J., Smith, D.W., and Cameron, J.R.: The route of insulin administration in the management of diabetis mellitus. J. Pediatr., *64*, 547 (1964).

43. Schwartz, M.L., Covino, B.G., Narang, R.M., et al.: Blood levels of lidocaine following subcutaneous administration prior to cardiac catheterization. Am. Heart J., *88*, 721 (1974).

44. Cradock, J.C., Kleinman, L.M., and Davignon, J.P.: Intrathecal injections—a review of pharmaceutical factors. Bull. Parenter. Drug. Assoc., *31*, 237 (1977).

45. Saal, W., Glowania, H.-J., Hengst, W., and Happ, J.: Pharmacodynamics and pharmacokinetics after subcutaneous and intramuscular injection of human chorionic gonadotropin. Fert. Ster., *56*, 225 (1991).

46. Salmonson, T., Danielson, B.G., and Wikstrom, B.: The pharmacokinetics and recombinant erythropoietin after intravenous and subcutaneous administration to healthy subjects. Br. J. Clin. Pharmac., *29*, 709 (1990).

47. Abraham, P.A., St. Peter, W.L., Redic-Kill, K.A., and Halstenson, C.E.: Controversies in determination of epoetin (recombinant human erythropoietin) dosages. Clin. Pharmacokinet., *22*, 409 (1992).

48. Sobel, B.E., et al.: Coronary thrombolysis with facilitated absorption of intramuscularly injected tissue-type plasminogen activator. Proc. Natl. Acad. Sci. USA, *82*, 4258 (1985).

49. Tosti-Croce, C., et al.: Intramuscular and subcutaneous administration of atrial natriuretic factor in the rat. Clin. Invest. Med., *12*, 381 (1989).

50. Chaffee, S., et al.: IgG antibody response to polyethylene glycol modified adenosine deaminase in patients with adenosine deaminase deficiency. J. Clin. Invest., *89*, 1643 (1992).

51. Sobel, B.E., Sarnoff, S.J., and Nachowiak, D.A.: Augmented and sustained plasma concentrations after intramuscular injections of molecular variants and deglycosylated forms of tissue-type plasminogen activators. Circulation, *81*, 1362 (1990).

52. Woodle, M.C., et al.: Prolonged systemic delivery of peptide drugs by long-circulating liposomes: Illustration with vasopressin in the Brattleboro rat. Pharm. Res., *9*, 260 (1992).

53. Arakawa, E., et al.: Application of drug-containing liposomes to the duration of the intramuscular absorption of water-soluble drugs in rats. Chem. Pharm. Bull., *23*, 2218 (1975).

54. Jackson, A.J.: Intramuscular absorption and regional lymphatic uptake of liposome-entrapped insulin. Drug Met. Disp., *9*, 535 (1981).

55. Ohsawa, T., et al.: Fate of lipid and encapsulated drug after intramuscular administration of liposomes prepared by the freeze-thawing method in rats. Chem. Pharm. Bull., *33*, 5103 (1985).

56. Csernus, V.J., Szende, B., and Schally, A.V.: Release of peptides from sustained delivery systems (microcapsules and microparticles) in vivo. Int. J. Peptide Protein Res., *35*, 557 (1990).

57. Omotosho, J.A., Whateley, T.L., and Florence, A.T.: Release of 5-fluorouracil from intramuscular w/o/w multiple emulsions. Biopharm. Drug Disp., *10*, 257 (1989).

58. Hershfield, M.S., and Chaffee, S.: PEG-enzyme replacement therapy in adenosine deaminase deficiency. *In Treatment of Genetic Diseases.* R.J. Desnick, Editor. New York, Churchill-Livingstone Inc., p. 169 (1991).

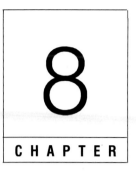

CHAPTER

8

Large-Volume Sterile Solutions

Large-volume intravenous solutions refer to injections intended for intravenous use, and they are packaged in containers holding 100 ml or more. Other sterile large-volume solutions include those used for irrigation or for dialysis. These may be packaged in containers designed to empty rapidly and contain a volume of more than 1000 ml. They are packaged in single-dose units in suitable glass or plastic containers and, in addition to being sterile, are pyrogen-free and free of particulate matter. Because of the large volumes administered, bacteriostatic agents are never included, since toxicity may result from administering large quantities of bacteriostatic agent.

Large-Volume Solutions for Intravenous Use

Large-volume parenterals intended to be administered intravenously are frequently called "intravenous" (I.V.) fluids or "infusion" fluids (Fig. 8–1). The most common uses of intravenous fluids include the correction of serious disturbances in electrolyte and fluid balances in the body and a means of providing basic nutrition. In recent years, they have been used as vehicles for other drugs and as a method of providing parenteral hyperalimentation. Infusion or intravenous fluids are packaged in containers having a capacity of 150 to 1000 ml. Mini-type infusion containers of 250-ml capacity are available with 50- and 100-ml fills for the dilution of drugs when used in the the "piggyback" technique (Fig. 8–2). This technique refers to the administration of a second solution through a Y-tube or gum rubber connection with the administration set of the first intravenous fluid, avoiding the need for another injection site. Special automatic piggyback sets are now available and are described later in this chapter.

Solutions to be administered intravenously or by infusion (venoclysis) must be clear and contain substances that can be assimilated and utilized by the circulatory system, such as ethyl alcohol, amino acids, dextrose, electrolytes,

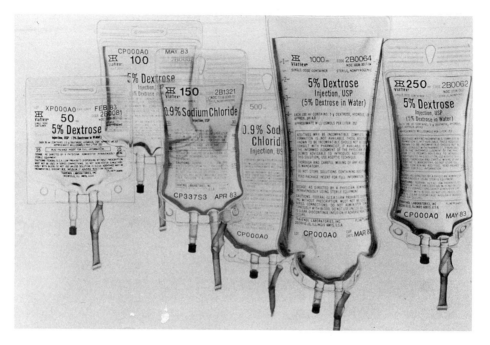

Figure 8–1. Large-volume intravenous solutions. (Courtesy of Baxter Healthcare Laboratories, Inc., Deerfield, IL.)

and vitamins. Manufacturers have made available many different kinds and combinations of intravenous solutions. The most commonly used are listed in Table 8–1.

Although it is desirable that intravenous fluids be isotonic to minimize trauma to the blood vessels, hypertonic or hypotonic solutions can be administered successfully. Highly concentrated hypertonic nutrient solutions are being used in parenteral nutrition. To minimize vessel irritation, these solutions are administered slowly with a catheter in a large vein such as the subclavian.

On rare occasions, intravenous fluids are administered into the subcutaneous tissues. This type of administration is called "hypodermoclysis" and is used in infants or obese patients, in whom veins are inaccessible (Fig. 8–3), and it has been used in the past to reduce speed shock. The potential for speed shock has been reduced with the advent of new types of intravenous administration devices. Administration of solutions by this route requires that they be isotonic and of low molecular weight. Hypertonic solutions cause body fluids and electrolytes to be drawn into the interstitial areas, resulting in edema. Suitable solutions for hypodermoclysis include Sodium Chloride Injection, Dextrose (2.5%) and Sodium Chloride (0.45%) Injection, and Ringer's Injection. Although Dextrose Injection, 5%, is isotonic, it has been shown to cause plasma volume loss. In a volume-depleted patient, this may result in vascular collapse. Solutions to be administered are infused slowly through a Y-type administration set employing two needles to facilitate absorption. A needle is usually inserted subcutaneously into each thigh. The rate of administration depends on many factors, including the individual's ability to absorb the fluid. Most large-volume parenteral solutions are given by the intravenous route,

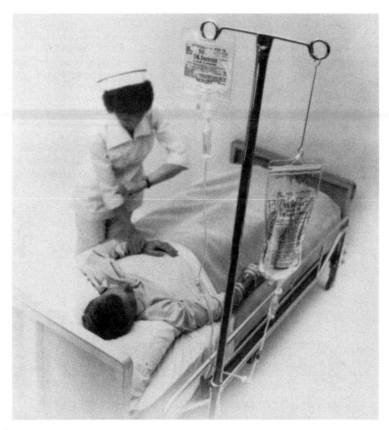

Figure 8–2. Intravenous administration using the automatic piggyback technique. (Courtesy of Baxter Healthcare Laboratories, Inc., Deerfield, IL.)

but a few are administered by hypodermoclysis. Intraosseous fluid adminis-tration in emergency situations was reported to have been successful, with no serious complications.[1]

Basic Nutrition

In addition to the need to maintain normal body functions, hospitalized patients require adequate caloric intake to survive the insults of illness or operation. Adequate caloric intake is a requirement for wound healing. For those patients who are not able to satisfy their food requirement orally, nu-trition must be supplied by the intravenous route. Administration of proteins, carbohydrates, and vitamins can be accomplished in this way. Various protein solutions containing amino acids are available commercially. These solutions are used to supply the body's nitrogen requirements. Recommended daily allowances of protein are approximately 0.9 g/kg of body weight for a healthy adult and 1.4 to 2.2 g/kg for healthy growing children and infants. Protein requirements may be higher for traumatized or malnourished patients. To supply adequate protein parenterally, various kinds of solutions and combinations of amino acids are available as synthetic amino acids. Proteins are used when oral feeding is not possible or when gastrointestinal absorption is impaired. Protein is available as 5% or 10% solutions.

TABLE 8–1. Large-Volume Solutions for Intravenous Use

Injection	Common Name	Concentration (%)	pH	Therapeutic Use
Dextrose	Glucose	2.5	3.5–6.5	Hydration, calories
	5 D/W	5		Hydration, calories
		10		Insulin shock, calories
		20		Insulin shock, calories
		50		Insulin shock, calories
Sodium Chloride	Normal Saline N.S.S.	0.9	4.5–7.0	Extracellular fluid replacement
	½ Normal Saline	0.45		Dehydration
		3		Hyponatremia
		5		Hyponatremia
Ringer's	Ringer's		5.0–7.5	Fluid and electrolyte replacement
NaCl		0.86 ⎫		
KCl		0.03 ⎬		
CaCl$_2$		0.033 ⎭		
Lactated Ringer's	Hartmann's		6.0–7.5	Fluid and electrolyte replacement
NaCl		0.6 ⎫		
KCl		0.03 ⎪		
CaCl$_2$		0.02 ⎬		
No lactate		0.3 ⎭		
Sodium Bicarbonate		1.4	8	Metabolic acidosis
		5		Metabolic acidosis
Ammonium Chloride		2.14	4.5–6.0	Metabolic alkalosis, hypochloremia
Sodium Lactate	M/6 Sodium Lactate	⅙ molar	6.0–7.3	Metabolic acidosis
Fructose	Levulose	10	3.0–6.0	Calories, fluid replacement
Fructose w/Electrolytes		10		
Invert Sugar		5	4	Calories, fluid replacement
		10		
Mannitol		5	5.0–7.0	Osmotic diuresis
also in combination with		10		
dextrose or		15		
sodium chloride		20		
Alcohol				
with 5% D/W		5	4.5	Sedative, analgesic, calories
with 5% D/W in N.S.S.		5		Sedative, analgesic, calories
Dextran 40				Priming fluid for extracorporeal circulation
in N.S.S.		10	5	Priming fluid for extracorporeal circulation
in 5% D/W		10	4	Priming fluid for extracorporeal circulation
Dextran 70				
in N.S.S.		6	5	Plasma volume expander
in 5% D/W		6	4	Plasma volume expander
Multiple electrolyte solutions				
varying combinations of electrolytes, dextrose, fructose, invert sugar			5.5	Fluid and electrolyte replacement

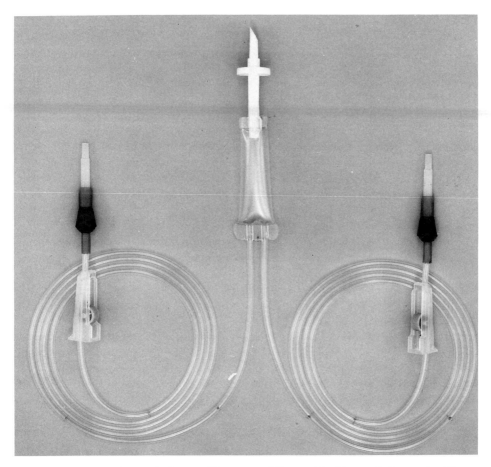

Figure 8–3. Hypodermoclysis set. (Courtesy of Baxter Healthcare Laboratories, Deerfield, IL.)

Because 1 g of dextrose provides 3.4 cal, 1000 ml Dextrose Injection, 5%, containing 50 g dextrose, supplies 170 cal, or approximately 200 cal. Traditionally, 1 g of dextrose has been calculated to provide 3.75 cal. Commercial dextrose is in the monohydrate form, however, and a 0.91 correction factor is indicated: 3.75 cal × 0.91 = 3.4 cal. The body utilizes dextrose at a rate of 0.5 g/kg of body weight/hour. Therefore, 1000 ml of Dextrose Injection, 5%, requires 1 1/2 hours for assimilation. The *U.S.P.* pH range for Dextrose Injection, 5%, is 3.5 to 6.5. The low pH is caused by the sugar acids present. Some practitioners believe that the acidity of dextrose solutions and other acid intravenous solutions may cause vein irritation and phlebitis. A few investigators have advocated the addition of sodium bicarbonate to neutralize the acid pH of intravenous solutions. One per cent sodium bicarbonate solution packaged in 20-ml containers is available for this purpose (Neut, Abbott; Buff,. Baxter Healthcare). An acid pH is essential to ensure stability of the dextrose solution during sterilization and storage. As the pH increases, caramelization occurs, and the dextrose solutions darken in appearance.

Other sources of calories include ethanol solutions supplying about 7 cal per g of ethyl alcohol. When administered too rapidly, ethanol solutions elicit depressant effects on the central nervous system. Fructose is available, and in combination as invert sugar (fructose and dextrose), it has the claimed advantage of more rapid utilization by the body. The dangers of administering fructose have been described. During the infusion of fructose solution, the rate of formation of lactate has been noted to exceed the rate of disposal of lactate, resulting in high levels of lactic acid in the blood.

Suitable forms of fat are available for intravenous feeding. To be administered intravenously, the fats or oils must be emulsified. In the past, difficulty with fat emulsions was related to untoward reactions believed to have been caused by the emulsifier used. Fat emulsions for intravenous administration are being used both in Europe and in the United States (Fig. 8–4). A sterile fat emulsion used in Sweden (Intralipid, Vitrum) contains 10 to 20% of fractionated soybean oil, 1.2% of fractionated lecithin from egg yolk, 2.5% of glycerin, and Water for Injection. Intralipid is supplied in the United States by KabiVitrum.

The Food and Drug Administration released Intralipid for use in the United States early in 1976. Intralipid contains 10% wt/vol of purified soybean oil, 1.2% egg yolk phospholipid, the emulsifier, and 2.25% glycerin, making the emulsion isotonic. Sodium hydroxide is added to adjust the pH between 5.5 and 9.0; the suspending water is pyrogen-free. Soybean oil comprises a number of neutral triglycerides, most of which are largely unsaturated fatty acids— linoleic (54%), oleic (26%), palmitic (9%), and linolenic (8%). These, together with the glycerin and egg lecithin, provide 1.1 kcal per ml emulsion.

The osmolality of Intralipid 10% is 280 milliosmols, comparable to that of blood. The diameter of its lipid particles ranges from 0.1 to 0.5 μm, which is comparable to the size of physiologic blood chylomicrons. Intralipid 10% is

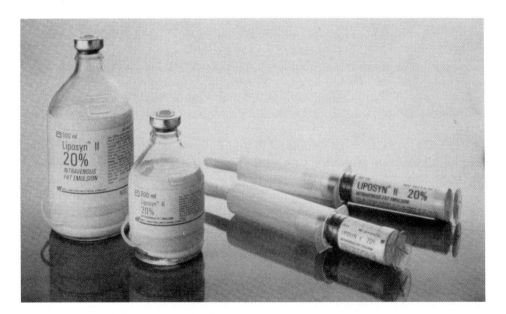

Figure 8–4. Liposyn II (20% intravenous fat emulsion). (Courtesy of Abbott Laboratories, North Chicago, IL.)

bottled under nitrogen and stored under refrigeration; so protected, the milky emulsion can be considered stable for 1 year following its manufacture.

Given intravenously, artificial fat droplets are distributed in the blood and metabolized in essentially the same pathways as are chylomicrons. Most of this lipid or lipoprotein is hydrolyzed by lipoprotein lipase, and the hydrolytic products—free fatty acids and monoglycerides—are taken up by cells and metabolized. The metabolism of 1 g of fat provides 9.1 kcal of energy, compared to 3.4 kcal provided by the metabolism of 1 g of glucose.

In addition to its value as a partial source of calories in a balanced program of total parenteral nutrition (TPN), including amino acids, dextrose, minerals, vitamins, and electrolytes, a lipid emulsion is useful in treating or preventing essential fatty acid deficiency (EFAD).

Frank studied the microscopic and macroscopic effects of 25 parenteral drugs combined with Intralipid.[2] Four of these combinations resulted in unacceptable admixtures. Calcium gluconate and tetracycline hydrochloride produced a cracked emulsion. Hyprotigen produced creaming in an unrefrigerated sample of Intralipid. Phenytoin precipitated as crystals. Although many drugs retain their stability in Intralipid, their bioavailability may be altered in such mixtures. Lynn reported that carbenicillin and cloxacillin provoked aggregation of the emulsion.[3] After 24 hours in Intralipid, methicillin crystallized. Ampicillin did *not* alter the character of the emulsion and was *not* altered itself by the chemical association.

Low toxicity and high stability depend, in large part, on the presence and preservation of small particles (<1 μm) in a fat emulsion. The brownian movement of small particles protects the emulsion. A change in pH, hydrolysis of the emulsifier, or the presence of a dissociated electrolyte (e.g., NaCl) or of any of a number of macromolecules tend to increase particle size and thus lead to creaming or breaking of the emulsion, or to complete separation of the oil. Aggregation of globules into particles over 6 μm in diameter greatly increases the risk of such serious side effects as emboli.

Restoration of Electrolyte Balance

Electrolyte disturbances can be caused by a variety of clinical conditions: trauma, injury, burns, shock, diarrhea, vomiting, and electrolytic shifts in body compartments. When they occur and the oral route cannot be used to correct the difficulty, electrolytes are administered intravenously. The condition of the kidneys must be considered before electrolyte replacement is initiated. Urinary depression may be the result of decreased fluid volume or renal impairment. A hydrating solution such as 5% D/W in 0.2% sodium chloride is administered. Urinary flow is restricted if the retention is functional. The most frequently used solution is Sodium Chloride Injection, an isotonic solution containing 154 mEq each of sodium and chloride ions. Ringer's Injection and Lactated Ringer's Injection contain small quantities of calcium and potassium ions. Deficits of these ions require additional supplementations. Lactated Ringer's Injection contains sodium lactate, which is metabolized to sodium bicarbonate and is useful for correcting metabolic acidosis. Solutions with multiple electrolytes are available commercially to simplify therapy (Isolyte, McGaw; Normosol, Abbott). These solutions closely resemble the composition of plasma electrolytes.

Fluid Replacement

Dehydration requires fluid replacement. As basic solutions, sodium chloride and dextrose injections can be used for fluid replacement when needed. Excessive use of large volume solutions can cause edema and water intoxication.

Blood and Blood Products

Blood and blood products can only be administered intravenously. In cases of shock, hemorrhage, blood protein loss, these products are used. No drug should be mixed with blood prior to administration (see Chapter 9, Blood Components and Plasma Expanders).

Drug Carriers

Because of convenience, the irritation potential of the drug, and the desire for continuous drug therapy, intravenous fluids are frequently used as vehicles for the intravenous administration of drugs. In some instances, the combination of one or more drugs in an intravenous fluid results in conditions not favorable for drug stability and may promote parenteral incompatibilities.

Parenteral Nutrition

One of the most exciting developments in parenteral nutrition has been the concept of parenteral. Parenteral nutrition is the long-term intravenous feeding of protein solutions containing high concentrations of dextrose (approximately 20%), electrolytes, vitamins, and in some instances insulin. The need to maintain adequate caloric intake while keeping the volume of solution required to a minimum necessitates the use of this hypertonic solution. The basic solution can be prepared by the combination of commercially available dextrose and amino acid (AA) solutions. These solutions are usually combinations of 50% dextrose and AA solution. At present, synthetic amino acids are commonly used. They are supplied as FreAmine III, McGaw; Aminosyn, 3.5%, 7%, Abbott; Travasol 5.5% and 8.5%. After mixing, they supply approximately 1 cal per ml of solution. Required supplements such as electrolytes and vitamins are frequently added to the basic solution. Many manufacturers provide the solutions in ready-to-mix kits. The solutions are administered via a large vein, such as the subclavian, over 8 to 24 hours. The purpose of using this vein and slow administration is to minimize adverse effects that may occur with such a hypertonic solution. The subclavian vein is large and close to the heart; therefore, the solution is diluted rapidly by the large volume of blood in the heart. Numerous references in the literature fully describe the methods of preparation and parenteral implications.

Specialized TPN solutions are illustrated in Figure 8–5.

Special Uses

Several large volume solutions are recognized more readily as drugs and are used for specific clinical conditions.

1-Arginine Hydrochloride Injection (R-Gene). This amino acid is effective in stimulating the utilization of ammonia by the body. Elevated levels of ammonia correlate with cerebral dysfunction and occur in liver damage, high protein feedings, excessive intake of ammonium chloride, and intestinal tract

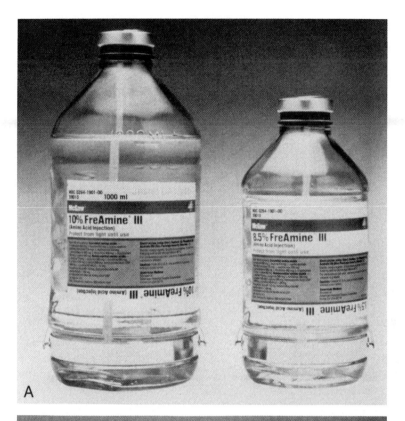

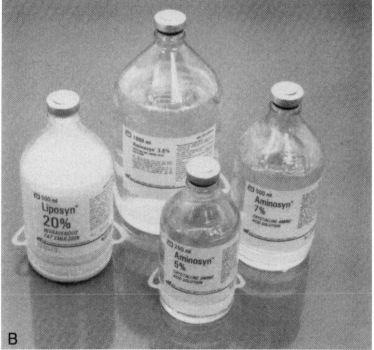

Figure 8–5. A, Freamine III amino acid injection. (Courtesy of McGaw, Irvine, CA.) B, Total parenteral solutions (I.V. fat and amino acid). (Courtesy of Abbott Laboratories, North Chicago, IL.)

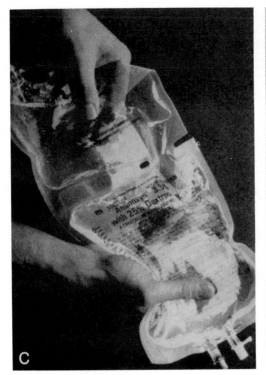

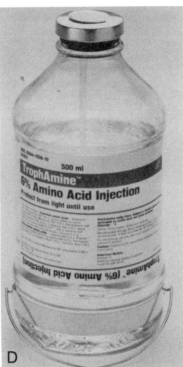

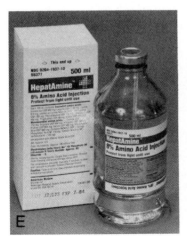

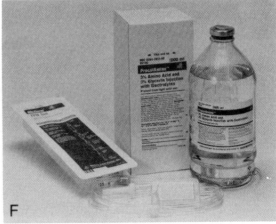

Figure 8–5 (*Continued*). C, Dual-compartment container of Nutrimix, an Aminosyn and dextrose mixture. (Courtesy of Abbott Laboratories, North Chicago, IL.) D, TrophAmine amino acid injection. (Courtesy of McGaw, Santa Ana, CA.) E, HepatAmine. (Courtesy of McGaw, Irvine, CA.) F, ProcalAmine (TNP set). (Courtesy of McGaw, Irvine, CA.)

bleeding in liver disease. It is believed that 1-Arginine enhances the formation of urea and thus reduces the ammonia level; however, clinical results are poor. R-Gene was removed from the market, but was subsequently reintroduced as R-Gene 10 (KabiVitrum). The official indications for this product are as an I.V. stimulant to the pituitary and as a diagnostic test for human growth hormone (HGH).

Urea—Lyophilized Form (Urevert, Baxter Healthcare). Solutions of urea are administered intravenously to reduce edema associated with operation, trauma, burns, and especially in the reduction of intracranial and intraocular pressure. Urea is not metabolized by the body. The administration of this concentrated solution causes osmotic diuresis.

Mannitol (Osmitrol, Baxter Healthcare). The intravenous administration of mannitol solutions results in osmotic diuresis. The solution is eliminated by the body almost entirely unmetabolized. Mannitol is of value in the prophylaxis of oliguria from tubular necrosis, in the treatment of cerebral edema, and in the promotion of diuresis. Dosage consists of 50 to 200 g as a 5%, 10%, or 20% solution. Twenty percent solutions of mannitol are saturated solutions. A decrease in room temperature may cause crystallization of the mannitol. If this occurs, the injection should be warmed prior to its administration to place the mannitol back into solution. Administration of the 20% injection requires the use of a blood filter set to ensure against infusion of mannitol crystals.

Dextran 70, Dextran 40 (Macrodex, Pharmacia; Rheomacrodex, Pharmacia; Gentran, Baxter Healthcare) (Fig. 8—6). Dextrans are polymolecular polysaccharides composed of glucose units formed by culturing a sucrose-containing medium. The average molecular weight of Dextran 70 is 70,000, and the average molecular weight of Dextran 40 is 40,000. When administered intravenously, Dextran 70 is an effective plasma volume expander. It is used in the treatment of trauma, hemorrhage, burns, and surgical shock. Owing to its lower molecular weight, Dextran 40 has less effect as a plasma volume expander than has Dextran 70. It is used as a priming fluid in pump-oxygenators during extracorporeal circulation. Studies have also shown that Dextran 40 has value as a prophylactic agent against thrombus formation. The drug prevents rouleau formation of red blood cells.

Sodium Bicarbonate Injection. In addition to its availability in ampuls, vials, and prefilled syringes, sodium bicarbonate, 5% injection, is also packaged in 500-ml bottles. This solution is used to combat acidosis by supplying a ready source of bicarbonate ion, and it can be administered as an intravenous fluid. The pH of sodium bicarbonate solutions is in the area of 8. Although an uncomplicated compound, sodium bicarbonate has presented problems in manufacture and administration. It decomposes to sodium carbonate with the liberation of carbon dioxide; if this occurs, the bicarbonate ion is not available. Sodium Bicarbonate Injection is usually packed in large ampuls; removal of the contents is time-consuming and difficult. Its availability in vials increased its convenience. For a short time, the injection was available in convenient aluminum screw-cap-covered vials; however, this container was withdrawn because metal filings from the closure fell into the solution when the vial was opened. This infusion fluid is packaged in a Type 1 glass container sealed with a rubber closure and requires a special administration set. Sodium bicarbonate

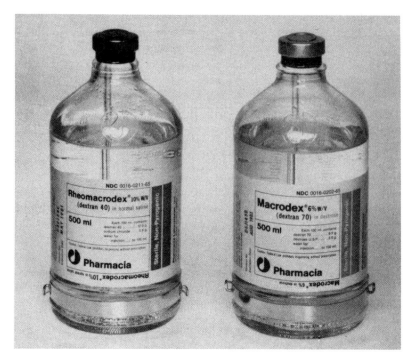

Figure 8–6.   Dextran 40, Dextran 70. (Courtesy of Pharmacia Laboratories, Inc., Piscataway, NJ.)

packaged in this manner has the disadvantages of requiring an additional intravenous site and being incapable of serving as a vehicle for other drug additives. The infusion fluid is available in 500-ml containers as 1.4%, $^1/_6$ molar, and 5% solutions. The injection has been made available in disposable prefilled syringes.

Sodium Lactate Injection ($^1/_6$ molar). Containing 167 mEq sodium and lactate ions per liter, this injection provides an immediate source of sodium for the elevation of bicarbonate level in severe acidosis. The lactate portion is metabolized by the liver into glycogen. This solution is used in the emergency treatment of metabolic acidosis.

Ammonium Chloride Injection (2.14%). Solutions are available containing 400 mEq per liter of ammonium and chloride ions and are used in the treatment of metabolic alkalosis and hypochloremia.

Large-Volume Solutions Not Administered Intravenously

Although solutions for irrigation and dialysis resemble intravenous fluids in many respects, they are not administered directly into the venous system. Their manufacture is subject to the same stringent controls as is that for intravenous fluids, but they may be packaged in containers that are larger than 1000-ml capacity and that are designed to empty rapidly.

Irrigation Solutions

Surgical Irrigating Solutions (Splash Solutions). Surgical irrigating solutions (Uromatic, Baxter; Urogate, Abbott) are used to bathe and moisten body tissue (Fig. 8–7). They may be used topically for moistening dressings, for wound irrigation, or as soaking or washing fluids for instruments. Sodium Chloride for Irrigation and Sterile Water for Irrigation are commonly used for these purposes. They are available commercially in screw-cap containers known as "pour" bottles. More recently, irrigating solutions have become available in rigid plastic pour bottles (Uromatic, Baxter; McGaw; Aqualite, Abbott) (Fig. 8–8).

Urologic Irrigation Solutions. It is common for surgeons performing urologic procedures to use a considerable amount of irrigation solutions during operations (Fig. 8–9). The solutions help to maintain the integrity of the tissue, to remove blood, and to provide a clear field of view for the surgeon. Urologic solutions require an administration set and are used with Foley catheters by connection to a cystoscope. Sterile Water for Irrigation and Sterile Glycine Solution are commonly used. Antibiotics are sometimes added, as in the case of Neosporin G.U. Irrigant.

Glycine Solution. Glycine, a relatively nontoxic amino acid, is commonly used to eliminate the risk of intravascular hemolysis during transurethral resection. It is supplied as a 1.5% solution in Water for Injection and packaged in 1000-, 1500-, and 3000-ml pour bottles. Fifteen per cent solution concentrates are available for dilution. The 1.5% solution is slightly hypotonic. Glycine solution is nonconducting and does not cause dispersion of high frequency current and loss of electrosurgical cutting efficiency.

Sorbital Solution. Sorbital solution 3% is a nonhemolytic urologic irrigant used for transurethral resection.

Urologic Solution G (Suby's Solution). Urologic solution G is an infrequently used solution containing citric acid, magnesium oxide, and sodium carbonate, and is designed to provide a non-operative treatment for urinary lithiasis by dissolution of calculi within the urinary tract. It contains sufficient citric acid to give a pH of 4. With the aid of hydrogen ion, insoluble calculi composed of calcium carbonate or phosphate are converted into soluble phosphoric acid. In addition, citrate ions combine with calcium ions to form soluble complexes.

Dialysis Solutions

Peritoneal Dialysis Solutions. Peritoneal dialysis solutions (Dianal, Baxter; Inpersol, Abbott) are not administered directly into the circulatory system, but rather into the peritoneal cavity (Fig. 8–10). Peritoneal dialysis is used to remove toxic substances normally excreted by the functioning kidney. In cases of poisoning or renal shutdown, or in patients awaiting renal transplants, dialysis is a lifesaving measure used to remove toxic substances, excessive body waste, and serum electrolytes. The composition of these commercially available solutions resembles that of potassium-free extracellular fluid. Solutions are available containing 1.5% and 4.25% dextrose and electrolytes. Solutions are made hypertonic to plasma with dextrose to avoid absorption of water into the intravascular compartment. By osmosis and diffusion, the peritoneal cavity

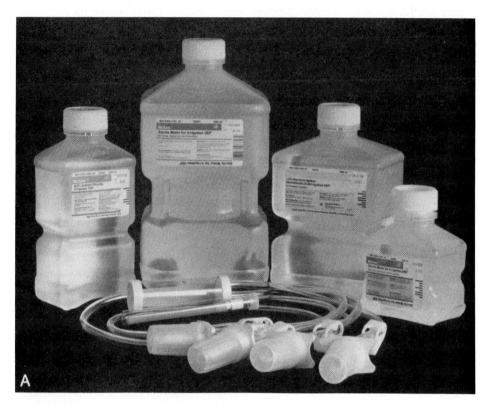

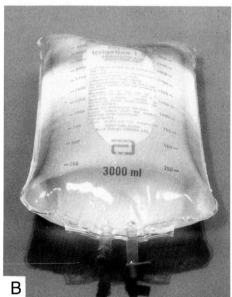

Figure 8–7. Surgical irrigating solutions. (A, Courtesy of McGaw, Santa Ana, CA. B, Courtesy of Abbott Laboratories, North Chicago, IL.)

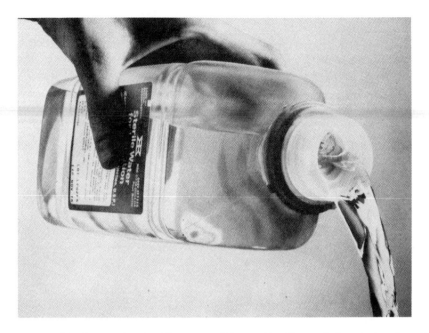

Figure 8–8.   Plastic-pour bottle. (Courtesy of Baxter Healthcare Laboratories, Inc., Deerfield, IL.)

behaves as a semipermeable membrane. Catabolites and other substances may be removed from the body. An incision is made on the linea alba (midline), and a trocar connected to a catheter attached to the container of the dialysis solution is inserted. The solution is permitted to flow into the abdominal cavity. The solution remains in the cavity for 30 to 90 minutes and is drained by a siphon. The procedure is repeated many times and may require 30 to 50 L of solution for daily treatment. Common additives to peritoneal dialysis solutions include tetracyclines, heparin, and potassium chloride.

Hemodialysis. Hemodialysis utilizes the same principles as peritoneal dialysis. In this procedure, the blood leaves the artery via a polyethylene catheter and passes through a disposable dialyzing membrane unit. This unit is bathed in an ideal electrolytic solution simulating body fluids. One important difference with hemodialysis bath solutions is that their method of use does not require the solution to be sterile, pyrogen-free, or free of particulate matter. Concentrated solutions of electrolytes can be purchased and are added to water in a tank containing the disposable dialyzing membrane through which the blood is flowing. After cycling through the dialyzer, the blood enters the body by vein.

Intravenous Fluid Administration Systems

Systems for administering intravenous fluids were classified as either the open system (nonvacuum) or the closed system (vacuum). The open system, marketed by Abbott Laboratories, utilized a screw-capped bottle packaged at atmospheric pressure. A tamper-proof metal overseal with a tear-away tab was removed, the screw cap was removed, and the administration set was attached

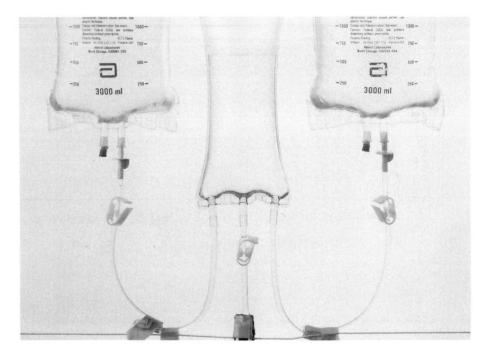

A

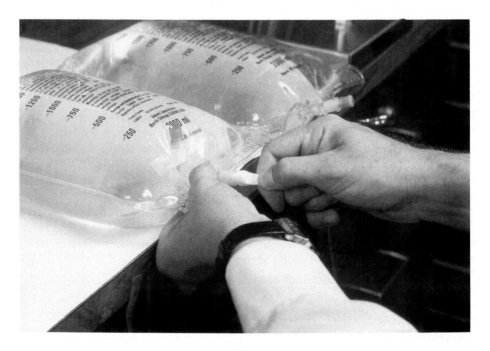

B

Figure 8–9. A, Urologic solution. B, Dialysis solutions. (A, B, Courtesy of Abbott Laboratories, North Chicago, IL.)

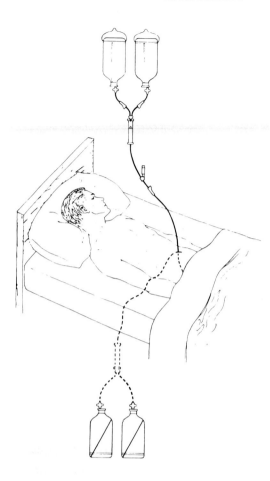

Figure 8–10. Peritoneal dialysis technique. (Courtesy of Baxter Healthcare Laboratories, Inc., Deerfield, IL.)

to the container. Because of problems of contamination with the open system, this type of packaging was removed from the market. Abbott Laboratories now manufactures a closed system container. All the presently available intravenous solutions packaged in glass are closed systems with a vacuum. Although there are variations in the types of sets used, all systems have common characteristics (Fig. 8–11) (Table 8–2).

All systems packaged in glass bottles require the entrance of air for operation. The vacuum present in the container after autoclaving must be released before the fluid can flow. These containers are Type II glass, with the exception of Sodium Bicarbonate Injection, which is packaged in Type I. All systems are for one-time use and all containers should be discarded after use. Intravenous fluids are packaged with approximately 3% excess in volume. The excess allows for priming the administration set and permits the labeled volume to be delivered from the container. The containers are graduated at 20-ml increments on scales that permit the volume in the container to be readily determined whether the bottle is inverted or in an upright position. A metal band around the container facilitates hanging it for use. Although these solutions are relatively stable, manufacturers date each solution to ensure proper rotation and to minimize stability problems resulting from prolonged or improper storage. Extreme temperatures are to be avoided during storage. Until

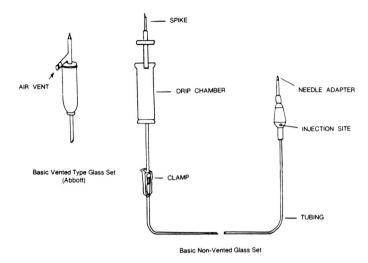

Figure 8–11.   Basic intravenous fluid administration sets. (Baxter, McGaw)

1971, all intravenous fluids in the United States were packaged in glass; plastic containers have been introduced by Baxter Healthcare Laboratories (Viaflex), Abbott Laboratories (LifeCare), and McGaw Laboratories (Accumed), and are discussed later in this chapter.

Administration sets, or devices used to administer intravenous fluids, are disposable, sterile, and free of pyrogens and particulate matter. The basic sets contain a spiked plastic device to enter or pierce the rubber closure on the container. A sight, or drip, chamber is present to allow setting of the rate of flow; the sight chamber allows uninterrupted air-free flow. The chamber leads to a length of polyethylene tubing with an attached gum rubber injection port. At the tip of the port is a rigid plastic device that accepts the needle hub. A clamp-like device on the tubing pinches the internal diameter of the tubing to regulate flow.

Before the container is pierced, the contents should be inspected to ensure that they are clear and free from particulate matter; then the container is pierced aseptically with the appropriate administration set. Air is removed from the tubing by pinching the sight chamber and allowing the fluid to flow

TABLE 8–2.   Intravenous Fluid Systems

System	Source
Glass, no air tube, vacuum, air filter on set	Abbott Laboratories
Glass, air tube, vacuum, no air filter	McGaw Laboratories
	Baxter Healthcare Laboratories·
Plastic, no air tube, nonvacuum	Baxter Healthcare Laboratories (Viaflex)
Plastic, no air tube, nonvacuum	Abbott (LifeCare)
Plastic, no air tube, nonvacuum	McGaw (Accumed)
Plastic, no air tube, nonvacuum	McGaw (EXCEL)

until air is removed. When air has been removed, the pinched clamp is closed. The venipuncture is made, the pinch clamp is opened, and the rate of flow is regulated.

It is of extreme importance to check the container to ensure that it is not cracked. Fine hairline cracks are difficult to see; however, they present a real hazard. The fact that they do occur is indicated by a lawsuit involving the death of a patient caused by septicemia from contamination of a cracked bottle.

Abbo-Vac (Abbott) System

The containers in the Abbo-Vac system have a vacuum and are closed with a solid rubber closure protected by a tear-off aluminum seal (Fig. 8–12). The set is equipped with a spike, which is forced through the solid closure. Air entering through a sidearm Teflon filter permits dissipation of the vacuum, and the solution is ready for use. As the solution leaves the container, air enters through the filter, producing a rising stream of air bubbles which indicates proper functioning. The Abbo-Vac set delivers 15 drops per ml.

Medication may be added to the system in several ways. By using syringe and needle, it may be added to the container fluid by insertion through the self-sealing rubber closure. With aseptic technique, medication may be added directly intravenously, if necessary, by injection through the gum rubber self-sealing injection site. Medication may also be added by use of a syringe with no needle attached by removing the Teflon air filter and injecting the solution into the intravenous fluid through the filter site and then replacing the filter. Additives packaged in convenience containers equipped with a spike may be used with these systems (Fig. 8–13). With either a Y-setup or secondary attachment, two containers may be set up simultaneously; however, secondary arrangements are not without hazards.

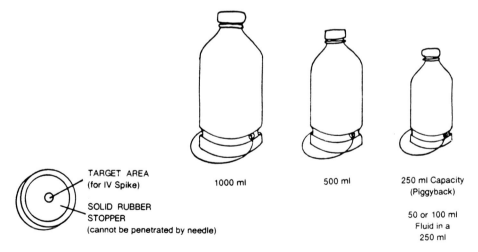

TARGET AREA
(for IV Spike)

SOLID RUBBER
STOPPER
(cannot be penetrated by needle)

1000 ml   500 ml   250 ml Capacity
(Piggyback)

50 or 100 ml
Fluid in a
250 ml

Figure 8–12. Abbott's intravenous glass container. The air venting is provided for in the intravenous set rather than the bottle. Thus, the bottles do not have integral air-venting tubes. Air enters the system through a bacteriologic air filter in the spike adapter of the intravenous set.

HOW TO USE ABBOTT'S NEW PINTOP VIAL

On your job you'll be encountering this helpful new Abbott additive container. It's called the Pintop Vial. The Pintop Vial makes it easy for you to add supplemental I.V. solution concentrates before setting up your I.V. bottles.

The Pintop Vial saves nursing time. For example, once you've plugged into the I.V. bottle, a 10 ml. fluid transfer is complete in less than two seconds!

The Pintop Vial is designed to be an important part of the Abbo-Vac® system. However, it is also compatible with other I.V. vacuum-container systems, and is also adaptable to syringe technique.

Examples of widely prescribed additives being supplied are *Potassium Chloride 20 mEq. (No. 4932), 30 mEq. (No. 4933), and 40 mEq. (No. 4934).* Your Abbott Hospital Representative will gladly give you the complete listing of medications available in the Pintop Vial.

Tamperproof metal seal tells at a glance that contents are intact. Tears away easily.

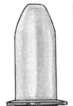

Rigid plastic hood protects sterile integrity of piercing pin. And (unlike some overseals) it's easy to remove.

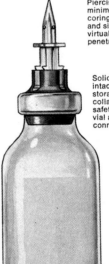

Piercing pin design minimizes chance of coring. Extremely sharp and siliconized for virtually frictionless penetration.

Solid stopper remains intact throughout storage. "Highrise" collar affords a sterile safety zone between vial and bottle when connected.

A slight overfill is included. This compensates for residual solution that remains after transfer.

Figure 8–13.   Pintop vial. (Courtesy of Abbott Laboratories, North Chicago, IL.)

Baxter and McGaw Systems

These systems differ basically from those previously described in that the rubber closures contain two openings (Fig. 8–14). One opening leads directly into a long plastic airway tube which permits air to enter the container above the solution as it is being administered. A second opening is present to receive the spike of the administration set. A thin rubber diaphragm maintains the integrity of the closure after removal of the aluminum tear-tab. The diaphragm is removed with a quick snap, dissipating the vacuum. The administration set may now be plugged into the container. The container is inverted. The flexible sight chamber may need to be pinched to achieve a level of the fluid. The pinch clamp is opened to allow flow to remove air from the system. The pinch clamp is closed, the venipuncture is performed, and the flow rate is adjusted. The standard Baxter and McGaw sets deliver 10 and 15 drops per ml, respectively.

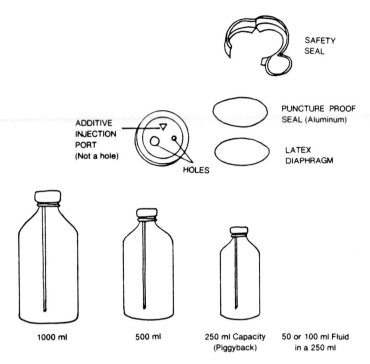

Figure 8–14. Baxter Healthcare and McGaw intravenous glass systems. LVP bottles have internal plastic venting tubes, which allow air to enter the bottles as fluid is infused into the patient.

Medication may be added by means of a needle and syringe through a target area marked on the rubber stopper, or through the opening that receives the spikes of the administration set before insertion. If this is done with the diaphragm intact, this area should be swabbed with alcohol. Medication also may be added after the removal of the gum rubber diaphragm. If the administration set is not placed in the bottle immediately, additive caps should be used to protect the fluid from contamination. If necessary, medication also can be injected through the gum rubber injection port while fluid administration is in progress. Additives may be placed directly into the container during administration, using a needle and syringe, by penetrating the target area in the rubber closure.

Prior to dissipating the vacuum, additive solutions in convenience packages (Pintop, Abbott) may be placed in the administration set opening and drawn into the container, utilizing the vacuum present (Fig. 8–13). A pumper-type convenience device may be used for sterile solids. The device is placed into the administration set opening; the infusion bottle is inverted; with pumping action, the infusion fluid is drawn into the device's container; and solution of the sterile solids is effected. The infusion fluid container is placed in an upright position, and with a pumping action the contents of the device are forced into the intravenous fluid. Convenience devices may be left in place to indicate that a drug has been added, or the supplied supplemental label may be used.

Plastic Intravenous Fluid Containers

Owing to the large volumes of intravenous fluid administered to some patients, the particulate matter found in them has been of special concern. Sources of this particulate matter, as discussed previously, include the packaging components themselves. The glass bottle and the rubber closure of the standard intravenous fluid container can contribute particulates, not only from their improper preparation before use, but also from their potential reaction with the solution and the chemicals present.

In the search for other packaging material, plastic was suggested as an alternative. Reports from abroad indicated that its use for intravenous fluids did result in the reduction of particulate material. As discussed in Chapter 4, however, plastic packaging is not necessarily totally inert and can present problems, including the leaching of chemicals from the plastic by the solution, the absorption of substances from the solutions, and the permeability of the plastic to moisture transfer. These problems have to be considered for any plastic used as a packaging material, especially for solutions.

In the United States, several intravenous fluids are packaged in plastic (Viaflex, Baxter Healthcare) (Fig. 8–15). The plastic container or bag is prepared from transparent plasticized polyvinyl chloride. For shipment and storage, the plastic container is inserted and sealed in a tear-off, translucent, heavy-duty

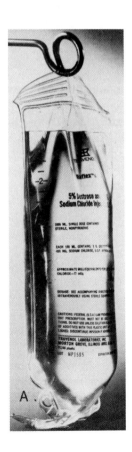

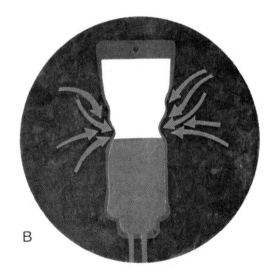

Figure 8–15. A, A plastic system offers several advantages over a glass bottle in intravenous therapy. The plastic bag is unbreakable, lightweight, easier to set up, and has a built-in hanger. B, The closed flexible plastic container does not require air venting to function; the bag collapses while the solution is being administered. (Courtesy of Baxter Healthcare Laboratories, Inc., Deerfield, IL.)

polyethylene case. The inner container or bag is designed with a plastic tab with an opening that permits it to be hung from an intravenous pole. On the opposite end are two sleeve ports. The plastic covering over one port can be removed to permit the insertion of the spike of the administration set. The other sleeve, with a gum rubber covering, permits addition of other medication to the intravenous fluid. When adding medication in this manner, the sleeve port should be milked to diffuse the added solution into the intravenous fluid. Adding medication through the sleeve port must be done with care to prevent the needle from puncturing the plastic. Because plastic material is not inherently resealing, puncturing it with a needle results in a hole.

The flexible plastic container functions physically by the forces of gravity and atmospheric pressure; as the fluid leaves the container, the bag collapses because it is not vented. Collapse of the bag precludes outside air from entering the container and eliminates the possibility of airborne contamination. In addition, the possibility of air embolism occurring from this collapsible system is reduced; however, the possibility of air embolism is greater when flexible plastic units are connected in a series of containers. Therefore, this type of hook-up is not recommended with plastic bags. Other advantages claimed for plastic packaging include reduction in breakage, economy in space during storage, simplified disposal, and reduction in weight and noise. Flexible and semi-rigid plastic containers are shown in Figure 8–16.

The use of convenience devices with the plastic container requires an appliance designed to place a vacuum within the bag. This equipment is available commercially under the name "Viavac" and consists of a plexiglass chamber in which the bag is placed. When vacuum is applied to the chamber, the contents of convenience devices, as well as other forms of medication, can be added. Its use is designed for a centralized intravenous admixture location. Tamper-proof seals are available for the sleeve ports, once medication has been added to the intravenous fluids. When adding other medication to intravenous fluids packaged in plastic, the same precautions must be observed as with other admixtures, with consideration of compatibility and clarity. Provided continued progress is made in using plastics that have been shown to be nonreactive with the solutions, the trend in packaging intravenous fluids in the immediate future is toward the plastic container (Fig. 8–17).

LifeCare System (Abbott)

(Fig. 8–18). LifeCare is similar in many respects to Baxter Healthcare's Viaflex system. This flexible polyvinylchloride container has a resealable additive port on the upper side of the bag. This position reduces the potential for "welling" of additive medication in the outlet port and possible delivery of an undiluted bolus. It is also claimed to facilitate aseptic technique. Normal syringes or specially designed syringes can be used to inject medication into this port.

Additive caps are available to protect the port after the addition of medication or during transportation, and they also serve as indicators that additives are present. A "Vacu-add" unit can be utilized to create a vacuum in the LifeCare bag to facilitate transfer of additives from small volume parenteral containers.

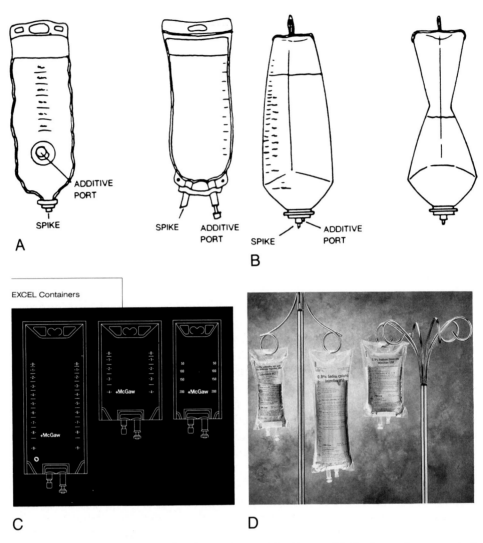

Figure 8–16. A, Abbott (LifeCare) and Baxter Healthcare (Viaflex) supply nonvented polyvinylchloride flexible plastic containers. These containers require nonvented sets. B, McGaw (Accumed) offers a nonvented semi-rigid polyolefin plastic container. C, D, McGaw is now offering the new non-PVC, nonphthalate EXCEL container. C is a diagram and D a photograph of this container.

Accumed System (McGaw)

Accumed (McGaw) plastic intravenous fluid administration system, utilizes a polyolefin plastic material (Fig. 8–19). This semi-rigid container has no plasticizer. The claim for virtually no extractibility or leachability is made. This plastic is also impermeable to vapor transmission. The system is not dependent on air and is programmed to produce predictable collapsibility and complete disposability. Combustible by-products of this container are water and carbon dioxide.

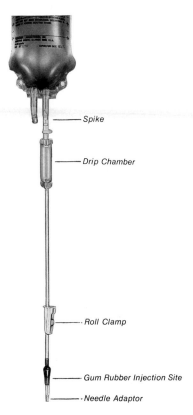

Figure 8–17. Basic intravenous administration set for flexible plastic container. (Courtesy of Baxter/Healthcare Laboratories, Inc. Deerfield, IL.)

Excel (McGaw)

As of the writing of this text, the Accumed semi-rigid polyolefin plastic container is being phased out of production in favor of a new non-PVC, non-phthalate flexible container termed EXCEL (Fig. 8–16C and D).

Incinerated PVC products produce hydrogen chloride gas as a toxic pollutant. Diethylehexyl phthalate (DEHP), a component of PVC containers, may leach into the soil in landfills. Several drugs absorb to PVC containers, notably nitroglycerin. Some substances (fat emulsions, blood, taxol) are known to leach DEHP.

It is claimed that the EXCEL 4 container eliminates or minimizes the above problems. The plastic film contains no plasticizers and exhibits no leachability. The container's solution contact layer is composed of a rubberized compolymer of ethylene and propylene, which are claimed to be clear, non-toxic and biologically inert. The EXCEL container is available in 250, 500, and 1 liter sizes. Smaller sizes (25, 50, and 100 ml) are available. They are known as PAB containers

The new Mini-Bag Plus container, a ready-to-mix system (Fig. 8–20) that accommodates standard 20 mm drug vials, is now available from Baxter Healthcare Corporation's I.V. Systems Division. The Mini-Bag Plus container is used in conjunction with the ReConPlus adapter.

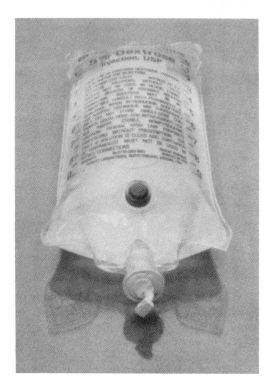

Figure 8–18. Plastic LVP bag. (Courtesy of Abbott Laboratories, North Chicago, IL.)

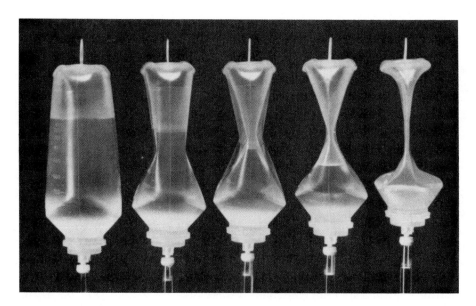

Figure 8–19. Accumed semi-rigid polyolefin containers. (Courtesy of McGaw, Inc. Irvine, CA.)

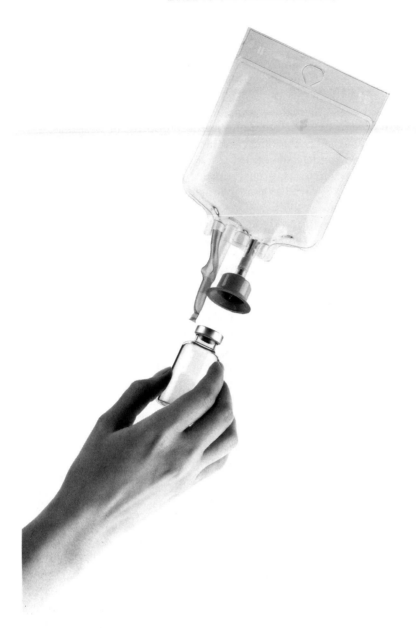

Figure 8–20.   Mini-Bag Plus container. (Courtesy of Baxter Healthcare Laboratories, Inc., Deerfield, IL.)

The Mini-Bag Plus container consists of a Mini-Bag container filled with diluent solution, a port tube that encloses a breakaway seal, a vial adapter with foil cover, and an I.V. tubing port with protector. To assemble the Mini-Bag Plus container, the adapter is aseptically placed over the prepared drug vial to reconstitute the drug, and the breakaway seal is snapped. Solution is squeezed from the bag to half-fill the vial, the bag is inverted, the drug vial shaken, and the bag squeezed and shaken to transfer the solution to dissolve and mix the drug.

Storage of Intravenous Fluids

Attention should be given to the storage conditions for large-volume solutions. Often, the storage of these solutions has low priority in hospitals. Overheated rooms and cold areas should be avoided because they accelerate discoloration, precipitation, and leaching.

In some instances, admixtures prepared several hours or more prior to administration are stored in a refrigerator. Refrigeration retards bacterial growth and drug deterioration. One study has shown that at reasonable administration rates a refrigerated admixture quickly approaches room temperature when the bottle is hung. It has been demonstrated that the incidence of cardiac arrest during massive blood replacement dropped from 58% to 7% when cold banked blood was warmed to body temperature before infusion.

Because infusions are packaged in single-use containers and no bacteriostatic agents are added, once they have been violated they should be used as soon as possible. Manipulated infusion fluids should always be used within 24 hours or be discarded. A more conservative recommendation is that I.V. mixtures be used within 1 hour after mixing, or if not, refrigerated and used within 24 hours. This safeguard minimizes contamination and does not allow sufficient time for incubation, if the solution inadvertently becomes contaminated.

Expiration dating on labels helps to rotate the stock of intravenous fluids in a manner that assures that the material will be used in order of its receipt. In addition, placing a 24-hour expiration date on an infusion that contains an additive lessens problems with stability.

Methods of Intravenous Administration

Drugs can be introduced intravenously in small or large volumes. An intravenous injection refers to a small volume of drug administered intravenously with a needle and syringe. Large volumes of solutions containing drugs given intravenously are administered in a variety of ways. Different methods are used to obtain the desired speed of achieving blood levels of the drug and to minimize the degree of irritation from the drug's administration. House staff availability, in addition to a particular hospital's policy as to what routes and classes of drugs may be administered by a nurse, can influence the methods of drug administration. The desire to achieve constant, prolonged blood levels also affects the mode of administration. The formulation of the injection that influences the manufacturer's recommendation as to the rate of injection is a factor to be considered. Except for Intralipid emulsion, only drugs in aqueous solution are given intravenously.

Drugs may be administered by the continuous or the intermittent technique. According to some authorities, either method of administration will be clinically effective in the majority of cases. Figure 8–21 depicts a "decision tree" for various modes of I.V. administration and lists various drugs and equipment that are to be explained in this chapter.

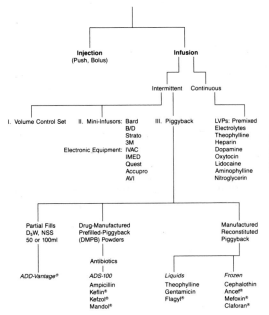

Figure 8–21. Decision tree for various modes of intravenous administration.

Continuous Therapy

Intravenous Infusion. A common method of administering drugs is to add the drug directly to an infusion container. The drug becomes diluted in the infusion fluid and is dripped slowly into the vein. This method permits the physician to accomplish fluid therapy and drug therapy simultaneously and achieves continuous, constant blood levels of the drug. In many instances, drug therapy is accomplished initially by intravenous push and then maintained slowly and constantly by intravenous infusion (Fig. 8–22). A possible disadvantage of this method of therapy is delayed incompatibility occurring in the infusion container. The drug remains in contact with the vehicle for several hours or longer. If the solution is contaminated during preparation or administration, there is an additional disadvantage in not administering the solution immediately with an intravenous push; the consequences of administering a contaminated product are more severe as the organisms proliferate.

Hook-ups. Hook-ups (Solution Series Set, Baxter; Secondary, Abbott; I.V. Series Set, McGaw) allow fluid to be added or solutions to be changed while the infusion continues (Fig. 8–23). A tube with a clamp is connected to the two containers. The air vent in the primary container is closed, and the air vent in the second container is opened, allowing the second container to empty first.

This type of hook-up has several disadvantages. An unintended increase in flow, if not noticed, will cause a double volume of fluid to be infused, which may produce circulatory overload. Physicians and nurses may have varying opinions as to the order of emptying. A layering effect may take place with solutions and drugs of varying viscosities, which may increase or decrease administration time. This type of I.V. administration should be avoided.

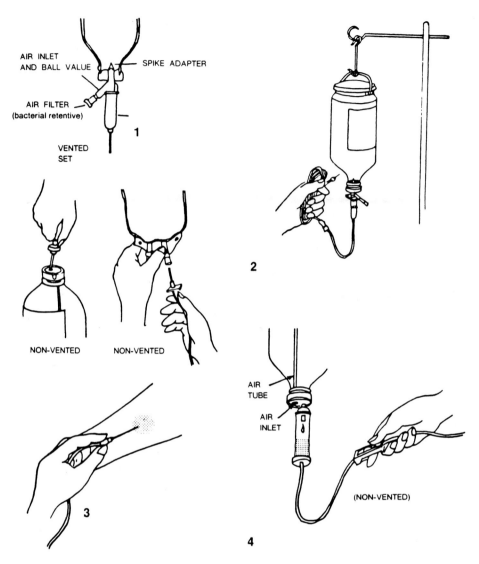

Figure 8–22. Process of starting LVP infusion continuous therapy. 1, Spike adapter of intravenous set is inserted into stopper of LVP container (bottle or plastic). 2, LVP container is hung on stand at bedside, and air is purged from the intravenous set by opening clamp until fluid comes out of needle. Set is then clamped off. 3, Venipuncture is made by intravenous team, or floor nurse. 4, Infusion rate is adjusted by slowly opening and closing clamp until desired drip rate, viewed in drip chamber, is obtained. The usual running time is 4 to 8 hours. (Usually, 125 ml is delivered in 1 hour.) Set is calculated to deliver 10, 15, 20, 50, or 60 drops per ml, depending on manufacturer.

Intermittent Therapy

In intermittent therapy, the drug is given at spaced intervals. Three possibilities for handling intermittent therapy have been suggested: (1) use of a mini-bottle with the already hanging administration set; (2) injection of the solution slowly by needle and syringe directly into a vein or injection site of an already hanging large-volume administration set (true intravenous push); or

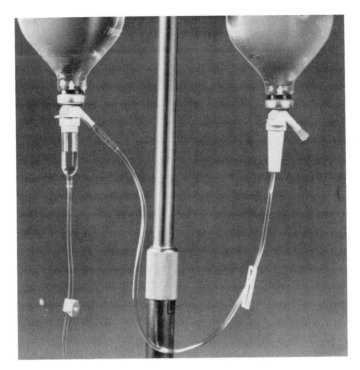

Figure 8–23.   Secondary hook-up provides a means of adding more fluid or of changing fluid without interrupting infusion. (Courtesy of Abbott Laboratories, North Chicago, IL.)

(3) addition of the drug to a predetermined volume of fluid in a volume-control device.

Piggyback Method. The piggyback method refers to the intermittent intravenous drip of a second solution, the reconstituted drug, through the venipuncture site of an established primary I.V. system (Figs. 8–24, 8–25). With this setup, the drug can be thought of as entering the vein on "top" of the primary I.V. fluid (hence, the designation "piggyback"). The piggyback technique not only eliminates the need for another venipuncture but also achieves drug dilution and peak blood levels within a relatively short time, usually 30 to 60 min. Drug dilution helps to reduce irritation, and early high serum levels are an important consideration in serious infection requiring aggressive drug therapy. These and other advantages have served to popularize the piggyback method of I.V. therapy, especially for the intermittent administration of antibiotics. At present, two possibilities exist for piggybacking.

Piggyback administration may be accomplished with any basic administration set, but the nurse must reestablish flow of the primary fluid after infusion of the piggyback drug solution. Special administration sets can be used; however, they contain pressure-sensitive valves that sense when the piggyback drug container is empty; at that point, the primary flow begins automatically, owing to a height (gravitational pull) difference between the primary fluid and piggyback drug containers (Fig. 8–26). Automatic piggyback administration sets are supplied by Abbott (Automatic Drug Delivery System), McGaw (IV Additive Set), and Travenol (Continu-Flo Set).

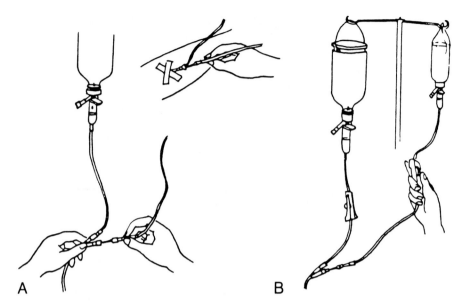

Figure 8–24. Process of starting piggyback infusion. A, The secondary set is purged of air, and its needle is inserted into a Y injection site of the primary set, or into the injection site at the end of the primary set. B, The piggyback infusion is started. Once it is completed, the primary fluid infusion will be restarted.

Prefilled Partial-Fill Containers (Underfills, Mini-bottles). Commercially supplied partial-fill containers used for piggybacking are 250-ml capacity infusion bottles or bags underfilled with 50 or 100 ml of 5% D/W or normal saline solution. The drug to be administered is first reconstituted in its original parenteral vial and then added by needle and syringe to the "underfill," which receives an administration set complete with needle. The needle of this piggyback delivery system is inserted into the Y-site or gum rubber injection port of a hanging primary infusion set. Flow of the primary intravenous fluid is stopped while the drug solution in the partial-fill container is administered (30 to 60 min). After the drug solution has been totally infused, the primary fluid flow is reestablished. When the next dose of drug is required, the piggyback procedure is repeated, replacing the prefilled partial-fill container and, in some cases, its administration set as well.

Prefilled Piggyback Units (Manufactured Prefilled Drug Containers). A more recent innovation by which piggybacking can be accomplished is the piggyback unit, a mini-bottle (100-ml capacity) prefilled with a specific amount of dry drug. Several manufacturers (Lilly, Roerig, SmithKline Beecham, Wyeth-Ayerst, Bristol) have introduced mini-bottles prefilled with various antibiotic products; each manufacturer's container is provided with either a plastic bag or a plastic hanger for direct suspension from an I.V. pole as the piggyback solution is administered through the resealable gum rubber injection site or Y-type facility of an existing I.V. system. Reconstitution of drug in a piggyback unit requires only the addition of a small volume of compatible diluent. Because the drug is reconstituted in and administered from the same bottle, no drug transfer is involved; transfer syringes and additional I.V. containers are

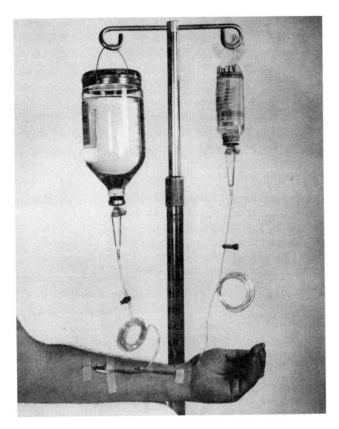

Figure 8–25. Piggyback infusion technique. (Courtesy of Abbott Laboratories, North Chicago, IL.)

not necessary. Prefilled piggyback units, therefore, offer greater ease in handling and considerable reduction in inventory costs than do either prefilled partial-fill containers or volume-control sets, for which prior reconstitution and subsequent transfer of the drug to be administered are essential.

Direct Intravenous Push (Bolus). In direct intravenous push the solution of the drug is placed into a syringe and administered in a short period of time directly into a vein (Fig. 8–27), or through the gum rubber injection site of the administration set (Fig. 8–28). The injection time is a matter of minutes and varies with different drugs according to the manufacturer's recommendations. Many drugs given by direct intravenous push are diluted further with the vehicle, using a larger syringe, to reduce the irritability of the drug on the vein. Table 8–3 lists the recommended times for a number of drugs.

The determination of which method and at what speed a drug may be given I.V. is associated with the physicochemical properties of the drug and bioavailability factors. Not all drugs may be pushed I.V. Those drugs that can are usually diluted sufficiently to minimize toxicity. Almost always, drugs pushed I.V. have recommended injection times established by the manufacturer. For example, phenytoin and diazepam injections must be given by I.V. push. When these drugs are diluted and given by other I.V. methods, the instability of the drugs causes precipitation. Therefore, they must be pushed at a specified

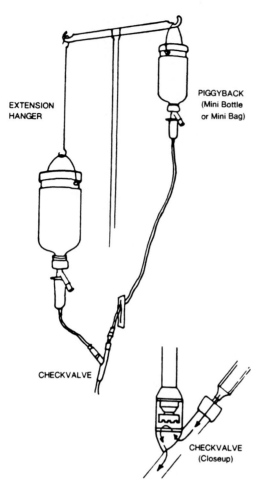

EXTENSION
HANGER

PIGGYBACK
(Mini Bottle
or Mini Bag)

CHECKVALVE

CHECKVALVE
(Closeup)

Figure 8–26. Automatic piggyback set with built-in checkvalve.

rate that is slow enough to prevent toxicity. In contrast to phenytoin and diazepam, because of its toxicity, gentamicin may not be given by push, but must be given well diluted (1 mg/ml) and must be administered piggyback or by volume-control method over a period of at least 1 hour to minimize renal and ototoxicity and neuromuscular blockade. Many drugs can be given I.V. by push or diluted in volume-control or piggyback units. Such is the case with ampicillin; however, direct I.V. push in less than 100 mg/min may cause seizures. The package insert for furosemide has been revised. Ototoxicity[5] is usually seen when the drug is given rapidly by push to patients with renal impairment. This is particularly associated with large doses and often when it is combined with other ototoxic drugs. An infusion rate of not more than 4 mg/min is suggested (formerly 10 mg/min).

On occasion, manufacturers suggest I.V. push but may not give definite injection time recommendations. Diazoxide (Hyperstat) is particularly unusual in that it must be pushed I.V. in less than 30 seconds. This is done to prevent the drug from becoming inactivated by plasma proteins. One publication[6] suggested administration in 10 seconds. When drugs are given by the I.V. push method, the manufacturers' recommendations must be followed. Grotting et

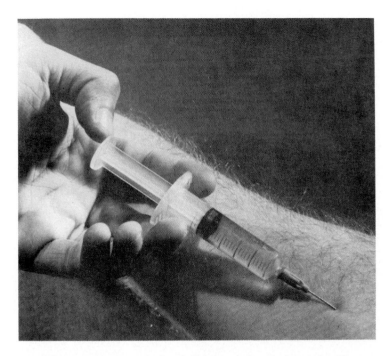

Figure 8–27. Direct intravenous push administered directly into vein. (Courtesy of Travenol Laboratories, Inc., Deerfield, IL.)

al.[7] published I.V. push rates of cancer chemotherapy drugs. A publication by Rapp et al.,[8] "Guidelines for the Administration of Commonly Used Intravenous Drugs," is also most valuable. The rationale and procedures for intermittent and direct I.V. push were reviewed by Godwin.[9] "How to Develop an I.V. Push Service" was published by Grotting et al.[10] A manual for the preparation and administration of drugs for I.V. is available through the Canadian Society of Hospital Pharmacists.[11]

Volume-Control Sets. Volume-control sets (Metriset, McGaw; Soluset, Abbott; Buretrol, Baxter) are calibrated plastic fluid chambers used as measuring devices in conjunction with intravenous bottles (Figs. 8–29, 8–30). These devices permit administration of drug solutions in precise quantities. Drugs in solution are added directly through the gum rubber injection port or the volume-control unit into a predetermined volume of fluid from the primary intravenous fluid. Four reasons have been suggested for using a volume-control set: (1) the chamber provides a means for critical measurement of infused fluid; (2) the chamber provides a vehicle for intermittent intravenous medication therapy, as opposed to continuous therapy; (3) unstable drugs may be administered quickly in a minimum volume of fluid; and (4) the chamber limits the volume of fluid that may be infused accidentally. Many potential problems exist with these devices because of their misuse, overuse, and abuse in hospitals.

Volume-Control Sets Versus Piggyback Method. The previously discussed disadvantages of volume-control sets and the microbiologic hazards (i.e., nosocomial infections as a result of bacterial colonization) associated with these devices have been repeatedly documented by numerous investigators.[12–14] The

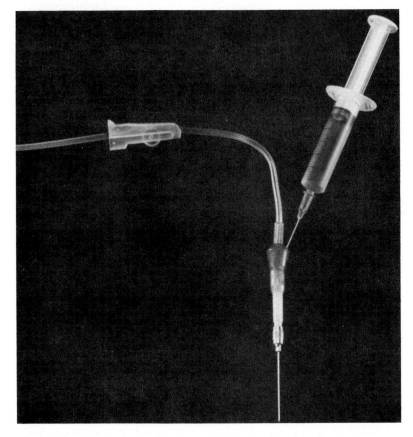

Figure 8–28. Direct intravenous push administered through gum rubber injection site of administration set. (Courtesy of Baxter Healthcare Laboratories, Inc., Deerfield, IL.)

National Coordinating Committee on Large Volume Parenterals (NCCLVP) states that "volume-control sets (Buretrol, Soluset, Volu-trol) should not be used for the routine administration of intermittent drug therapy in adults." The same NCCLVP panel "does not recommend volume-control sets as devices for injections of intermittent IV medication . . . (but) does recommend the use of partially-filled bags or bottles for this."

Prefilled partial-fill containers have many advantages over volume-control sets: Underfills are easier and faster to use, so nurses can better meet the

TABLE 8–3.   Recommended Push Times for Certain Drugs

Injection	Concentration	Time
Valium	5 mg/ml	Not less 3. mg/min
Keflin	100 mg/ml	Not less 200 mg/min
Ancef	100 mg/ml	Not less 200 mg/min
Aminophylline	500 mg/20 ml	Slowly
Dilantin	50 mg/ml	Not less 1 minute
Hyperstat	15 mg/ml	Within 10–30 seconds

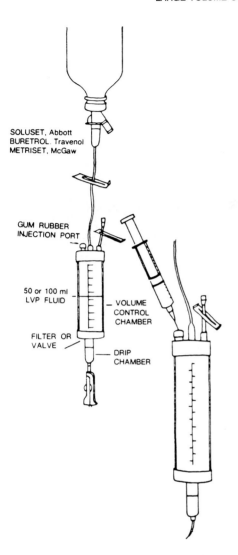

SOLUSET, Abbott
BURETROL, Travenol
METRISET, McGaw

GUM RUBBER
INJECTION PORT

50 or 100 ml
LVP FLUID

VOLUME
CONTROL
CHAMBER

FILTER OR
VALVE

DRIP
CHAMBER

Figure 8–29. Intermittent infusion system for antibiotics and other drugs.

demands of crowded work schedules; they are properly labeled for one-time unit-dose use only, lessening the chances of medication error, admixture incompatibility, and solution contamination; and they foster use of the proper diluent in the right amount.

All the aforementioned features apply equally well to prefilled piggyback units, which provide even greater convenience, economy, and patient safety in I.V. therapy than partial-fill containers. In obviating the need for transfer of reconstituted drug, easy-to-use piggyback units improve the quality of patient care through reduced potential for solution contamination. Self-contained reconstitution and administration capabilities also eliminate expenditure for parenteral drug vials, transfer syringes, and the more costly partial-fill containers; this reduced inventory with proven dollar savings in turn releases shelf storage needed for other purposes. In short, prefilled piggyback units truly represent a new dimension in unit dose; that is, a unique, sophisticated packaging for direct administration of drug.

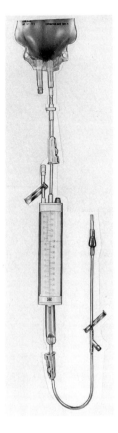

Figure 8–30. Buretrol volume-control set permits the administration of intravenous fluids in limited amounts and precise volumes. (Courtesy of Baxter Healthcare Laboratories, Inc., Deerfield, IL.)

Flow Rates of Intravenous Infusion Fluids

The rate of flow of intravenous fluids is determined by the prescribing physician whose judgment is based on a variety of factors, such as the patient's body surface area and age, and the composition of the fluid to be administered. The rate of administration and total volume are often limited by the patient's ability to assimilate the fluid. Patients with congestive heart failure or pulmonary difficulties can react adversely to infusion fluids. Extreme caution is exercised when administering fluids to patients with any degree of renal impairment.

The physician may want rapid or slow infusion, depending on his objective. He may want fluids, or perhaps his interest is in administering electrolytes. His primary interest may be in the administration of a drug and not necessarily with fluids. The usual or normal flow rate of low-viscosity isotonic solutions (5% D/W, normal saline, Ringer's lactate) is approximately 125 ml/ hour or 1 L every 8 hours. This amounts to 2 ml/min. Highly hypertonic solutions such as hyperalimentation solutions are administered at a rate not exceeding 1 L every 8 hours or 3 L every 24 hours. Only in exceptional cases (blood loss, shock, or administration of anesthesia) would the rate be in excess of 1 L every 1 $\frac{1}{2}$ hours. This amounts to 11 ml/min. Often, orders are written as "KVO" (keep vein open), in which case, the rate of administration would be slow. The objective is to keep the intravenous fluid running in an-

Body Surface Area
In Square Meters

This nomogram, on which may be based the desired
dosage of intravenous fluid, is derived from the
formula for surface of DuBois and DuBois,
Log A = Log H X 0.725 + Log W X 0.425 + 1.8564

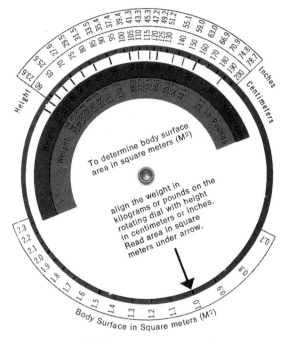

Surface Area (S.A.) of infants and children
in square meters from body weight in kilograms

Wt. Kg.	S.A.	Wt. Kg.	S.A.	Wt. Kg.	S.A.
1.0	.10	6	.33	14	.61
1.5	.12	7	.38	15	.64
2.0	.15	8	.42	16	.71
2.5	.18	9	.45	17	.74
3	.20	10	.49	18	.76
4	.25	11	.52	19	.79
5	.29	12	.55	20	.82
		13	.58		

Figure 8–31.   Nomogram used to calculate body surface area. (Courtesy of Abbott Laboratories, North Chicago, IL.)

ticipation of future therapy. Gravity-fed intravenous flow rates below 10 ml/ hour reduce pressure to the point at which blood will regurgitate through the needle and tubing, and a clot may form. When solutions are administered too rapidly, speed shock occurs. Side reactions caused by rapid infusion vary with the drug. Nomograms are used to calculate body surface area (Fig. 8–31).

The physician, having decided on the volume to be administered, may prescribe his order in one of several ways: (1) 1000 ml every 8 hours, (2) 1000 ml at 50 ml/hour, (3) 30 drops (gtt)/min, or (4) KVO with 5 D/W.

Gravity Flow

To administer fluids from an intravenous container by gravity, the container must be supported above the patient in order for the solution to flow. The inverted container with the administration set in place is hung approximately 1 meter above the patient. Flow will not begin until the pinch clamp is opened and air is allowed to enter the container. For a plastic infusion container, however, air is not required for the solution to flow. As the solution leaves the container, it drops into a drip chamber (sight chamber). By collecting in this chamber, the solution can flow without allowing air to enter the length of administration tubing. The rate can be adjusted by counting the drops that enter the drip chamber. The clamp on the tubing is then adjusted to regulate flow (Fig. 8–32).

To determine the rate of flow requested, one must know the number of drops per milliliter delivered by the administration set being used; this varies with the commercial source. For example, if a set delivers 10 drops/ml and

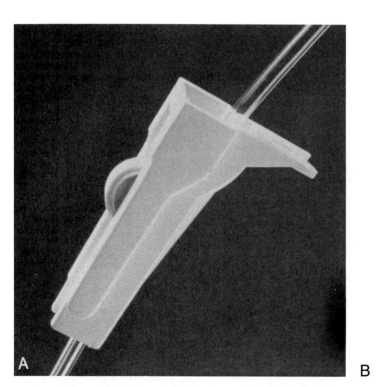

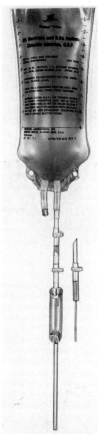

Figure 8–32. A, Abbott Cair Clamp used to regulate flow in infusion fluid. (Courtesy of Abbott Laboratories, North Chicago, IL.) B, Administration set adapter for reducing drop size to $1/50$ ml inserted into drip chamber of administration set. Set delivers 50 drops per ml, enabling the patient to receive a slow infusion. (Courtesy of Baxter Healthcare Laboratories, Inc., Deerfield, IL.)

1000 ml are to be infused over 480 minutes, then 1000 ml ÷ 480 = 2.08 ml/ min × 10 gtt/ml = 20.8 gtt = 21 gtt/min. If 50 ml/hour are to be infused, 0.83 ml/min × 10 = 8.3 gtt = 8 gtt/min. All manufacturers of intravenous fluids distribute calculators and charts for determining rates of flow (Fig. 8–33).

A needle is attached to the needle adaptor and the administration set is cleared of air by allowing the solution to fill the tubing. The clamp is closed and the venipuncture is made. The desired rate is now regulated. When stainless steel cannulas are used for intravenous administration, an 18- to 21-gauge, 1 1/2-in. needle is commonly used. Smaller scalp-vein needles are being used with increasing frequency, as are plastic needles.

Positive Pressure

The majority of infusion fluids are administered by the gravity method. Medical emergencies do arise, presenting situations in which fluids must be administered rapidly. For example, rapid infusion of blood is necessary in hemorrhage. Positive pressure administration sets that enable external pressure to be applied for rapid administration are available (Fig. 8–34).

Inaccuracies in Intravenous Flow Rates

Intravenous systems and administration sets are not precision devices. Fortunately, precision is not always required in the administration of I.V. fluids. When accurate and precise flow rates are required, however, other methods must be followed (see Pumps and Controllers, p. 158).

Accurate infusion rates ensure patient safety and drug efficiency. Inaccurate rates are contrary to rational drug therapy and can lead to delayed or toxic response in the patient, increased risk of phlebitis and thrombophlebitis, pulmonary edema, speed shock, and metabolic problems.

Gravity-flow I.V. systems are affected by the following factors, which may alter the flow during administration:

Volume.[15,16] Flow rate problems begin immediately upon arrival of the I.V. bottle into the hospital: (1) The liter container has, as a minimum, a rec-

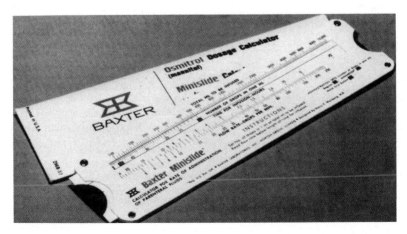

Figure 8–33. Calculator for determining rate of flow for a given volume of fluid over a set period of time. (Courtesy of Baxter Healthcare Laboratories, Inc., Deerfield, IL.)

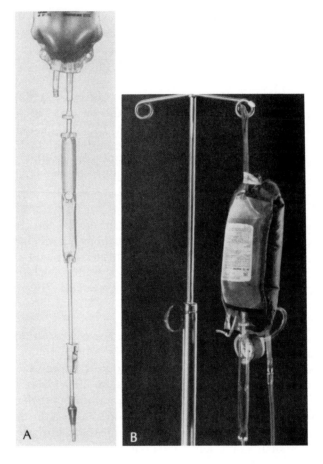

Figure 8–34. A, Positive pressure set permits fluids to run by gravity with a pressure unit available for rapid infusion should an emergency arise. B, Blood cuff with external pressure provides rapid infusion of blood. (Courtesy of Baxter Healthcare Laboratories, Inc., Deerfield, IL.)

ommended excess of 2 to 3%; (2) additives may be used at least 50% of the time. In the case of hyperalimentation, these additives may account for an additional 50 ml or more. Most often, these excesses in volume are not considered when flow rate calculations are made.

Variations in Size of Drip Chamber Orifice.[17,18] To be consistent and re-productive in flow, the orifices of the different drip chambers must be identical. Mass-produced administration sets are not precision instruments; therefore, some variances can be expected in flow.

Viscosity of Solution.[19,20] When a manufacturer states that an administration set delivers a specified number of drops per milliliter, viscosities of the various solutions have not been considered. The sets are calibrated for distilled water.

Twenty drops of 5% D/W will not deliver into a patient's vein the same volume as 20 drops of hyperalimentation solution. The viscosity of the solution will affect the size of the drop (and hence the volume) as it forms and leaves the orifice of the drip chamber. For example, parenteral hyperalimentation solutions have a greater specific gravity and form smaller-sized drops than do other I.V. solutions.

Plastic (Cold Flow).[19–21] Adjusting the rate of flow with a screw or roller clamp causes distortion of the plastic tubing. The nurse, leaving the administration set after flow rate is adjusted, has only to return in minutes to find the adjustment off 100% owing to changes in the bore diameter of the plastic tubing (cold flow).

Fonkalsrud et al. reported on the design of a new clamp.[21] In this study, the decrease in flow rate over the first hour was over 50%; whereas, the newly designed clamp (ARDL), a roller-type clamp, allows the tubing to be compressed at the edges. Thus, the area of tubing through which the fluid flows is under less stress. This clamp is patented by Abbott Laboratories under the name of CAIR (constant accurate infusion rate) clamp. A number of publications suggest that Silastic tubing may cause a lesser degree of error.[20]

Slipping of Clamps. To some small degree, the possibility exists for the force of gravity to reposition a set clamp. The result of the pull of gravity, of course, affects the rate of flow, and can result in a runaway I.V. injection.

Final Filters.[22] The use of final filters in the I.V. system may cause flow rates to decrease or even cease, depending on the degree of particulate matter blocking the filter surface.

Patient's Blood Pressure and Movements.[23] One study has shown clearly that body movements and blood pressure during I.V. therapy can affect the rate of flow.

Extravasation. Infiltration causes a decrease in flow rate because of the increased resistance to flow of the subcutaneous tissue.

Movement of Patient for Diagnostic Test. Often flow is interrupted by non-nursing personnel, or changed when patients are subjected to testing. Frequently, the established flow rate is not readjusted to the pretest rate. Additionally, when patients are transported, the solution container should be maintained at the same height, or the speed of the solution should be readjusted to the prescribed rate of flow.

Height of I.V. Container. I.V. fluids flow because of gravity. Any change in gravity caused by raising or lowering the container alters the rate of flow. Once the rate has been established, changes in the height of the container in relation to the patient will alter fluid flow.

Clot Formation.[19] Clot formation in the lumen of the cannula may alter or completely stop flow. Clot formation may occur when increased venous pressure results from blood pressure cuffs or restraints above the needle.

Kinked Tubing. Flow may be interrupted by patients lying on tubing. Complete blockage may occur if tubing is completely kinked. An innovation used to prevent kinked tubing of venipuncture sets has been developed.

Pressure Changes in I.V. Container.[19,21] As fluid is administered to the patient, pressures within the container change. This changing head pressure causes changes in rates in flow.

Rate of Flow.[17,24] An increase in drop rate results in the formation of larger drops. Rapid rates mean drop size can increase as much as 25%.

Obstructed vents and airway tubes on I.V. fluid can alter flow.

Shunting in the drip chamber[19,25] may cause drops to flow down the side of the drip chamber instead of dripping clearly.

Changes in needle position[26] may push the bevel of the needle against or away from wall of vein.

Temperature and Nature of Solutions.[26] Stimulation of vasoconstriction resulting from cold (blood) or irritating solutions may cause venous spasm with resultant changes in flow.

Trauma to Vein.[26] Injuries such as phlebitis or thrombosis reduce the lumen of the vein and decrease flow.

Y-sets and Multiple Solutions.[26] The rates should be reestablished when the patient receives two solutions simultaneously.

Demoruelle et al.,[27] in an extensive study of administration set flow rates, showed a percent change in flow rate at the end of the first hour of flow for 7 different sets to have a range of -63.1% to a $+50.5\%$. They suggested that the United States Pharmacopeial Convention establish standards for administration sets:

1. The average volume of fluid delivered should be within $\pm10\%$ of the theoretical volume.
2. The maximum number of flow rate adjustments necessary in 24 hours should be 10.
3. The maximum change in flow rate at the end of the first hour of operation should be $\pm33\%$.

Pumps and Controllers. Several manufacturers have developed pumps and controllers. When accurate constant flow rate is critical, as for parenteral nutrition solutions, pediatric therapy, or special drug therapy, mechanical devices are essential. The extensive use of infusion pumps in one hospital has been reported.[28] Several excellent evaluations of pumps have also been published.[29,30]

Manufacturers of I.V. systems have redesigned clamps and explored the development of more precise flow devices in an effort to achieve greater accuracy and efficiency in I.V. flow rates.

Flow Control in I.V. Therapy

Administration Sets

Currently, about 160 million I.V. administration sets are used to administer about 400 million I.V. fluids. They are *sterile, pyrogen-free,* relatively *inexpensive,* and basically simple to use. Their major drawback is lack of accuracy. With most I.V. fluid administration, some degree of error can be tolerated; however, when *accuracy* is required in I.V. administration such as TPN, drug therapy, and pediatric therapy, other methods must be considered. With *intra-arterial* therapy, methods other than gravity must be used.

Who Needs Control I.V. Flow?

Accurate infusion rates ensure patient safety and optimum drug efficacy; they promote physician compliance and conformance and ensure the desired drug response. Inaccurate rates are contrary to rational drug therapy and fail to comply with the physician's treatment. Inaccurate flow rates can:

1. lead to delayed or toxic patient response to drug therapy or I.V. therapy,
2. increase the possibility of phlebitis and thrombophlebitis,
3. complicate infiltrations,
4. cause pulmonary edema, which may lead to impaired renal and cardiac function,
5. cause speed shock,
6. create metabolic problems.

One of the primary functions of an I.V. therapist is to *maintain constant accurate flow rate.* This is a difficult order when one considers the problems confronted by the nurse. The demands of the workload from physicians, patients, and administration, and of laboratory, dietary, and other clinical activities, make it difficult to meet the above requirement. Above all, the nurse can be defeated from the very start by the myriad of mechanical and physical problems associated with current I.V. delivery systems, which have already been discussed.

Although various infusion pumps and controllers are used in hospitals across the country, only a limited number of publications attest to their desirability. This is understandable considering their recent appearance in hospitals. The use of pumps with heparin,[31-33] parenteral hyperalimentation,[34-37] lidocaine,[38] and oxytocin[39] has been reported. Their use with hyperalimentation of the newborn[40] and in aircraft[41] has also been reported. Several publications[42-44] reported on the use of I.V. controllers, and one publication[45] described the utility of pumps in reducing the volume of fluid infused. Several excellent evaluations[46,47] of various pumps have been published, including one[48] concerning inspection and preventive maintenance of infusion pumps.

Pumps

Turco[49] stated, "Disadvantages of pumps are extra cost and personnel training required for their use, in addition to bedside clutter and electrical hazards." Kopezynski[41] commented "consequently a simple form of treatment such as I.V. infusion is apparently to be made more complicated for the medical crew member with the introduction of a new form of equipment. This problem cannot be avoided; however, it is not serious enough to prevent acceptance of this device." Martinez[40] found pumps satisfactory when used for parenteral hyperalimentation of the newborn; however, when used in adults for whom less nursing care was available, the lack of consistency and accuracy and the absence of safety features created many problems. Some of these problems, such as air embolism despite the use of filters, I.V. solution bags running dry, and clotted catheters, were catastrophic. Monahan and Webb[45] suggest that, with the use of pumps, infiltration can be more serious than the gravity flow system, i.e., the hazard of air emboli is more significant. In a survey,[50] users of infusion pumps reported a variety of problems including "inaccurate flow rate and volume delivered, nonconstant flow rate, a lag time between change of setting and change of drop rate, inadequate alarms, complexity of operation, placing tubing in wrong way, possibility of contamination with use of syringe pumps, air in cassette of a small piston pump, possible damage to blood being pumped, possible overload of fluid if device fails, required use of special tubing, possible damage to tubing if the pump head is dirty, patients may 'play with the pumps,' change the settings, and turn off the alarms and others." Emergency Care Research Institute (ECRI)[51] reported on one type of pump and the electrical hazard it presented if not grounded properly. Electrical hazards can also be present with the use of electrosurgical equipment.[52] ECRI[53] reported on the potential shock hazard associated with a battery charger of one pump. Bubble formation in a roller type pump has been reported;[54] the source of air was the pumping element material. Insertion of Luer connectors into pump chambers[55] has precipitated rupture. Croke et al.[56] reported on pseudoarrhythmia as a result of a defective infusion pump and ECG monitor; a defective pump connecting pin caused artifact. ECRI set an error limit of 10% for delivery of fluid to the critically ill; however, in several studies[46,47] of 9 infusion pumps, 6 had an error rate of greater than 10%.

Many of the problems or potential problems in pump technology were resolved by the manufacturer as they were reported.

ECRI[46,47] has evaluated infusion pumps in their application to parenteral nutrition and listed 26 factors of performance and safety criteria.

Robinson et al.[57] reviewed a pharmacy-based infusion pump program and outlined plans for use, quality control, selection, economic justification, and revenue generation. An excellent review[58] of I.V. pumps described a nurse's viewpoint of the various pumps available.

Rapp et al.[59] reported on the cost savings and safety of electronic infusion control. Emergency Care Research Institute completed an in-depth evaluation of infusion controllers.[60] Kelly et al.[61] attempted to classify electronic controllers and pumps according to the type of drug used and the clinical condition of the patient. This paper presented a logical method for instrument selection. A recently published sourcebook[62] on control-drug delivery presents the potential complications and problems associated with electronic equipment as well as the proper use and selection of the equipment in hospitals. An annual buyers' guide[63] of pumps and controllers has been published, illustrating all those available and their specifications.

We have seen a proliferation of pump devices for the general administration of I.V. fluids (Fig. 8–35). Although pumps have been available for many years for intraarterial pressure infusions, we are led to believe that they should also be used for general I.V. use. Eliminating the consideration of pumps for pressure infusions where they are an absolute necessity, the major claim for them is a greater degree of accuracy (most manufacturers claim accuracy ±2%). This degree of accuracy, however, has been questioned. Other advantages claimed by some pump manufacturers are savings of nurses' time and the detection of infiltrations or occlusions and air.

In general, two pumping mechanisms are employed: piston-cylinder and peristaltic.

1. *Piston-Cylinder.* Movement of a piston in a cylinder produces a pressure sufficient to expel the fluid contents of the cylinder. Moving diaphragm pumps are also included here. The terms "syringe pump" and "volumetric pump" are often used to describe devices having this pumping action.

2. *Peristaltic.* Movement of the wall of the pumping chamber as a result of an externally applied force produces a pressure sufficient to expel fluid contents of the pumping chamber. The lumen of the tubular pumping chamber

is totally or nearly totally occluded by the external force; as the point of occlusion moves along the tube, the fluid is propelled by the resultant increases of pressure.

The peristaltic pumping mechanism can be further classified in two subdivisions: *rotary* and *linear*. In rotary peristaltic pumping, the tubular pumping chamber is arranged in a somewhat semicircular shape and the point of contact, usually provided by a roller, moves around the semicircular pumping chamber, making contact with the chamber at the beginning of the semicircle and breaking contact at the opposite end, thus propelling fluid through the pumping chamber. In some rotary peristaltic pumps, the lumen of the pumping chamber is occluded by forcing the tubing against a stationary, semicircular backing plate. In other designs, the lumen is occluded by forcing the roller against one side of the tubing and allowing tension in the tubing to provide the resistance necessary to allow occlusion. In linear peristaltic pumping, the tubular pumping chamber is straight and the point of contact moves along the pumping chamber. Most of these pumps have a row of "fingers," which sequentially press the tubing against a stationary backing plate; thus, a wave-like motion of the wall propels fluid through the pumping chamber.

There is some concern with the administration of blood utilizing infusion pumps (Fig. 8–36) and the effect of the pumping mechanism upon red blood cells (RBCs). Strayer et al.[64] studied the effect of a multipurpose infusion pump (MMT-9500) on RBCs. This particular pump had no effect upon the integrity of whole blood, packed red blood cells, and platelets.

In another study, Burch et al.[65] used a linear peristaltic pump on a variety of blood products and a range of infusion rates. No substantial degree of hemolysis was found.

Gibson et al.[66] reported a tenfold higher concentration of plasma-free hemoglobin infused by means of a peristaltic pump.

With the increasing use of portable infusion pumps, studies of stability in these devices are appearing in the literature. Stiles et al.[67] studied three cephalosporins and penicillin G in the Pharmacia Deltec CADD-VT portable infusion pump. Cefazolin sodium, cefoxitin sodium, cefatazidime, and penicillin G sodium in admixtures with sterile water for injection were found to be stable when stored in the reservoirs and frozen at $-20°$ C for 30 days and then refrigerated for 4 days at $5°$ C. With the exception of penicillin G sodium, no significant loss of activity was observed after the drugs were pumped at body temperature for one day.

In a follow up study, Stiles et al.[68] studied the stability of fluorouracil in four different portable infusion pumps (Pharmacia Deltec CADD-I, Cormed II, Med Fusion Provider). Fluorouracil was stable in all pump systems over a 7-day period at $37°$ C.

Tu et al.[69] studied the stability of Gentamicin Sulfate administered by Pharmacia Deltec CADD-VT pump. No significant concentration changes occurred throughout a 36-day period.

Altman et al.[70] studied the stability of Morphine Sulfate in Cormed III intravenous bags. This study showed that solutions of Morphine Sulfate 0.5 to 60 mg/mL stored at 5 or $37°$ C were stable for 14 days in Kalex bags, except for 60 mg/mL solutions stored at $5°$ C for 9 days or longer.

Allen[71] found Fentanyl Citrate in 0.9% sodium chloride solution stable for

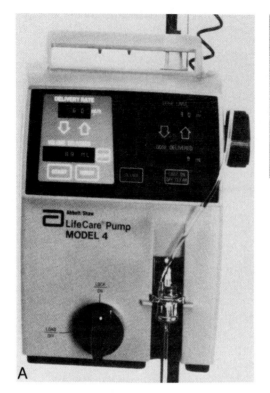

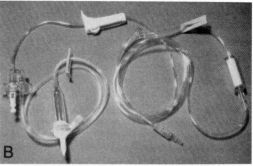

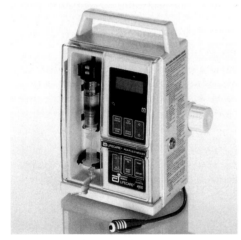

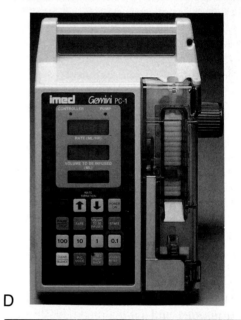

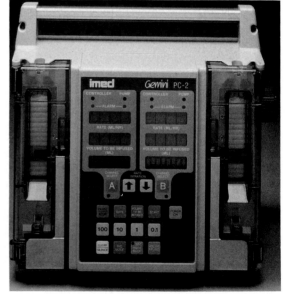

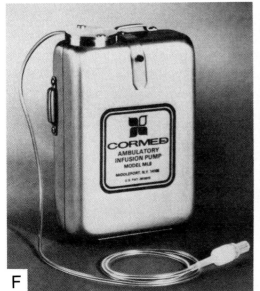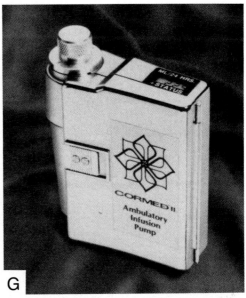

Figure 8–35. Infusion pumps. A, Abbott/Shaw LifeCare Model 4 pump. B, Administration set for A. C, Abbott Lifecare PCA 4100 infusor. (A–C courtesy of Abbott Laboratories, North Chicago, IL.) D, E, Gemini PC-1 and PC-2 controllers. (D and E courtesy of IMED Corporation, San Diego, CA.) F, G, Cormed ambulatory infusion pumps. (F and G courtesy of Cormed Inc., Medina, NY.)

30 days in PVC reservoirs for portable infusion pumps. Tu[72] found Fentanyl Citrate and Bupivacaine in an admixture with 0.9% Sodium Chloride injection stable when stored for 30 days at 3° or 23° C with or without overwraps in portable pump reservoirs. Rochard et al.[73] studied Fluorouracil Cytarabine and Doxorubicin Hydrochloride in Ethylene Vinylacetate portable infusion pump reservoirs and found these drugs relatively stable. Stiles[74] et al. studied Ondansetron Hydrochloride and found stability when it was stored for 30 days at 3° C and then administered by portable infusion pump over 24 hours at 30° C.

The increasing use of portable infusion pumps will necessitate continual compatibility studies.

Controllers

Many individuals are not able to differentiate between pump devices and controllers. Controllers work on the concept of gravity and exert no pressure; they count drops electrically or extrude volumes of fluid mechanically and electronically (Fig. 8–37). They are less complex than pump devices and usually less expensive. They have no *moving components*, which could mean fewer maintenance problems. They are generally less sophisticated, but they achieve ±2% drop rate accuracy (as stated by the manufacturer) in a gravity-type I.V. flow. They present difficulty with the administration of viscous solutions such as blood or oral alimentation. With one company, IVAC, any standard administration set can be used; the Burron Epic requires a special set that contains a chamber housing a ball bearing that electronically and magnetically deter-

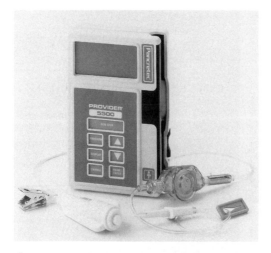

A

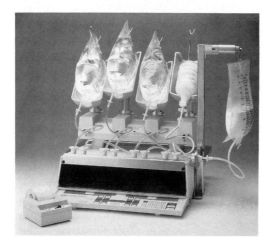

Figure 8–36.   Pumps. A, The Lifecare Provider 5500 Portable Infusion Pump can be used for continuous epidural administration. B, The Abbott Nutrimix Macro Compounder for Automated TPN Compounder for automated TPN compounding. C, The Abbott/Omni-Flow 4000 4-channel Programmable Multiple Medication Infusion System. (Courtesy of Abbott Laboratories, North Chicago, IL.)

B

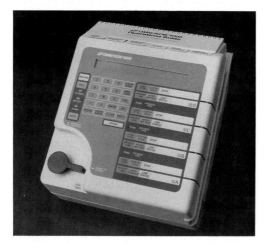

C

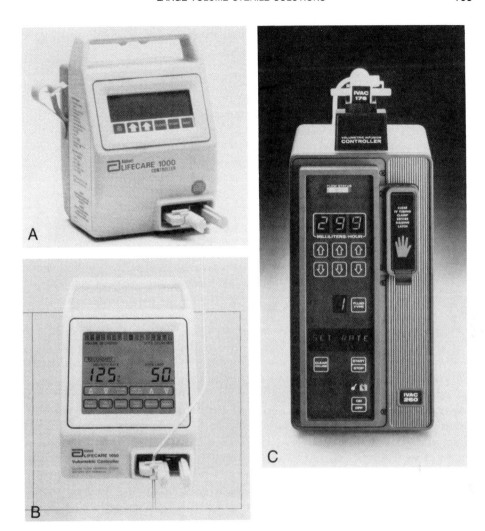

Figure 8–37. Controllers. A, Abbott LifeCare 1000 Controller. B, Abbott LifeCare 1050 Volumetric Controller. C, IVAC 260 Volumetric Infusion Controller. (A, Courtesy of Abbott Laboratories, North Chicago, IL. C, Courtesy of IVAC Corporation, San Diego, CA.)

mines the movement of the ball. It would seem logical that controllers that cost less, require less training, have fewer problems mechanically, and achieve reasonable accuracy (±2% drop rate as stated by manufacturer's brochure) be the device of choice. This could be the case with uncomplicated therapy when some degree of inaccuracy can be tolerated with minimal safeguards.

Requirements of Ideal Pumps and Controllers

These devices should be:
1. Mechanically sound.
2. Mechanically reliable. Flow rate should be accurate within ± 10%, repeatable, and constant.
3. Of a maximum output pressure that will not damage injection site or cause extravasation.

4. Equipped with battery option when power failures occur.
5. Compact.
6. Portable.
7. Reasonably priced.
8. Easy to operate.
9. Constructed to permit cleaning and sterilizing.
10. Equipped with alarm to signal depletion of I.V. solution and stop pump.
11. Equipped with other alarms to detect malfunction, battery depletion, infiltration, and excessive output pressure.
12. In compliance with all electrical safety standards for hospital use. (See Appendix 5)

Selection of Infusion Devices

Many hospitals that have acquired infusion devices have failed to develop an organized approach to the utilization of such devices. Often, infusion devices are chosen for specific purposes. Later, as the devices become commonplace in the institution, they are used in a greater variety of ways. As with any new procedure, there may be some justification for trial and error experimentation, but an organized approach for the use of devices will allow full and effective usage of the equipment in the safest manner possible.

It is no small wonder that some confusion currently exists regarding the selection of the appropriate device. A rapidly growing technology has produced shifts in thinking among the users as to the choice of device for a particular use. It is generally accepted that most infusion device problems originate from a poor understanding of the device on the user's part rather than from the instrument itself. Those contemplating the selection and purchase of instruments should give immediate consideration to at least the following:

1. Infusion devices introduce technologic complexity and demand a greater degree of user understanding.
2. Personnel must be trained in the use of the equipment.
3. Apparent operational costs (the cost of the devices and sets) may increase. Total institutional cost may actually decrease, however, because problems associated with conventional I.V. therapy are often reduced or eliminated.
4. The equipment must be maintained.
5. In a rapidly changing technical area such as infusion devices, the equipment can soon become outdated.
6. There may be a limitation on the number of infusion devices any one institution is capable of purchasing. Therefore, patient selection is a factor for consideration.

Justification for Infusion Devices

As reported in the literature, infusion devices:

Provide accurate and timely delivery of fluids and drugs.
Can change the flow rate when needed.
Provide controlled limitation of fluid intake.

Minimize the number of I.V. infusion checks required of the nurse.

Reduce infiltration rates.

Reduce the occurrence of infusion phlebitis.

Reduce the cost of I.V. therapy.

Save nursing time.

Allow intra-arterial administration of drugs.

Reduce the incidence of runaway I.V.s, plugged needles, and empty bottle conditions.

Reduce the incidence of dehydration caused by insufficient fluid replacement.

Permit accurate small-volume delivery of drugs and fluids.

Permit accurate large-volume delivery of drugs and fluids.

Simplify I.V. therapy.

Enable the hospital staff to meet pharmaceutical companies' recommendations on many selected drugs, e.g., nitroprusside, streptokinase, dopamine.

Reduce the incidence of infection by maintaining catheter patency and by avoiding occluded catheters.

Avoid gastric distension, emesis, and aspiration in enteral nutrition.

Permit the administration of a constant rate of flow of vasopressin, counteracting volume depletion while bleeding is controlled in life-threatening hemorrhage from peptic ulcer.

Permit patients to undergo arterial infusions of chemotherapeutic agents directly into the target organ while leading a more normal life.

Committee for Instrument Selection

A hospital committee for the selection of proper infusion devices should be established.[75] The committee should have representation from nursing service, biomedical, medical staff, anesthesia, purchasing, and administration. The nursing service representatives should include nursing specialists from the intensive care, emergency room, and medical and surgical units. If enteral instruments are used, representation from the dietary department is needed.

The committee should define the problems associated with I.V. therapy in the institution. Incident reports can be a source of information. Reports of phlebitis, infiltrations, restarts, inaccurate drug delivery, and other related I.V. problems often can help determine the type of infusion equipment needed.

Once the problems experienced in the institution are pinpointed, input regarding solutions to the problems can be gathered. Careful consideration of the following factors might help identify needs.

Requirements for rate control with high pressure.

Requirements for rate control without high pressure.

Pressure required for arterial lines.

Capabilities of pumps and controllers.

Intensity of drug therapy, type of patient, and length of hospital stay.

Hospital mix of equipment.

Small-volume infusion delivery needs.

Hospital occupancy rate.

Average daily I.V.s

Number of pediatric beds.
Special care beds.
Who monitors I.V.s: floor nurse or I.V team.
Consultation with other institutions for information and experiences.

The committee may invite a manufacturer to give a presentation. At the presentation, consideration should be given to such equipment factors as:

Simplicity of operation.
Weight.
Ease of use.
Hospital compatibility of instrument.
Hazards associated with instrument.
Cost considerations; lease versus purchase.
Company ability to respond to service, inservice programs for life of the instruments.

Once the equipment has been purchased, inservice of equipment through-out the hospital is performed. Responsibility for and control of the equipment must be established; control may be a nursing service, I.V. team, or pharmacy responsibility. Responsibility for maintenance, cleaning, and care of the equipment must be established.

Criteria For Using Infusion Devices

General Use

When a greater degree of accuracy is desired than is achievable using gravity-fed manual clamp methods:

When positive pressure is required to override vessel pressure, such as with intra-arterial therapy, or additive resistances in the I.V. line.
When significant morbidity is associated with drug extravasation.
Where a danger of fluid overload exists.
For complicated drug dosage regimens.
When there is a specification from a pharmaceutical manufacturer.
When instrumentation provides an effective method of risk reduction.

Nutrition

Total parenteral nutrition.
Enteral alimentation: stomach or jejunum.
I.V. fat.
Vitamin/mineral preparation.
Pediatric formulas.

Fluid Administration

Critical care fluid management.
Pediatric fluid management.
Restricted fluid situations.
Blood and blood products.
Controlled clinical trials.
General electrolyte administration.

Drug Therapy

Continuous drug therapy.
Chemotherapy.
Intra-arterial infusions.
Oxytocic agents.
Regional heparinization.
Antiarrhythmic agents.
Pressor agents.
Bronchoactive agents.
Hypoglycemic agents.
Anticoagulants.
Cardiovascular drugs.
Neonatology drug therapy.
Corticosteroids.
I.V. anesthetics.
Anti-infective agents.
Muscle relaxants.
Antihypertensives.

Other Uses

Closed wound irrigation.
Keep-vein-open (KVO) for central lines, e.g., cardiac catheter, intra-arterial infusions.
Peritoneal dialysis.

Home Use

Parenteral and enteral nutrition.
Insulin therapy.
Oncology therapy.
Antibiotic therapy.

Patient Complications

Restarts.
Infiltration morbidity with drug extravasation.
Runaways.
Phlebitis.
Fluid overload.
Complicated drug dosage regimens.

On some occasions, not enough infusion instruments may be available for every potential use. The following priority list may be used for determining which drugs or nutritional products receive priority to be administered by means of an infusion instrument. When such an occasion arises, infusion instruments will be removed from patients receiving the drugs/nutrition, starting at the bottom of the list (5) with the oral alimentation group.

1. Drugs administered by constant infusion that require frequent dose adjustments and have a small therapeutic:toxic ratio. These drugs must be administered by an infusion pump or controller: dobutamine, dopamine, isoproterenol, lidocaine, nitroglycerin, nitroprusside, procainamide, ri-

todrine, and vasopressin. Improper infusion rates for these drugs may become life-threatening within minutes.

When it is necessary to remove an infusion pump from a patient for a higher priority infusion, the intravenous infusion bottles should contain no more than a 6- to 8-hour supply of solution. They should be labeled with the appropriate rate and time for the infusion.

2. Drugs that are administered at a fixed hourly rate that, when properly used, may have the dose changed every few hours. Improper infusion rates may be life-threatening within hours. These drugs include aminocaproic acid, antineoplastics, heparin, insulin, morphine, naloxone, oxytocin, streptokinase, I.V. solutions given by Hickman catheter, and total parenteral nutrition by a central line.

3. Drugs that are administered at a fixed hourly rate that, when properly used, may require a dose adjustment every few days. Because of drug toxicity, the use of an infusion pump is strongly recommended. Aminophylline falls into this category.

4. I.V. fluids administered to patients with severe fluid restrictions.

5. Oral alimentation preparations that are administered at a fixed hourly rate that, when properly used, may require a rate change every few days. If they are administered without an infusion pump, the immediate threat to the patient is minimal.

Standardized Concentration For Drugs Administered By Constant Infusion

Standardized concentration of drugs used for instrumentation can simplify procedures and help minimize errors. An example from one hospital is reproduced below:[76]

> Various concentrations of drugs are frequently prescribed for the administration of drugs by constant infusion. This leads to confusion when the rates of infusion must be changed.
>
> The following drugs given by constant infusion, and their recommended concentrations, have been approved by a hospital staff committee. These concentrations can be changed if the clinical situation requires a more concentrated solution. Charts indicating flow rates for each concentration are available from the department of pharmacy. A similar list should be adopted in each hospital as a safety and quality assurance measure.
>
> aminophylline 1 g/250 ml and 1 g/500 ml
> dobutamine 250 mg/ml
> dopamine 400 mg/250 ml
> isoproterenol 1 mg/250 ml
> lidocaine 1 g/500 ml and 2 g/500 ml
> heparin 20,000 units/L and 30,000 units/L
> morphine 50 mg/250 ml
> insulin 50 units/500 ml
> nitroprusside 50 mg/250 ml and 100 mg/250 ml
> vasopressin 100 units/250 ml
> ritodrine 150 mg/500 ml
> epinephrine 2 mg/250 ml
> norepinephrine 4 mg/250 ml

The department of pharmacy provides constant flow charts for all of these standard drug solutions to expedite dosage calculation as well as changes in flow rate.

The following are the Recommendations of Practice for the National Intravenous Therapy Association as they relate to infusion devices.[77]

Mechanical Controlling Devices

Mechanical controlling devices are used to provide minimal deviation from the prescribed medical order in the delivery of solutions and/or medications, thus reducing the risk of possible I.V. complications.

Recommendations For Infusion Devices

1. Delivery of all aspects of I.V. therapy shall be controlled with minimal deviation from the prescribed rate ordered.
2. The use of gravity-feed mechanical devices (I.V. controllers) is advocated for the majority delivery of I.V. therapy.
3. The use of pressure-feed mechanical devices (I.V. pumps) is recommended for controlling I.V. delivery when a specified accuracy of I.V. delivery is mandatory due to patient risk.
4. I.V. pumps should maintain I.V. delivery without stringent deviation from the prescribed medical order, and their accuracy or deviated limit (plus or minus) shall be stated by the manufacturer.
5. All I.V. electronic devices shall be routinely cleaned and checked for possible malfunctions.
6. The use of electronic mechanical controlling infusion devices shall be prioritized and stated by hospital policy in the I.V. Policy and Procedures Manual.
7. The registered professional I.V. nurse shall be proficient and knowledgeable in the use of mechanical controlling devices within the health care facility.
8. Operating instructions for electronic mechanical I.V. controlling devices shall be affixed to the device.
9. Audible and visible alarms to detect air, deviated flow, occlusion, and any other deviations placing the patient at risk shall be integrated within the mechanical infusion device.
10. If the mechanical controlling device is battery operated, the life and potency of the battery should be ascertained and changed accordingly.
11. Mechanical electronic controlling devices should be patient-tamperproof.

Methods for emulating the accuracy of flow-regulatory devices have been described by Carleton et al.[78]

Patient-Controlled Analgesia (PCA)

Pain Management

Usually and traditionally, the acute or chronic pain experienced by patients in selected diseases is treated initially by oral narcotics and analgesics. However, many clinical situations preclude oral administration. Typically, pain from disease has been treated by parenteral analgesics given by the I.M. or S.C. route.

This medication cycle from patient complaint to pain relief can often be lengthy. Frequently, the dose administered can be too large or too small, resulting in either sedation or poor pain relief.

Parenteral drugs given I.V. offer rapid distribution in the body and fast onset of action. The drug undergoes no biotransformation or inactivation, and therefore allows more precise dose management.

PCA

Patient-controlled analgesia (PCA) is a system for delivery of intravenous or SC narcotics by direct patient intervention. This therapy utilizes a mechanical electronic infusion control device. This device gives the patient the ability to self-administer analgesics in proportion to the degree of relief desired.

Several of these devices have been developed and are undergoing development at Bard, Abbott, Pharmacia Deltec, Baxter Healthcare, and Becton Dickinson. The early initial device allowed patient-triggered I.V. doses; later, refinement in the microprocessors allowed tailoring of infusions so that additional bolus doses could be given to a baseline infusion. Additional developments have led to ambulatory PCA devices that are small enough to be worn on a belt. An additional design being used is a balloon-powered device that operates mechanically from an inflated balloon, this device is disposable (Baxter Healthcare, Becton Dickinson).

In its simplest terms, PCA allows a patient to initiate an intravenous infusion of a prescribed narcotic analgesic and maintain a self regulated small amount of an incremental dose needed for controlling a variety of pain associated medical problems.

The success and popularity of PCA are based upon the inadequacy of conventional IM and IV dosing (Fig. 8–38) such as variables that effect absorption and distribution.[79] Conservative nursing practices and inherent procedure cause delays in securing medications and ultimate administration to the patient (Fig. 8–39).[80] The perception and sensation of pain in any one patient depend upon individual levels of endorphins and other biochemicals in cerebrospiral fluid.[81] The last several years, have seen the increasing use of infusion devices for epidural or intrathecal administration.

Patient-controlled analgesia (PCA) eliminates the peak-and-valley effects of traditional drug therapy. Epidural or intrathecal therapy of PCA allows a longer duration of drug action.

Kwan[82] has reviewed the use of infusion devices for epidural or intrathecal administration.

Future Trends For Infusion Devices

The quality of patient care has been improved by the increasing use of sensitive infusion devices. With proper use of these devices, flow rates can be maintained, and parenteral and enteral nutrition can be safely conducted. Technical advances have come quickly in the field of electronic infusion devices, and progress shows no sign of slowing. Research is being done on closed-loop infusion, where drug response or body chemical concentrations is coordinated by the infusion device. The future promises ever-greater safety and efficiency.

Plastic Medical Components

Early experiments with parenteral packaging material utilized such materials as pigs' bladders and goat skins. The disadvantages of these materials are obvious.

Glass appeared to solve the packaging problems for parenteral products. Glass is a relatively inexpensive, clear, stable material that can be shaped, sterilized, sealed, and handled; however, it is still far from being the ideal container. Breakage, disposability, weight, and increased cost have led to the increased development and use of "plastic" for parenteral packaging. "Plastic" is a term used generally to describe a variety of compounds of high molecular weight that can be molded to shape, hardness, and clarity.

Devices and Materials Used in Parenteral Medical Practice

Plastic devices used for parenteral medical practice include
1. Disposable syringes (polyethylene, polypropylene, polycarbonate).
2. I.V. solution administration sets (polyvinylchloride [PVC]).
3. Plastic I.V. catheters (Teflon, polypropylene).
4. Blood containers (polyvinylchloride).
5. I.V. solution containers (polyvinylchloride, Viaflex, LifeCare, polyolefin, Accumed).
6. Irrigating solutions, (polyolefins, polyethylene, polypropylene) (McGaw, Baxter Healthcare, Abbott).

Plastic components, like rubber formulations, may contain a variety of additives to enhance the quality desired for their use. The basic polymer (plastic) may contain *plasticizers* to give flexibility to the package, as in the LifeCare or Viaflex containers. *Antioxidants* are added to prevent discoloration. Plastic devices are produced with heat and pressure, which may result in the need for *stabilizing agents. Fillers* may be added to enhance the formulation. *Antistatic agents* are sometimes needed to prevent clinging of the material. *Colorants* may be necessary for some devices. *Lubricants* are added to facilitate removal from the production molds.

Some common plastic materials used in medical devices are listed below:

Polyethylene. Various densities are available (low, medium, high). A relatively inert, opaque material containing no plasticizer. A common ingredient of plastic syringes.

Polypropylene. Similar to polyethylene, it is relatively inert. Many grades are sterilizable. A common ingredient of plastic syringes.

Polyvinylchloride. Available in a variety of formulations. Available in a relatively clear, inert, sterilizable container. When 30 to 40% of a phalate ester is added to the formula, this product can be flexible. Polyvinylchloride formulations are used to manufacture plastic I.V. bags (Viaflex, LifeCare). All I.V. tubing administration sets are polyvinylchloride formulations.

Polystyrene. An inexpensive, rigid clear type of plastic material; however,

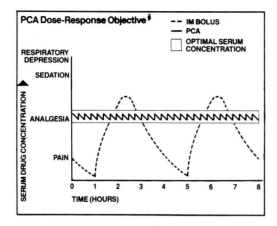

Figure 8–38. Characteristic pattern comparison of IM bolus serum concentration vs PCA

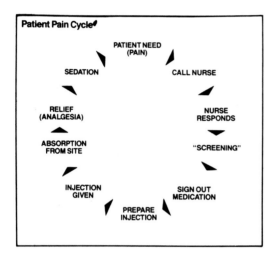

Figure 8–39. Patient pain cycle—sequence of events

not very inert. Will react with paraldehyde and other materials. Has a low melting temperature and cannot be heat sterilized.

Nylon. A stable, inert, generally opaque material. Can be made and used where hardness is necessary (e.g., spike I.V. sets, filters in blood sets).

Polymethylmethacrylate (Lucite). A relatively expensive, stable, hard material used to make needle adapters on I.V. sets.

Polyolefins (polyethylene and polypropylene). A mixture of two compounds produces a rigid or semi-rigid formulation. Contains no plasticizer. Available in use for McGaw, Baxter Healthcare, and Abbott irrigation containers. Currently available in McGaw I.V. container (Accumed).

A common I.V. administration set may combine a variety of plastic components tailored to suit a particular need. For example, an administration set contains a nylon spike, a Lucite Y-site, a polyvinylchloride tube, and a polypropylene clamp.

Medical Considerations of Plastic Containers for Parenteral Use

Numerous factors are involved in considering plastic material for parenteral use: vapor transmission, sterilization qualities, texture, clarity, weight, aging, ease of production, ease of destruction, ultimate method of use, inertness, chemical reactivity of the plastic material with the drug, binding, leaching and, probably most important, biologic safety. Medical uses of plastic materials are increasing at an accelerated pace as a result of the many advantages of plastics, such as disposability, lightness, cost. Current technology, however, does not permit the formulation of the ideal container (whatever that may be) for a particular medical use. Usually, a compromise of one or some of the desired qualities and attributes must be made.

A new concept in the packaging of intravenous fluids, Viaflex, was introduced into the United States in 1971 by Travenol (now Baxter Healthcare) Laboratories. Abbott Laboratories introduced a similar container, LifeCare. These soft, flexible plastic bags have some advantages over the traditional glass containers. The most outstanding feature of this type of container is its ability to respond to normal outside atmospheric pressure, with the result that no venting is required. Because of its rigidity, a glass container must be vented to allow solution to flow. The closed system of bags may mean that the threat of contaminating air entering by the usual methods is eliminated. Hansen and Hepler[83] studied glass systems and the Viaflex and concluded that the Viaflex system offered significantly better protection against contamination by airborne microbes than did other systems. Paretz et al.,[84] however, found the incidence of contamination with Viaflex containers to be 5 times greater than that with glass (6.9% for Viaflex, 1.3% for glass). The source of contamination was unclear but "touch" appeared to play an important role. The possibility of air embolism is significantly reduced in the use of flexible plastic containers; however, the possibility of air embolism is greater when flexible plastic units are connected in a series of containers. Therefore, this type of hook-up is not recommended.

Flexible containers are nonbreakable; however, accidental punctures can create a point of entry for microorganisms.[85] Additions of drugs through the additive port with a needle can cause puncture of the plastic.[86] Flexible plastic containers are lighter and consume less space than glass. They are thought to be easier to handle and dispose of, although this point has been questioned.[86,87] Some workers suggest that the lack of rigidity presents problems when manipulation is required. Studies have shown that plastic I.V. containers have less particulate matter than do glass containers.[88] Other studies have shown generation of colloidal-sized material after agitation and unusual manipulation. Needham and Luzzi[89] have identified this material as di-2-ethylhexylphthalate (DEHP), although the labeled maximum of 5 ppm was not exceeded.

Incomplete mixing of drugs[90] added to intravenous solutions is more likely to occur with plastic bags than with glass. This poor mixing is partly a result of pooled drug at the injection site, and the manufacturer has taken steps to correct this. Proper mixing precautions are noted in the manufacturer's brochure. Significant amounts of some drugs may be adsorbed to the bag. Several drugs are known not to be adsorbed, but for many the amount of adsorption is unknown.[90] The Medical Letter, commenting on flexible plastic I.V. bags, noted that they are convenient but can adsorb some drugs out of solution and may introduce chemicals into solution, and summarized that plastic containers have not proven more reliable than glass in protecting against contamination of I.V. fluids. The reader is referred to the last published review of plastic containers.[87]

I.V. Teams

In past years, intravenous therapy was generally uncomplicated, consisting chiefly of supplying simple fluids to fasting patients. With better understanding of fluids and drug therapy and parenteral nutrition, intravenous therapy has become increasingly complex. A better understanding of the problems associated with intravenous therapy (e.g., contamination, particulation) has also enlightened medical care workers so that specialized expert training is required for those who administer injections. This has led to the development of specialized groups: the American Association of I.V. Therapists and the Intravenous Nursing Society. The sole concern of these groups is to provide expert patient care in intravenous therapy. To accomplish these goals, educational meetings, journal publications, and *The Journal of Intravenous Nursing*, which is the official publication of the Intravenous Nursing Society, have been utilized. The concept of intravenous teams has evolved from these specialty groups. Sophisticated medicine requires sophisticated I.V. therapy. The initiation and justification for I.V. teams have been reported by Kelly et al.,[91] Kimmell,[92] and Godfrey.[93] Willett[94] describes the development of an I.V. team in a small hospital. The nature of parenteral medication will require the growth and proliferation of I.V. teams in the future. The complex legal and ethical nature of parenteral therapy will demand that specialized groups of trained individuals perform intravenous therapy.

National Coordinating Committee on Large Volume Parenterals

The National Coordinating Committee on Large Volume Parenterals (NCCLVP), a group cosponsored by the U.S.P. and the FDA, is financed by an FDA contract. This committee was established in 1971 to deal with problems of concern in large-volume parenterals. Those concerns were partly precipitated by a national outbreak of contaminated I.V. fluids.[95] Representation on the committee was drawn from many national organizations, including the four manufacturers of LVPs. The initial research was to determine the problems. The bibliography and literature review on the ecology of LVPs in hospitals was completed in August, 1973.[96] A master list describing 167 problems associated with LVPs was generated from a national sample of 26 hospitals. Identification of the component procedures and techniques used by hospital personnel in preparing and administering LVPs was also established by this committee, as were guidelines to the type of personnel and training for those who give LVPs in hospitals. From the list of 167 problems, 39 were targeted as top priority. Four expert working subcommittees dealt with these problems: Microbial and Pyrogenic Contamination; Particulate and Chemical Contamination; Incompatibilities and Stability, Delivery, and Recall; and the Dissemination of Information and TPN. A list of 35 top priority problems and recommendations was published.[97]

Other important accomplishments of the NCCLVP were the development and publication of a document entitled "Recommended Methods for Compounding Intravenous Admixtures in Hospitals."[98] This detailed set of procedures[98] was sent to all hospitals with the purpose of instructing how to compound and administer LVPs so that the quality built into the product by the manufacturer is maintained all the way to the bedside. A third document produced and published was a "Recommended System for Surveillance and Reporting of Problems with Large Volume Parenterals in Hospitals."[99] This is an early-warning system of procedures that is designed to detect problems of LVPs immediately and to transmit the alert to FDA, CDC, and state and local health authorities. It interphases with the Drug Product Defect Reporting System.

The committee also developed "Test Methods for Particulate Matter in LVPs." An expert panel recommended the standards that became official in the first supplement to *U.S.P. XIX*. A report[100] approved by the Subcommittee on Incompatibilities and Instabilities of the NCCLVP discussed recommendations to hospitals, manufacturers, pharmacists, physicians, and FDA and/or USP concerning the problems associated with incompatibilities. Additional discussion included problems with formulation, administration, and packaging material. The literature concerning incompatibilities was also presented. Two additional documents were published concerning labeling and testing of LVPs.[101,102]

Trends and Developments in I.V. Delivery Systems

The hospital pharmacy's potential involvements in the dissemination of parenteral products can be envisioned using one of three different scenarios. Deciding which roles the hospital pharmacist will play in the process of delivering parenteral drugs suitable for a patient's needs—whether the roles are related to the parenteral drug's procurement, storage, accounting, distribution, preparation or manufacture—is dictated by many factors, including the presence and amount of trained personnel and the space in which to store and mix the drug products; the hospital administration's commitment to such pharmacy functions as the intravenous admixture service; and the availability of adequate pharmacy programs and services and the willingness of the hospital's pharmacists to participate in the manipulation of parenteral drugs.

The final product—the parenteral drug that is injected or infused into the patient—must be appropriate in its concentration, dilution, and rate.

Three Scenarios

Procurement, Storage, Accountability, Distribution

In this, the scenario of minimum involvement, the pharmacist is required to purchase, properly store, maintain adequate records, and ultimately distribute the drug to the nursing unit, where it will be injected by either a nurse or a physician.

In this scenario, the nurse is charged with removing the sterile dosage form from an ampul, vial, or syringe (a solution ready for injection). Alternatively, the dry parenteral would have to be reconstituted by the nurse, who would select the diluent and its concentration.

In some situations, the nurse may be required to perform further manipulations of the parenteral drug.

The parenteral drug may require only a limited amount of manipulation; for example, with a unit-dose syringe, the nurse would be required to simply remove the needle's sheath and administer the injection.

Although the type of system outlined in this first scenario is considered undesirable by professional organizations and most pharmacists, this type of parenteral distribution still exists in some hospitals in the United States.

Procurement, Storage, Distribution, Preparation

Hospital pharmacists in this distribution scenario present to either the nurse or physician the completed parenteral dosage form, which is ready for injection. It therefore requires only a minimal amount of manipulation by the nurse or physician.

The hospital pharmacy department must be dedicated to and capable of handling and preparing parenteral products for this scenario to be justified.

It requires technical knowledge, skill, adequate personnel, proper equipment, and a hospital administration supportive of such centralized pharmacy areas as I.V. admixture and reconstitution services.

According to one survey, over 54% of the general hospitals in the United States reported conducting an I.V. admixture service, and over 66% of specialized hospitals reported that they had such a service.[103]

Of all the survey's respondents, fully 89% said they purchased as many drugs in unit-dose packages as possible. The survey also disclosed that, of the hospitals with more than 500 beds, the average number of I.V. admixtures performed and dispensed on a weekly basis was over 1000, and reconstituted I.V. piggyback containers numbered over 2000 per week.

The preparation of parenteral drug products may be as simple as drawing the parenteral drug into a syringe from an ampul or vial or as complex as preparing a total parenteral nutrition (TPN) solution. The hospital pharmacy must be capable of handling all preparation situations.

The heart of such a distribution system is the pharmacy's program of I.V. admixtures and piggybacking.

In this scenario, the hospital pharmacist requires syringe prefilling and reconstitution programs, and may well require freezing abilities.

Bulk and As-Needed Parenteral Manufacturing

Some hospital pharmacies offer a manufacturing service that prepares the parenteral dosage forms. In this scenario, the pharmacy starts with the raw chemicals needed to mix the parenteral drug and transforms them into a final sterile product.

Manufacturing can be done in smaller amounts of a unit or two to satisfy parenteral drug needs as they arise, or in large-bulk groups consisting of many units for long-term needs.

Whether a hospital pharmacy should manufacture its own parenteral drug products depends on several factors. To cite several examples, does the medical staff require certain drug products that are not commercially available, or do they require unavailable dosage strengths of existing products? Are the proper manufacturing equipment and personnel available, and does the hospital pharmacy possess the appropriate knowledge of manufacturing techniques?

The need for this type of function in hospital pharmacies has waned in recent years because of the increasing commercial availability of numerous parenteral dosage forms.

In 1976, infusion devices accounted for $185 million in sales. Such sales amounted to $585 million in 1982. By 1988, device sales may amount to $1 billion or more.[104] Further innovations in packaging systems will increase this growth. Although hospitals have experienced a trend toward cost containment and pressure has been placed on hospitals to hold the line on costs, this has had and will continue to have a minimal effect on the expansion of I.V. therapy. As much as 70 to 80% of hospital costs are labor costs. Thus, significant pressures in the cutting of material costs (i.e., those costs reflected in goods and supplies) will offer only insignificant savings. Cost constraints will have to be achieved through systems that reduce labor. The onus on the I.V. manufacturers will be to refine the I.V. systems (both electronic and mechanical) and I.V. packaging in an effort to reduce labor costs. Drugs will be packaged in systems that will reduce any necessary manipulations in hospitals to a minimum.

I.V. drug delivery systems have attracted the attention of almost every major pharmaceutical firm as well as members of the medical device industry. Intense research in this field enforces the belief that new uses and methods of administration will be found for established drugs. A better understanding of pharmacokinetic and pharmacodynamic principles of drugs has opened the door to the development of new concepts in I.V. delivery systems. Newer delivery systems can provide

For the Patient:
Round-the-clock administration of drugs and nutritional formulas.
Continuous pain relief.
Reduced dosage and frequency of administration.
Reduced cost through decreased labor.
Increased convenience and safety.

For the Manufacturer:
New uses for approved, established drugs.
Reduced regulatory approval time.
Increased revenue.
Maintenance of current revenue and market shares.

The medical staffs of most hospitals recognize the problems associated with intravenous drug administration and impose limitations on their nursing personnel regarding the administration of drugs by I.V. push. This limitation has led to the hospital-wide use of various types of intermittent infusion devices—such as volume-control units, minibags and minibottles—for the administration of scheduled intravenous medications. This, in turn, has satisfied the requirement for dilution and prompted hospitals to allow their nurses to give intravenous medications. This has also resulted in clinical decision-making by the nurses and pharmacist concerning which medications can be given effectively using such intermittent infusion devices.

A review of intermittent drug administration systems is in order. With the advent of antibiotics, particularly cephalothin, volume-control units gained wide hospital use in the 1960s and 1970s. These devices provided a method for intermittent drug administration.[8]

In 1971, Duma et al.[12] noted the hazards associated with these devices. Henry and Harrison[13] also noted problems associated with these devices.

The early 1970s saw the introduction of the minibottle and, eventually, minibag containers (underfills, piggyback containers). These containers supplied diluent of D_5W and normal saline in 50-ml or 100-ml containers. They allowed dilution and preparation of the drug by pharmacists.

Minicontainer diluents offered many advantages. McAllister et al.[105] reported on the safety of minibags over in-line burettes. Paxinos et al.[106] studied volume-control sets, piggyback systems, and a combination of the two in intermittent I.V. therapy. They concluded that the piggyback system is safe and effective, although costly. They found that an alternate system they devised (a combination volume-control unit and piggyback) was safe, effective, and less costly than the piggyback systems alone.

In 1975, the National Coordinating Committee on Large Volume Parenterals (NCCLCPs)[98] stated "The use of volume control sets is discouraged for intermittent drug therapy in adults."

Grey[107] compared methods and costs preparing I.V. piggyback solutions for diluent use in piggyback containers and noted that manufacturers' prefilled drug containers offered significant cost savings.

Several manufacturers responded to the hospital pharmacist's needs by supplying a variety of antibiotics in manufacturer's prefilled piggyback glass containers. In addition, drug manufacturers supplied bulk prefilled containers to accommodate I.V. reconstitution and admixture programs.

In an evaluation of ampicillin, Gibbs[108] noted that, for hospitals using glass systems, the prefilled 1-g piggyback bottle was best; for hospitals using I.V. bags, the 10-g "bulk" container was best. Hand et al.[109] also reported on the cost effectiveness of manufacturer's prefilled piggyback containers.

Paxinos et al.[110] studied the contamination rates and costs associated with the use of four intermittent infusion systems. They noted that the piggyback using the minibag was the most expensive; the piggyback with the Buretrol was the least expensive; and the piggyback using the drug manufacturer's prefilled piggybacks was the most efficacious.

Yarborough et al.[111] compared four admixture procedures for intermittent therapy. This group found no significant differences in the contamination rates between systems (1.3 to 2.5%). They also noted that no system worked best in all categories, and that hospital considerations affect the final choice of a system.

Dreiman[112] compared six methods of preparing piggyback doses of cephalothin and considered labor, equipment, and material costs for each of the six methods studied. The personnel cost proved the lowest for partial-fill bottles and drug prefilled manufacturer's bottles. Material costs were lowest for both manufacturers' prefilled bottles using a pressure infusor and for partial-fill bottles with the Pharm-Aid fluid dispensing system. The preferred systems, however, included the drug manufacturers prefilled bottle, using the pressure infusor, as well as gravity flow method in conjunction with the drug manufacturers prefilled bottle.

Lu et al.[113] studied a new vacuum-filling method for reconstitution of most drug-manufacturers prefilled containers and noted that the vacuum diluent method was both effective and safe.

Fraterigo et al.[114] studied the accuracy and efficiency of three methods of preparing piggyback admixtures.

1. Pharm Aid fluid dispensing system
2. Valleylab I.V. Formulator
3. Viavac vacuum unit

This group noted that the I.V. Formulator required the least amount of time. The cost was nearly identical for all three systems, however, and no one system was best for all situations.

Pohorylo et al.[115] studied the time and cost associated with four methods of filling piggyback bottles.

1. Traditional vacuum method
2. Wheaton Unispense Model II
3. Valleylab I.V. 6500 Formulator
4. Instafil Method

This group concluded that for small batches the Instafil method was best, and for larger batches methods 2 and 3 were best.

Markowsky et al.[116] compared six methods for preparing cefazolin sodium for intermittent injection.

1. Manual Syringe and Stopcock
2. Multi-Ad System
3. Wheaton Unispense
4. Valleylab I.V. Formulator
5. Faspak ADS-100
6. Prefilled Manufacturer's Piggyback Bottles (DMPB)

Systems 1 through 4 used bulk 10-g vials added to partial fills, and systems 5 and 6 used DMPBs. It was concluded from this study that the Faspak ADS-100 system achieved the lowest personnel cost and the DMPB system achieved the lowest annual cost.

The decade from the 1970s through the early 1980s explored using methods other than volume-control units for intermittent I.V. drug administration. The partial-fill diluent piggyback containers were accepted and became widely used. Over 100 million piggyback containers are used yearly in the United States today. Introduction of powdered DMPBs in the early 1970s along with bulk containers expedited I.V. piggyback administration.

Large-Volume Parenterals (LVPs) With Manufactured Additives (Premixes)

In the late 1970s, the industry recognized the need to add simple electrolytes during manufacture. It has been estimated that considerable amounts of LVPs contain potassium chloride (40 to 60%). With over 300 million units of LVPs used yearly in the United States, millions of small-volume parenterals (SVPs) with potassium chloride had to be added to LVPs.

Turco[117] studied the cost and time required to add KCl to LVPs using three systems:

1. Ampul KCl—needle and syringe.
2. Vial transfer and needle method.
3. Pintop method.

The pintop method proved the most convenient and the fastest, but was also the most expensive.

In a second study, Turco[118] studied a comparison of manufacturers' "premixed" and "non-premixed" potassium chloride LVPs and noted that the purchase of "premixed" KCl solutions from the manufacturer proved the most logical choice so long as the medical and nursing staffs can be taught to recognize the contents of the container.

Premixed LVPs containing KCl have gained wide use. Other LVP premixes have become available, e.g., lidocaine, heparin, theophylline, and dopamine (Fig. 8–40).

Premixed drug solutions and containers offer significant advantages to hospitals: They are less demanding of time, and they have less potential for error and contamination. It is significant that drug and fluid manufacturers have combined efforts to achieve optimal packaging for hospital use.

An innovation in prefilled I.V. piggyback containers has been the introduction of ready-to-use plastic containers of solutions that require no manipulation or dilution and thus are ready for direct intravenous infusion. The antibiotic metronidazole (Flagyl, Searle & Co.) is marketed in ready-to-use Viaflex plastic I.V. containers from Baxter Healthcare Labs.

I.V. Flagyl was originally introduced in 500-mg vials of lyophilized drug requiring reconstitution and buffering. Later it was introduced in 100-ml ready-to-use glass containers and, eventually, in Viaflex containers.

In early 1982, Travenol (now Baxter Healthcare) announced agreements to package I.V. drugs produced by Schering, Bristol, SmithKline, Hoechst-Roussel, and Merck in Viaflex containers. These provide additional ready-to-serve antibiotics in convenient packaging and, more importantly, will serve to generate systems for premixing oncolytic drugs.

Frozen Premixes

Currently Baxter Healthcare delivers to hospitals frozen drug products packaged in polyvinylchloride containers. These frozen products are stored in a freezer in the hospital's pharmacy and thawed and used when needed. Available are frozen cefazolin (Ancef), cephalothin, cefoxitin (Mefoxin), cimetidine (Tagamet), and cefotaxime (Claforan) (Fig. 8–41).

Under new agreements with drug manufacturers, Baxter Healthcare packages premixed solutions of Hoechst-Roussel's Claforan (cefotaxime sodium). These third-generation cephalosporins will be distributed by Baxter Healthcare to hospitals in frozen form. Double-bag Viaflex has been introduced by Baxter Healthcare, offering the convenience of incompatible drugs in liquid form.

Faspak/ADS-100 System

Eli Lilly supplies a non-PVC plastic piggyback container, named "Faspak," which contains the dry, powdered form of certain drugs (Keflin, Kefzol, Man-

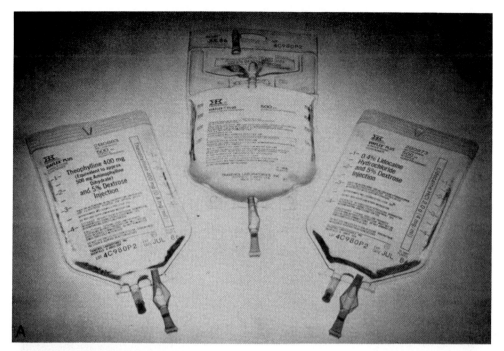

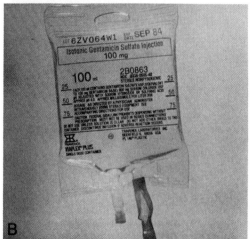

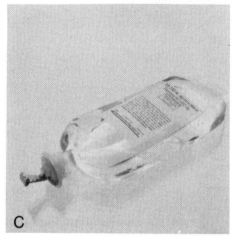

Figure 8–40. Premixed LVPs. (A, B, Courtesy of Baxter Healthcare Laboratories, Inc., Deerfield, IL. C, Courtesy of Abbott Laboratories, North Chicago, IL.)

dol, and ampicillin), which upon reconstitution with the appropriate diluent, allows direct administration of the diluted drug. This avoids a transferring step that normally takes place when reconstituting a powdered drug. To help in the reconstitution step, a specialized dilution pump named the ADS-100 system is supplied.

The package design eliminates the need for transferring between containers after reconstitution, and the Faspak acts as a final delivery container.

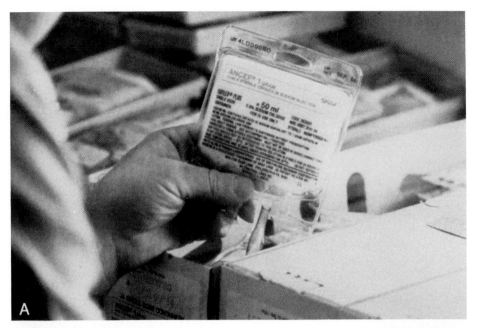

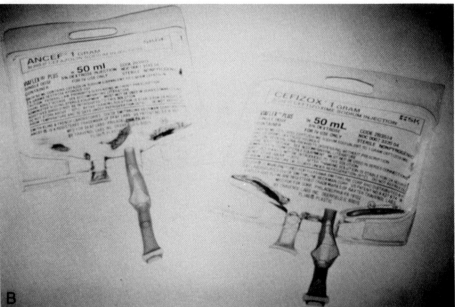

Figure 8–41. A, B, Frozen premixes. (Courtesy of Baxter Healthcare Laboratories Inc., Deerfield, IL.)

Abbott/ADD-Vantage System

Introduced in 1985, the Abbott ADD-Vantage system has two parts: a plastic I.V. bag sold by Abbott that is filled with solution, and a separate glass vial of powder or liquid drug sold by a drug maker. The vial is encased by a plastic cover that is removed prior to use. The user locks the vial holding the drug into a chamber at the top of the plastic bag and mixes the drug and solution by externally removing the vial's stopper. Abbott claims ADD-Vantage saves both labor and material costs and minimizes drug waste. SmithKline Beecham, Wyeth, Upjohn, Lilly, Burroughs Wellcome, and Roche have made available vials designed for the ADD-Vantage system (Table 8–4, Figs. 8–42 and 8–43).

Foltyn et al.[119] studied the costs associated with seven methods of preparing and administering small-volume injections. The study was completed at 13 hospitals. The systems included the minibag, frozen, syringe pump, volume control set, ADD-vantage, and CRIS systems. When labor and material cost were considered, the CRIS system was the least expensive method of administration.

Mini-Infuser Pumps for Intermittent I.V. Drug Delivery

A novel concept in intermittent drug delivery, introduced several years ago, was the Bard-Harvard Mini-Infuser System. This instrument was designed for the administration of antibiotics and other medications delivered intermittently in 40 minutes or less. This battery-generated, lightweight instrument uses standard disposable syringes and microbore disposable extension sets. Different models are available, depending on volume-to-be-delivered selection. This instrument provides accuracy, constant flow, convenience, and safety for intermittent drug delivery.[120–122]

Introduced and designed for intermittent I.V. drug delivery, Becton Dickinson's 360 infusor allows drug delivery intermittently over 60 minutes or less in a volume dilution of up to 50 ml. This instrument is currently undergoing hospital evaluations.

Abbott Laboratories, IVAC Corporation, and Pancretec, Inc. all manufacture syringe pumps as well. AVI, Inc. makes a syringe device called Medifuse, which uses a constantly applied force, instead of the usual battery power, to propel the syringe plunger.

Larger Electronic Equipment

We have recently seen the introduction of electronic equipment for automated administration of intermittent secondary medications (piggyback). Four manufacturers supply this equipment as part of a system that uses an electronic pump.

These systems allow the programming of the secondary infusion (piggyback); at the time of completion, the systems automatically revert back to the desired primary fluid flow rate. These devices save time, offer nursing convenience, and reduce intravenous sites lost as a result of dry secondary bottles (if no check valve set is normally used), and also reduce the possibility of the primary solution infusing at the secondary rate. One system can limit the volume infused from the secondary container, introducing the possibility of cost savings by compounding the secondary container to contain more than one dose. These systems also reduce the need for using multiple electronic equipment devices. These instruments can increase the precision of drug

TABLE 8–4. ADD-Vantage Marketed Products

COMPANY	BRAND NAME
Abbott Laboratories DILUENTS	
Abbott Laboratories DRUGS	A-methaPred® 500 mg A-methaPred® 1,000 mg
	Aminocaproic Acid 5 g
	Clindamycin 300 mg Clindamycin 600 mg Clindamycin 900 mg
	Erythrocin® 500 mg Erythrocin® 1 gram
	Gentamicin 60 mg Gentamicin 80 mg Gentamicin 100 mg
	Methyldopate 250 mg Methyldopate 500 mg
	Nitropress® 50 mg

Abbott Laboratories
  KITS
	Erythrocin® 500 mg
	  and 100 mL D5W
	Erythrocin® 1 g
	  and 250 mL D5W

	Nitropress® 50 mg and 250 mL D5W

	Pentothal® 2.5 g
	  and 100 mL 0.9% NaCl
	Pentothal® 6.5 g
	  and 250 mL 0.9% NaCl

Bristol	Polycillin-N® 1 g Polycillin-N® 2 g
	Nafcil™ 1 g Nafcil™ 2 g
	Prostaphlin® 1 g Prostaphlin® 2 g
	Cefadyl® 1 g Cefadyl® 2 g
Burroughs Wellcome	Septra® 5 mL Septra® 10 mL
Hoechst-Roussel	Claforan® 1 g Claforan® 2 g
Lederle	Pipracil® 2 g Pipracil® 3 g Pipracil® 4 g

TABLE 8–4. (*Continued*)

Lilly	Keflin® 1 g Keflin® 2 g
	Kefurox® 750 mg Kefurox® 1.5 g
	Kefzol® 500 mg Kefzol® 1 g
	Mandol® 1 g Mandol® 2 g
	Nebcin® 60 mg Nebcin® 80 mg
	Tazidime® 1 g Tazidime® 2 g
	Vancocin® 500 mg Vancocin® 1 g
Merck	Mefoxin® 1 g Mefoxin® 2 g
	Primaxin® 250 mg Primaxin® 500 mg
Miles	Mezlin® 3 g Mezlin® 4 g
Roche	Rocephin® 1 g Rocephin® 2 g
Roerig	Unasyn® 1.5 g
Smith Kline-Beecham	Bactocill® 1 g Bactocill® 2 g
	Nallpen® 1 g Nallpen® 2 g
	Tagamet®
	Ticar® 3 g
	Timentin® 3.1 g
	Totacillin-N® 1 g Totacillin-N® 2 g
Upjohn	Cleocin® 600 mg Cleocin® 900 mg
Wyeth	Omnipen®-N 500 mg Omnipen®-N 1 g Omnipen®-N 2 g
	Unipen® 500 mg Unipen® 1 g Unipen® 2 g

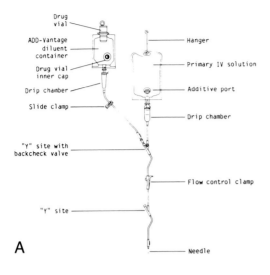

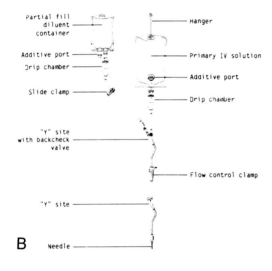

Figure 8–42. Overview of intravenous admixture systems. A, ADD-Vantage system. B, Partial-fill diluent container. C, Drug manufacturer's partial-fill piggyback (DMP). D, Frozen partial fill. E, Syringe pump. F, Burette set. G, CRIS infusion system. (A through G Courtesy of Abbott Laboratories, North Chicago, IL.)

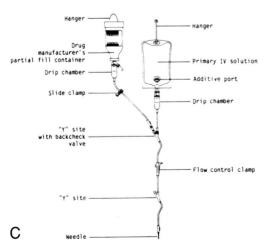

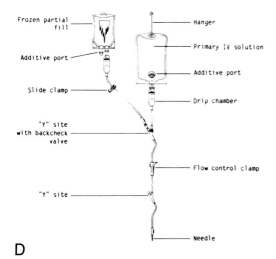

D

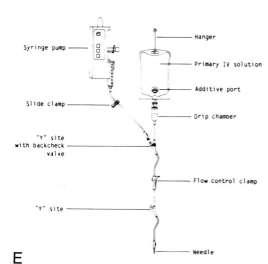

E

Figure 8–42. (*Continued*)

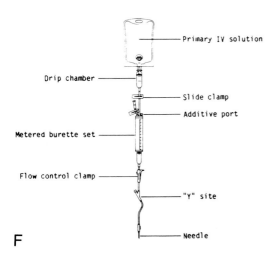

F

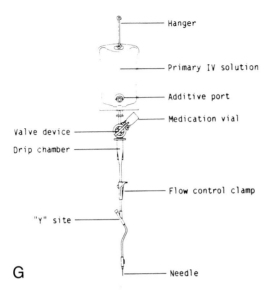

Figure 8–42. (*Continued*)

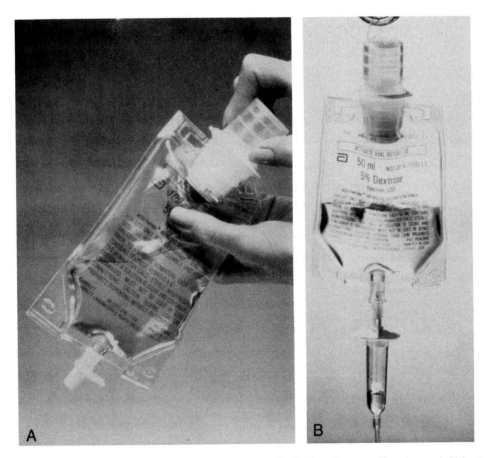

Figure 8–43. A, Abbott ADD-Vantage system. B, System in use. (Courtesy of Abbott Laboratories, North Chicago, IL.)

administration and allow optimal interpretation of serum drug level concentrations.

Baxter Healthcare Infusor

The Infusor is a continuous infusion system. Drug is injected into the infusor, which then inflates a balloon reservoir, creating constant internal pressure. As the reservoir deflates, medication is delivered through an orifice of controlled size that regulates the infusion at a constant rate of 2 ml/hr. When infusion is completed, the empty infusor is discarded. Rates of drug administration can be varied from 1 to 24 hr/infusor, depending on the solution concentration. An excellent review of high-technology I.V. infusion devices can be found in the literature.[123]

Reconstitution and Admixture Service

McGaw has established Central Admixture Pharmacy Services (CAPS). CAPS admixes, dispenses, and delivers patient-specific sterile solutions to the hospital pharmacist. Thus far, eight centers are operating in the U.S.

References

1. Valdis, M.M.: Intraosseous fluid administration in emergencies. Lancet, 1, 1235 (1977).
2. Frank, J.T.: Intralipid compatibility study. Drug. Intell. Clin. Pharm., 7, 351 (1973).
3. Lynn, B. (Letter to the Editor): Intralipid compatibility study. Drug Intell. Clin. Pharm., 8, 75 (1974).
4. McGaw Inc. 2525 McGaw Ave., Irvine, CA: Changing Solutions Booklet.
5. Dorr, R.T.: Furosemide administration recommendations—patients with renal failure. Am. J. I.V. Ther., Aug.–Sept. (1976).
6. Shrrard, D.J.: Treatment of hypertensive crisis with diazoxide. N. Engl. J. Med., 292, 266 (1975).
7. Grotting, M.A., et al.: Putting RNs in the I.V. push chemotherapy picture. Am. J. I.V. Ther., Oct.–Nov. (1976).
8. Rapp, R.P., Wermeling, D.P., and Piecoro, J.J., Jr.: Guidelines for the administration of commonly used intravenous drugs—1984 update. Drug Intell. Clin. Pharm., 18, 218 (1984).
9. Godwin, H.N.: Intermittent and direct I.V. push: rationale and procedures. Am. J. I.V. Ther., Jan. (1975).
10. Grotting, M.A., et al.: How to develop an I.V. push service. Am. J. I.V. Ther., Apr.–May (1976).
11. Naylor, M.J.V., et al.: Manual for the Preparation and Administration of Drugs for Intravenous Use. Toronto, Canadian Society of Hospital Pharmacists, Toronto General Hospital (1976).
12. Duma, R.J., Warner, J.F., and Dalpon, H.P.: Septicemia from intravenous infusions. N. Engl. J. Med., 284, 257 (1971).
13. Henry, R.H., and Harrison, W.L.: Problems in the use of volume control sets for intravenous fluids. Am. J. Hosp. Pharm., 29, 485 (1972).
14. Ravin, R.L.: Intermittent Intravenous Therapy. Syracuse, N.Y., Bristol Laboratories, 1973.
15. The United States Pharmacopeia Convention Inc., 19th Revision. July 1, 1975, p. 583.
16. Wuest, J.R.: Staffing and I.V. additive service. Drug Intell. Clin. Pharm., 4, 25 (1970).
17. Ferenchak, P., et al.: Drop size and rate in parenteral infusion. Surgery, 70, 674–677, Nov. 1971.

18. Turco, S.: Unpublished work.
19. Qundersen, J.: Pitfalls in drop-infusion technique—a newer device for automatic control of infusion rates. Acta Anaesthesiol. Scand., *16*, 17 (1972).
20. Susser, A.: Unique concept in clamping affords precise control of I.V. flow rates. Nation's Hosp., *3*, 1 (1971).
21. Fonkalsrud, E.W., et al.: A new even-flow intravenous infusion clamp. Arch. Surg., *102*, 530 (1971).
22. Turco, S., and Davis, N.M.: Comparison of commercial final filtration devices. Hosp. Pharm., *8*, 137 (1973).
23. Temple University Hospital Pharmacy Seminar, Philadelphia, PA, 1974.
24. La Coure, D.: Drop size in intravenous infusion. Acta Anesthesiol. Scand., *24* (Suppl.), 35 (1966).
25. Hutchinson, B.R.: The performance of intravenous drip sets. N.Z. Med. J., *70*, 91 (1969).
26. Plumer, A.L.: Principles and Practices of I.V. Therapy. Boston, Little, Brown & Co., 1970.
27. Demoruelle, J.L., et al.: Flow rate maintenance and output of intravenous fluid administration sets. Am. J. Hosp. Pharm., *32*, 177 (1975).
28. Monahan, J.J., et al.: Intravenous infusion pumps—an added dimension to parenteral therapy. Am. J. Hosp. Pharm., *29*, 54 (1972).
29. Health Devices, Dec. (1972).
30. Health Devices, June (1975).
31. Swanson, M., et al.: Heparin therapy by continuous intravenous infusion. Am. J. Hosp. Pharm., *28*, 792 (1971).
32. Annual R$_x$ For Heart Disease. Newsletter, Memorial Hospital Medical Center of Long Beach. Summer (1972).
33. Salzman, H.W., et al.: Management of heparin therapy. N. Engl. J. Med., *292*, 1046 (1975).
34. Sherman, J.O., et al.: Parenteral hyperalimentation. Surg. Clin. North Am., *51*, 37 (1971).
35. Dudrick, S.J., and Wilmore, D.W.: Long term parenteral feeding. Hosp. Pract., *3*, 65 (1968).
36. Dudrick, S.J., and Rhoads, J.E.: New horizons for intravenous feeding. JAMA, *215*, 939 (1971).
37. Dudrick, S.J., and Rhoads, J.E.: Total intravenous feeding. Sci. Am., *226*, 73 (1972).
38. Fibrillation deaths cut with lidocaine regimen. Med. World News, March 31 (1972).
39. Hamlett, J.D.: A new electronic pump for oxytocin infusion. Br. J. Clin. Pract., *26*, Feb. (1972).
40. Martinez, D.R.: Peripheral hyperalimentation of the newborn. Eighth Annual ASHP Midyear Clinical Meeting, Washington, D.C. Dec. 10, 1973.
41. Kopezynski, H.D.: Inflight intravenous therapy: a new dimension. Aviat. Space Environ. Med., *1305*, Oct. (1975).
42. Coggin, S.: Modern I.V. technology. Med. Electron. Data, Jan.–Feb. (1975).
43. Eshuk, E., et al.: New I.V. instrument regulates flow and eliminates up to 75% of restarts. Nation's Hosp., Spring (1972).
44. Schwerman, E.A., et al.: New electronic I.V. control found accurate, safe, economical. Nation's Hosp., Spring (1977).
45. Monahan, J.J., and Webb, J.: Intravenous infusion pumps—an added dimension to parenteral therapy. Am. J. Hosp. Pharm., *29*, 54 (1972).
46. *ECRI: Infusion pumps. Health Devices, Dec. (1972).
47. ECRI: Infusion pumps. Health Devices, June (1975).
48. ECRI: Inspection and preventive maintenance of infusion pumps. Health Devices, July (1975).

*Emergency Care Research Institute
5200 Butler Pike
Plymouth Meeting, PA 19462.

49. Turco, S.J., et al.: A comparison of commercial final filtration devices. Hosp. Pharm., *8*, 137 (1973).
50. Yates, W.G., et al.: Safety and performance of angiographic injections and infusion with withdrawal pumps. University of Utah Research Institute, April 22, 1977.
51. ECRI: IVAC 400 infusion pump. Health Devices, July (1971).
52. ECRI: IVAC infusion pumps. Health Devices, Sept.–Oct. (1972).
53. ECRI: Battery charger for halter pumps. Health Devices, July–Aug. (1972).
54. Hanneman, R.E., et al.: Bubble formation in the roller infusion pump. Am. J. Dis. Child., *125*, 706 (1973).
55. Younes, R.P.: Halter infusion pump. J. Pediatr., *79*, 344 (1971).
56. Croke, R.P., et al.: Pseudoarrhythmia due to defective infusion pump and ECG monitor. JAMA, *235*, 705 (1976).
57. Robinson, L.A., et al.: Pharmacy-blood infusion pump program. Am. J. Hosp. Pharm., *34*, 697 (1977).
58. Beaumont, E.: The new I.V. infusion pumps. Nursing, 77, July (1977).
59. Rapp, R.P., et al.: Effects of electronic infusion control on the efficacy, complications and cost of I.V. therapy. Hosp. Form., *14*, 953 (1979).
60. ECRI: Evaluation: Infusion Controllers. Health Devices. *14*, 219 (1985).
61. Kelly, W.N., et al.: Selective patient criteria for the use of electronic infusion devices. Am. J. I.V. Ther. Clin. Nutr., *10*(3), 18 (1983).
62. Sourcebook for I.V. Therapy. IVAC Corporation, San Diego, CA, Dec. 1985.
63. Second Annual Buyer's Guide to Electronic Pumps and Controllers. Pharm. Pract. News, *13*(7), 17 (1986).
64. Strayer, A.H., et al.: Administration of whole blood, packed red blood cells, and platelets using a multipurpose Infusion Pump. Am. J. Hosp. Pharm., *48*, 1970 (1991).
65. Burch, K.J., et al.: Effect of an infusion device on the integrity of whole blood and packed red blood cells. Am. J. Hosp. Pharm., *48*, 92 (1991).
66. Gibson, J.S., et al.: Effects of intravenous delivery systems on infused red blood cells. Am. J. Hosp. Pharm., *41*, 468 (1984).
67. Stiles, M.L., et al.: Stability of cefazolin sodium, Cefoxtin sodium, ceftzidime, and penicillin G sodium in portable pump reservoirs. Am. J. Hosp. Pharm., *46*, 1408 (1989).
68. Stiles, M.L., et al.: Stability of fluorouracil administered through four portable infusion pumps. Am. J. Hosp. Pharm., *46*, 2036 (1989).
69. Tu, Y.H., et al.: Stability study of gentamicin sulfate administered via pharmacia deltec CADD-VT pump. Hosp. Pharm., *25*, 843 (1990).
70. Altman, L., et al.: Stability of morphine sulfate in Cormed III (Kalex) intravenous bags Am. J. Hosp. Pharm., 1990; *47*, 2040 (1990).
71. Allen, L.V., et al.: Stability of Fentanyl citrate in 0.9% sodium chloride solution in portable infusion pumps. Am. J. Hosp. Pharm., *47*, 1572 (1990).
72. Tu, Y.H., et al.: Stability of Fentanyl Citrate and Bupivacaine Hydrochloride in portable pump reservoirs. Am. J. Hosp. Pharm., *47*, 2037 (1990).
73. Rochard, E.B., et al.: Stability of fluorourocil, cytabrine, or doxorubicin hydrochloride in ethylene vinylacetate portable infusion pump reservoirs. Am. J. Hosp. Pharm., *49*, 619 (1992).
74. Stiles, M.L., et al.: Stability of ondansetron hydrochloride in portable infusion pump reservoirs. Am. J. Hosp. Pharm., *49*, 1471 (1992).
75. Coggin, S.: The selection and use of intravenous pumps and controllers: the nursing viewpoint. NITA, *4*, 16 (1981).
76. Temple University Hospital Pharmacy Department, Philadelphia, PA.
77. Annual Recommendations of Practice NITA, Revised November 1981.
78. Carleton, B.C., et al.: Methods for emulating drip-rate accuracy of intravenous flow-regulating devices. Am. J. Hosp. Pharm. 48, 244 (1991).
79. Bennett, R.L., Griffen, W.O.: Patient controlled analgesia. Contemp. Surg., *23*, 75, (1983).
80. Graves, D.A., et al.: Patient controlled analgesia. Ann. Intern. Med., *99*, 360, (1983).

81. Bivins, B.A., and Baumann, T.J.: Patient controlled analgesia (PCA): A clinical evaluation of safety and efficacy in hospitalized trauma/surgery patients. Departments of Surgery and Pharmacy, Henry Ford Hospital, Detroit, Michigan, 48210, December 1984.

82. Kwan, J.W.: Use of infusion devices for epidural or intrathecal administration of spinal opioids. Am. J. Hosp. Pharm., 47, 18 (1990).

83. Hansen, J.S., and Hepler, C.D.: Contamination of intravenous solutions by airborne microbes. Am. J. Hosp. Pharm., 30, 326 (1973).

84. Paretz, D.M., et al.: Microbial contamination of glass bottle (open vented) and plastic bag (closed non-vented) intravenous fluid delivery systems. Am. J. Hosp. Pharm., 31, 726 (1974).

85. Viaflex containers. Med. Lett. Drug. Ther., 14, 19 (1972).

86. Turco, S., and King, R.E.: Sterile Dosage Forms. Philadelphia, Lea & Febiger, 1974, p. 140.

87. Petrick, R.J., et al.: Review of current knowledge of plastic intravenous fluid containers. Am. J. Hosp. Pharm., 34, 357 (1977).

88. Turco, S.J., and Davis, N.M.: Particulate matter in intravenous fluids—phase 3. Am. J. Hosp. Pharm., 30, 611 (1973).

89. Needham, T.E., and Luzzi, L.A.: Particulate matter in polyvinylchloride intravenous bags. N. Engl. J. Med., 209, 1256 (1973).

90. Plastic Containers for Intravenous Solutions. Med. Lett. Drug Ther., 17, 10 (1975).

91. Kelly, W.N., et al.: Initiating and justifying an I.V. team. Am. J. I.V. Ther., Oct.–Nov. (1975).

92. Kimmell, R.: How to start an I.V. team: dream to working reality. Am. J. I.V. Ther., Feb.–Mar. (1977).

93. Godfrey, D.: How to Set Up an I.V. Team. Baltimore, Johns Hopkins Hospital. Inservice Document (1977).

94. Willett, R.D.: Developing an I.V. therapy team in a small hospital. Am. J. I.V. Ther., Aug.–Sept. (1976).

95. U.S. Dept. Health, Education and Welfare: Nosocomial Bacteremias Associated With Intravenous Fluid Therapy. Atlanta, CDC, March 12, 1971.

96. Brown, T.R., et al.: The Ecology of Large Volume Infusions in Hospitals, U.S.P. Contract No. 00001, Dept. Health Care Adm., School of Pharmacy, University of Mississippi.

97. Recommendations to pharmacists for solving problems with large volume parenterals. Am. J. Hosp. Pharm., 33, 231 (1976).

98. Recommended methods for compounding intravenous admixtures in hospitals. Am. J. Hosp. Pharm., 32, 261 (1975).

99. Recommended system for surveillance and reporting of problems with large volume parenterals in hospitals. Am. J. Hosp. Pharm., 32, 1251 (1975).

100. Bergman, H.D: Incompatibilities in large volume parenterals. Drug Intell. Clin. Pharm., 11, 345 (1977).

101. Recommendations for labeling of large volume parenterals. Am. J. Hosp. Pharm., 35, 49 (1978).

102. Recommended procedures for in-use testing of large volume parenterals suspected of contamination or of producing a reaction in a patient. Am. J. Hosp. Pharm., 35, 678 (1978).

103. Lilly Hospital Pharmacy Survey 1984. Eli Lilly Company, Indianapolis, IN.

104. Financial Analysts Federation Meeting: Health care seminar. December 1, 1983, Franklin Plaza, Philadelphia, PA.

105. McAllister, J.C., et al.: Comparison of the safety and efficiency of three intermittent intravenous therapy systems—the minibottle, the minibag and the in-line burette. Am. J. Hosp. Pharm., 31, 961 (1974).

106. Paxinos, J., et al.: Combined volume control set—piggyback system for intermittent I.V. therapy. Am. J. Hosp. Pharm., 32, 892 (1975).

107. Grey, C.: Comparison of methods and costs of preparing intravenous piggyback solutions. Hosp. Pharm., 6, 10 (1976).

108. Gibbs, C.W.: Evaluation of methods of preparing ampicillin for intermittent I.V. administration. Hosp. Pharm., 12, 409 (1977).

109. Hand, J., et al.: Pressure filling of I.V. piggyback solutions. Hosp. Pharm., *12*, 274 (1977).

110. Paxinos, J., et al.: Contamination rates and costs associated with the use of four intermittent I.V. infusion systems. Am. J. Hosp. Pharm., *36*, 1497 (1979).

111. Yarborough, M.C., et al.: A comparison of four admixture procedures for intermittent I.V. therapy. Hosp. Pharm., *15*, 179 (1980).

112. Dreiman, R.K.: Comparison of six methods of preparing piggyback doses of cephalothin sodium. Am. J. Hosp. Pharm., *37*, 1342 (1980).

113. Lu, A., et al.: A new vacuum filling method for mass reconstitution of manufacturers' IVPBs. Hosp. Pharm., *17*, 380 (1982).

114. Fraterigo, C.C., et al.: Accuracy and efficiency of three methods of preparing piggyback admixtures. Am. J. Hosp. Pharm., *39*, 1920 (1982).

115. Pohorylo, E.M., et al.: Time and cost comparison of four methods of filling piggyback bottles. Am. J. Hosp. Pharm., *40*, 88 (1983).

116. Markowsky, S.J., et al.: Comparison of six methods of preparing cefazolin sodium for intermittent injection. Am. J. Hosp. Pharm., *40*, 1653 (1983).

117. Turco, S.J.: Cost and time required to add potassium chloride to large volume parenterals. Hosp. Pharm., *14*, 718 (1979).

118. Turco, S.J.: A comparison of premixed and non-premixed potassium chloride large-volume parenterals. Hosp. Pharm., *14*, 720 (1979).

119. Foltyn, C.S., et al.: Comparison of seven methods of preparing and administering small-volume injections. Am. J. Hosp. Pharm. *45*, 1896, (1988).

120. Cologelo, A., et al.: Implementation and cost analysis of a syringe pump system for intermittent I.V. drug delivery. Am. J. Hosp. Pharm., *42*, 581 (1985).

121. Bousquet, J., et al.: Pharmacy-initiated implementation of an infusion type pump. Am. J. Hosp. Pharm., *42*, 584 (1985).

122. Reilly, R.T., et al.: Cost comparison of two systems for intermittent I.V. administration of small-volume injections. Am. J. Hosp. Pharm., *42*, 323 (1985).

123. Kwan, J.W.: High-technology I.V. infusion devices. Am. J. Hosp. Pharm. *46*, 320 (1989).

PCA—Selected Bibliography

Buchanan, C.: Development of a patient controlled analgesia pump system. Parenterals, *4*, 27 (1986).

Graves, D.A., et al.: Morphine requirements using patient-controlled analgesia; Influence of diurnal varation and morbid obesity. Clin. Pharm., *2*, 49, (1983).

White, P.F.: Patient controlled analgesia: A new approach to the management of postoperative pain. Semin. Anesth. *4*, 255 (1985).

Williamson, J. et al.: Implementation of an IV morphine infusion program in a community hospital. Hosp. Pharm., *21*, 1098 (1986).

CHAPTER

Blood Components and Plasma Expanders

Clyde Buchanan

This chapter reviews the composition, clinical applications, and adverse reactions of blood derivatives, plasma expanders, clotting factors, and intravenous immune globulins. Biologic products used for active or passive immunization against specific diseases are not within the scope of this chapter. Blood products are grouped under four general uses: tissue oxygenation, plasma volume expansion, coagulation, and immunodeficiency.

Tissue Oxygenation

In the United States, the only products commercially available to carry oxygen to body tissues are whole blood and red blood cells. Although artificial blood substitutes are being tested, none have satisfied the Food and Drug Administration (FDA) as to their safety and effectiveness for tissue oxygenation.

Whole Blood U.S.P.

Whole blood is obtained from suitable human blood donors who have tested negative for anemia and infectious agents: human immunodeficiency virus (HIV-1 and 2), hepatitis viruses B and C, and syphilis.[1] A unit of whole blood aseptically drawn from a single donor contains about 500 ml of anticoagulated blood with a red cell (erythrocyte) composition of 35 to 40%. Whole blood is indicated only for a symptomatic deficit in oxygen carrying capacity plus a volume deficit associated with shock.[1] The primary risks from blood transfusions are listed in Table 9–1. Whole blood can transmit, albeit rarely, hepatitis, syphilis, malaria, Chagas' disease, brucellosis, cytomegalovirus, human immunodeficiency viruses, and other infections.[2,3] Whole blood preserved with CPDA can be stored up to 35 days at 4°C with good viability of red cells (Table 9–2).

Red Blood Cells U.S.P.

Red blood cells (RBCs) are derived from whole blood by sedimentation or centrifugation and are stored at 1 to 6°C.[4] A unit of RBCs contains a volume of about 300 ml with a red cell composition of 65 to 80%.[1] RBC's are indicated for patients with a symptomatic deficit of oxygen-carrying capacity as determined by good clinical judgment.[5] Besides providing more oxygen-carrying capacity in a smaller volume, RBCs are safer than whole blood because they contain less sodium, potassium, acid, ammonia, and citrate.

Plasma Volume Expansion

Although whole blood and red cells are often needed in hemorrhagic shock, resuscitation is usually initiated with crystalloid and/or colloid solutions. Crystalloids are electrolyte solutions such as lactated Ringer's and sodium chloride 0.9%. Colloids are solutions of large molecules such as albumin or hetastarch. Much controversy exists as to whether crystalloids or colloids are preferred as first-line agents to treat hemorrhagic shock.[6,7] Crystalloids replenish interstitial as well as intravascular fluid and are much less expensive than colloids. Colloids persist longer and hold fluid better within the bloodstream, but may or may not cause less pulmonary edema than crystalloids.[8] Fresh-frozen plasma should not be used to treat hemorrhagic shock because of its ability to transmit infectious diseases.[9] Dextran products and plasma protein fraction are declining in use as plasma expanders because of coagulation and laboratory interferences of the dextrans[7] and hypotension caused by certain lots of plasma protein fraction.[10]

Crystalloids

Crystalloids are represented by sodium chloride 0.9% and lactated Ringer's injection (LRI). LRI (or Hartmann's solution) is an isotonic solution of sodium chloride, potassium chloride, calcium chloride, and sodium lactate. Except for the lactate content and absence of bicarbonate, LRI closely approximates the composition of extracellular fluid. Lactate is ultimately metabolized to bicarbonate. The absence of bicarbonate in LRI prevents precipitation of calcium bicarbonate and calcium carbonate. Upon intravenous administration, the ions of LRI are distributed both intravascularly and interstitially; thus its effect as a plasma expander is transient. LRI is somewhat hypo-osmolar and contains no readily available energy substrate (Table 9–3).

Because the body's response to hypovolemia is to draw interstitial fluid into the bloodstream to restore circulation volume, LRI has become widely used to replenish extracellular fluid compartments.[11] Laks et al. determined that LRI used alone in surgery as a blood replacement was required in a volume 2.7 times that of shed blood to maintain stable hemodynamic status and intravascular volume.[12]

Table 9–1. Adverse Reactions to Blood and Blood Derivatives

Blood Derivative	Hepatitis Risk*	Microbial Contamination	Allergic Reaction	Febrile (Pyrogenic) Reaction
Whole blood	Rare (<1% per unit)	Very rare	Occasional (1%)	Occasional (0.5–1%)
Red blood cells	Rare	Very rare	Occasional	Occasional
Albumin	None reported	None reported	Very rare	Rare
Plasma protein fraction	None reported	None reported	Rare	Rare
Fresh frozen plasma (single donor)	Rare	Very rare	Occasional	Occasional
Cryoprecipitate	Occasional	Very rare	Common	Occasional
Platelets concentrate	Occasional	Very rare	Common	Occasional
Antihemophilic factor	Common	Rare	Very common (5–20%)	Common
Factor IX complex	Common	Occasional	Very common	Common
Anti-inhibitor coagulant complex	Common	Rare	Very common	Common
Anti-thrombin III	None reported	None reported	Rare	None reported
Intravenous immune globulin	None reported	Occasional	Rare	None reported

*Risk of Hepatitis B transmission is in the range of 1:200 to 1:300 per unit.[5] Hepatitis C transmission risk is 1:3333 per unit (From Donahue et al. N. Engl. J. Med., 327:369 1992). HIV transmission risk is 1:40,000 to 1:1,000,000 per unit.[5]

Table 9–2. Properties of Blood and Red Cells Stored in CPDA-1*

	Whole Blood		Red Cells	
	0 Days	35 Days	0 Days	35 Days
pH	7.6 ± 0.13	6.98 ± 0.16	7.55 ± 0.12	6.71 ± 1.5
Plasma hemoglobin mg/L	8.2 ± 9.5	46.1 ± 28	7.8 ± 8.4	658 ± 81.7
Plasma potassium mEq/L	4.2 ± 1.8	27.3 ± 4.6	5.1 ± 6.2	78.5 ± 21.5
mg/dl	16.4 ± 7	106.7 ± 18	20 ± 24.3	307 ± 84
Plasma sodium mEq/L	169 ± 9	155 ± 9	169 ± 15	111 ± 21.5
mg/dl	388 ± 21	356 ± 21	388 ± 34.5	255 ± 49
Dextrose mmol/L	24.4 ± 3.2	12.7 ± 2.8	22.7 ± 4.2	5.2 ± 3.4
mg/dl	440 ± 57	229 ± 51	409 ± 75	93 ± 62
ATP†(μmol/g hb)	4.18 ± 0.68	2.4 ± 0.76	4.2 ± 0.82	1.9 ± 0.75
2,3 DPG (μmol/g hb)	13.2 ± 0	0.7 ± 1.6	12.7 ± 1.8	0.35 ± 0.37
% Survival		79 ± 10%		71 ± 16%
Blood ammonia μmol/L	41.8 ± 25.8	1118 ± 27 [1]		
μg/dl	71.23 ± 44	1904 ± 46		
Cholinesterase	87% at 21 days in CPD			
Lymphocytes	8×10^8 at 21 days			
T lymphocytes	10% in 72 hours			

*CPDA-1 = citric acid, sodium citrate, dextrose, and adenine.
†ATP = adenosine triphosphate; 2,3-DPG = 2,3 diphosphoglycerate; Adapted from Moore, G.L., et al.: Some properties of blood stored in anticoagulant CPDA-1 solution. A brief summary. Transfusion, 21:135 1981.

Table 9–3. Composition of Plasma Volume Expanders

Blood Substitute	Albumin (g/dl)	Globulins (g/dl)	Sodium (mEq/dl)	Potassium (mEq/dl)	Chloride (mEq/dl)	Calories (per dl)	mOsm/L
Fresh-frozen plasma	3.2–5.6	1.3–3.2	13.8–14.8	0.35–0.5	9.8–10.6	30	280–290
Albumin, 25%	24+	<1.0	14.5 ± 1.5	—	12 ± 1	100	1500
Albumin, 5%	4.8+	<0.2	14.5 ± 1.5	0.1	12 ± 1	20	300
Plasma protein fraction, 5%	4.4	0.6	14.5 ± 1.5	0.2	12 ± 1	20	290
Dextran 40, 10% in D5W	—	—	—	—	—	20	277
Dextran 40, 10% in NS	—	—	15.4	—	15.4	Almost 0	308
Dextran 70, 6% in D5W	—	—	—	—	—	20	277
Dextran 70, 6% in NS	—	—	15.4	—	15.4	Almost 0	308
Hetastarch, 6% in NS	—	—	15.4	—	15.4	Almost 0	300
Lactated Ringer's injection*	—	—	13	0.4	10.9	Almost 0	273

*Lactated Ringer's Injection also contains 0.25 mEq calcium/dl and 2.8 mEq lactate/dl.

In adults, 1 to 2 L of LRI may be infused rapidly in the initial treatment of hypovolemic shock. Thereafter, patient status must be monitored to maintain normal serum electrolytes, hematocrit, coagulation factors, and colloid osmotic pressure. Abnormalities (or suspected abnormalities) of these parameters require added electrolytes, RBCs, plasma or coagulation factors, and possibly a colloid solution, respectively.

Albumin Human U.S.P.

Albumin is a 96+% pure albumin fraction extracted from the plasma of healthy donors tested for syphilis, hepatitis and human immunodeficiency viruses. This and heat treatment render albumin free of hepatitis or HIV risk. Albumin is available as a 5% concentration and as 25% albumin, which is osmotically equivalent to five times its volume of plasma. Regardless of the albumin concentration, the sodium chloride concentration is between 13 and 16 mEq/dL. The term "salt-poor," referring to 25% albumin, is misleading and not permitted by the FDA in labeling (Table 9–3).

When given intravenously, albumin 25% draws $3^1/_2$ times its own volume intravascularly from the interstitial and intracellular spaces in normally hydrated subjects.[13] Therefore, albumin 25% is contraindicated in hypovolemic patients unless enough additional fluids are given. Albumin 5% is the better concentration to treat a volume deficit, whereas the 25% solution may be preferred for an oncotic deficit.

Besides emergency treatment of hypovolemic shock, the FDA-approved labeling for albumin includes preventing plasma and sodium losses that usually follow serious burns and treating hypoproteinemia.[14] Other FDA-approved indications are adult respiratory distress syndrome, cardiopulmonary bypass procedures, acute liver failure, neonatal hemolytic disease, acute peritonitis, pancreatitis, or other conditions involving compartmentalization of protein-rich fluids, dilution of red cells, acute nephrosis, and renal dialysis.[15–17]

Excessive volumes of albumin solution can cause red cell dilution and hypocoagulability.[18] Other side effects are rare (see Table 9–1).

Hetastarch

Hetastarch is a waxy starch primarily composed of amylopectin, which is treated with sodium hydroxide and ethylene oxide. Hetastarch (or hydroxyethyl starch) has been heavily promoted as a cost-effective substitute for albumin 5%. The viscosity and the osmotic and clinical properties of hetastarch 6% are similar to those of albumin 5%.[19]

Because hetastarch molecules exist over a molecular weight range of 10,000 to 1,000,000, their excretion is multiphasic. Molecules with a molecular weight under 50,000 are passively excreted by the kidneys. Larger molecules are more slowly metabolized by enzymes until they are small enough to undergo kidney elimination or to be assimilated as glucose.[20] Thirty-three percent of a 30 g hetastarch dose is renally eliminated within 24 hours of administration.[21] However, the apparent intravascular half-life of hetastarch is about 17 hours because of metabolism in the bloodstream (by amylase), liver and the reticuloendothelial system.[19]

Like albumin, hetastarch is approved by the FDA for the treatment of hypovolemia when volume expansion is desired. But unlike albumin, hetastarch's adjunctive use in leukapheresis is FDA-approved to increase the yield of granulocytes by centrifugal means.[21] In 1989, DuPont introduced a modification of hetastarch called pentastarch, that is only indicated as an adjunct in leukapheresis.[22] Pentastarch 10% is administered intravenously in a 500 ml volume to improve the harvesting and increase the yield of leukocytes and has the same contraindications as hetastarch.[23]

Hetastarch has low antigenicity[24] and does not impair renal function, but is contraindicated in severe renal failure or severe congestive heart failure. Caution is recommended in administering hetastarch to patients with hepatic dysfunction. As with large doses of albumin, hetastarch may significantly reduce hematocrit and cause hypocoagulability.[25]

Coagulation

Bleeding disorders may be caused by a deficiency of any of 13 coagulation factors in the blood. Hemophilia A (a deficiency of Factor VIII) accounts for about 85% of the patients with bleeding disorders. Factor IX deficiency (Hemophilia B or Christmas disease) accounts for almost 15% of hemophiliacs. A small percentage of hemophiliacs have hemophiloid conditions such as von Willebrand's disease, a deficit in von Willebrand's factor.[26]

Fresh-Frozen Plasma

Fresh-frozen plasma (FFP) is the fluid portion of one unit of whole blood that has been separated and frozen within 8 hours of collection.[1] FFP is indicated for: (1) replacement of known factor deficiencies like II, V, VII, X and XI; (2) rapid reversal of warfarin anticoagulation; (3) massive blood transfusion (greater than total body blood volume within several hours); (4) antithrombin III deficiency; (5) treatment of immunodeficiencies (although intravenous immune globulin is usually a better choice) and (6) treatment of thrombotic thrombocytopenic purpura. FFP should not be used when a coagulopathy can be corrected with vitamin K, cryoprecipitate, Factor VIII or Factor IX complex.[9]

FFP was the mainstay of hemophiliac therapy until the mid-1960s, when Factor VIII concentrate became available. FFP has a low hepatitis risk, but may cause chills, fever, allergic reactions, or circulatory overload (see Table 9–1).

Cryoprecipitated Antihemophilic Factor U.S.P.

Cryoprecipitated antihemophilic factor (cryoprecipitate) is Factor VIII prepared from a single unit of whole blood by slowly thawing fresh frozen anticoagulated plasma between 1 and 6°C.[1] It is then removed from the plasma by centrifugation and refrozen. Cryoprecipitate is widely used for hemophilia A and is also indicated for von Willebrand's disease or for replacement of fibrinogen or Factor XIII.

Cryoprecipitate is not indicated unless there is laboratory confirmation of a deficiency of a factor contained in cryoprecipitate. It can transmit hepatitis and other infectious diseases and may cause febrile or allergic reactions.[1]

Table 9–4.   Units of Factor VIII in Blood Components*

	Average Volume (ml)	Factor VIII Units/ml	Factor VIII Units/ Container
Fresh whole blood	517	0.5	258.5
Fresh plasma	225	1.0	225
Fresh-frozen plasma	200	0.8	180
Cryoprecipitate	10	8.0	80
Factor VIII concentrate	6–30	10–40	60–250

*One unit of factor VIII is defined as the amount of factor VIII in 1 ml of normal fresh plasma.

Platelet Concentrate U.S.P.

Platelets are harvested from single donors by plateletapheresis (single donor platelets) or separated from whole blood by pooling of platelets from multiple donors (platelets, pooled) to achieve a therapeutic dose.[27] Depending on the method of separation, the concentrate may contain significant numbers of lymphocytes and a few erythrocytes.[1] Plastic bags containing harvested platelets must be agitated gently and continuously and stored at 20 to 24°C. With new storage bags, federal regulations now allow storage of up to 5 days.[28]

The product is indicated for the treatment of (1) active bleeding if a platelet disorder has reduced platelet counts below $50,000/mm^3$; and (2) thrombocytopenia or functionally abnormal platelets to prevent bleeding when platelet counts are below 10,000 to $20,000/mm^3$.[27] Platelets may also be useful in thrombocytopenia secondary to chemotherapy or cancer.[1] Platelets are usually ineffective in treating idiopathic or immune thrombocytopenia purpura (ITP) or disseminated intravascular coagulation (DIC). Platelets are not generally recommended during massive transfusion or cardiac surgery.[27]

Chills, fever, or allergic reactions may occur after administration of platelets. Hepatitis or other infectious diseases are risks. Repeated platelet transfusions alloimmunize some patients to HLA antigens so that the patients may then respond only to HLA-matched platelets.

Antihemophilic Factor U.S.P.

Antihemophilic Factor (AHF) is a commercial preparation containing large amounts of nearly pure Factor VIII in liquid or dry lyophilized products (Table 9–4). These products are much more expensive than cryoprecipitate, but have the advantage of stability at 4°C and portability by a patient who is traveling.

There are at least four manufacturers of AHF who use a variety of methods in preparation leading to annual treatment costs ranging from $20,000 to over $60,000 per year. Those products that are pasteurized and treated with an organic solvent and detergent are least likely to transmit hepatitis and other communicable diseases, including the HIV virus.[29] Rarely, antihemophilic factor causes hemolytic anemia, or thrombosis or fibrinolysis.[30]

One manufacturer, using a monoclonal murine antibody on a sepharose column, has produced a purified AHF (Monoclate) that has about four times the activity per mg of protein as older AHFs.[29] In the future, recombinant DNA

Table 9–5. Immune Globulin Classes*

Class	Plasma Concentration (g/dL)	Molecular Weights	Monomeric Subunits	Primary Biologic Activity
IgG	1.3	150,000	One	Major antibody directed against infectious agents through complement activation and opsonization; anti-Rh specificity
IgA	0.4	325,000	Two	Major antibody in external secretions; initial protective mechanism at the mucous membrane against viruses and toxins
IgM	0.12	900,000	Five	Initial response to a new antigen; first antibody to form; anti-ABO specificity, complement activation, opsonization
IgD	0.003	160,000	One	Found on the surface of lymphocytes, particularly B cells
IgE	<0.0005	170,000	One	Found on mast cells; role in anaphylactic reactions and release of histamine; immunity to some parasitic diseases

*Modified from Wordell, C.J.: Use of intravenous immune globulin therapy: An overview. *D.I.C.P. Ann. Pharmacother., 25*:805 (1991).

technology may provide a source of pure coagulation factors such as AHF, which are free of disease transmission and transfusion reaction possibilities.[30]

Factor IX Complex U.S.P.

Factor IX complex U.S.P. or prothrombin complex concentrate is produced from pooled plasma and also contains Factors II, VII, and X. Factor IX complex is indicated in patients who cannot tolerate the volume required with doses of FFP in the treatment of hemophilia B. A relatively high risk of hepatitis must be weighed against the benefits of Factor IX complex. This product may also cause DIC or generalized thrombosis.[31]

Anti-Inhibitor Coagulant Complex

Anti-inhibitor coagulant complex is prepared from pooled human plasma and contains varying amounts of other clotting factors as well as components of

Table 9–6.   Immune Globulin G Subclasses*

Subclass	Plasma Concentration (g/dL)	Primary Biologic Activity
IgG$_1$	0.9	Antibody to tetanus, measles; tissue protection; strong affinity for Fc receptor on macrophages; passive cutaneous anaphylaxis; complement activation
IgG$_2$	0.3	Activity against polysaccharide-containing bacteria; complement activation
IgG$_3$	0.1	Complement activation; strong affinity for Fc receptor on macrophages; passive cutaneous anaphylaxis
IgG$_4$	0.05	Passive cutaneous anaphylaxis; antibody to factor VIII

*Modified from Wordell, C.J. Use of intravenous immune globulin therapy: An overview. *D.I.C.P. Ann. Pharmacother., 25*:805 (1991).

the kinin-generating system. Anti-inhibitor coagulant complex is used in hemophilia A patients who have antibodies that inhibit Factor VIII. It is estimated that 5 to 20% of hemophilia A patients exhibit such antibodies. It is contraindicated in patients with signs of fibrinolysis or DIC.[31]

Adverse reactions include fever, chills, hypo- or hypertension, and allergy. Also, headache, flushing, and changes in pulse rate may be caused by anti-inhibitor coagulant complex. Its risk of causing hepatitis is relatively high.

Antithrombin III (Human)

Antithrombin III is prepared from pooled human plasma of normal donors and is purified by affinity chromatography; it contains no preservatives.[32] Antithrombin III is also heat-treated in solution to prevent contamination with pathogens. It is not known whether antithrombin can transmit hepatitis or HIV.

Antithrombin III is indicated for treating patients with hereditary antithrombin III deficiency in connection with surgical or obstetric procedures or when they suffer from thromboembolism. Antithrombin III plasma levels should be monitored during therapy to achieve at least 80% of normal levels.[33]

Immunodeficiency

Immune globulins are a very important part of the body's immune system. There are five classes, all produced by mature B cells (plasma cells).[34] The five classes of immunoglobulins and their characteristics are shown in Table 9–5.[35] Immune globulin G (IgG) is the major antibody class against infectious organisms. Although IgG was first extracted from human plasma in the 1940s, a commercial, safe intravenous form was not available until the early 1980s.[36]

Table 9–7. Characteristics of the Preparations of Intravenous Immune Globulin Available in the United States*

Brand Name	Manufacturing Process	Additives	Approximate IgA Content (µg/ml)	Form Supplied	Storage Temp. (°C)	Manufacturer
Gamimune N	pH 4.25, diafiltration	10% maltose	270	5% liquid, pH 4.25	2–8	Cutter Biological, Miles Laboratories
Gammagard	Polyethylene glycol, DEAE-Sephadex, ultrafiltration	2% maltose, 0.2% polyethylene glycol, 0.3 M glycine, 0.15 M sodium chloride, 3% albumin	0.4–1.9	Lyophilized, 5%, pH 6.8	<25	Hyland Division, Baxter Healthcare
Gammar-IV	Low-ionic-strength ethanol	5% sucrose, 2.5% albumin, 0.5 sodium chloride	20	Lyophilized, 5%, pH 7.0	< 30	Armour Pharmaceutical
IVEEGAM	Immobilized trypsin, polyethylene glycol	5% glucose, 0.3% sodium chloride, 0.5 polyethylene glycol	5	Lyophilized, 5%, pH 6.8	2–8	Immuno-US
Sandoglobulin	pH 4.0, 1:10,000 trypsin	5% or 10% sucrose (sodium chloride in diluent)	720	Lyophilized, 3% or 6%, pH 6.6	<25	Sandoz Pharmaceutical
Venoglobulin-I	Polyethylene glycol, DEAE-Sephadex	2% D-mannitol, 1% albumin, 0.5% sodium chloride, <0.6% polyethylene glycol	24	Lyophilized, 5%, pH 6.8	<30	Alpha Therapeutic

*Modified from Buckley, R.H., and Schiff, R.I.: The use of intravenous immune globulin in immunodeficiency diseases. N. Engl. J. Med., 325:110 (1991).

Table 9–8. Summary of Blood Products and Plasma Expanders*

Product	Major Indications	Contraindications	Special Precautions
Whole blood	Symptomatic anemia with large volume deficit	Conditions responsive to specific component	Must be ABO-identical Labile coagulation factors deteriorate within 24 hours after collection
Red blood cells	Symptomatic anemia	Pharmacologically treatable anemia Coagulation deficiency	Must be ABO-compatible
Red blood cells, leukocytes removed	Symptomatic anemia, febrile reactions from leukocyte antibodies	Pharmacologically treatable anemia Coagulation deficiency	Must be ABO-compatible
Red blood cells, adenine-saline added	Symptomatic anemia with volume deficit	Pharmacologically treatable anemia Coagulation deficiency	Must be ABO-compatible
Fresh frozen plasma	Deficit of labile and stable plasma coagulation factors and TTP	Condition responsive to volume replacement	Should be ABO-compatible

Table 9–8. *Continued*

Product	Major Indications	Contraindications	Special Precautions*
Liquid plasma and plasma	Deficit of stable coagulation factors	Deficit of labile coagulation factors or volume replacement	Should be ABO-compatible
Cryoprecipitated AHF	Hemophilia A von Willebrand's Disease Hypofibrinogenemia Factor XIII deficiency	Conditions not deficient in contained factors	Frequent repeat doses may be necessary
Platelets: platelets, pheresis	Bleeding from thrombocytopenia or platelet function abnormality	Plasma coagulation deficits and some conditions with rapid platelet destruction (e.g. ITP)	Should not use some microaggregate filters (check manufacturer's instructions)
Granulocytes	Neutropenia with infection	Infection responsive to antibiotics	Must be ABO-compatible, do not use depth-type microaggregate filters

*Modified from American Red Cross, Council of Community Blood Banks and American Association of Blood Banks: Circular of Information for the Use of Human Blood and Blood Components. American Red Cross, August 1, 1992.

Intravenous Immune Globulin U.S.P.

IgG is comprised of four subclasses (IgG_1–IgG_4), each of which has a different primary plasma concentration and biologic activity (Table 9–6).[35] Six commercial intravenous IgGs are currently available, and they differ as to their manufacturing process, additives, contamination with IgA and dosage formulation (Table 9–7).[37]

Because of the broad biologic immune activity of intravenous immune globulin (IVIG), this product has been used for many diseases.[38] Labeled indications for IVIG include chronic lymphocytic leukemia, primary immunodeficiency disorders and idiopathic thrombocytopenic purpura (ITP).[39] Non-FDA labeled indications are many and controversial, because of conflicting or inadequate studies to support the indications and because of the high expense of the inappropriate use of IVIG. Non-labeled indications include Kawasaki syndrome, neonatal sepsis, autoimmune diseases like myasthenia gravis and systemic lupus erythematosus, IgG subclass deficiencies, cystic fibrosis, thermal injury, cytomegalovirus infection, HIV infection, and oral use for inadequate gastrointestinal tract production of IgG.[39]

Adverse reactions to IVIG are primarily related to infusion rate, activation of complement complexes and anaphylactic reactions to a component of the product.[35] Infusion rate-related reactions most commonly seen are headache, nausea, vomiting and (rarely) fever. Complement activation reactions include: facial flushing, chest tightness, chills, fever, abdominal pain, syncope, nausea, diaphoresis and hypotension or hypertension. IgA contamination is a significant cause of anaphylactic reactions in some patients. Therefore, such patients should use the low-IgA products.[35]

The risk of viral transmission by IVIG products is somewhat controversial. However, IVIG products currently on the market do not transmit hepatitis[40] or human immune viruses.[41]

Summary

The use of natural and synthetic components of blood is summarized in Table 9–8. In general, resuscitation for hemorrhagic shock should begin with a crystalloid solution such as lactated Ringer's injection or sodium chloride 0.9% injection. After 1 to 2 L are given, colloid solution may be administered to provide oncotic support. Thereafter, the clinician must monitor patient parameters to provide oxygenation of tissues with whole blood or packed red cells and for proper coagulability with the appropriate clotting factors. Hemophilia requires selection of the blood product that provides the deficient factor(s), causes the fewest risks, and optimizes use of a limited community blood supply. Some primary and secondary immune globulin deficiencies may be replaced with an intravenous immune globulin product. It may be appropriate to use intravenous immune globulins for other autoimmune diseases as well as to prevent infections in immunocompromised patients.

References

1. American Red Cross, Council of Community Blood Banks and American Association of Blood Banks: Circular of Information For the Use of Human Blood and Blood Components. American Red Cross, February 15, 1991, First Printing.

2. Welch, H.G., Meechan, K.R., and Goodnough, L.T.: Prudent strategies for elective red blood cell transfusion. Ann. Intern. Med., 116:393 (1992).

3. Aach, R.D., et al.: Hepatitis C virus infection in post-transfusion hepatitis: an analysis with first- and second-generation assays. N. Engl. J. Med., 325:1325 (1991).

4. Silberstein, L.E., et al. Strategies for the review of transfusion practices. JAMA, 262:1993 (1989).

5. National Institutes of Health Consensus Conference. Perioperative red blood cell transfusion. JAMA, 260:2700 (1988).

6. Ross, A.D., and Angaran, D.M.: Colloids vs. crystalloids—A continuing controversy. Drug Intell. Clin. Pharm., 18:202 (1984).

7. Griffel, M.I., and Kaufman, B.S. Pharmacology of colloids and crystalloids. Crit. Care Clin., 8:235 (1992).

8. Moss, G.S., and Gould, S.A.: Plasma expanders: An update. Am. J. Surg., 155:425 (1988).

9. N.I.H. Consensus Conference: Fresh-frozen plasma: Indications for use. JAMA, 253:551, (1985).

10. Heinonen, J.H., et al.: Correlation of hypotensive effect of plasma protein fraction with prekallikrein activator activity: A clinical study in patients having open heart surgery. Ann. Thorac. Surg., 33:244 (1982).

11. Rush, B.F., and Steward, R.A.: More liberal use of a plasma expander. N. Engl. J. Med., 280:1202 (1969).

12. Laks, H., et al.: Crystalloid versus colloid hemodilution in man. Surg. Gynecol. Obstet., 142:506 (1976).

13. Heyl, J.T., et al.: Studies on the plasma proteins. V. The effect of concentrated solutions of human and bovine albumin on blood volume after acute blood loss in man. J. Clin. Invest., 22:763 (1943).

14. Package labeling: Albumin (Human) 5%, U.S.P. (Plasbumin-5). Cutter/Miles, February 1992.

15. Package labeling: Albumin (Human) 25%, U.S.P. (Plasbumin-25) Cutter/Miles, March 1991.

16. Tullis, J.L.: Albumin-2 guidelines for clinical use. JAMA, 237:460 (1977).

17. Alexander, M.R., et al.: Therapeutic use of albumin: 2. JAMA, 247:831 (1982).

18. Lucus, C.E., et al.: Altered coagulation protein content after albumin resuscitation. Ann. Surg., 196:198 1982.

19. Nakasato, S.K.: Evaluation of hetastarch. Clin. Pharm., 1:509 (1982).

20. Hulse, J.D., and Yacobi, A.: Hetastarch: An overview of the colloid and its metabolism. Drug Intell. Clin. Pharm., 17:334 (1983).

21. Package labeling: 6% Hetastarch in 0.9% sodium chloride (Hespan). DuPont, October, 1991.

22. Strauss, R.G., et al. A multicenter trial to document the efficacy and safety of a rapidly excreted analog of hydroxyethyl starch for leukapheresis with a note on steroid stimulation of granulocyte donors. Transfusion, 26:258, 1986.

23. Package labeling: 10% pentastarch in 0.9% sodium chloride injection (Pentaspan). DuPont, 1988.

24. Ring, J., and Messmer, K.: Incidence and severity of anaphylactoid reactions to colloid volume substitution. Lancet, 1:466 (1977).

25. Strauss, R.G.: Review of the effects of hydroxyethyl starch on blood coagulation system. Transfusion, 21:299 (1981).

26. Rodvold, K.A., and Friedenberg, W.R.: Coagulation disorders. In DiPiro, J.T., et al. (eds.): Pharmacotherapy A Pathophysiologic Approach. New York, Elsevier, 1989, pp. 1003–17.

27. National Institutes of Health Consensus Conference. Platelet Transfusion Therapy. JAMA, 257:1777 (1987).

28. Nacht, A. The use of blood products in shock. Crit. Care Clin., 8:255 1992.

29. Monoclate: A purified antihemophilic factor. Med. Let. Drugs Ther., 29:1 (1988).

30. Johnson, A.J.: Approaches to plasma fractionation for improved recovery and the development of potentially useful clinical factors. Clin. Haematol., 13:3 (1984).

31. Kransnoff, A.R., and Mangione, R.A. Blood products used in the treatment of hemophilia. Hosp. Pharm., 17:598, 1982.

32. Package Labeling: Antithrombin III (Human) (Thrombate III). Cutter/Miles, January 1992.
33. Package Labeling: Antithrombin III (Human) (ATnativ). Baxter, April 1990.
34. Dwyer, J.M. Manipulating the immune system with immune globulin. N. Engl. J. Med., *326*:107 (1992).
35. Wordell, C.J. Use of intravenous immune globulin therapy: An overview. D.I.C.P. Ann. Pharmacother., *25*:805 (1991).
36. Immune Globulin, Intravenous. Med. Let. Drugs Ther. *24*:81, 1982.
37. Buckley, R.H., and Schiff, R.I.: The use of intravenous immune globulin in immunodeficiency diseases. N. Engl. J. Med., *325*:110 (1991).
38. Knapp, M.J., and Colburn, P.A. Clinical uses of intravenous immune globulin. Clin. Pharm., *9*:509 (1990).
39. ASHP Commission on Therapeutics: ASHP therapeutic guidelines for intravenous immune globulin. Clin. Pharm., *11*:117 (1992).
40. Gutteridge, C.N., Veys, P., and Newland, A.C. Safety of intravenous immunoglobulin for treatment of auto-immune thrombocytopenia. Acta Haematol., *79*:88 (1988).
41. Centers for Disease Control: Safety of therapeutic immune globulin preparations with respect to transmission of human T-lymphotropic virus type III-lymphadenopathy-associated virus infection. M.M.W.R., *35*:231 (1986).

CHAPTER

Fundamentals of Fluid and Electrolyte Therapy

Murray M. Tuckerman

Mortality and morbidity of patients caused by imbalance of water and electrolytes, blood carbohydrates, and proteins have decreased with increasing understanding of the balances involved. Nearly all solutions required to treat imbalances are available from manufacturers of parenteral products.

The proportions between water and electrolytes, carbohydrates, and proteins normally is maintained within a narrow range through a combination of dietary intake, metabolism, and excretion. Abnormalities can be produced by disease or injury. The physiology of the various systems is known. The imbalances can be determined by blood analysis. Methods for correcting the imbalances are available; nevertheless the therapy frequently is perplexing because of constraints of impaired function of kidney, liver, respiration, or hormones. A program for fluid therapy for correction of imbalance includes consideration of water, electrolytes, carbohydrates, and proteins (Table 10–1).

Measurement of Solute Concentration

The concentration of the solutes in parenteral therapeutic fluids and in blood or plasma may be stated in a variety of ways. Each of these ways is related to a particular property that may be of interest. Prepared fluids may be multiply labeled in several of these ways to provide information in convenient form or to provide information for a particular purpose. Sometimes the label refers to information originally obtained on the basis of units of solute per unit weight of solvent. This has been transformed into units of solute per unit

Table 10–1. Fundamentals of Body Water and Electrolytes

Electrolyte	Calculated as	At. Wt. (or Mol Wt.)	Valence	Eq. Wt. (or Eq. Vol.)	Normal Adult Ranges (mEq/L)
Sodium	Na	23	1	23	135–147
Potassium	K	39	1	39	3.8–5.0
Calcium	Total Ca	40	2	20	4.3–5.5
	Ionized Ca^{++}	40	2	20	2.4–2.8
Magnesium	Mg	24.3	2	12.2	1.7–2.3
Bicarbonate	CO_2 content	(44)	—	(22.26)	26–30
Chloride	Cl	35.5	1	35.5	100–106
Phosphate, inorganic	P	31	2.0	17.2	1.7–2.3
Sulfate, inorganic	S	32	2	16	0.3–1.3
Organic acids	Lactic acid	(90)	1	90	0.9–1.9
	Total organic acids	—	—	—	2–10
Proteinate	Plasma proteins	—	—	—	14.6–19.0

From Fundamentals of Body Water and Electrolytes. Deerfield, Ill., Baxter Laboratories, Inc., 1967, p. 47.

volume of solution for purposes of labeling. The method of transforming information is not always simple or noncontroversial.

The ways of labeling therapeutic fluids are as follows:
1. Weight per unit volume
2. Molecules per unit volume
3. Number of electrical charges per unit volume
4. Number of particles per unit volume unable to diffuse through a membrane
5. Tonicity: isotonic, hypotonic, or hypertonic

Each of these is discussed in detail:
1. Weight per unit volume is usually expressed using the metric system. The units which are frequently encountered are:
   a. Grams per liter (g/L)
   b. Milligrams per liter (mg/L)
   c. Milligrams per milliliter (mg/mL), sometimes incorrectly stated as milligrams per Cubic centimeter (mg/cc)
   d. Milligrams per deciliter (mg/dL), used in laboratory reports, sometimes incorrectly stated as milligram percent (mg %). This last designation arose because a dL is 100 mL and anything per 100 might be considered as percent.

Solutions labeled in percent can be readily converted to metric concentration as one (1) percent is 10 g/L. Thus a 5% dextrose solution contains

$$5\% \times 10 \text{ g/L}\% = 50 \text{ mg/L} \qquad \text{(Eq. 10–1)}$$

but not of $C_6H_{12}O_6$, anhydrous dextrose. It is customary to label parenteral fluids in terms of the highest stable hydrate of the solute, without regard to the degree of hydration of the substance actually used in the compounding of the solution. Dextrose is labeled as the monohydrate. A 5% dextrose solution contains 50 g/L of $C_6H_{12}O_6 \cdot H_2O$.

Laboratory reports, however, are for the concentration of the anhydrous substance. This difference adds to the complexity of calculating the amount of solution to be administered for therapy.

2. The measurement of molecules per unit volume is usually expressed as molarity, the number of moles per unit volume. A mole (mol) is the number of grams of a substance numerically equivalent to its molecular weight. A millimole (mmol) is one thousandth of a mole, or the molecular weight expressed in milligrams. Units frequently encountered are moles per liter (mol/L) and millimoles per liter (mmol/L). A solution that contains one (1) mole per liter may also be designated as a one molar (1 M) solution. Equimolar solutions of undissociated substances contain equal concentrations of particles.

The molecular weight of a substance is calculated by summing the atomic weights of the individual atoms. The current international atomic weights are based on the assignment of a weight of 12 atomic mass units (amu) to the carbon-12 isotope.

An atomic mass unit weighs 1.6604×10^{-24} g. Note that the numeric value of the atomic mass unit and the number of molecules in a mole (Avogadro's number) are necessarily reciprocals. The actual atomic weight of naturally occurring isotope mixtures of an element may vary according to geologic origin.

3. The number of electrical charges is usually expressed as equivalents. The concentration is expressed as the number of moles of electric charge per unit volume.

Equivalents refer only to charged particles. One (1) equivalent is the atomic or molecular weight of the ion in grams divided by the number of electrical charges it carries. Positively charged ions are cations; negatively charged ions are anions. The unit most frequently encountered is milliequivalents per liter (mEq/L).

Measuring ion concentrations in milliequivalents per liter emphasizes that ions associate to maintain electrical neutrality. There must be equal concentrations of cations and anions in body fluids. This requirement is important in determining ion transport in the kidney and in movement of ions between cell and extracellular fluid. The relationships cannot be easily followed using any other units of concentration.

A problem in the use of equivalents is that elements of interest can exist in both ionized and undissociated forms, or in ions bearing different numbers of electrical charge. The concentration of an ion in equivalents can be calculated from the following equation:

$$\text{mEq/L} = \frac{\text{mg}}{\text{dL}} \times \frac{10\ \text{dL}}{\text{L}} \times \frac{1\ \text{mEq}}{\text{mol wt (mg)}} \times \frac{\text{no. of electrical charges}}{\text{ion}} \quad \text{(Eq. 10–2)}$$

Calcium, for example, has a total concentration in the blood of about 10 mg/dL. For this calcium concentration, the calculation is (mol wt Ca = 40.0):

$$\text{mEq/L Ca}^{++} = 10\ \text{mg/dL} \times 10\ \text{dL/L} \times 1\ \text{mEq/40.0 mg} \times 2 \quad \text{(Eq. 10–3)}$$
$$= 5.0\ \text{mEq/L}$$

Actually, only 40 to 50 percent of the total calcium is ionized, so that the concentration of calcium ion is only 2.0 to 2.5 mEq/L. The remaining calcium is bound to albumin and, to a lesser extent, to blood citrate. Only the concentration of the ionized calcium influences the rate of the physiologic processes in which it participates.

The *United States Pharmacopeia XXII* (U.S.P.) requires that "The concentration and dosage of electrolytes for replacement therapy (e.g., sodium chloride or potassium chloride) shall be stated on the label in milliequivalents (mEq). The label of the product shall also indicate the quantity of ingredient(s) in terms of weight or percentage concentration."

Phosphorus presents a further problem. Not only is it present in both bound (organic) and ionized (inorganic) forms, but the ionized forms carry different amounts of charge. At the usual blood pH of 7.4, the ionized forms are principally $H_2PO_4^{-1}$ and HPO_4^{-2}. The ratio of these two forms can be calculated from the ionization constant for the equilibrium:

$$H^+ + HPO_4^{-2} \leftrightarrow H_2PO_4^{-1} \qquad \text{(Eq. 10–4)}$$

$$K_i = [H^+] [HPO_4^{-2}]/[H_2PO_4^{-1}] = 6.2 \times 10^{-8} \qquad \text{(Eq. 10–5)}$$

(The square brackets indicate concentrations in moles per liter.)
The ratio $[HPO_4^{-2}]/[H_2PO_4^{-1}]$ is calculated as follows:

$$pH = \log 1/[H^+] \qquad \text{(Eq. 10–6)}$$

For pH 7.4, $[H^+]$ = antilog -7.4 (Eq. 10–7)
$$= \text{antilog } 0.6 \times 10^{-8}$$
$$= 3.98 \times 10^{-8}$$

Substituting this value in equation 10–5, and rearranging, one obtains the following:

$$[HPO_4^{-2}]/[H_2PO_4^{-1}] = 6.2 \times 10^{-8}/3.98 \times 10^{-8} \qquad \text{(Eq. 10–8)}$$
$$= 1.5$$

The average charge of a phosphorus-containing anion can be calculated as follows:

$$\text{av charge/ion} = \frac{(\text{charge ion } 1 \times \text{rel conc}) + (\text{charge ion } 2 \times \text{rel conc})}{(\text{rel conc ion } 1 + \text{rel conc ion } 2)} \qquad \text{(Eq. 10–9)}$$

(av = average, rel = relative, conc = concentration).
Solving the above, using the relative concentrations of equation 10–8, one obtains the following:

$$\text{Average charge per ion} = (2 \times 1.5) + (1 \times 1)/(1.5 + 1) \qquad \text{(Eq. 10–10)}$$
$$= 1.6$$

Blood phosphorus is usually reported as inorganic phosphorus. A normal inorganic serum phosphorus value is 3.5 mg/dL. Substituting in equation 10–2 (at wt Phosphorus = 31.0), one obtains the following:

$$\text{mEq/L phosphate} = 3.5 \text{ mg/dL} \times 10 \text{ dL/L} \times 1 \text{ mEq/31.0 mg} \times 1.6 \qquad \text{(Eq. 10–11)}$$
$$= 1.8 \text{ mEq/L}$$

From these complex relationships, it can be seen that prescribing phosphorus or phosphate in terms of milliequivalents is literally meaningless and may be hazardous. Phosphorus (or phosphate) should always be prescribed on a molar basis, as millimoles.

Equivalents should never be used to refer to entire compounds but only to single ions. An order for 40 mEq of potassium phosphate raises the question of whether this is for 40 mEq of potassium and the accompanying phosphate or whether it means something else.

If it is filled with monobasic potassium phosphate, N.F., KH_2PO_4 (mol wt. 136.09), the 40 mEq will be supplied as follows: because each mole of KH_2PO_4 contains I atom of potassium and the charge on the potassium ion is +1, 1 mole of KH_2PO_4 contains 1 equivalent of K^+. The 40 mEq is then 40 × mol wt (mg), that is, 40 × 136.09 mg or 5.444 g. Each molecule of KH_2PO_4 contains 1 atom of P. The mol wt of P is 31.0. The 40 millimoles of KH_2PO_4 that provide 40 mEq of K^+ also provide 40 millimoles of P, that is, 40 × 31.0 mg or 1.24 g of P.

If the order is filled with dibasic potassium phosphate, U.S.P., K_2HPO_4 (mol wt 174.18), the 40 mEq will be supplied as follows: Because each mole of K_2HPO_4 contains 2 atoms of potassium and the charge on the potassium ion is +1, 1 mole of K_2HPO_4 contains 2 atoms of K^+. The 40 mEq is then 40/2 × mol wt (mg), that is, 40/2 × 136.09 mg or 3.584 g. The 20 millimoles of K_2HPO_4 provides 20 millimoles of P, that is, 20 × 31.0 mg or 0.62 g of P.

If Potassium Phosphates Injection, U.S.P. is used, the amount of phosphorus depends on the brand. The Abbott brand provides in each ml 4.4 mEq of K^+ and 3 mM of phosphorus; McGaw, 3 mEq of K^+ and 2.15 mM of P; Baxter, 2 mEq of K^+ and 1.12 mM of P. Using the Baxter product requires 20 ml, which is 0.695 g of P. Using the McGaw product requires 13.3 ml, which is 0.889 g of P. Using the Abbott product requires 9.09 mL, which is 0.845 g of P.

4. The concentration of particles unable to diffuse through a membrane is usually expressed as osmolarity. The unit most frequently encountered is milliosmoles per liter (mOs/L). This value is most often needed to assess the work required to be done by the kidneys in excreting the solute.

If solutions at two different concentrations are separated by a membrane which is permeable to the solvent but not to the solute (a semipermeable membrane), solvent will flow through the membrane from the solution of lower solute concentration to the solution of higher solute concentration. This flow of solvent is osmosis.

If increasing static pressure is applied to the solution of higher solute concentration, a pressure will be found that just stops the flow of solvent. This pressure is the osmotic pressure of the system. It is a measure of the free energy difference that provides the driving force for the solvent flow. It is also the excess pressure that would have to be applied to a solution to increase its activity to that of pure solvent at the same temperature.

Osmotic pressure is a property of the system containing the semipermeable membrane. If the two solutions of different concentrations were carefully layered, as could be done because of their difference in density, there would be solvent transfer to make the system homogeneous, but no osmotic pressure.

Assuming that the solution of lower concentration is pure solvent, the dependency of osmotic pressures on concentration and temperature is given by the van't Hoff equation:

$$\pi = MRT \qquad \text{(Eq. 10–12)}$$

π = osmotic pressure (atmospheres)
M = molar concentration of particles unable to diffuse
R = proportionality constant (liter-atmospheres per degree Kelvin)
T = absolute temperature (degrees Kelvin)

The proportionality constant R has the value 0.082, identical within experimental error with the value of R in the ideal gas law.

It is difficult to make direct measurement of osmotic pressure. Other properties of solutions that depend on the concentration of particles (colligative properties) are usually measured and the osmolarity calculated. The properties usually measured are depression of the freezing point and the difference in temperature between a solution and pure solvent at the same vapor pressure.

The measurements initially yield values in osmolality. This concentration is expressed in units of milliosmoles of solute per kilogram of solvent (mOs/kg). In very dilute solutions, the difference between osmolarity and osmolality is negligible, but in some of the more concentrated electrolyte solutions, the difference may be several percent. Methods for converting osmolality to osmolarity have been developed and are discussed in the following section.

The use of freezing-point depression gives particle concentrations near the freezing point of the solvent. The values usually desired are those at body temperature. Temperature corrections for volume changes and dissociation are not easily made, so that freezing-point depression values are of limited utility. Vapor pressure measurements are more difficult to make and involve comparison with appropriate standards but have the advantage of being able to be made at the temperature of interest.

Practically, the utility of physical measurements is restricted by the fact that biologic membranes do not behave as perfect semipermeable membranes. In addition, solute is transferred across biologic membranes by processes other than diffusion. These processes are discussed later under "Transport Across Biological Membranes."

5. Tonicity is a property of systems that is not easily quantified. If two solutions, each of a different solute, are separated by a membrane permeable to solvent only and there is no flow of solvent, the solutions are termed iso-osmotic. If the membrane is a cell membrane separating the natural cell contents from an aqueous solution and there is no net flow of water, the solution is termed isotonic. If water flows out of the cell, as shown by cell shrinkage,

the solution is termed hypertonic. If water flows into the cell, causing swelling or rupture (hemolysis of red blood cells), the solution is termed hypotonic.

Osmolality and Calculation of Osmolarity

Unfortunately for the workers in fluid therapy who need the particle concentration in numbers per unit volume, the physical chemists, to avoid the temperature dependency of tabulated values, have determined the colligative properties (properties dependent upon the concentration of solute particles) of solutions on the basis of numbers of particles per kilogram of solvent. That is, the physical chemists report values in osmolality, milliosmoles per kilogram (mOs/kg), whereas the fluid therapist needs the values in osmolarity, milliosmoles per liter (mOs/L). The similarity in sound and spelling between "osmolarity" and "osmolality" creates confusion. The fact that for extremely dilute solutions the two are nearly equal numerically sustains the confusion. Authors have used the two terms interchangeably when referring to the results of calculations from freezing-point data, thus compounding the confusion and requiring references to be read very carefully.

Molal solutions prepared at one temperature have the same molal concentration at any other temperature. Molar solutions prepared at one temperature change molarity with change in temperature because the volume of the solution changes with temperature.

To further add to the difficulty, real solutions deviate from the properties predicted on the assumption of ideal behavior. It is thus necessary to refer to tables of properties for particular concentrations of particular solutes rather than relying on calculations assuming ideal behavior.[1,2]

The need for knowing the osmolarity of parenteral fluids is shown by the labeling requirement in the United States Pharmacopeia XXII. "Where an osmolarity declaration is required in the individual monograph, the label states the total osmolar concentration in milliosmoles per liter. Where the contents are less than 100 mL, or where the label states that the article is not for direct injection but is to be diluted before use, the label alternatively may state the total osmolar concentration in milliosmoles per milliliter." A list of injections requiring such labeling is given in Table 10–2. General Chapter 785 of the U.S.P., unfortunately, is unclear as to how the value is to be determined, leading to differences in labeling of the same solutions by different manufacturers.[3]

An assumption is made in the preparation of parenteral fluids that, for most substances of interest, a solution iso-osmotic with plasma is also isotonic. The first problem, then, is determining the osmolarity of plasma. The commonly accepted value of the freezing point of the plasma of a normal, hydrated person is −0.56°C. Using the Scientific Tables, this gives a real osmolality of 302 mOs/Kg. This may be converted to osmolarity by multiplying by an appropriate factor, which is tabulated as 0.940 for plasma with a specific gravity of 1.026 (1 liter of plasma of specific gravity 1.026 contains 940 g of water). This gives the commonly accepted osmolarity of plasma of 284 mOs/L.

It should be noted that the commonly accepted value for the freezing point of plasma has been challenged. Thus Lund et al. give −0.52°C and Hendry gives −0.53°C.[4,5]

Table 10–2. Official Injections Requiring Osmolarity Labeling by the *United States Pharmacopeia XXII*, U.S. Pharmocopeial Convention, Inc., Rockville, MD., 1989.

Alcohol in Dextrose Injection
Ammonium Chloride Injection
Arginine Hydrochloride Injection
Calcium Chloride Injection
Calcium Gluceptate Injection
Calcium Gluconate Injection
Calcium Levulinate Injection
Dextrose Injection
Dextrose and Sodium Chloride Injection
Fructose Injection
Fructose and Sodium Chloride Injection
Magnesium Sulfate Injection
Mannitol Injection
Mannitol in Sodium Chloride Injection
Potassium Acetate Injection
Potassium Chloride Injection
Potassium Chloride in Dextrose Injection
Potassium Chloride in Dextrose and Sodium Chloride Injection
Potassium Chloride in Sodium Chloride Injection
Potassium Phosphates Injection
Protein Hydrolysate Injection
Ringer's Injection
Lactated Ringer's Injection
Sodium Acetate Injection
Sodium Bicarbonate Injection
Sodium Chloride Injection
Sodium Lactate Injection
Sodium Phosphates Injection

If the freezing point of plasma is taken as $-0.53°C$, its real osmolality is 285.8 mOs/Kg (as contrasted to its calculated ideal osmolality of $0.53/1.86 = 284.9$ mOs/L). This value is corrected for the high specific volume of plasma protein and the volume occupied by inorganic constituents of plasma by making use of the specific gravity of the plasma as was done above. Using again the factor of 0.940 for plasma with a specific gravity of 1.026 gives an osmolarity of 269 mOs/L.

The osmolality calculated by osmometry using freezing point or vapor pressure is required to be converted to osmolarity. The methodology, which rests on the most secure theoretic base, is given by Streng et al.[6] This shows that

$$\text{osmolarity (mOs/L)} = \text{osmolality (mOs/Kg)} \, [d_1^0 (1 - 0.001020 \, v_0^2]$$

d_1^0 = density of pure solvent   Eq. (10–13)

v_0^2 = partial molar volume of the solute at infinite dilution.

For multiple solutes, a summation over all the species is necessary. This involves defining a standard reference state, a problem which has not been satisfactorily resolved. Factors needed for this calculation, as given by the authors,[6] are:

$$\text{Potassium Chloride } v_0^2 = 25.74 \text{ ml/mole, } K = 0.99704$$
$$\text{Sodium Chloride } v_0^2 = 16.63 \text{ ml/mole, } K = 0.98049$$

$$K = d_1^0 (1 - 0.00102 \, v_0^2), \text{ with } d_1^0 = 0.99707 \text{ g/ml at } 25°C.$$

Sodium Chloride Injection, 0.9% w/v, is listed as 286 mOsm/Kg and 280 mOs/L.

A difficulty with the method is obtaining values for the partial molar volumes for the substances of interest in fluid therapy.

A method with a less secure theoretical base makes use of the density of the solution.[7] By this method,

$$\text{mOsm/L} = \text{mOsm/Kg (density} - \text{grams solute/ml)} \qquad \text{Eq. (10–14)}$$

Strictly, the density is that of the solution at the freezing point. This can be approximated from tabulated values of $\rho = D_4^{20}$. The grams of solute/ml is taken at temperature of 25°C, the official temperature for labeling of U.S.P. solutions. For various solutions of calcium chloride, dextrose, mannitol, potassium chloride, sodium bicarbonate and sodium chloride, the authors give the osmolality calculated from their own freezing point measurements; the corresponding osmolarity calculated from their equations; the osmolality gathered from the literature; and osmolarity assuming ideal behavior. Again, the difference in freezing points reported by these authors and elsewhere in the literature can only add to the confusion in labeling. Sodium Chloride Injection, 0.9% w/v is listed as 292 mOs/Kg and 291.4 mOs/L. Using the literature value of 287 mOs/Kg and a density of 1.0046, equation 10–14 gives 286 mOs/L.

There is an additional consideration. Determination of freezing point or vapor pressure of plasma measures total effective particles. This gives too high an estimate of the osmocity of solutions expected to be isotonic with plasma because the urea content of the plasma adds to its osmocity but has no effect on tonicity. A correction for urea content of plasma could be made if the data are to be used for estimating concentration of substances for isotonic solutions. By comparison with experimental errors in the determination of the colligative properties of plasma and the assumptions required to convert osmolality to osmolarity, this correction is negligible. The work involved in the calculation is not rewarded by increased confidence in the accuracy of the results.

In summary, controversy exists about the exact freezing point of parenteral fluids. The method of converting mOs/Kg calculated from physical measurements to mOs/L is not simple. What is known is that the assumption of ideal behavior is inadequate and can lead to grossly incorrect results.

Transport Across Biological Membranes

Membranes are the primary barriers to the movement of solute in the body. All the membranes are permeable to water, which passes through freely by simple diffusion or osmosis. When water moves across a membrane, it may carry with it solutes to which the membrane is permeable. This is known as solvent drag and is independent of solute concentration or other processes affecting movement of solute across the membrane.

Small solutes may diffuse through all membranes, but at a rate slower than that of water. The ability to cross the lipoprotein membrane depends in part upon the lipid solubility of the solute. Lipid-soluble gases, oxygen and carbon dioxide, and lipid-soluble urea pass through rapidly. Small hydrophilic ions and glucose diffuse only through the aqueous channels of the membrane and thus move more slowly than lipophilic substances. The process is passive diffusion from a region of higher concentration to a region of lower concentration.

When an ion moves across a membrane, it carries its electrical charge, thus setting up an electrical potential on the membrane. This potential repels ions of the same charge sign, inhibiting their passage through the membrane, and attracts ions of opposite charge sign (counter-ions). Because of active transport mechanisms (to be discussed later), charges are separated to varying degrees across all living biologic membranes. This causes a persistent membrane potential, so that strict electrical neutrality is not maintained. This electrostatic charge is too small to be detected clinically.

An interesting form of passive transport, co-transport, takes place when an active carrier combines with its specific substrate and the combination then drags with it another solute. The total combination makes for more efficient transport of both solutes. The net effect is such that it appears that the presence of either solute enhances the transport of the other.

An example of this is at the brush border of the renal proximal tubules. The fundamental process is sodium transport from the tubule lumen into the cell. The actual transport is sodium-glucose, sodium-phosphate, and sodium-amino acids. Sodium thus enhances the reabsorption of the co-transports and the organic substances enhance the reabsorption of sodium. Note that one of the solutes may move against a gradient. In that case, the process is called secondary active transport. Energy must eventually be provided.

Countertransport is closely related to co-transport. In countertransport, a carrier moves ions across a membrane in one direction and an ion of like electrical charge moves in the opposite direction. The two phenomena, co-transport and countertransport, are forms of coupled transport.

Moving a solute against a gradient is called active transport or pumping, which requires energy. An example of this is the relationships between sodium and potassium ions in muscle cell and in the interstitial fluid surrounding the cell. Because the extracellular concentration of sodium is higher than the cellular concentration, sodium tends to diffuse passively into the cell. The reverse relationship holds for potassium, which tends to diffuse out of the cell. The concentration gradients are maintained, however, by active transport of sodium ion out of the cell and potassium ion into the cell, against the concentration gradients.

The activity of this sodium ion-potassium ion pump seems to be regulated by an enzyme, sodium-potassium-activated adenosine triphosphatase, which catalyzes the hydrolysis of higher energy adenosine triphosphate (ATP) into

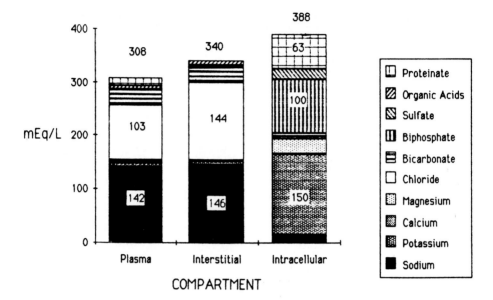

Figure 10–1.   Electrolytes in body water compartments.

lower energy adenosine diphosphate (ADP) to release the energy required by the pump.

Macromolecules that are too large to cross cell membranes are moved by a process called endocytosis. The macromolecule is first surrounded by cell membrane, then drawn into the cell and pinched off. The former cell membrane is now an intracellular membrane forming the boundary of a vesicle, which can then release the macromolecule. Endocytosis is the mechanism for tubular reabsorption of large polypeptides such as insulin.

Water Balance

Total body water is 45 to 50% of body weight of adult females but 55 to 60% of body weight of adult males. Individual and gender-specific variability is mostly a result of variations in skeletal weight and proportion of adipose tissue.

The body water is divided into two compartments, the intracellular fluid, water within the cells, and extracellular fluid, water not in cells. The extracellular fluid is further subdivided. The largest subdivision is interstitial/lymph water, the fluid which bathes all cells, and plasma, water which circulates rapidly. These two are in equilibrium across the walls of capillaries. There are another three small extracellular water compartments; water in dense connective tissue such as tendons and cartilage, water in bones, and the transcellular water of cerebrospinal, synovial, pleural and intraocular fluids, digestive secretions, and sweat. Electrolytes in body water compartments are represented by the graph in Figure 10–1.

Total body water cannot be measured directly. It is estimated by dilution techniques using either deuterium oxide or antipyrine. The calculation is sim-

Table 10–3. Representative Distribution of Water in a 70 kg Male

Compartment	Volume (Liters)
Total body water*	42
Intracellular water[†]	25
Interstitial/lymph	8
Plasma	3
Dense connective tissue	3
Bone	2
Transcellular	1

*Total body water = 60% of body weight
[†]Intracellular water = 60% of total body water

ple but requires knowledge of the amount of these substances that is excreted and the final concentration in the water.

$$\text{Volume of distribution} = \frac{\text{amount given} - \text{amount excreted}}{\text{concentration}} \qquad \text{Eq. (10–15)}$$

In the same way, extracellular volume has been measured using sulfate or a nonmetabolizable sugar such as inulin or mannitol. Plasma volume has been measured using Evans blue, a dye which is plasma bound, or radioiodinated albumin. Intracellular water cannot be determined directly but is estimated as the difference between total body water and extracellular water. Although there are significant variations with age, weight, and gender, and with time for a given individual, representative distribution might be as given in Table 10–3.

Water moves freely across all body membranes. The distribution of water between cellular and extracellular fluid depends upon the number of osmotically active particles in each compartment. Most of these particles are K^+ in the cellular fluid and Na^+ in the extracellular fluid. The divalent ions are mostly protein-bound and osmotically inactive. The osmotically active ions are restricted to their compartments by the $Na^+ - K^+$ pump in the cell membrane. The ratio of the volume of cellular to extracellular fluid is determined, then, mainly by the exchangeable Na^+/K^+ ratio. Assuming adequate water intake, water balance in the body is regulated by kidney excretion of water in response to the blood level of antidiuretic hormone (ADH) released from the supraoptic nucleus of the hypothalamus and the neurohypophysis of the pituitary. Factors affecting the levels of this hormone are shown in Table 10–4. The homeostatic mechanism is closely regulated so that normal variation is less than 2% and usually less than 1% per day. Antidiuretic hormone acts by increasing water resorption in the distal portion of the kidney tubule.

Water imbalance can be divided into extracellular fluid volume (ECF) deficit and extracellular fluid volume excess, each of which can be subdivided. Primary water deficit (primary dehydration, hypotonic dehydration, hypovolemia) is caused whenever water intake is inadequate, or by inability of the patient to slake thirst because of loss of consciousness or physical disability. It can be caused by oversecretion, such as in diabetes insipidus or in patients

Table 10–4. Factors Affecting Release of Antidiuretic Hormone

Stimulation	Inhibition
Hyperosmolar extracellular fluid	Hypo-osmolar extracellular fluid
Decreased aortic blood pressure	Elevated blood pressure increase in pressure in left auricle
Decreased carotid artery blood pressure	
Decrease in distention of left atrial wall	Lying down, back downward
Decrease in distention of pulmonary veins	Cold, with a drop in blood temperature
	Drugs
Emotional stress	alcohol
Pain	atropine
Standing without much movement	diphenylhydantoin
Elevated temperature	epinephrine
Low plasma volume	
Drugs	
acetylcholine	
barbiturates	
meperidine	
morphine	
nicotine	

given concentrated tubal feedings, or by increase in water loss from the lungs during rapid respiration.

Water and electrolyte deficits are caused by loss of body fluids as a result of vomiting, diarrhea, edema, intestinal obstruction, excessive gastrointestinal drainage (fistulous drainage or nasogastric suction), paracentesis or thoracentesis, burns, peritonitis, ascites, pleural effusion, excessive sweating due to fever or high ambient temperatures, chronic renal insufficiency or uremia with acidosis, and acidosis of starvation or diabetes. Loss of water and sodium can be overwhelming if mineralocorticoid levels are low, such as in chronic adrenocortical insufficiency (Addison's disease) or sudden withdrawal of steroid therapy.

Laboratory findings in ECF deficit are:
1. Concentrated urine
2. Elevated hematocrit
3. Elevated hemoglobin
4. Elevated red blood count
5. High blood nitrogen (azotemia)
6. Absence of urinary chloride, if renal function is normal
7. Urinary sodium absent or very low, if there is water and electrolyte deficit

Clinical observations in ECF deficit are:
1. Large output of urine (oliguria) or no urine (anuria)
2. Acute weight loss, more than 5% of body weight
3. Dryness of skin and mucous membrane
4. Longitudinal wrinkling of tongue
5. Hypotension

6. Tachycardia
7. Lowered body temperature

One type of extracellular fluid volume excess is hypotonic volume excess (dilution hyponatremia) owing to retention of water without retention of sodium, such as occurs in some cases of bronchogenic carcinoma, adrenal insufficiency and inappropriate antidiuretic hormone secretion (IADH) caused by hypothalamic injury as sometimes occurs in intercranial aneurysms. The chief cause, however, is iatrogenic. If too much 5% glucose is given over a long period of time, water intoxication can occur. A surgical procedure no longer used called for a patient to be fully hydrated before surgery by starting intravenous infusion of 5% glucose the night before and continuing during surgery and recovery, in the belief that postoperative patients were intolerant of electrolyte solutions. Because the concentration of antidiuretic hormone is high during surgery and in the early postoperative period (pain increases release of ADH), the intravenous fluid was retained.

The progressive symptoms of water intoxication are
1. Confusion
2. Bizarre behavior
3. Fixed stare
4. Inability to talk
5. Nausea and vomiting, sometimes
6. Periods of violence and noisiness
7. Delirium
8. Muscular weakness
9. Drowsiness
10. Coma

Note that there are no gross physical symptoms, since there is no edema or increase in skin turgor. Although water intoxication is rare, it can happen during long operative procedures and when administration of fluids has been ordered by several physicians without any one recognizing the magnitude of the total intake. It can also happen when a thirsty person drinks too much water without replacing the lost electrolytes. It formerly happened when infant diarrhea was treated with water and carbohydrate only, without electrolyte replacement.

In the hospitalized patient, water balance is usually checked by measuring water intake and urinary output, estimating fecal loss and insensible loss through sweat and respiration. The patient is generally checked by daily weighing, since changes in weight of a fully hydrated patient signify a change in the water balance.

The need for water is based on the value of 1600 ml/m^2 of body surface/day. Body surface is estimated from nomograms which relate height and weight of the patient to body surface. The weight is not the actual weight, but is an estimate of the lean muscle mass weight which may run from 94% of total weight in an athlete, through 75% of total weight for the average woman, to 60% or less for the obese or edematous patient. Table 10–5 shows some normal values relating to water balance.

A second type of extracellular fluid volume excess is isotonic volume excess. Some of the causes are

Table 10–5.   Normal Values Relating to Water Balance

	Losses
Adult urinary output	1000–2500 ml/day
Minimal urinary output	400–600 ml/day of sp. gr. above 1.030 and 1000–1400 milliosmolar
Fecal loss	100–200 ml/day
Respiratory loss	From 300 to 500 ml/day in females, up to 750 ml/day for males
Surface evaporation and sweat	300 to 500 ml/m²/day
Loss during fever	About 300 ml/°C above normal/day
	Gains
Drink	1000–2500 ml/day
Food	100–1500 ml/day
Metabolism	200–400 ml/day

1. Edema from congestive heart failure
2. Excessive administration of adrenal corticoid hormone, or presence of large amounts of these hormones in the immediate postoperative phase of surgery
3. Hyperaldosteronism, which stimulates renal retention of sodium, which, in turn, stimulates production of ADH
4. Kidney disease
5. Chronic liver disease with portal hypertension
6. Plasma protein deficit because of dietary deficiency, which reduces osmotic pull at the venous end of the kidney capillary
7. Excessive dietary intake of salt
8. Excessive infusion of isotonic sodium chloride, thus causing a chloride excess

Laboratory findings in isotonic volume excess are:
1. Low hematocrit
2. Low hemoglobin
3. Low erythrocyte count

Clinical symptoms are:
1. Acute weight gain, in excess of 5% of body weight
2. Pitting edema
3. Moist rales in lung
4. Puffy eyelids
5. Shortness of breath (dyspnea)
6. Bounding pulse, as a result of increase in plasma volume

The goal of therapy is to remove the excess sodium and water without producing abnormal changes in osmolarity or composition of the body fluids. This generally requires correction of the underlying cause. Sometimes abdominal paracentesis or thoracentesis or phlebotomy is done. In other instances a hypotonic solution balanced with respect to electrolyte proportions is infused slowly to aid in the excretion of excess sodium.

The tonicity of plasma, which is one way of evaluating body hydration, may be estimated adequately by equating the osmolarity of plasma with twice the number of milliequivalents per liter of sodium ion found by blood analysis. This simple relationship has no theoretical basis, but is due to a fortuitous balancing of factors. First, sodium ion is the predominant osmotically active substance in plasma. Small contributions are made by potassium, calcium and magnesium ions and by blood glucose. Urea is osmotically inactive in the body. Secondly, the apparent osmotic activity of sodium ion is about 90% of that expected from its concentration; but the water content of plasma is about 93%, so that the osmotically active concentration of sodium in plasma water is higher than that calculated from the concentration in plasma.

Sodium Balance

About 90% of the total body sodium is in the extracellular fluid. The normal plasma concentration of Na^+ is 135 to 145 mEq/L.

Sodium excess is usually caused by water loss from the extracellular fluid not accompanied by loss of salt (sodium chloride). The fluid becomes hypertonic, and water moves into it from the interstitial fluid. This causes a total body water deficit, or dehydration. Adequate water intake is usually ensured by the sensation of thirst, which is partially controlled by the hypothalamus. Deficient water intake can occur in patients who cannot communicate the feeling of thirst and those unable to swallow. Sodium excess can also be caused by excessive water output, such as in sweating in hot weather or prolonged high fevers, in severe vomiting, and in prolonged copious diarrhea. A less usual cause is lack of antidiuretic hormone, causing diabetes insipidus. In infants, who generally have a reduced capacity to excrete solutes, the excess can be produced by excessive intake through feeding of soup or skimmed milk that has been overly concentrated by boiling or by inadequate dilution with water when prepared from concentrates. The symptoms are those of water deficit. The deficit can be calculated from the value for serum sodium. For each 1% increase in serum sodium above normal values, there is a 1% deficit in total body water. Thus, for the 70-kg male with a total body water of 42 L, each 1% increase requires replacement of 0.42 L, either orally or with intravenous 5% dextrose.

Sodium deficit with normal sodium serum concentrations is caused by simultaneous loss of water and electrolytes. This has been discussed under "Water Balance" as "water and electrolyte deficit."

Sodium deficit with hyponatremia is frequently found in cirrhosis as a result of many factors: inadequate dietary intake, sequestration of sodium in the perineal ascites, increased absorption levels because of decreased inactivation by the liver, and inappropriate secretion of antidiuretic hormone. Findings in hyponatremia may include

1. Hypotonic extracellular fluid (not reliable in hyperglycemia, hyperlipidemia or hyperproteinemia)
2. Decrease in interstitial and plasma volumes
3. Serum sodium value less than 137 mEq/L (normal is 142) and serum chloride less than 98 mEq/L (normal is 103)
4. Muscle weakness
5. Agitation, apprehension, or anxiety
6. Cloudy sensorium and convulsions

7. Abdominal cramps
8. Oliguria or anuria
9. "Fingerprinting" of the sternum

Treatment for the problems depends on the underlying cause.[8]

Fluid and electrolyte disorders can be classified as follows:
1. Hypervolemia and edema (sodium and water excess, plasma sodium less than 10 mEq/L)
   a. congestive heart failure
   b. cirrhosis of the liver
   Treatment: water restriction to less than the calculated daily loss
2. Hypovolemia (plasma sodium less than 10 mEq/L)
   a. gastrointestinal losses without urinary loss of bicarbonate
   b. excessive sweating
   c. other losses, not involving the kidneys
   Treatment: Intravenous isotonic saline; in emergencies, hypertonic saline administered slowly and limited to 300 ml/4 hours
3. Hypervolemia (plasma sodium greater than 10 mEq/L)
   a. diuretic overuse
   b. adrenal insufficiency
   c. chronic kidney failure (renal salt wasting)
   d. vomiting with metabolic alkalosis and bicarbonaturia
   Treatment: water restriction. The negative fluid balance can be calculated by the method which requires an estimate of total body water
4. Hypervolemia without edema
   a. primary hypothyroidism (myxedema)
   b. syndrome of inappropriate antidiuretic hormone (SIADH)
   Treatment: water restriction and an initial dose of furosemide, 1 mg/kg, with replacement of electrolytes lost in the urine, followed by subsequent doses to achieve the desired negative water balance.

Potassium Balance

Serum potassium levels do not necessarily indicate the intracellular concentration of potassium. In patients with anoxemia, low insulin levels, or low blood glucose, potassium may not move into the cells. The kidneys may excrete potassium even when total body potassium is low. In the cells of the renal tubules, sodium is absorbed from the fluid in the lumen and potassium is excreted in its place.

Potassium deficit, hypokalemia, defined as serum potassium values of less than 3.5 mEq/L (normal range is 3.5 to 5.0 mEq/L), causes movement of potassium from cells into the intracellular fluid while hydrogen ion moves into the cell. In the renal tubules, sodium is exchanged for hydrogen ion instead of potassium. The hydrogen ions are then excreted, and bicarbonate ion is consequently retained, causing alkalosis. Thus, in hypokalemia, the urine is acid, plasma levels of potassium and chloride are low, plasma levels of bicarbonate are high, and so is plasma pH.

Potassium deficit may be shown by:
1. Paralytic ileus

2. Fatigue
3. Decreased deep tendon reflexes
4. Weak pulse
5. Increased cardiac sensitively to digitalis
6. Abnormal electrocardiogram (not useful for diagnosis of hypokalemia, but useful for monitoring therapy)
   a. P wave flattened or inverted
   b. ST segment depressed
   c. U wave may follow T wave

Hypokalemia may be caused by:
1. Thiazide diuretics in large amounts over prolonged periods for treatment of hypertension
2. Volume contraction, causing aldosterone increase
3. Protracted vomiting or diarrhea
4. Mineralocorticoid activity of therapy with cortisone or adrenocortico-tropic drugs
5. Hyperaldosteronism associated with cirrhosis of the liver
6. Severe burns
7. Excessive sweating (sweat contains about 9 mEq K^+/L)
8. Inadequate dietary intake (usually accompanying severe illness)
9. Overtreatment of hyperkalemia with ion exchange resins
10. Treatment of diabetic acidosis with insulin
11. Decrease of renal tubule absorption of potassium, caused by some antibiotics such as penicillins
12. Metabolic alkalosis caused by administration of sodium bicarbonate or sodium lactate

Treatment of hypokalemia is usually complicated by the underlying disease process. In patients receiving thiazide diuretics and digitalis for whom hypokalemia is life-threatening, therapy must not be started until serum potassium levels have been determined and adequate kidney function shown by creatinine clearance evaluation. Treatment must be extremely cautious if there is impaired kidney function.

In the presence of acidosis or aldosterone deficiency, such as in Addison's disease or the first postoperative day, and in chronic or acute kidney disease, potassium-containing solutions are contraindicated unless serum levels are low and there are clinical signs of deficit, because the conditions are expected to produce hyperkalemia.

If intravenous potassium salts are used to replenish extracellular stores, they should not be given in glucose solution because glucose causes movement of potassium into cells. Isotonicity is produced through addition of sodium salts. The concentration of potassium should be about 40 mEq/L and never more than 80 mEq/L. It can be administered at rates up to 30 mEq/hour.

Potassium excess, hyperkalemia, may occur in kidney failure as a result of inability to excrete excess potassium, and in aldosterone deficiency. Other causes of hyperkalemia are extensive tissue damage in which cellular potassium is released, rapid transfusion of banked blood containing high concentrations of potassium, or other excessive potassium administration.

Potassium excess may be shown by:

1. Paresthesia in the fingers
2. Weakness, muscle pain, muscle cramps
3. Diarrhea
4. Abnormal electrocardiogram
   a. T waves very narrow
   b. S wave increase
   c. QRS interval widening
   d. P wave disappearance

Therapy for hyperkalemia is directed to the removal of the excess. The regimen may include:

1. Potassium-free diet to decrease intake
2. Intravenous sodium chloride, to promote excretion, if the kidneys are fully functional
3. In the nondiabetic patient, intravenous insulin with dextrose and bicarbonate to provide movement of potassium into the cells. A popular mixture is made by the addition of 15 units of regular insulin and 44 to 88 mEq of (sodium) bicarbonate added to 500 ml of 10% Dextrose in Water
4. Acetazolamide, for carbonic anhydrase inhibition, to cause an increase in urine volume and output of potassium, sodium, and bicarbonate
5. Ion exchange resins have been used to remove dietary potassium at doses of 15 g, three times a day. The sodium form of the resin is usually chosen, as the hydrogen form might add to acidosis and the calcium form might contribute to hypercalcemia. The sodium form does add about 2 g/day to sodium intake and requires concomitant administration of an osmotic laxative, usually 30 ml of 70% sorbitol, to prevent fecal impaction.
6. In mineralocorticoid deficiency, fludrocortisone seems to be the current choice. It is less expensive than the formerly used desoxycorticosterone acetate. Carbonic anhydrase inhibitors are not effective for prolonged therapy.

Calcium Balance

Calcium is present in serum as calcium ion (43 to 49% of the total), complexed to anions such as phosphate or citrate (5 to 7%), or bound to serum protein, primarily albumins (44 to 52%). The ionized and complexed forms diffuse easily through body membranes. The ionized form only is biologically active in regulatory hormonal control mechanisms and other biologic functions such as neuromuscular excitation threshold, myocardial contraction, and blood coagulation. Decreases in serum albumin concentration, such as occur in nephrotic syndrome, cirrhosis, or malnutrition, decrease total serum calcium (about 0.8 mg/dL for each 1 g/L decrease in serum albumin) without affecting the concentration of ionized calcium. Ionized calcium levels in plasma are maintained through dynamic equilibrium with calcium in bone. The mechanisms are not well defined, but are known to involve gastrointestinal absorption and kidney tubule reabsorption, parathyroid hormone, 1,25-dihydroxycholecalciferol, and calcitonin. Disturbances of the hormone levels may disturb absorption or equilibrium.

Calcium excess, hypercalcemia, may be caused in a variety of ways:
1. Excessive dietary intake of vitamin D, causing increased absorption of dietary calcium.
2. Excessive intake of milk or calcium salts, especially with sodium bicarbonate
3. Multiple myeloma or other osteolytic bone malignancies.
4. Leukemia.

Hypercalcemia may cause the following:
1. Lassitude
2. Anorexia
3. Constipation
4. Nausea and vomiting (serum levels above 12 mg/dL)
5. Polyuria and polydipsia, in reduced kidney function
6. Cardiac arrhythmia and death (serum levels above 15 mg/dL)

Therapy is usually based on the following considerations:
1. Restriction of dietary calcium, but this is not expected to be effective if bone is the source of the excess calcium.
2. Adequate hydration to maintain kidney elimination of calcium.
3. Use of glucocorticoids (prednisone, 40 mg/day) may be effective in mild cases.
4. Use of intravenous Sodium Chloride Injection to produce sodium diuresis. Sodium inhibits tubule reabsorption of calcium. The sodium load must be appropriate for patients with other conditions such as congestive heart failure.
5. Loop diuretics, such as ethacrynic acid and furosemide increase kidney excretion of calcium. These may be given intravenously in the Sodium Chloride Injection. Thiazide diuretics cause calcium retention.
6. Phosphate administration, orally, causes deposition of calcium in bone. Intravenous and rectal administration have also been used.
7. Mithramycin, in about one tenth of the antineoplastic dose, 25 mg/kg/day, for 1 to 3 days, repeated at weekly or longer intervals as the patient responds, probably prevents resorption of calcium from bone. Serum calcium concentration usually drops in 1 to 2 days following the start of treatment.

Calcium deficit, hypocalcemia, is a rare problem because of the large calcium reserves present in bone; however, hypocalcemia may be found in the following conditions:
1. Intestinal malabsorption, such as in:
   a. steatorrhea
   b. pancreatitis
2. Vitamin D deficiency, caused by:
   a. inadequate intake or exposure to sunlight (primary deficiency)
   b. malabsorption due to chronic use of oily laxatives (mineral oil or castor oil, although no cases have been reported in the literature)
   c. anticonvulsant therapy, particularly with diphenylhydantoin or phenobarbital, which increase liver microsomal activity thus increasing the rate of metabolism of 25-dihydroxycholecalciferol, lowering its

concentration, and consequently lowering the concentration of the biologically active 1,25-dihydroxycholecalciferol that is made from it.
3. Parathyroid hormone deficiency, caused by:
    a. gland malfunction
    b. surgical removal of the gland
4. Phosphate depletion, caused by
    a. chronic, long-term use of aluminum-containing antacids, which bind phosphate
    b. intravenous therapy with low-phosphate solutions
    c. hemodialysis with low-phosphate solutions

Therapy is directed toward remedying the causes. Vitamin D can be provided in many forms. Ergocalciferol is available as tablets, capsules, oral liquids, or injection. Cholecalciferol is available in fish liver oils. A vitamin D analog, dihydrotachysterol, Hytakerol, is available as tablets, capsules and an oral solution. It may be more effective than vitamin D in increasing serum calcium values. Calcifediol, 25-hydroxycholecalciferol, Calderol, is available in capsules. Calcitriol, 1,25-dihydroxycholecalciferol, Rocaltrol, is available in capsules. Synthetic calcitonin, Calcimar, is available as a parenteral for subcutaneous or intramuscular injection.

Oral calcium is best absorbed from its fully ionized form. Calcium carbonate appears to be the preferred source, but like all inorganic calcium compounds, frequently causes constipation. Calcium lactate and calcium gluconate, by comparison, may produce less constipation and reduced but adequate absorption.

Phosphorus Balance

Hypophosphatemia, serum phosphate less than 2.5 mg/dL, is known to produce the following conditions:
1. Depression of serum calcium levels, as discussed under Calcium Balance
2. Neuromuscular irritability, weakness, and malaise
3. Anorexia
4. Skeletal aches
5. Confusion
6. Hyperventilation
7. Hemolysis

The symptoms are reversible when adequate dietary phosphorus is provided. Because of the serious consequences of phosphate depletion, it is recommended that phosphate be added to dextrose solutions and particularly hyperalimentation solutions. For adults with no active disease, a recommended maintenance dose is 0.15 mM/Kg/day.

Magnesium Balance

Magnesium ions are efficiently absorbed from dietary sources and highly conserved. Magnesium deficit, hypomagnesemia, is defined as serum levels less than 0.45 mEq/L (0.55 mg/dL).

Hypomagnesemia may cause

1. Neuromuscular disturbances
    a. ataxia
    b. tremors
    c. tetany
    d. convulsions
2. Behavioral disturbances
    b. irritability
    c. psychosis
3. Cardiac disturbances similar to those produced by hypocalcemia or hypokalemia

Magnesium excess, hypermagnesemia, is defined as serum levels above 2.5 mEq/L (3.0 mg/dL). It is very rare except in kidney failure.
Hypermagnesemia may cause
1. Loss of the patellar reflex
2. Depression of deep tendon reflexes (flaccid paralysis)
3. Heart block, leading to death
4. Respiratory depression, caused by profound central nervous system depression, leading to death.

Therapy of hypermagnesemia might include
1. Intravenous administration of 10 to 20 mL of 10% calcium gluconate
2. Intravenous administration of loop diuretics, ethacrynic acid or furosemide, along with maintenance of adequate hydration in order to increase urinary excretion of magnesium
3. Peritoneal dialysis or hemodialysis, in extreme cases

Bicarbonate Balance

Bicarbonate balance includes acid-base balance and acidosis and alkalosis. Bicarbonate in the extracellular fluid forms part of a buffer system as shown by the following equations:

$$H^+ + HCO_3^- \leftrightarrow H_2CO_3$$

$$H_2CO_3 \xrightarrow[\text{anhydrase}]{\text{carbonic}} CO_2 + H_2O$$

The carbon dioxide is excreted through the lungs. Normal plasma bicarbonate is 23 to 29 mEq/L. Normal carbon dioxide partial pressure in venous blood is 35 to 40 mm Hg. Since the carbonic acid/bicarbonate system is the major buffer system present in plasma, it essentially establishes blood pH.

The bicarbonate buffer system of blood can be described using the Henderson-Hasselbalch equation:

$$pH = pK + \log\{[HCO_3^-]/[H_2CO_3]\} \qquad \text{Eq. (10–16)}$$

Assuming the usual blood pH of 7.4 and pK = 6.37 at 25°C for the equilibrium $H_2CO_3 \leftrightarrow H^+ + HCO_3^-$

$$\log\{[HCO_3^-]/[H_2CO_3]\} = pH - pK$$
$$= 1.03$$
$$[HCO_3^-]/[H_2CO_3] = 10.7$$

The concentration of carbonic acid is regulated by the amount of breathing (ventilation). The concentration of bicarbonate ion is regulated by the kidneys. Bicarbonate may be excreted in the urine with sodium and potassium ions or the kidney may secrete hydrogen ion, returning bicarbonate to the plasma.

Primary bicarbonate excess, defined as plasma bicarbonate values above 30 mEq/L in adults or 25 mEq/L in children and blood pH above 7.45, is called metabolic alkalosis. The usual cause is chloride ion loss (generally accompanied by potassium ion loss) caused by vomiting, gastric suction, or excessive diuretic use. It may be caused by excessive alkali intake. Bicarbonate excess may produce:

1. Respiratory depression
2. Muscle hypertonicity, hyperactive reflexes, tetany
3. Convulsions, occasionally

Note that intracellular potassium deficit produces a similar metabolic alkalosis which does not respond to administration of chloride alone.

Therapy is directed toward the replacement of potassium chloride given in 0.9% Sodium Chloride Injection, Ringer's Injection, or, in severe alkalosis, 0.9% Ammonium Chloride Injection.

Primary carbonic acid deficit, defined as plasma bicarbonate below 20 mEq/L and plasma pH above 7.45, is called respiratory alkalosis. This deficit is caused by hyperventilation, resulting in excessive respiratory depletion. The hyperventilation may be caused by:

1. Hypoxia
2. Fever
3. Encephalitis
4. Salicylate poisoning

Respiratory alkalosis may produce:
1. Deep, rapid breathing when there is no exertion
2. Hyperactive tendon reflexes
3. Positive Chvostek's sign (unilateral facial spasm elicited by a slight tap over the facial nerve)
4. Positive Trousseau's sign (latent tetany, shown by a characteristic attitude of the hand when the upper arm is compressed, as by a blood pressure cuff)
5. Convulsions, in severe deficit

Primary bicarbonate deficit, defined as plasma bicarbonate less than 20 mEq/L and plasma pH below 7.35, is called metabolic acidosis. It may be caused by:

1. Prolonged diarrhea, especially in infants; fistulas or other gastrointestinal drainage that causes excessive bicarbonate loss
2. Diabetes mellitus or starvation causing accumulation of ketones

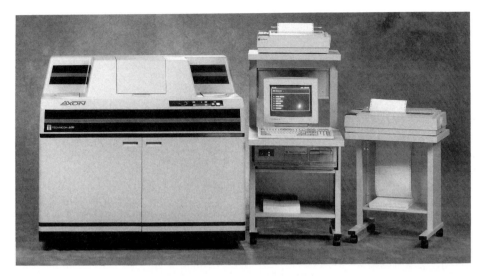

Figure 10–2. The measurement of electrolyte and other biochemical values in blood or urine has been facilitated by analytic automated equipment such as the SMA 6/60. Test configuration for this equipment includes four electrolytes (sodium, potassium, carbon dioxide, and chloride) plus glucose and blood urea nitrogen (BUN). (Courtesy of Technicon Instruments Corporation, Tarrytown, NY.)

3. Renal insufficiency, causing accumulation of phosphate and sulfate
4. Shock
5. Excessive therapy with ammonium chloride (hyperchloremic acidosis)
6. Congestive heart failure, producing tissue anoxia and subsequent decrease in serum carbon dioxide and increase in serum lactic acid

Metabolic acidosis may be accompanied by:
1. Weakness
2. Warm skin and flushing
3. Progressive increase in the rate and depth of respiration
4. Disorientation, progressing to coma

Therapy is directed toward restoration of normal plasma pH by correcting the underlying pathophysiology, if possible, and by providing alkali in the form of bicarbonate precursors such as sodium acetate or sodium lactate. Obviously, if lactate accumulation is part of the problem, sodium acetate would be used. In ketosis due to starvation, carbohydrate is also needed. If serum potassium values are not elevated and there is adequate urinary output, potassium is also given to replace cellular potassium losses which accompany acidosis.

Primary carbonic acid excess, defined as plasma bicarbonate above 30 mEq/L in adults or 25 mEq/L in children and plasma pH below 7.35, is called respiratory acidosis. It is caused by inadequate ventilation. Hypoventilation may be caused by:
1. Obstructive dyspnea
2. Respiratory muscle weakness or paralysis
3. Pneumonia

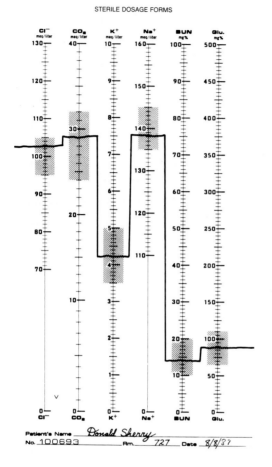

Figure 10–3. Results from the SMA 6/60 are reported as shown. The shaded areas in each column represent normal values. (Courtesy of Technicon Instruments Corporation, Tarrytown, NY.)

4. Chronic pulmonary disease
    a. emphysema
    b. extensive bronchiectasis
    c. pulmonary fibrosis
5. Poisoning by respiratory depressants
    a. morphine
    b. barbiturates
    c. carbon dioxide

Respiratory acidosis may be accompanied by
1. Reduced respiration causing weakness and cyanosis
2. Confusion progressing to coma

Therapy is directed to correction of the underlying pulmonary pathology.

Anion Balance

If the concentration of cations in milliequivalents per liter is summed and compared with the sum of anions, the sum of the anions will be less. The difference is called the anion gap. It represents the lactate, acetate, pyruvate,

Table 10–6. Selected Reference Values for Serum

Substance	Normal Range Minimum	Normal Range Maximum	Units
Bicarbonate	23	29	mEq/L
Calcium, ionized	2.1	2.6	mEq/L
	4.25	5.25	mg/dL
	1.05	1.30	mmol/L
Calcium, total	4.5	5.5	mEq/L
(varies with protein concentration,	9.0	11.0	mg/dL
slightly higher in children)	2.25	2.75	mmol/L
Carbon dioxide			
(includes bicarbonate and carbonic acid)			
Adult	24	30	mmol/L
Infant	20	28	mmol/L
Carbon dioxide, tension, pCO_2	35	45	mm Hg
Chloride	96	106	mEq/L
Magnesium	1.5	2.5	mEq/L
	1.8	3.0	mg/dL
Phosphate, inorganic			
Adults	3.0	4.5	mg/dL
	1.0	1.5	mmol/L
Children	4.0	7.0	mg/dL
	1.3	2.3	mmol/L
Potassium	3.5	5.0	mEq/L
Sodium	136	145	mEq/L

NOTE: The number of figures shown indicates the expected precision of the laboratory data.

and other anions not measured in the typical battery of electrolyte tests. The value in normal patients depends on the methods of analysis used in the particular laboratory. A reasonable value is 12 to 15 mEq/L.

The measurement of electrolytes (and other biochemical values) has been greatly facilitated by sophisticated, multichannel, automatic analyzers (Fig. 10–2). Results are usually superimposed on normal values for each substance, thus easing interpretation and allowing rapid detection of abnormalities (Fig. 10–3). Reference values, representing 95% confidence limits, are given in Table 10–6. These values vary with each laboratory; standard deviations on individual determinations may vary from 1 to 20%.

References

1. Diem, K., and Lentner, C. (eds.): Documenta Geigy. Scientific Tables. 7th Ed. Basle, Switzerland, Ciba-Geigy, 1970.
2. Weast, R.C. (ed.): Handbook of Chemistry and Physics. 65th Ed., Boca Raton, Fl., CRC Press, Inc., 1984.
3. Turco, S.J., and Schott, M.: Osmoles, osmolarity, osmolality, confusion. Hosp. Pharm., *15*:260 (1980).
4. Lund, C.G., et al.: Danish Pharmacopeial Commission, Copenhagen, Munksgaard, 1947; extracted from Siegel, F.P.: Tonicity, osmoticity, osmolality, and osmolarity. *In* Remington's Pharmaceutical Sciences. 17th Ed. Edited by A.R. Gennaro. Easton, PA, Mack Publishing Co., 1985, p. 1463.

5. Hendry, E.B., Osmolarity of human serum and of chemical solutions of biologic importance. Clin. Chem., 7:156 (1961).
6. Streng, H., Huber, H.E., and Carstensen, J.T.: Relationship between osmolarity and osmolality. J. Pharm. Sci., 67:384 (1978).
7. Murty, B.S.R., Kapor, J.N., and DeLuca, P.P.: Compliance with U.S.P. osmolarity labeling requirements. Am. J. Hosp. Pharm., 33:546 (1976).
8. Lindeman, R.D., and Papper, S.: Therapy of fluid and electrolyte disorders. Ann. Intern. Med., 82:64 (1975).
9. Hantman, D., et al., Rapid correction of hyponatremia in the syndrome of inappropriate secretion of antidiuretic hormone. Ann. Intern. Med., 78:870 (1973).

Bibliography

1. Alberty, R.A.: Physical Chemistry. 6th Ed. New York, Wiley, 1983.
2. Baxter Guide to Fluid Therapy, Baxter Laboratories, Morton Grove, IL, 1970.
3. Goldberger, E.: A Primer of Water, Electrolyte and Acid-Base Syndromes. 7th Ed. Philadelphia, Lea & Febiger, 1985.
4. Goodhart, R.S., and Shills, M.E.: Modern Nutrition in Health and Disease. 6th Ed., Philadelphia, Lea & Febiger, 1980.
5. Guide to Parenteral Fluid Therapy, McGaw Laboratories, Glendale, CA, 1963.
6. Mason, E.E.: Fluid, Electrolyte and Nutrient Therapy in Surgery. Philadelphia, Lea & Febiger, 1974.
7. Reference Handbook, The Medical Letter, New Rochelle, NY, Jan., 1973.
8. Rose, B.D.: Clinical Physiology of Acid-Base and Electrolyte Disorders, 2nd Ed. New York, McGraw-Hill, 1984.

CHAPTER

Parenteral Admixtures and Incompatibilities

The physical, chemical, and therapeutic problems that arise when parenteral drugs are combined and administered by injection are called "parenteral incompatibilities." The tendency of practitioners to prescribe several drugs combined and administered together is prompted by the convenience and time-saving features of the practice, the reduction in the number of injections necessary, an attempt to treat several conditions simultaneously, and the ability to give the drugs in controlled increments. Although problems have probably existed since the acceptance of the parenteral method of administration, only recently have they become a concern to practitioners, owing to the number of parenteral drugs available, the increasing use of parenteral drugs, and the increasing use of large-volume parenteral fluids as vehicles for other drugs. The increased use of parenteral drugs is revealed in surveys that show that, in the average hospital, 24% of the total dosage forms dispensed to inpatients are in the form of an injection.[1] In one study in a large university hospital, over 39% of patients received a daily injection.[2]

Many hospitals have established pharmacy intravenous additive programs which have centralized the responsibility, increased the uniformity, and improved the safety of combining drugs for parenteral administration. Such services have been a contributing factor in improving patient care.

Admixtures

The combination of parenteral dosage forms for administration as a single entity is called an "admixture." Because of convenience, intravenous fluids are frequently used as vehicles, or carriers, for other parenteral drugs. The drug placed in solution in another parenteral dosage is the additive (Fig. 11–1).

239

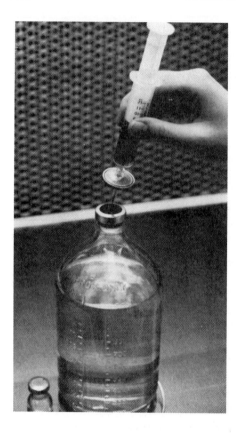

Figure 11–1. In the preparation of admixtures, sterile disposable filter units can be used to remove extemporaneous particulate matter and to ensure sterility during manipulation. Small-volume additives can also be sterilized with this procedure. (Courtesy of Millipore Corporation, Bedford, MA.)

Numerous studies have been done to determine the extent of admixture use. Studies at the National Institutes of Health (NIH) and the University of Michigan showed that 50 to 70% of the intravenous fluids administered contained additives. Other surveys showed that the majority of orders received contained 1 or 2 additives, and a small percentage required as many as 6 additives to be administered in the same intravenous fluid (Fig. 11–2).[3–4]

Theoretically, the number of possible combinations of parenteral drugs in intravenous fluids is staggering. A group at the University of Chicago calculated that 24 drugs added in groups of 2 to 5% D/W produced 276 unique pairs.[4] In this particular hospital, there was the possibility of using any one of 36 different intravenous fluids as the vehicle, thus bringing the number of possibilities to over 9000. If the 24 drugs were used in combinations of twos, threes, and fours when added to 5% D/W, these combinations produced 11,000 unique admixtures. When varied with the 36 different intravenous solutions, these 24 drugs could produce over 396,000 possible combinations. The inclusion of any of the other hundreds of parenteral drugs available with the 24 used in this study rapidly increases the number of possibilities. Recognizing the extent of possible combinations is important in seeking a reasonable and practical solution to a problem.

Other important factors in considering the number of combinations possible include brand variations, drug concentration, added substances, order of mixing, and time elapsing prior to administration.

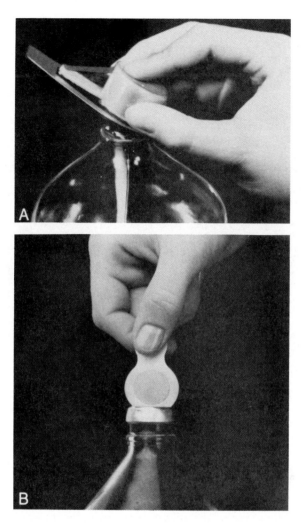

Figure 11–2. After the addition of other drugs, additive caps can be used to maintain the integrity of the admixture until time of use. A, Travenol cap. (Courtesy of Travenol Laboratories, Morton Grove, IL.) B, The IVA Seal III, a new paper seal, offers color coding and tamper-evident construction to enhance control in the preparation of intravenous admixtures. (Courtesy of U.S. Clinical Products, Inc., Richardson, TX.)

Selected equipment used in preparing intravenous admixtures is shown in Figures 11–3 through 11–8.

Incompatibilities

Large-volume fluids have their own therapeutic uses; they were not necessarily formulated to act as carriers or vehicles for other drugs. Likewise, parenteral drugs used as additives were not necessarily formulated to remain stable and active when added to one of a variety of large-volume fluids. Nevertheless, current medical practice results in this use for these solutions, and the potential problem of parenteral incompatibilities arises.

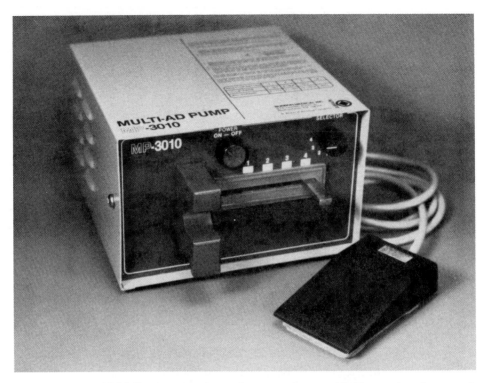

Figure 11–3. Multi-AD Pump reconstitutes drug manufacturers' bottles and performs such other tasks as medication injection into minibags or bottles and intravenous or oral syringe prefilling. (Courtesy of Burron Medical Inc., Bethlehem, PA.)

The NCCLVP has defined incompatibility as a phenomenon that occurs when one drug is mixed with others to produce, by physicochemical means, a product unsuitable for administration to the patient. The patient may not receive the full therapeutic effect of the mixture, or toxic decomposition products may result. The precipitated incompatibility may irritate the veins or cause occlusion of vessels.

Incompatibilities can be divided into three categories: therapeutic (pharmacologic), physical, and chemical.[5] Therapeutic incompatibilities occur when two or more drugs administered concurrently result in undesirable antagonistic or synergistic pharmacologic action. Examples of incompatibilities are the antagonism between chloramphenicol and penicillin and the possibility that penicillin or cortisone may antagonize the effect of heparin and produce a misleading picture of the anticoagulant effect of heparin. Antagonism of folic acid to methotrexate and of warfarin to phytonadione have been reported, as has a synergism between calcium ion and digoxin.

When the combination of two or more drugs in solution results in a change in the appearance of the solution, such as a change in color, formation of turbidity or precipitate, or the evolution of a gas, it is called a "physical incompatibility." Physical incompatibilities are the easiest to detect and represent the types most familiar to hospital pharmacists. They can frequently be predicted from the chemical characteristics of the drugs involved. For ex-

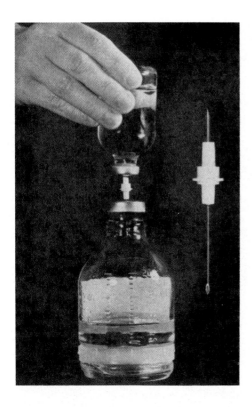

Figure 11–4. Double-ended, filtered transfer needle offers one-step filter and transfer of medication and eliminates the need for a separate syringe. (Courtesy of Burron Medical Inc., Bethlehem, PA.)

ample, the sodium salts of weak acids such as sodium diphenylhydantoin or sodium phenobarbital precipitate as free acids when added to intravenous fluids having an acidic pH. Calcium salts precipitate in the presence of sodium bicarbonate, and acid salts such as dimenhydrinate precipitate when added to an alkaline medium. When mixed together, cephalothin and gentamicin produce a yellow precipitate. Injections that require a special vehicle for solubilization, such as diazepam, precipitate when added to aqueous solutions because of their low water solubility. Available compatibility charts attempt to outline this type of incompatibility.

Degradation of drugs in solution resulting from the combination of parenteral dosage forms is called "chemical incompatibility." This is an arbitrary classification because physical incompatibilities also result from chemical changes. Most chemical incompatibilities result from hydrolysis, oxidation, reduction, or complexing and can be detected only with suitable analytic methods.

Probably the greatest single factor in causing an incompatibility is a change in acid-base environment. Results of this type of change were illustrated in the discussion of physical incompatibilities. The solubility and stability of a drug may vary as the pH of the solution varies. A change in the pH may be a clue in predicting an incompatibility, especially one involving drug stability, since it is not necessarily apparent physically.

Penicillin provides a good example of the effect of pH on drug stability. The antibiotic in solution remains active for 24 hours at pH 6.5, but at pH 3.5 is destroyed in a short time. Potassium penicillin G contains a citrate buffer; therefore, the injection is buffered at pH 6.0 to 6.5 when reconstituted

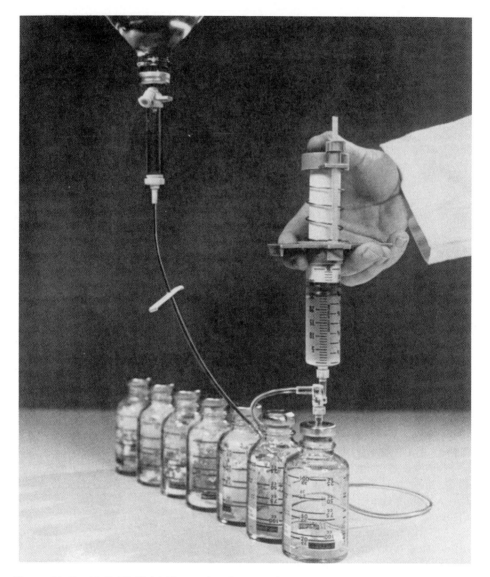

Figure 11–5. Multi-AD Fluid Dispensing System offers a streamlined method of injecting additives into intravenous containers. (Courtesy of Burron Medical Inc., Bethlehem, PA.)

with Sterile Water for Injection, 5% D/W, or Sodium Chloride Injection. When this reconstituted solution is added to an intravenous fluid such as Dextrose Injection of Sodium Chloride Injection, the normal acid pH of the solutions is buffered at pH 6.0 to 6.5, thus ensuring the antibiotic's activity. Carbenicillin should not be admixed in the same bottle with gentamicin. The latter loses its activity when present in the same solution as carbenicillin. Adding other drugs, such as metaraminol bitartrate, ascorbic acid, or tetracycline hydrochloride, that have a low pH to the intravenous fluid containing the penicillin may lower the pH to a point at which the penicillin may be inactivated. The same can happen if the reconstituted penicillin solution is

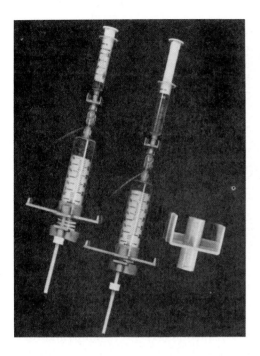

Figure 11–6. Burron's Fluid Dispensing Connector facilitates the prefilling of unit-dose syringes from a larger master syringe. (Courtesy of Burron Medical Inc., Bethlehem, PA.)

added to intravenous fluids of high buffering capacity that have a pH below 6.0, such as Lactated Ringer's Injection or protein hydrolysates.

In a similar manner, the addition of the reconstituted penicillin to solutions in the alkaline range can be deleterious. Dilute sodium bicarbonate solutions are sometimes added to 5% D/W to reduce the incidence of phlebitis, or the bicarbonate ion may be used for treating acidosis (Chapter 10). Studies have shown that penicillin present in solution at pH 8.5 retains only 25% of its activity after 6 hours and 1% after 24 hours. With higher temperatures or higher pH, the inactivation of the antibiotic is accelerated.

The stability of the antibiotic sodium ampicillin is also pH dependent. When reconstituted sodium ampicillin is added to 5% D/W at the concentration of 30 mg per ml, its period of stability under the prevalent acid conditions is 4

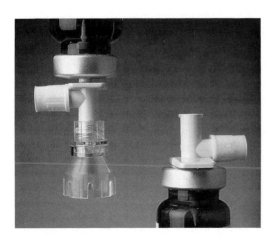

Figure 11–7. Mini-Spike I.V. Additive Dispensing Pin. (Courtesy of Burron Medical Inc., Bethlehem, PA.)

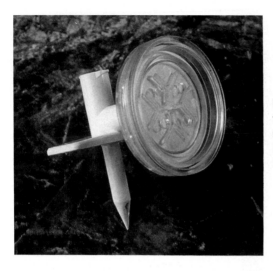

Figure 11–8. Chemo-Dispensing Pin for reconstituting and dispensing chemotherapeutic drugs packaged in rubber-stoppered vials. (Courtesy of Burron Medical Inc., Bethlehem, PA.)

hours. When added to Sodium Chloride Injection, however, its loss in activity is less than 10% in 8 hours. For this reason, Sodium Chloride Injection is the intravenous fluid of choice for sodium ampicillin.

As the number of additives increases, the likelihood of creating conditions unfavorable for the stability of one or more of them also increases. Aminophyllin Injection added to Sodium Chloride Injection already containing vitamin B complex and vitamin C as additives results in an alkaline solution unfavorable to the stability of the vitamins.

Complexation can occur between drugs, rendering them inactive. Tetracycline in the presence of calcium ions forms a complex that reduces the tetracycline activity.

When formulating a drug into a suitable parenteral dosage form, a manufacturer uses adjuvants or added substances to obtain a stable solution (Chapter 2). When a drug is added to an intravenous fluid, the conditions of the drug are changed. Drugs packaged under an inert atmosphere such as nitrogen, because of their ease of oxidation, lose this protection and the value of any antioxidant present when they are added to the intravenous fluid. The added substances in one injection may not be compatible with the drug and added substances in another when they are placed together in an intravenous fluid. Placing two injections together in the same syringe may accentuate the problems because of the concentrations involved and the difficulty in thoroughly mixing the injections, creating what is called a "layering effect."

Many injections have special storage requirements such as protection from light or refrigeration. Using these solutions with intravenous fluids, not administering them immediately, or administering them for prolonged periods may produce conditions not favorable to the drug's stability. Administration bottles of intravenous fluids containing light-sensitive drugs such as amphotericin B or vitamin K_1 should be covered with aluminum foil during administration to reduce decomposition from light.

The primary I.V. fluid is usually a carbohydrate, electrolyte, or amino acid solution. Carbohydrate solutions are not usually a problem with additives; although they are acidic, they have negligible buffer capacity, and the additive determines the pH. The monovalent cations are sodium and potassium and are usually compatible; however, divalent cations (calcium, magnesium) can be troublesome in the presence of bicarbonate, citrate, and phosphate. Calcium and phosphate in TPN solutions require special care in mixing. Lactate, acetate, and gluconate present as salts can act as buffers and resist changes in pH that may make the additive insoluble. Amino acid-containing I.V. solutions may degrade acid-labile drugs, bind drugs, or form complexes. No drug additive should be mixed with fat emulsion (Intralipid).

Frequency of Occurrence of Incompatibility

Determining the frequency of incompatibility occurrence is difficult and complex. Few, if any, valid studies have been undertaken. Wilmore and Dudrick, in a study of filters used for TPN fluids, found that 14 filters became obstructed by occlusion of the filter pores by drug precipitates. Thus, in this study, at least 5.6% of the infusions had physical incompatibility. Considering that an estimated 100 million admixtures are prepared yearly, the probability of incompatibility is great.

Minimization of Incompatibilities

Although it may be impossible to predict and prevent all parenteral incompatibilities, practicing the following general principles is helpful in minimizing the difficulties:

1. Use freshly prepared solutions if possible; periodically observing the running of the intravenous fluid to detect changes in appearance. Discard any unused solution after 24 hours. Refrigeration may be required if it is necessary to prepare admixtures in advance. Proper storage temperatures must be maintained. Admixtures should be returned to room temperature prior to infusion. Although furosemide (Lasix) does not require refrigeration, it is sometimes stored under refrigeration in prefilled syringes to reduce the effects of light. This can cause crystallization and should not be done. Cephaloridine (Loridine) injections become milky white during refrigeration and should be returned to room temperature prior to use.

2. Encourage the use of as few additives as possible in infusion fluids. As additives increase, so do the number of potential problems. When one considers that vitamin B complex with vitamin C may contain up to 10 drug substances in addition to the pharmaceutic adjuvants present, the potential of problems occurring becomes clear. Mixing thoroughly after each additive prevents concentrated layering effects.

Dilution may prevent incompatibility; for example, erythromycin lactobionate is incompatible with electrolytes in concentrated form; however, it is compatible when properly diluted. It will form a solid gel in a small vial of 0.9% sodium chloride; in a liter bottle of 0.9% sodium chloride, it will dissolve completely.

3. Become knowledgeable about parenteral therapy. The practitioner can become aware of incompatibilities through the literature. Numerous references are available for sources listing and discussing parenteral incompatibilities. Attempt to answer and to explain the incompatibilities that come to your attention as part of the daily routine.

4. Make physicians and others aware of possible incompatibilities and always be ready to suggest alternate approaches to avoid the difficulties. In some instances, incompatibilities can be avoided by selecting another route or site of administration for one of the drugs involved.

5. The preparation of the admixture should be accomplished using aseptic technique in a proper area. The containers of the injections to be used should be examined for acceptability in all aspects, such as clarity, absence of cracks in the glass, and presence of vacuum if the system requires it.

6. Keep a file of available data and add to it from your own experience and the literature.

7. Utilize available compatibility charts. Although these charts have limitations, the proper use of this information can be helpful in predicting incompatibilities. Most charts list only physical incompatibilities; they cannot be used for chemical or therapeutic incompatibilities. The chart used should relate to the system of intravenous fluids used in the hospital. Charts for other systems can be helpful, but they cannot be depended on categorically to rule out a problem. The same injections prepared by different companies may differ in pH values. If the brand or source of additive varies from the one used in compilation of the chart, the results may differ because different substances are used by various companies to prepare the additives. If the concentration of the drug in a specific problem is different from that used in compiling the chart, the results may also be different. The data in the chart are concentration-dependent and the concentration per unit volume is frequently specified. Charts are updated from time to time; thus the age of the data can influence results. If your order of mixing is different from the order used in preparing the chart, the results can be different. Most charts specify a definite period of observation, usually 24 hours. If your solutions are stored longer than this (a questionable practice), the results may differ.

8. It is impossible to chart or discuss every possible admixture. Instead, principles must be learned and applied. For example, no drug should ever be added to blood or blood products. According to the charts, almost every type of additive causes an incompatibility when added to protein hydrolysates, yet it is common practice to combine several additives in hyperalimentation solutions. Penicillins form potentially allergenic conjugates with proteinaceous materials. Therefore, it is not advisable to add them to protein hydrolysate solutions. Other general principles to remember are that penicillins are inactivated at either low or high pH values; sympathomimetic amines are especially sensitive when added to intravenous fluids; and therapeutic large-volume solutions such as sodium bicarbonate, urea, mannitol, dextran, and L-arginine should never contain additives.

Parenteral Incompatibility

The stability of Sodium Ampicillin Injection has been shown to be affected by pH.[6] Results of one study indicate the pH to be most stable at 7.5. Degradation increases as the pH varies above or below 7.5. Dextrose solutions should be avoided. In ampicillin preparations,[7,8] ampicillin is stable for 8 hours at room temperature and 48 to 72 hours under refrigeration when reconstituted with Sterile Water for Injection or Sodium Chloride Injection.

Reports concerning the compatibility of metaraminol,[9] norepinephrine (Levophed),[10] dopamine,[11,12] and isoproterenol[13] have been published.

There has been a publication of heparin stability in 5% dextrose and 0.9% sodium chloride[14] in addition to heparin stability in 5% dextrose.[15]

Cephalosporin,[16] cefazolin,[17] oxacillin,[18] sodium nafcillin (Unipen),[19] and carbenicillin[20] stability studies have been published.

McRae and King[21] discuss the compatibility of antineoplastic, antibiotic, and corticosteroid drugs in intravenous admixtures. Parker[22] has reported on methyldopa (Aldomet). The stability of tobramycin[23] has been reported on, as has the stability of aminophylline in 5% dextrose.[24] Stability of erythromycin gluceptate in sodium chloride and dextrose injection has also been published.[25] A comparative stability study of several antibiotics admixed in minibags and minibottles has been published by Dinel et al.[26] The subject of parenteral admixture stability continues to be a perplexing one, however; since the previous edition of this text was published, several new stability studies have appeared in the literature.

Lee et al.[27] studied the stability of bretylium in common large-volume parenteral solutions. Bretylium was found to be compatible in all 11 large-volume parenteral solutions studied.

Parke-Davis, the manufacturer of Dilantin (phenytoin) recommends that phenytoin injection be given by I.V. push because dilution of phenytoin injection causes crystalization. Direct I.V. push of phenytoin is inconvenient and on some occasions not practical. Carmichael et al.[28] suggest that phenytoin may be infused over a period of not more than 1 hour with no more than 50 ml of normal saline. Cloyd et al.[29] also found normal saline to be a suitable vehicle for phenytoin. Newton et al.[30] noted that the time required for crystallization was not predictable.

Incompatibility between carbenicillin and promethazine has been reported.[31]

Continuous intravenous infusion of diazepam is not an approved method of administration. Mixtures of diazepam in plastic I.V. containers significantly reduce the diazepam concentration.[32] In a study by Parker et al.,[33] no visual incompatibility was observed when diazepam was infused in glass I.V. bottles; 90% of the original potency was retained after 4 hours. When it was administered in plastic burette chambers, over 38% loss in potency was noted in 2 hours. Tung et al.[34] studied the stability of 5 antibiotics in plastic I.V. solution containers of 5% dextrose and normal saline. These stability studies reveal that amikacin, methicillin, vancomycin, and ticarcillin were stable for 24 hours. Erythromycin lactobionate was also stable for 24 hours in normal saline; however, the addition of sodium bicarbonate 4% was required to assure stability in dextrose 5%.

The visual and chemical compatibility of verapamil hydrochloride injection in 10 commonly used large-volume solutions packaged in glass, polyolefin, or polyvinyl chloride containers showed that no significant degradation of verapamil HCl had taken place in the solutions or through contact with the containers.[35] Carmustine stability was studied in the presence of sodium bicarbonate in dextrose 5% and normal saline.[36] It was shown that sodium bicarbonate accelerated the decomposition of carmustine.

Lidocaine hydrochloride was found to be stable for up to 120 days at room temperature in 5% dextrose injection in plastic infusion bags.[37]

The stability of trimethoprim-sulfamethoxazole injection in 5% dextrose and sodium chloride injection was studied:[38] Dextrose was found to be the preferred diluent for trimethoprim-sulfamethoxazole injection if a dilution of 1:10 volume/volume (v/v) is desired. Either 5% dextrose or normal saline may be used if a dilution of 1:25 v/v is desired.

The stability of cefamandole nafate and cefoxitin sodium solutions in D5W and NS were studied.[39] The cefamandole solutions were stable for 5 days at 24° C and 44 days at 5° C. The cefoxitin solutions were stable for 24 hours at 24° C and 13 days at 5° C.

Newton et al.,[40] studying amine-type drugs in 5% dextrose, noted that epinephrine HCl, norepinephrine bitartrate, and isoproterenol HCl should not be combined with aminophylline or other alkaline drugs in LVP solutions. As a sole additive, these drugs were stable for at least 48 hours in 5% dextrose injection. It was also noted that visual inspection failed to detect drug degradation and stability, indicating assays were necessary to detect degradation.

Cutie[41] studied the visual compatibility of a number of small-volume parenterals and verapamil HCl in 5% dextrose injection and 0.9% sodium chloride. A transient precipitate was noted with aminophylline.

Henderson et al.[42] studied the in vitro inactivation of gentamicin, tobramycin, and netilmicin by carbenicillin, azlocillin, and mezlocillin. Inactivation occurs with aminoglycosides and penicillins and mixing should be avoided.

Yuhas et al.[43] studied the stability of cimetidine HCl admixtures at room temperature with a variety of drugs. This study suggested that incompatibility may be expected when cimetidine HCl is combined with some antibiotics. Precipitates occurred with amphotericin B, cefamandole nafate, cefazolin sodium, and cephalothin sodium.

Cummings et al.[44] studied the stability of propranolol HCl in plastic containers with 5 commonly used large-volume parenteral liquids. Propranolol HCl was found to be visually and chemically compatible for 24 hours when mixed in LifeCare, Viaflex, or Accumed plastic containers.

Lee et al.[45] studied the compatibility of bretylium tosylate admixtures with dopamine, lidocaine, procainamide, and nitroglycerin in glass and plastic containers of 5% dextrose and sodium chloride as the diluents. There was no degradation of bretylium in any of the solutions studied. Dopamine and lidocaine were also stable; however, nitroglycerin was not stable in plastic, and procainamide concentrations decreased under all storage conditions.

Johnson et al.[46] studied the effects of containers, diluent, temperature, and illumination on the stability and compatibility of azathioprine sodium. No solution of admixture differed significantly from the initial concentration up to 16 days of constant illumination. Mixtures with 5% dextrose and water precipitated by day 16. Reconstituted solutions stored in the original manufacturer's vial or plastic syringe at 4° C formed a precipitate by day 4.

Benvenuto et al.[47] studied several antitumor agents for stability in underfilled plastic and glass administration containers. From these studies, they concluded that carmustine and bleomycin should be administered in glass containers. Continuous infusions of doxorubicin and fluorouracil are more completely delivered from plastic containers. Mitomycin should not be dissolved in 5% dextrose injection.

Townsend et al.[48] studied the stability of methylprednisolone sodium succinate in some volumes of 5% dextrose and 0.9% sodium chloride injections. Solutions were stable for 12 hours.

Yuhas et al.[49] studied cimetidine hydrochloride compatibility and stability at room temperature in 19 different I.V. fluids. They found it visually and chemically compatible for 1 week in concentrations of 120 and 500 mg/dl.

Poochikian et al.[50] studied the stability of anthracycline antitumor agents in four infusion fluids, and found that the stability of those compounds was pH dependent.

Newton et al.[51] studied the characteristics of diazepam in aqueous admixture solutions and corroborated early reports by recommending against less than a 1:100 volume dilution of diazepam injection when compounding I.V. mixtures.

The compatibility of netilmicin[52] sulfate injection with commonly used intravenous injections and additives illustrated that netilmicin sulfate injection at a concentration of 3 mg/ml was stable for at least 7 days with 37 I.V. fluids and 22 different drugs.

Pfeifle et al.[53] suggested the dextrose solutions are not suitable as vehicles for phenytoin sodium; however, sodium chloride and lactated Ringer's solution were acceptable with those concentrations studied.

In a study[54] of sorption of diazepam in I.V.-fluid containers and sets, it was shown that no sorption problems occurred with diazepam in glass or polyolefin containers but that volume-control sets or flexible plastic bags should be avoided.

Calcium and phosphorus compatibility[55] in parenteral nutrition solutions were shown to be affected by many variables: temperature, amino acid concentration, pH, and others.

Haloperidol[56] was found to be stable in 5% dextrose injection for at least 38 days.

Moxalactam disodium[57] solutions maintained at least 90% of initial potency for up to 96 hours when stored in a refrigerator; at room temperature, the reconstituted solutions should be used within 24 hours.

Cefamandole nafate[58] was found stable in 26 of 37 parenteral solutions studied for at least 3 days at 25° C and 10 days at 5° C; however, storage limits of 24 and 96 hours, respectively, are recommended because of the potential for microbial growth.

Cimetidine HCl[59] in a concentration of 30 mg/10 ml was found to be visually and chemically stable in total parenteral nutrition solutions containing various additives over a 24-hour period at both room temperature and 4° C.

Kowaluk et al.[60] stated that sorption can be minimized by administering infusions through short lengths of small-diameter tubing, particularly if the tubing is made of inert plastic.

The stability and compatibility of lidocaine HCl with selected large-volume parenteral solutions and drug additives were studied by Kirschenbaum et al.[61] Lidocaine was stable in the solutions studied for 14 days at 25° C and compatible visually for 24 hours in admixtures with drugs. The exception was phenytoin sodium.

Souney et al.[62] found that vitamin B complex and ascorbic acid had no effect on the antimicrobial activity of cefazolin sodium over a 24-hour period.

Trimethoprim-sulfamethoxazole was studied[63] in 5 large-volume parenteral solutions and found to be stable for at least 12 hours at room temperature.

Diazepam[64] was found to be stable when repackaged in glass disposable syringes for up to 90 days when stored at 4° C or 30° C.

Digoxin[65] injection was found to be compatible with five commonly used I.V. fluids.

Hydromorphone HCl[66] was found to be compatible in 17 different I.V. fluids for at least 24 hours at 25° C.

Dobutamine HCl[67] was found to be stable for a minimum of 48 hours in a variety of admixtures.

Zatz et al.[68] studied refrigerated aminophylline in 5% Dextrose and stated it was stable for up to 96 hours.

Aminophylline[69] injection was found to be stable in parenteral nutrition solutions for 24 hours in concentrations up to 1.5 mg/ml.

Cutie[70] studied the visual compatibility of verapamil HCl with 68 admixtures; visual compatibility was present with all the drugs studied.

Methylprednisolone sodium succinate[71] in 5% dextrose and 0.9% sodium chloride admixtures produced adequate stability from 8 to 24 hours, depending on drug concentrations.

Kirschenbaum et al.[72] studied dobutamine HCl with large-volume parenteral solutions and selected additives. This group found dobutamine to be compatible with a number of additives. Dobutamine was found to be incompatible with sodium bicarbonate-containing solutions.

Labetalol HCl[73] was studied in 11 large-volume parenteral fluids for compatibility and stability. It was found to be stable for 72 hours at 4° C and 25° C in all I.V. solutions except 5% sodium bicarbonate injection.

Clindamycin phosphate[74] was found to be stable and compatible in commonly used large-volume parenteral solutions for 8 weeks at −10° C, 32 days at 4° C, and 16 days at 25° C in glass and polyvinyl chloride containers.

Droperidol[75] is stable in glass containers for 7 to 10 days at room temperature with 5% dextrose and 0.9% sodium chloride injection, but undergoes sorptive loss from admixtures in lactated Ringer's injection when stored in flexible polyvinyl chloride bags.

Newton et al.[76] studied the solubility and sorption of lorazepam in I.V. admixtures. Lorazepam was soluble and stable in 5% dextrose, with a maximum 5% sorption up to 5 hours.

Bretylium tosylate[77] was stable for 4 weeks in glass and plastic containers of common large-volume parenteral solutions. Those admixtures studied with other drugs were visually compatible, with the exception of phenytoin.

Nahata[78] found ceftriaxone sodium stable in commonly selected I.V. fluids up to a period of 48 hours at room temperature and 72 hours in the refrigerator.

Cytarabine, methotrexate, and hydrocortisone sodium succinate[79] were found to be stable for up to 24 hours in 3 common I.V. fluids.

Combinations of dobutamine HCl and verapamil HCl[80] in 0.9% sodium chloride and 5% dextrose were found to be stable for 48 hours at 24° C and 7 days at 5° C.

Amiodarone HCl,[81] when combined with various other drugs, showed visual compatibility for 24 hours with all of the drugs studied except aminophylline.

Fluorouracil[82] is stable in 5% dextrose injection for at least 16 weeks when stored at 5° C in 2 types of plastic containers.

Succinylcholine Chloride Injection U.S.P.[83] should be stored in the refrigerator. If unbuffered succinylcholine chloride injection must be stored at room temperature, it should not be stored for longer than 4 weeks.

Ranitidine HCl[84] in total parenteral nutrient solutions was stable up to 48 hours at room temperature.

Cytarabine[85] at a concentration of 50 mg/ml was stable for at least 48 hours in the parenteral nutrient solution studied.

Solutions of morphine sulfate or meperidine HCl[86] in polyvinylchloride (PVC) bags containing total parenteral nutrition solutions or 5% dextrose injection are visually and chemically compatible as well as stable and available for 36 hours when stored at 21.5° C with no protection from environmental light.

Storage of 2-drug admixtures of aztreonam and ampicillin[87] at the concentrations studied in 0.9% sodium chloride injection should not exceed 48 hours at 4° C or 24 hours at 25° C. For 2-drug admixtures prepared in 5% dextrose injection, storage should not exceed 2 hours at 25° C or 8 hours at 4° C.

Furosemide[88] precipitates when added to admixtures containing either gentamicin sulfate or netilmicin sulfate in 5% dextrose or 0.9% sodium chloride injection; therefore, furosemide should be administered separately.

Clindamycin and gentamicin[89] mixed together in 5% dextrose injection are stable for 24 hours.

Unbuffered admixtures of mitomycin[90] should not be prepared in advance; buffered mitomycin is stable in 5% dextrose injection for 15 days at room temperature and 120 days at refrigerated temperature.

Intravenous admixtures of aztreonam and clindamycin phosphate[91] in studied concentrations were stable for at least 48 hours at 22° C and at least 7 days at 4° C.

Tobramycin sulfate[92] is stable in 5% dextrose injection alone and in the presence of calcium gluconate for at least 1 hour. Tobramycin and calcium gluconate can be infused through the same intravenous line.

When reconstituted with Sterile Water for Injection and with commonly used I.V. fluids, cefonicid sodium[93] vials and small-volume infusions are chemically stable for 24 hours at room temperature and for 72 hours at 5° C. If desired, reconstituted cefonicid sodium vials can be frozen for as long as 8 weeks, thawed, and then kept at room temperature for 24 hours or at 5° C for 72 hours.

Clindamycin[94] was found to be stable for at least 48 hours when mixed with cefoxitin sodium, cefamandole nafate, or cefazolin sodium in either 5% dextrose injection or 0.9% sodium chloride injection and for at least 24 hours when mixed with ceftizoxime sodium in 0.9% sodium chloride injection.

Cimetidine HCl[95] in concentrations up to 1.8 g/1.5 L was stable and did not affect the fat emulsion for at least 24 hours.

Dandurand et al.[96] studied the effects of light irradiation upon the stability of Dopamine hydrochloride. 1000 μg/ml of Dopamine HCl in 5% dextrose injection was found to have clinically acceptable stability for 36 hours.

In a study of frozen stability of Amoxicillin Sodium, Concannon[97] found Amoxicillin sodium injection to be unstable in aqueous solutions stored between 0° C and −20° C. The t90 of the frozen solution decreased from 2 days to 1 hour between 0° C and −7° C, however, the t90 at −30° C increased to 13 days.

The leaching effect of diethylhexyl phthalate (DEHP) from polyvinyl chloride bags mixed with cyclosporin shows significant leaching within 48 hours (33 mg DEHP).[98] It is recommend the intravenous cyclosporin be prepared in glass containers to minimize DEHP leaking. If plastic I.V. bags are utilized, the admixture should be used immediately after preparation.

The stability of intravenous admixtures of doxorubicin and Vincristine[99] were found to be stable for at least 7 days at 37° C when mixed in 0.9% sodium chloride injection, 0.45% sodium chloride injection and 2.5% dextrose injection. This 7-day stability allows for continuous infusion with ambulatory patients via pump devices.

It has been shown that the absorption of diazepam is greater in PVC tubing than polyethylene or glass I.V. containers.[100]

Admixtures of levodopa in 5% dextrose injection, adjusted to a pH of 5 or 6 were found to be stable for 7 days.[101]

Stability of terbutaline sulfate[102] admixtures stored in polyvinyl chloride bags showed 168 hours of stability at room temperature when mixed in concentration of 30 μg/ml in 5% dextrose injection 0.9% and 0.45% sodium chloride injections.

Admixtures[103] of aztreonam and nafcillin, when mixed in 0.9% sodium chloride injection or 5% dextrose injection in glass or plastic containers, precipitate slowly. This incompatible combination should be administered separately.

Nahata et al.[104] studied the stability of phenobarbital sodium diluted in 0.9% sodium chloride injection. At a diluted concentration; 10 mg/ml taken from the commercially available product 65 mg/ml and added to 0.9% sodium chloride injection produced a stable product when stored over a 4-week period in the refrigerator.

The stability[105] of clindamycin phosphate with aztreonam, ceftazidime sodium, ceftriaxone sodium, or piperacillin sodium was studied. Clindamycin was compatible with aztreonam and piperacillin. Admixtures of clindamycin and ceftazidime in 5% dextrose injection should be used within 24 hours at room temperature. Clindamycin and ceftriaxone can be mixed in 0.9% sodium, chloride injection if administered within 8 hours. Ceftriaxone is stable for only 1 hour in combination with clindamycin in D5W.

Kuhn et al.[106] found netilmicin sulfate in admixture with calcium gluconate and aminophylline stable for at least 2 hours in 5% dextrose or 0.2% sodium chloride injection.

Cyclosporin is stable in D5W in glass containers or polyvinyl chloride minibags for 24 hours and in normal saline for 6 to 12 hours in glass containers. However, these authors[107] suggest that, due to the potential for leaching of plasticizers, cyclosporin admixtures should be stored in glass or used within 6 hours if stored in polyvinyl chloride minibags.

Tu et al.[108] studied the stability of papaverine hydrochloride and phentolamine mesylate alone and combined in injectable mixtures. All solutions and combinations were found stable for up to 30 days when stored at 5° C or 25° C.

Visor et al.[109] studied the stability of Ganciclovir sodium in 5% dextrose or 0.9% Sodium chloride injections. Ganciclovir was found to be stable under all storage conditions for up to 5 days.

Pentamidine[110] injection was found to be stable for 48 hours in either 5% dextrose injection or 0.9% Sodium chloride injection in PVC bags.

Gentamicin[111] stored in glass syringes after dilution from 40 mg/ml to 10 mg/ml in 0.9% sodium chloride injection was found stable for 12 weeks refrigerated.

Theophylline in 5% dextrose injection in a concentration of 4 mg/ml or less can be mixed with methylprednisolone sodium succinate in a final concentration of 2 mg/ml or less and administered within 24 hours after admixture.[112]

Nahata et al.[113] studied the stability of vancomycin hydrochloride in plastic syringes with dextrose injection. Vancomycin was stable for 24 hours in plastic syringes when stored in the refrigerator.

Ticarcillin, mezlocillin, and piperacillin were found to be stable for 24 hours in TPN solutions commonly used in adults.[114]

Fitzgerald et al.[115] found that calcium and phosphate solubility in neonatal parenteral nutrient solutions containing Aminosyn PF was decreased when compared to the amino acid solution Troph Amine.

Visual incompatibilities were reported by Nelson et al.[116] between heparin and dacarbazine. A white flocculent precipitate formed with the two drugs in the I.V. tubing.

These authors recommend that, after dacarbazine administration, the I.V. tubing should be flushed with 0.9% sodium chloride injection.

Raymond et al.[117] achieved stability for 24 hours by adjusting the pH of dextrose injection to 7.5 with the addition of procainamide hydrochloride injection.

Riley[118] studied the stability of milrinone and digoxin, furosemide, procainamide hydrochloride, propanolol hydrochloride, quinidine gluconate, or verapamil hydrochloride in 5% dextrose injection. Milrinone and furosemide were found to be incompatible in 5% dextrose injection. The remaining admixtures were found to be compatible for 4 hours at room temperature.

Behme et al.[119] found the bacteriostat in benzyl-alcohol-preserved bacteriostatic water for injection incompatible with concentrations of 100 mg/ml of Ifosfamide; at lower concentrations the incompatibility was not seen.

Verapamil hydrochloride injection in final concentrations of 0.1 to 0.4 mg/ml can be added to a commercial preparation of premixed theophylline in 5% dextrose injection in concentrations of 0.4 to 4 mg/ml and administered within 24 hours without loss of potency of either drug.[120]

Precipitation develops when verapamil hydrochloride is added to nafcillin sodium, oxacillin sodium, ampicillin sodium or mezlocillin sodium. It is recommended that the I.V. tubing be flushed before and after this drug is administered through a Y-injection site when the penicillins are utilized alone.[121]

Colucci et al.[122] studied the compatibility of a number of drugs in combination with labetalol hydrochloride, cefaperazone sodium, and nafcillin sodium and found these drugs to be incompatible.

Esmolol hydrochloride and sodium nitroprusside[123] were found to be compatible for 24 hours in admixtures containing both drugs in 5% dextrose injection.

The compatibility of ranitidine hydrochloride[124] was visually studied with a number of critical care drugs. No visual incompatibility was observed.

Esmolol hydrochloride[125] was visually compatible and chemically stable for at least 24 hours when mixed with aminophylline, heparin sodium, bretylium tosylate, or procainamide hydrochloride in PVC bags containing 5% dextrose injection.

Bleomycin[126] at concentrations of 0.3 and 3 units/ml in admixtures with 0.9% sodium chloride injection, can be stored at room temperature in glass or PVC containers for 24 hours. Bleomycin should not be diluted with 5% dextrose injection.

Ranitidine[127] is stable for 7 days at room temperature and 30 days at 4° C in a variety of I.V. fluids. Frozen admixtures were stable for 60 days and 114 days refrigerated.

Floy et al.[128] studied the compatibility of ketorolac tromethamine injection with common infusion fluids and administration sets. Ketorolac tromethamine injection was physically and chemically stable when mixed with a variety of commonly used infusion solutions and not absorbed to PVC set components or glass. Admixtures containing cisplatin and fluorouracil[129] are stable for only 1.5 hours and should not be mixed together for continuous infusion.

At least 86% of the original concentration of ranitidine[130] was retained at 48 hours in dextrose amino acid TPN solution.

Wilson et al.[131] found micrinone at 0.10 to 0.73 mg/ml compatible with atropine sulfate, morphine sulfate, lidocaine hydrochloride, epinephrine, calcium chloride and sodium bicarbonate stored at room temperature for 20 minutes in glass containers.

Enalaprilat[132] was found visually incompatible with phenytoin sodium and amphotericin B; several other drugs tested with enalaprilat injection showed visual compatibility.

Tripp et al.[133] studied the stability of TNA formulations made by adding fat emulsion and electrolytes to a Nutrimix container with amino acids and dextrose; under the conditions of this study stability was achieved for up to 10 days.

Amphotericin B[134] maintained its stability at 100 μg/ml in 5%, 10%, 15% and 20% dextrose injection for 24 hours at 15 to 25° C and protected from light.

Cefoperazone sodium[135] is stable in peritoneal dialysis solutions containing 1.5% and 4.24% dextrose injection for 14 days at 4° C, 8 days at 25° C, and 24 hours at 37° C.

Cefoperazone sodium[136] 10 mg/ml and furosemide 0.2 mg/ml in admixtures of 5% dextrose injection are stable for 2 days at 25° C and 5 days at 4° C.

Visual compatibility[137] of a variety of drugs in combination with meperidine hydrochloride and morphine sulfate were studied during simulated Y-site injection. Incompatibilities were found with Imipenem-Cilastatin sodium with meperidine hydrochloride; acyclovir and furosemide were incompatible with both morphine sulfate and meperidine hydrochloride.

Miconazole[138] when mixed in PVC bags and peritoneal dialysis fluid is not chemically stable and must be mixed immediately before administration.

Cefoperazone sodium[139] 5 mg/ml and cimetidine hydrochloride 2 mg/ml in admixtures of 5% dextrose injection are stable for 48 hours at 4 and 25° C.

Ceftazidime[140] may be added directly to containers of parenteral nutrient solutions if the infusion time is less than 12 hours for a final drug concentration of 6 mg/ml, or less than 6 hours for a concentration of 1 mg/ml.

Nizatidine[141] in a concentration of 150 μg/ml was stable for 48 hours at 22° C in TNA solutions containing 3% and 5% Intralipid or Liposyn II.

Dobutamine hydrochloride[142] 5 and 7.5 μg/ml in 4.25% dextrose dialysis solution was stable for 24 hours. In concentrations of 2.5 μg/ml in 1.5% dextrose dialysate, stability is achieved for only 4 hours at room temperature.

Methylprednisolone sodium succinate[143] in concentrations equivalent to methylprednisolone 0.4 and 1.25 mg/ml was chemically stable and visually compatible in admixtures with cimetidine 3 mg/ml in 5% dextrose injection 100 ml at 24° C for 24 hours.

Amrinone[144] and sodium bicarbonate are incompatible in intravenous admixtures. Amrinone was found compatible with digoxin, propranolol hydrochloride, potassium chloride, and verapamil hydrochloride. Amrinone and procamide are compatible in 0.45% sodium chloride injection, but, not in 5% dextrose injection.

Lor et al.[145] studied the visual compatibility of Fluconazole with commonly used injectable drugs during simulated Y-site administration, a majority of the drugs studied were found to be visually incompatible with Fluconazole.

Amphotericin B[146] in 5% dextrose injection is stable at concentrations of 0.92, 1.20, and 1.40 mg/ml when stored at 6 and 25° C for up to 36 hours.

Zidovudine,[147] 4 mg/ml in admixture with 5% dextrose injection or 0.9% sodium chloride injection stored in polyvinyl chloride infusion bags, was stable for up to 192 hours at room temperature and under refrigeration.

Ciprofloxacin[148] injection was compatible with gentamicin, metronidazole, and tobramycin and incompatible with aminophylline and clindamycin. The compatibility of ciprofloxacin-amikacin admixtures depended on the I.V. solution and temperature.

Octreotide acetate[149] at a concentration of 45 μg/dl in TNA solution containing 3% lipids was physically compatible for 48 hours at room temperature and for 7 days under refrigeration.

Recombinant[150] interleukin-2 does not lose biologic activity when mixed with gentamicin sulfate, tobramycin sulfate, amikacin sulfate, ticarcillin disodium, piperacillin sodium, morphine sulfate, TPN solution, or fat emulsion.

To aid the pharmacist in admixture preparation, four texts have also been made available. A computerized listing, I.V. Additives and Pharmacy Technology of Sterile Products—1,[151] has been published. This source, covering the period 1970 to 1975, makes the search of the parenteral literature relatively easy. A combined industrial and professional effort produced Parenteral Drug Information Guide,[152] a text devoted to parenteral incompatibility data. A recently published text, Handbook on Injectable Drugs,[153] offers a compatibility guide of drugs with complete references. King's Guide to Parenteral Admixtures[154] provides an easy-to-read reference. An up-to-date guide to stability and reconstitution has been prepared by Kirschenbaum and Latiolais.[155]

For a complete discussion of parenteral incompatibility, the reader is referred to these texts.

The Stability of Frozen Antibiotics (Injectable Medication)

To increase the efficiency of I.V. admixture programs, a limited number of pharmacy I.V. admixture programs have found it efficient to freeze reconstituted drugs, particularly antibiotics. The stability of reconstituted drugs is somewhat limited. In some cases, stability is limited to only a few hours; in many cases, however, reconstituted liquid can be frozen and then thawed at the time of use. In the frozen form, the stability of the antibiotic can be increased. Often, the stability in the frozen form is known and the information is supplied by the manufacturer. In some cases, individual researchers have published reports on the frozen stability of drugs. It is unwise to freeze drugs arbitrarily without adequate stability studies for guidance. Additionally, the freezing temperature, storage conditions, and packaging parameters of published studies must be closely adhered to.

The package insert for sodium ampicillin[156,157] injections stated that, at room temperature, the reconstituted vial must be used within 1 hour and is stable for only 8 hours when added to normal saline solution and only for 4 hours when added to 5% dextrose injection at a very low concentration. Savello and Shangraw[158] studied the stability of frozen sodium ampicillin and concluded that freezing is not advised. In some cases, frozen sodium ampicillin was stable; however, 1% concentrations actually degraded more rapidly in the frozen state. Based on this study, there was no real advantage in freezing a reconstituted vial.

Shoup and Thur[159] reported that frozen buffered penicillin G potassium injection was stable for 12 weeks; however, the method of assay has been questioned.[160]

Stolar et al.[161] found frozen solutions of sodium methicillin to be stable for 10 weeks.

Boylan et al.[160] studied the stability of frozen sodium cephalothin and cephaloridine and concluded that solutions of sodium cephalothin (100 mg/ml and 230 mg/ml) or cephaloridine (200 mg/ml) in Water for Injection are stable for 6 weeks if frozen immediately after reconstitution. Water for Injection is the recommended diluent. Frozen solutions should be stored only in the original containers. Once thawed, solutions should not be refrozen.

Carone et al.[162] studied the stability of frozen solutions of cefazolin sodium in nine commonly used diluents at concentrations of 1 g with 2.5 ml, 500 mg with 100 ml, and 10 g with 45 ml in both glass and polyvinylchloride plastic containers.

The diluents were: Water for Injection U.S.P.; 0.9% Sodium Chloride Injection U.S.P.; 5% Dextrose Injection U.S.P. (D5W); D5W with 0.02% sodium bicarbonate; D5W in Lactated Ringer's Injection U.S.P.; Lactated Ringer's Injection U.S.P.; Ionosol B in D5W; Normosol M in D5W; and Plasma-Lyte in D5W.

Frozen cefazolin sodium solutions, containing Water for Injection U.S.P., 5% Dextrose Injection U.S.P. or 0.9% Sodium Chloride Injection U.S.P. as the diluent, retained more than 90% of labeled potency for up to 26 weeks when frozen within 1 hour after reconstitution and held at $-10°$ C or $-20°$ C.

Frozen cefazolin sodium solutions made with other diluents were stable for up to 4 weeks when frozen within 1 hour after reconstitution and held at $-10°$ C.

Parodi[163] studied the stability of frozen antibiotic solutions in Viaflex infusion containers. After frozen storage, ranging from 14 to 23 days, only clindamycin was unacceptable.

Solutions of cephapirin sodium[164] at concentrations of 50, 100, and 400 mg/ml in Sterile Water for Injection, normal saline, and 5% dextrose injection were prepared and frozen in the original vial within 1 hour after reconstitution. The vials were stored at $-15°$ C during the test period. After storage for 1, 3, 7, 14, 30, 45, and 60 days in the frozen state, the samples were allowed to thaw at room temperature.

Physical observations of the thawed solutions as a function of time indicated all samples to be clear, without the presence of a precipitate or insoluble material. There was no increase in color or any significant changes in pH or chromatographic zones from the original solutions. The frozen solutions were stable at least 60 days.

Knecht et al.[165] studied the stability of frozen solutions of cefazolin sodium packaged in glass and plastic disposable syringes. They concluded that, packaged thus, cefazolin sodium solution can be frozen for periods up to 6 weeks, thawed and stored for periods up to 96 hours at 5° C, and still be potent.

Dinel et al.[166,167] studied the stability of several antibiotics frozen in 50-ml minibags containing normal saline and 5% dextrose. Only ampicillin had significant loss in potency.

Some hospital pharmacists reconstitute and then freeze unstable antibiotic solutions such as the penicillins, to utilize staff time during slow periods. Freezing maintains the stability of the solution and, when the drug is required for use, it is removed from the refrigerator and allowed to thaw at room temperature. Not all unstable drugs should be considered stable in the frozen state. If documentation is not in the literature, stability studies must be done.

Table 11–1 lists drug-I.V. plastic stability studies that have been conducted during the past several years. Those drugs listed in the table in many cases were studied for a period of 24 hours; in some few cases, longer. The reader is referred to the references for a more detailed explanation and evaluation.

Effects of Microwave Radiation on Frozen Parenteral Antibiotics

Microwaves are part of the electromagnetic spectrum, with wavelengths longer than infrared waves and shorter than radio and television waves. A typical quantum of microwave energy is approximately 10^{-5} eV and cannot normally cause ionization. Within the microwave oven, the microwaves produce an alternating electric field. When any surface containing a polar compound (e.g., water) is introduced into the alternating electric field, the polar molecules also attempt to change their positions. This continuous molecular movement produces extensive, increased collisions (friction) between adjacent water molecules, and thus, a general heating of the entire medium. Substances such as glass, plastic, and paper are not generally heated by microwaves because their molecules are nonpolar.

In order to optimize the use of available labor, frozen parenteral products (particularly antibiotics) are utilized in a selected number of admixture pro-

Table 11–1.   Reported Drug Stability in Plastic* IV Fluid Containers—A Literature Review

	Incompatible	Compatible
Amikacin sulfate[34]		X
Amphotericin B[168]		X
Ampicillin sodium[166†]		X
Ascorbic acid[169]		X
Azathioprine sodium[46]		X
Bleomycin sulfate[47]	X	
Bretylium tosylate[45,77]		X
Carbenicillin disodium[166]		X
Carmustine[47]	X	
Cefazolin sodium[166]		X
Cephalothin sodium[166]		X
Clindamycin[74]		X
Clonazepam[170]	X	
Cloxacillin sodium[166]		X
Cyanocobalamin[169]		X
Cyclophosphamide[47]		X
Cytarabine[47]		X
Dacarbazine[47]		X
Dactinomycin[47]		X
Diazepam[32,33,54,171]	X	
Dobutamine HCl[67]		X
Dopamine HCl[45,172]		X
Doxorubicin HCl[47]		X
Droperidol[75‡]	X	X
d-Tubocurarine chloride[169]		X
Erythromycin gluceptate[166]		X
Erythromycin lactobionate[34]		X
Fluorouracil[47]		X
Gentamicin sulfate[166]		X
Haloperidol[56]		X
Heparin[173]		X
Hydrocortisone sodium[169]		X
Insulin[77,174§]	X	
Isoproterenol[175]		X
Leucovorin calcium[47]		X
Lidocaine HCl[37,45,61,169]		X
Lorazepam[76]		X
Menadiol sodium diphosphate[169]		X
Methicillin sodium[34]		X
Methohexital sodium[169]	X	
Mithramycin[47]		X
Mitomycin[47]		X
Netilmicin sulfate[52‖]		X
Niacin[169]		X
Niacinamide[169]		X
Nitroglycerin[45]	X	
Penicillin G K[166]		X
Pentobarbitol sodium		X
Procainamide[45]	X	
Propranolol HCl[44]		X

Table 11-1. *Continued*

	Incompatible	Compatible
Pyridoxine HCl[169]		x
Riboflavin[169]		x
Rolitetracycline base[166]		x
Thiamine HCl[169]		x
Ticarcillin[34]		x
Tobramycin sulfate[176]		x
Vancomycin HCl[34]		x
Vinblastine sulfate[47]		x
Vincristine sulfate[47]		x
Vitamin A (retinol acetate)[169,177,178]	x	
Vitamin E[169]		x
Warfarin sodium[169]	x	

*Polyvinylchloride
†Polyolefin
‡Loss occurs in lactated Ringer's only
§Occurs with glass also, adsorption of insulin to surface
‖PVC administration set only

grams. One manufacturer has begun shipment of frozen antibiotics to hospitals. These frozen antibiotics are ready to use after thawing. No mixing, diluting, or extemporaneous compounding is required. Methods of thawing have included room temperature, warm-water baths, and microwave radiation.

The following products have been evaluated or commented upon with regard to stability and activity *after freezing* and *microwave thawing*.

Cefazolin (Ancef, SmithKline Beecham; Kefzol, Lilly)

Tomecko et al.[179] demonstrated that cefazolin sodium minibag admixtures frozen and then thawed in a microwave oven retain at least 90% of their initial antimicrobial activity. These authors give recommendations for the proper use of microwave ovens and the hazards that may be associated with this method of thawing.

Holmes et al.[180] studied several antibiotics, including cefazolin admixtures, using microwave thaw. They found that the studied antibiotic admixtures, except ampicillin sodium, can be frozen at −20° C for up to 30 days and thawed by microwave radiation without affecting antibiotic activity.

One manufacturer[181] of cefazolin does not recommend microwave thawing and another[182] comments: "May use water bath but do not submerge during thawing."

Cimetidine (Tagamet, SmithKline Beecham)

Elliot et al.[183] studied the stability of cimetidine 300 mg/50 ml in 5% dextrose and 100 ml normal saline, which was frozen for 28 days. Samples were allowed to thaw at room temperature and compared with microwave thawing. The authors concluded that microwave thawing does not affect cimetidine stability.

The manufacturer[181] of cimetidine does not recommend the freezing of the diluted injection to avoid the possibility of a cimetidine precipitate forming upon freezing that may not completely redissolve at the time of administration.

Cefamandole (Mandol, Lilly)

The manufacturer[182] reveals that Mandol in Sterile Water for Injection, normal saline, or 5% dextrose can be frozen immediately after reconstitution and is stable for up to 6 months when stored at $-20°$ C. This applies to Mandol in the original container, glass partial-fills, or in Viaflex bags. Thawing of the product can be speeded up by the use of a water bath, warming slowly (37° C or less), and taking care to avoid heat after thawing is complete.

Cephalothin Sodium (Keflin, Lilly)

Solutions of Neutral Keflin in Sterile Water for Injection, normal saline, or 5% dextrose that are frozen immediately after reconstitution are stable for up to 12 weeks at $-20°$ C. This applies to vials, Faspaks, glass partial-fills, Viaflex bags, or B–D glaspak syringes.

The manufacturer[182] advises avoidance of microwave for thawing solutions of Neutral Keflin. Microwave ovens utilize a high-energy source that could cause structural alteration of the Keflin molecule. Also a possibility is that of leaching of substances from the rubber stopper when frozen ampuls of Neutral Keflin are thawed using microwave.

Cefotaxime Sodium (Claforan, Hoechst-Roussel)

Information from the package insert indicates Claforan in 5% dextrose, normal saline or Sterile Water for Injection maintains satisfactory potency for 24 hours at room temperature (25° C), for 10 days under refrigeration (below 5° C), and for at least 13 weeks in the frozen state. After reconstitution, Claforan may be stored in disposable glass or plastic syringes for 24 hours at room temperature, 5 days under refrigeration, and 13 weeks frozen.

Solutions of Claforan[184] in normal saline or 5% dextrose in Viaflex bags are stable for 24 hours at room temperature, 5 days under refrigeration, and 13 weeks frozen. Frozen samples should not be heated but should be thawed at room temperature before use. Any unused portions after the periods mentioned should be discarded; they should never be refrozen.

No data are available for microwave radiation.

Piperacillin (Pipracil, Lederle)

Extensive stability studies[185] have demonstrated the chemical stability of piperacillin (potency, pH, and clarity) through 24 hours at room temperature, up to 1 week refrigerated, and up to 1 month frozen. The manufacturer indicates little change in potency occurs (potency greater than 95%) after frozen and thawed by microwave.

Cefoxitin (Mefoxin, Merck, Sharpe & Dohme)

The package insert indicates that Mefoxin solutions in 5% dextrose, bacteriostatic water for injection, or normal saline maintains satisfactory potency for 24 hours at room temperature, 1 week under refrigeration and for at least 30 weeks in the frozen state. Direct communication from the manufacturer[186] indicated that after microwave thawing, the drug maintains full stability for 24 hours.

Other Drugs

Holmes et al.[187] studied the stability of 6 antibiotics in I.V. fluids in PVC containers after freezing and microwave thawing (tobramycin sulfate, amikacin sulfate, ticarcillin disodium, clindamycin phosphate, nafcillin sodium, and ampicillin sodium). All antibiotics except ampicillin sodium retained 90% or more potency under microwave thawing after storage at $-20°$ C for 30 days and after subsequent storage at room temperature for 24 hours.

Ampicillin sodium was stable in 0.9% sodium chloride when stored at $-30°$ C or $-70°$ C, microwave-thawed, and stored up to 8 hours at room temperature. Ampicillin sodium was stable in 5% dextrose when stored at $-70°$ C and microwave-thawed, but its potency declined to 70.5% after 8 hours storage at room temperature.

Ausman et al.[188] demonstrated no deleterious effect on parenteral nutrition solutions stored frozen for 60 days at $-20°$ C and microwave-thawed.

General Precautions Required with the Use of Microwave Ovens

• The possibility exists of radiation leakage; however, manufacturers of microwave ovens are required to comply with federal standards.

• Microwave ovens may interfere with cardiac pacemakers, requiring careful screening of personnel who are exposed to microwave ovens.

• Leaching of rubber stopper material is a possibility when exposing rubber material to microwave heating.

• The placement of a closed or sealed container in a microwave oven will cause an increase in internal pressure that may result in explosion.

• Microwave ovens offer heterogeneous heat; unequal distribution of heat can occur.

• Each hospital should develop its own protocol to ensure that the solution temperature does not exceed room temperature.

Nitroglycerin Adsorption in Administration Sets

The usefulness of intravenous nitroglycerin in a variety of cardiovascular disorders has been described.[189–191] In the past, pharmacists prepared nitroglycerin for I.V. infusion, using soluble nitroglycerin tablets. Since 1981, several pharmaceutical companies have marketed nitroglycerin solutions for I.V. administration (e.g., Parke Davis, Nitrostat; American Critical Care, Tridil; Abbott Labs, Nitroglycerin; Marion Labs, Nitro-BID I.V.). Nitroglycerin is a relatively unstable compound that is destroyed by heat (precluding heat sterilization) and degraded by light and oxidation. In addition, it is adsorbed to polyvinylchloride (PVC), a plastic that is used for all common administration-set components and some infusion containers. It has also been shown that final in-line I.V. filters adsorb significant amounts of nitroglycerin.[192] The amount of nitroglycerin adsorption varies depending on factors such as concentration, flow rate, surface area, and contact time. Assuming the worst case, for example, an 0.5 mg/ml solution prepared from 80% potent sublingual tablets (still within U.S.P. specifications), filtered through a membrane filter, then placed in a 250-ml plastic I.V. bag and delivered through a typical infusion set would result in less than 20% of the anticipated potency.

To avoid the portion of this major degradation that results from adsorption in polyvinylchloride, it is recommended that nitroglycerin solutions be infused through non-PVC administration sets. These special sets are made of or lined with polyethylene, another plastic. The polyethylene or "coextruded" sets are less pliable than those of polyvinylchloride. Specialty nitroglycerin sets are relatively expensive.

Intravenous nitroglycerin should be regulated by automatic infusion equipment (pumps or controllers) to ensure consistent dose administration; however, it was some time before infusion equipment manufacturers were able to develop non-PVC tubing and other set components (e.g., cassette pistons and drip chambers) that were compatible with their instruments. Straight, polyethylene tubing supplied by nitroglycerin manufacturers was tried by clinicians in some infusion devices that employ straight tubing. Unfortunately, this resulted in reports of health hazards,[193,194] because polyethylene tubing was stiffer than the PVC tubing the instruments were designed to use. Some pumps or controllers did not exert force adequate to fully occlude the less pliant polyethylene tubing. This can result in "flow too fast" alarms or excessive flow. In some cases, when the instrument is stopped, the nitroglycerin solution may flow by gravity around the compression points. One manufacturer recommended several complex solutions[195] to help decrease the potential for excessive flow. With some instruments, there is no way around using materials containing PVC in cassettes and component parts.

This problem is handled in several ways by practitioners. Some believe the best solution is to continue using PVC-containing administration sets; the sorption of nitroglycerin by PVC may be the easier problem to work around. Even though the loss to PVC is significant, the amount of drug the patient receives is based on hemodynamic functions;[196,197] however, when the previously used (saturated) set is changed, retitration of the drug is necessary. One report describes the loss of nitroglycerin in pulmonary artery delivery systems.[198] A polyethylene-lined (PEL) intravenous administration set has been developed that provides consistent delivery of I.V. nitroglycerin to patients.[199]

The Emergency Care Research Institute (ECRI) has published recommendations to follow when using a manufacturer-supplied non-PVC-containing administration set for infusion of nitroglycerin solution.[193,194] In addition to non-PVC-containing administration sets, several manufacturers have made available non-PVC-containing pump administration sets.

Phthalate Extraction From PVC-Containing Administration Sets When Used With Lipids

The tubing used in standard, commercially available administration sets is a medical-grade polyvinylchloride (PVC) plastic, formulated with added ingredients to provide a soft, flexible tubing, that is not degraded by heat, light, or oxidizing agents. Among these added ingredients is di(2-ethylhexyl)phthalate (DEHP).

The concern for the use of a set made of tubing plasticized with phthalate for giving I.V. fat has its origin in the fact that these phthalate compounds are more soluble in lipids than in water, and thus would be extracted into the emulsion. The possible toxicity of the phthalate remains a *theoretical* problem, however.

On the basis of information received from Abbott Laboratories (personal communications, 1983 and 1986), the clinical risk in the use of phthalate-plasticized sets for the administration of lipids appears to be negligible. Abbott supplies non-PVC-containing administration sets for those who wish to use them, as does Alpha-Therapeutic Corporation. Although this manufacturer does not actively promote this set, approximately 50% of its customers request and use the non-phthalate-containing set.

Travenol Laboratories conducted studies of the extraction of phthalate from PVC-containing administration sets and found insignificant amounts extracted. Travenol does not supply non-PVC-containing sets and, indeed, recommends the use of PVC sets with its own lipid emulsion.

Kabi-Vitrum, on the other hand, produces a phthalate-free fat emulsion administration set and recommends that it be used in any administration of lipid emulsion.

Adsorption of Insulin to Infusion Containers

No matter how precisely an insulin solution is prepared, if the drug becomes unavailable to the patient because of adsorption in the infusion system, patient care can be compromised. This has been found to be the case, especially with low-dose infusions. In the late 1950s, several investigators reported on the adsorption of insulin to glass containers.[200–202] Weisenfield et al.[203] reported that from 10 to 33% of insulin in solutions was adsorbed in infusion bottles and tubing. They also noted that this adsorption decreased with increasing concentrations of insulin.

Adsorption of insulin to glassware and tubing depends on the following factors:

1. Concentration of insulin
2. Contact time of insulin in glass and tubing
3. Flow-rate of infusion solution
4. Presence of other negatively charged proteins such as human serum albumin (HSA)

Administration of concentrated solutions of insulin from a syringe directly into a vein or tubing does not result in any significant insulin loss, because the solutions used are more concentrated. Studies of insulin adsorption in Viaflex containers, which utilized automated radioimmunoassay techniques, found that 23% of the total insulin was adsorbed during the first 30 minutes of infusion.[205]

Petty et al.[205] found adsorption of total insulin to glass containers was decreased from 52% to 28% by the addition of small amounts of HSA. They found that 50% of the total insulin adsorbed by glass and polyvinylchloride containers occurred within 15 seconds of filling. Of the remaining insulin in the infusion fluid, 50% more was adsorbed in the infusion set. They calculated that if 30 units of insulin in 1000 ml of lactated Ringer's are infused, by the time the solution reached the patient, only 6.36 units would be available.

Weber et al.[206] studied insulin adsorption in parenteral nutrition solutions and found that 40 to 60% of the 30 units per liter were lost to the equipment. In this study, the addition of HSA to the parenteral solutions reduced adsorption by 10%. Peterson et al.[207] reduced adsorption by flushing the infusion equipment with 50 ml of solution containing 50 units per liter of insulin. This permitted delivery of 75% of the insulin in the first 50 ml infused, and 100% (zero adsorption) thereafter.

Weber et al.[208] studied parenteral solutions made up of amino acids and protein hydrolysates in dextrose with 30 units of insulin per liter and found that 40 to 47% of the insulin was absorbed in the infusion equipment. Varying the concentration of insulin has a small but significant effect on insulin loss. The use of in-line filters and polyvinylchloride bags resulted in an even greater loss of insulin, while the addition of albumin, electrolytes, or vitamins decreased insulin loss. Stability studies[204] of various preparations of insulin in concentrated form in glass and plastic syringes showed that regular, NPH, and Lente insulin can be stored under refrigeration without loss of potency; however, mixtures of regular insulin with NPH or Lente must be administered immediately.

Hirsch et al.,[209] using a radiotracer technique to determine the adsorption of insulin to the internal surface of polyvinylchloride I.V. tubing, found the adsorption, especially at low-dose insulin levels, was enough to be clinically significant. Whalen et al.[210] studied the availability of insulin during continuous low-dose infusions and found that the degree of adsorption varied widely with the type of solution and the administration set used. Hirsch et al.[175] studied adsorption of insulin in polyolefin infusion containers and found that adsorption with this material was less than that which occurred with polyvinylchloride containers.

Twardowski et al.[211,212] studied the binding of insulin to peritoneal dialysis solution and found that insulin binding was an instantaneous phenomenon not influenced by time. Insulin was found to be more readily adsorbed to glass surfaces than to plastic surfaces. Adsorption is decreased with addition of HSA, blood, and gelatin. Insulin adsorption is greater in an electrolyte solution than in dextrose.

Kane et al.[213] also found that insulin binding occurs with continuous ambulatory peritoneal dialysis systems (CAPDs). These authors suggest that excess insulin be added to ensure delivery of the desired dose. Storage of the solution should be limited to 1 hour. In a clinical situation, Talbot[215] noted that insulin treatment may fail because the needle injecting insulin into the infusion bag may be shorter than the injection port dead space, and therefore, the insulin never reaches the infusion fluid.

Pretreatment with 0.9% sodium chloride and insulin has been suggested by Furberg et al.[214] to minimize insulin binding.

Handling and Disposal of Chemotherapeutic Agents for Cancer

In the early 1980s, concern developed among health care workers about environmental contamination when handling cytotoxic agents. The mutagenic and allergic responses of health care personnel began to receive attention.[216–222] In 1985, the American Society of Hospital Pharmacists published a technical assistance bulletin on handling cytotoxic drugs in hospitals.[223] OSHA also responded by publishing comprehensive guidelines for personnel dealing with

cytotoxic agents.[224] Precautions for health care personnel are now understood
and practiced.[225] The effort to minimize environmental and human contamination has also been extended to manufacturers of devices and drugs. Special
guards (Cytoguard, Mead Johnson), filters, and other devices became available
to minimize contamination. Specialized companies now supply clothing, waste
disposal systems, gloves and distinctive labeling that meet the OSHA guidelines.

Personnel handling antineoplastic agents may be at potential risk. Although
the evidence is not conclusive, it appears that measures should be taken to
minimize unnecessary exposure by implementing some basic concepts and following common sense.

1. Vertical laminar flow-hoods (or bacteriologic glove boxes) for preparation
   and reconstitution of neoplastic drugs.
2. Personnel reconstituting these drugs should wear gloves and mask.
3. Antineoplastic drugs should be handled and disposed of centrally. Disposal should be handled through specially designed waste containers and
   incineration.
4. Personnel involved in handling admixtures of antineoplastic drugs should
   have periodic testing of their blood (chemistry screen, complete blood
   count, and differential cell count).
5. Personnel handling antineoplastic drugs should be informed that a potential problem may exist.
6. Special labeling of containers should be instituted to ensure proper handling and disposal.

Crudi[226] noted the adverse effects of reconstituting antineoplastic agents in
unventilated areas. Among the symptoms he noted were light-headedness,
nausea, headache, and nasal mucosal sore; others reported hair loss and allergic sensitivity.

Falck et al.[221] reported an increase in mutagenicity in the urine of nurses
handling cytostatic drugs on oncology units.

Other side effects have been reported by pharmacists.[227] Others have reported side effects while preparing dacarbazine and cisplatin admixtures.[228,229]
One survey illustrated a definite lack of standardized practices in hospitals in
the handling of antineoplastic agents. Anderson et al.[230] studied the uptake of
mutagenic substances by persons handling injectable antineoplastic agents.
Mutagenicity was observed in the urine of all personnel during periods when
they prepared antineoplastic admixtures. Crudi et al.[231] studied possible occupational hazards associated with the preparation and administration of antineoplastic agents. Several excellent recommendations and guidelines have
become available.[232–241]

Admixture Programs

A survey by Stolar[242] indicated that 52% of hospitals with 300 beds or more
provided complete or partial admixture service and 25% of smaller hospitals
provided this service. The Joint Commission on Accreditation of Hospitals[243]
stated that pharmaceutical services provide the review and compounding of
large-volume parenterals. The Minimum Standards for Pharmacies in Hospitals, published by the American Society of Hospital Pharmacists, stated that

all preparations of sterile products be done by pharmacy personnel. The NCCLVP Committee on Large-Volume Parenterals recommended 24-hour I.V. admixture service.[244] The legal aspects of pharmacist involvement in I.V. admixture programs were discussed by Mitchell,[245] and the justification for such has been reviewed in the literature.[246,247] A variety of procedural manuals and guides have been published.[248–252] Training programs for pharmacy personnel have been published,[253,254] and pharmacy-nursing communications have been discussed.[255] Computer-assisted admixture programs[256,257] have aided in the implementation of such programs. Numerous publications supplying techniques are available,[258–264] as are excellent guidelines for the I.V. administration of drugs.[265,266] A thorough manual on centralized admixture program implementation and procedure is available from Abbott Laboratories.[267]

Approaches in policy and procedure in intravenous admixture programs vary from one hospital to another, creating modifications of the system and a certain amount of individuality in each ongoing program; however, the basic objectives and functions are common to all hospitals. The goal of an admixture program is to provide intravenous medication for the patient accurately and safely. The completed product can possess the desired qualities, regardless of the system implemented (Table 11–2).

To accomplish the basic goals, certain skills must be acquired. One must become familiar with the literature and attend conferences and workshops. Visits to ongoing programs in other hospitals are also helpful. An understanding of intravenous drug stability, sterility, and incompatibilities is also a part of the necessary knowledge. Dexterity with needle syringes and other devices must be acquired. A knowledge of milliequivalents and electrolytes is also a necessity. Aseptic technique must be acquired. These skills and knowledge can be gained during the planning stages of the admixture program.

Initial planning includes a study of the current system and the use of intravenous fluids and additives within the hospital. This provides helpful information in determining the additives ordered per day and the workload periods that develop. A formal committee can be established to determine policies and procedures pertaining to this service. The laboratory where this service is centralized will have to be planned and furnished with suitable equipment (Fig. 11–9).

Reconstitution of Sterile Solids

Drugs or substances that are not stable in solution are packaged as sterile, dry-filled solids or sterile lyophilized powders (Chapter 3). Prior to their use by either injection or addition to an intravenous fluid, the sterile solid must be reconstituted as a solution by using a suitable diluent in the proper volume to give the specified concentration. In reconstituting sterile solids, procedures that maintain sterility and freedom from pyrogens and particulate matter of the resulting injection are used. The stability of these injections depends on the drug substance and can vary greatly. The hospital pharmacist is dependent on the package insert as well as on recent references in the literature for the recommended storage period and conditions for a given injection.

Over the past several years, highly publicized incidents of morbidity and mortality have occurred associated with pharmacy-prepared sterile products.

Table 11–2. Flow Chart for Intravenous Admixture Preparation (Parenteral Prescription)

1. Physician writes or transmits to pharmacy via computer admixture order. R D5$^1/_2$ NSS Liter—Vits—20 mEq KCl Run at 120 ml/hr Start 8 AM, then DC	Order includes intravenous fluid wanted, additives and their concentrations, rate of flow, starting time, and length of therapy.
2. Order is transmitted to pharmacy.	Order is transmitted by technician, nurse, or pharmacist or computer. Orders may be phoned to pharmacy; verification with original order is made upon delivery of admixture.
3. Order is checked for dose compatibility, drug allergies, and stability.	The proper dose is checked; this requires a knowledge of milliequivalent calculations. Order is checked for compatibility. Admixtures are given maximum expiration period of 24 hours. Drugs such as ampicillin require shorter expiration periods.
4. Clerical work: label and profile work sheet.	Typed label contains bottle number, patient's name and room number, date prepared, and expiration date. Intravenous fluid and additives with the amounts are included on the label. The total time for the infusion, the milliliters per hour, and drops per minute are included. The label is affixed upside down in order that it can be read when hung. A profile work sheet is prepared so the admixture can be recycled if necessary. It is filed so that the pharmacist will be alerted when the next bottle is due for preparation. Charging the patient's account can be done at this point.
5. Preparation of admixture by pharmacist or supervised technician.	In handling the sterile products, the aseptic techniques involved must maintain the characteristics and integrity of the product. Additive caps may be affixed for storage (see Fig. 11–2).
6. Completed admixture is checked by pharmacist.	Label is checked with the original order. The empty containers are checked to confirm the additives. The admixture is checked for color change, coring, and other particulate matter.
7. Delivery to patient area.	Completed admixture may be delivered by messenger or by the pharmacist on a decentralized unit. STAT orders are usually picked up by nursing staff.
8. Storage in patient area.	If the admixture is not to be infused immediately, storage under refrigeration may be required.

Table 11–2. *Continued*

9. Administration to patient.	Nurse checks for correctness of patient's name, drug and concentration, solution, expiration date, and time started. Infusion of admixtures can run ahead of or behind schedule, necessitating that the pharmacists modify the preparation of continued orders.

These incidents precipitated concern and a subsequent review by the Food and Drug Administration (FDA). The FDA concern led to a memo sent to hospital pharmacists alerting those preparing sterile products to the potential hazards during preparation.[268]

Following these events, the American Society of Hospital Pharmacists established a survey review of practices by hospital pharmacists in preparing sterile products. This review revealed that sterile product preparation in hospitals was not uniform and had deficiencies that might compromise patient safety.[269] Subsequently proposed guidelines were drafted and published.[270] These guidelines are awaiting comments, and a final document will be published. The proposal guidelines[270] for pharmacy-prepared sterile products recommend that process validation be performed and that:

> "The aseptic technique of each person preparing sterile products should be observed and evaluated as satisfactory during orientation and training and on a

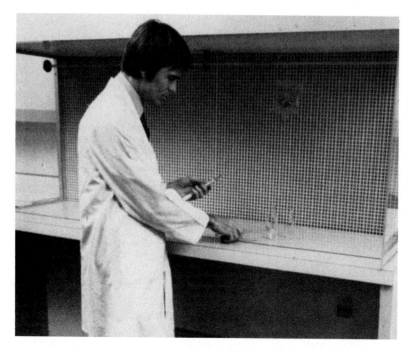

Figure 11–9. Preparation of admixture using a laminar flow hood. (Courtesy of Baxter Healthcare Laboratories, Inc., Deerfield, IL.)

regular basis by supervisory personnel. Competency for sterile product preparation should be reassessed and documented at least every six months or whenever unacceptable techniques are observed or detected. In addition to observation, methods of evaluating knowledge of aseptic technique and other issues might include written or practical test."

Stated in Risk Level II, further clarification of process validation suggests a successful complete process validation on technique to include an appropriate microbiologic growth monitoring procedure that involves periodic testing and evaluation of personnel based on process simulation.

Several reports have recommended or evaluated methods that permit "end Product Testing[271-275] End product testing serves as a valuable effective tool utilized in microbiologic quality assurance. Additional reports have been published that have evaluated process validation of personnel.[276-278]

References

1. Highlights of a Study on Single Unit Drug Dispensing. Toledo, Ohio, Owens-Illinois, 1968.
2. Turco, S.J., and Spoon, S.: Percentage of hospitalized patients receiving injections. Am. J. I.V. Ther., 4, 50 (1977).
3. Holysko, Sr., M.N., and Ravin, R.L.: A pharmacy centralized intravenous additive service. Am. J. Hosp. Pharm., 22, 266 (1965).
4. Dunworth, D., and Kenna, F.: Preliminary report: Incompatibility of combinations of medications in intravenous solutions. Am. J. Hosp. Pharm., 22, 190 (1965).
5. Parker, E.A.: Parenteral incompatibilities. Hosp. Pharm., 4, 14 (1969).
6. Raffanti, E.F., Jr., and King, J.C.: Effect of pH on the stability of sodium ampicillin solutions. Am. J. Hosp. Pharm., 31, 745 (1974).
7. Totacillin-N. Bristol, Tenn., Beecham Laboratories.
8. Omnipen. Philadelphia, Pa., Wyeth Laboratories.
9. Turner, F.E., and King, J.C.: Spectrophotometric analysis of intravenous admixtures containing metaraminol and corticosteroids. Am. J. Hosp. Pharm., 30, 128 (1973).
10. Parker, E.A.: Compatibility digest, Levophed bitartrate injection. Am. J. Hosp. Pharm., 32, 214 (1975).
11. Gardella, L.A., Zardsrinski, J.F., and Possley, L.H.: Intropin (dopamine hydrochloride) intravenous admixture compatibility. Part I. Am. J. Hosp. Pharm., 32, 575 (1975).
12. Gardella, L.A., Zardsrinski, J.F., and Possley, L.H.: Intropin (dopamine hydrochloride) intravenous admixture compatibility. Part 2. Am. J. Hosp. Pharm., 33, 537 (1976).
13. Leach, J.K., et al.: Biological activity of dilute isoproterenol stored for long periods in plastic bags. Am. J. Hosp. Pharm., 34, 709 (1977).
14. Mitchell, J.F., Barger, R.C., and Cantwell, L.: Heparin stability in 5% dextrose and 0.9% sodium chloride solutions. Am. J. Hosp. Pharm., 33, 540 (1976).
15. Turco, S.J.: I.V. Drug incompatibility. Heparin Sodium, USP. Am. J. I.V. Ther., 3, 16 (1976).
16. Mann, J.M., Coleman, D.L., and Boylan, J.C.: Stability of parenteral solutions of sodium cephalothin, cephaloridine, potassium penicillin G, and rancomycin hydrochloride. Am. J. Hosp. Pharm., 28, 760 (1971).
17. Bornstein, M., Thomas, P.N., Coleman, D.L., and Boylan, J.C.: Stability of parenteral solutions of cefazolin sodium. Am. J. Hosp. Pharm., 31, 296 (1974).
18. Chatterji, D., Hiranaka, P.K., and Galleui, J.F.: Stability of sodium oxacillin in intravenous solutions. Am. J. Hosp. Pharm., 32, 1130 (1975).
19. Parker, E.A., and Levin, H.J.: Compatibility digest, Unipen injection. Am. J. Hosp. Pharm., 32, 943 (1975).

20. Zost, E.D., and Yanchick, V.A.: Compatibility and stability of disodium carben-icillin in combination with other drugs and large volume parenteral solutions. Am. J. Hosp. Pharm., 29, 135 (1972).
21. McRae, M.P., and King, J.C.: Compatibility of antineoplastic, antibiotic and cor-ticosteroid drugs in I.V. admixtures. Am. J. Hosp. Pharm., 33, 1010 (1976).
22. Parker, E.A.: Compatibility digest, Aldomet injection. Am. J. Hosp. Pharm., 31, 1076 (1974).
23. Bergstrom, R.F., Fites, A.L., and Lamb, J.W.: Stability of parenteral solutions of tobramycin sulfate. Am. J. Hosp. Pharm., 32, 887 (1975).
24. Turco, S.J., et al.: Stability of aminophylline in 5% dextrose in water. Hosp. Pharm., 10, 374 (1975).
25. Bergstrom, R.F., and Fites, A.L.: Stability of erythromycin gluceptate in sodium chloride injection and dextrose injection. Letters, Am. J. Hosp. Pharm., 32, 241 (1975).
26. Dinel, B.A., et al.: Comparative stability of antibiotic admixtures in minibags and minibottles: Drug Intell. Clin. Pharm., 11, 226 (1977).
27. Lee, Y.C., et al.: Bretylium tosylate intravenous admixture compatibility. I: Sta-bility in common large-volume parenteral solutions. Am. J. Hosp. Pharm., 37, 803 (1980).
28. Carmichael, R.E., et al.: Solubility and stability of phenytoin sodium when mixed with intravenous solutions. Am. J. Hosp. Pharm., 37, 95 (1980).
29. Cloyd, J.C., et al.: Concentration-time profile of phenytoin after admixture with small volumes of intravenous fluids. Am. J. Hosp. Pharm., 35, 48 (1978).
30. Newton, D.W., et al.: Prediction of phenytoin solubility in intravenous admix-tures: physicochemical theory. Am. J. Hosp. Pharm., 37, 1247 (1980).
31. Otterman, G.E., et al.: Incompatibility between carbenicillin injection and pro-methazine injection. Am. J. Hosp. Pharm., 36, 1156 (1979).
32. Cloyd, J.C., et al.: Availability of diazepam from plastic containers. Am. J. Hosp. Pharm., 37:492, (1980).
33. Parker, W.A., and MacCara, M.E.: Compatibility of diazepam with intravenous fluid containers and administration sets. Am. J. Hosp. Pharm., 37, 496 (1980).
34. Tung, E.C., et al.: Stability of five antibiotics in plastic I.V. solution containers of dextrose and sodium chloride. Drug Intell. Clin. Pharm., 14, 848 (1980).
35. Cutie, M.R., et al.: Compatibility of verapamil hydrochloride injection in com-monly used large volume parenterals. Am. J. Hosp. Pharm., 37, 675 (1980).
36. Colvin, M., et al.: Stability of carmustine in the presence of sodium bicarbonate. Am. J. Hosp. Pharm. 37, 677 (1980).
37. Smith, F.M., et al.: Stability of lidocaine HCl in 5% dextrose injection in plastic bags. Am. J. Hosp. Pharm., 38, 1745 (1981).
38. Lesko, L.J., et al.: Stability of trimethoprim-sulfamethoxazole injection in two infusion fluids. Am. J. Hosp. Pharm., 38, 1004 (1981).
39. DasGupta, V., et al.: Stability of cefamandole nafate and cefoxotin sodium so-lutions. Am. J. Hosp. Pharm., 38, 875 (1981).
40. Newton, D.W., et al.: Stability of five catecholamines and terbutaline sulfate in 5% dextrose injection in the absence and presence of aminophylline. Am. J. Hosp. Pharm., 38, 1314 (1981).
41. Cutie, M.R.: Compatibility of verapamil HCl with other additives. Am. J. Hosp. Pharm., 38, 231 (1981).
42. Henderson, J.L., et al.: In vitro inactivation of gentamicin, tobramycin and ne-tilmicin by carbenicillin, azlocillin or mezlocillin. Am. J. Hosp. Pharm., 38, 1167 (1981).
43. Yuhas, E.M., et al.: Cimetidine hydrochloride compatibility III: Room temper-ature stability in drug admixtures. Am. J. Hosp. Pharm., 38, 1919 (1981).
44. Cummings, D.S., et al.: Compatibility of propranolol HCl with intravenous in-fusion fluids in plastic containers. Am. J. Hosp. Pharm., 39, 1685 (1982).
45. Lee, Y.C., et al.: Bretylium tosylate intravenous admixture compatibility. II: Do-pamine, lidocaine, procainamide, and nitroglycerin. Am. J. Hosp. Pharm., 38, 183 (1981).

46. Johnson, C.A., et al.: Compatibility of azathioprine sodium with I.V. fluids. Am. J. Hosp. Pharm., 38, 871 (1981).
47. Benvenuto, J.A., et al.: Stability and compatibility of antitumor agents in glass and plastic containers. Am. J. Hosp. Pharm., 38, 1914 (1981).
48. Townsend, R.J., et al.: Stability of methylprednisolone sodium succinate in small volumes of 5% dextrose and 0.9% sodium chloride injection. Am. J. Hosp. Pharm., 38, 1319 (1981).
49. Yuhas, E.M., et al.: Cimetidine hydrochloride compatibility and room temperature stability in intravenous infusion fluids. Am. J. Hosp. Pharm., 38, 879 (1981).
50. Poochikian, G.K., et al.: Stability of anthracycline antitumor agents in four infusion fluids. Am. J. Hosp. Pharm., 38, 483 (1981).
51. Newton, D.W., et al.: Solubility characteristics of diazepam in aqueous admixture solution: Theory and practice. Am. J. Hosp. Pharm., 38, 179 (1981).
52. Chaudry, I.A., et al.: Compatibility of netilmicin sulfate injection with commonly used intravenous injections and additives. Am. J. Hosp. Pharm., 38, 1737 (1981).
53. Pfeifle, C.E., et al.: Phenytoin sodium solubility in three intravenous solutions. Am. J. Hosp. Pharm., 38, 358 (1981).
54. Mason, N.A., et al.: Factors affecting diazepam infusion: Solubility, administration-set composition, and flow rate. Am. J. Hosp. Pharm., 38, 1449 (1981).
55. Eggert, L.D., et al.: Calcium and phosphorous compatibility in parenteral nutrition solutions for neonates. Am. J. Hosp. Pharm., 39, 49 (1982).
56. DasGupta, V., et al.: Stability of haloperidol in 5% dextrose injection. Am. J. Hosp. Pharm., 39, 292 (1982).
57. Bornstein, M., et al.: Moxalactam disodium compatibility with intramuscular and intravenous diluents. Am. J. Hosp. Pharm., 39, 1495 (1982).
58. Frable, R.A., et al.: Stability of cefamandole nafate injection with parenteral solutions and additives. Am. J. Hosp. Pharm., 39, 622 (1982).
59. Tsallas, G., et al.: Stability of cimetidine hydrochloride in parenteral nutrition solutions. Am. J. Hosp. Pharm., 39, 484 (1982).
60. Kowaluk, E.A., et al.: Interactions between drugs and intravenous delivery systems. Am. J. Hosp. Pharm., 39, 460 (1982).
61. Kirschenbaum, H.L., et al.: Stability and compatibility of lidocaine HCl with selected large volume parenterals and drug additives. Am. J. Hosp. Pharm., 39, 1013 (1982).
62. Souney, P.F., et al.: Effect of vitamin B complex and ascorbic acid on the antimicrobial activity of cefazolin sodium. Am. J. Hosp. Pharm., 39, 840 (1982).
63. Dean, K.W., et al.: Stability of trimethoprim-sulfamethoxazole injection in five infusion fluids. Am. J. Hosp. Pharm., 38, 1681 (1982).
64. Smith, F.M., et al.: Stability of diazepam injection repackaged in glass unit dose syringes. Am. J. Hosp. Pharm., 39, 1687 (1982).
65. Shank, W.A., et al.: Stability of digoxin in common large volume injections. Am. J. Hosp. Pharm., 39, 844 (1982).
66. Cutie, M.R., et al.: Compatibility of hydromorphone HCl in large volume parenterals. Am. J. Hosp. Pharm., 39, 307 (1982).
67. Kirschenbaum, H.L., et al.: Stability of dobutamine HCl in selected large volume parenterals. Am. J. Hosp. Pharm., 39, 1923 (1982).
68. Zatz, L., et al.: Stability of refrigerated aminophylline in 5% dextrose in water: A 96 hour study. Hosp. Pharm., 16, 548 (1982).
69. Niemiec, P.W., Jr., et al.: Stability of aminophylline injection in three parenteral nutrient solutions. Am. J. Hosp. Pharm., 40, 428 (1983).
70. Cutie, M.R.: Compatibility of verapamil HCl injection with commonly used additives. Am. J. Hosp. Pharm., 40, 1205 (1983).
71. Pyter, R.A., et al.: Stability of methylprednisolone sodium succinate in 5% dextrose and 0.9% sodium chloride injection. Am. J. Hosp. Pharm., 40, 1329 (1983).
72. Kirschenbaum, H.L., et al.: Compatibility and stability of dobutamine HCl with large volume parenterals and selected additives. Am. J. Hosp. Pharm., 40, 1690 (1983).
73. Yuen, P.C., et al.: Compatibility and stability of labetalol HCl in commonly used I.V. solutions. Am. J. Hosp. Pharm., 40, 1007 (1983).

74. Porter, W.R., et al.: Compatibility and stability of clindamycin phosphate with intravenous fluids. Am. J. Hosp. Pharm., *40*, 91 (1983).

75. Ray, J.B., et al.: Droperidol stability in intravenous admixtures. Am. J. Hosp. Pharm., *40*, 94 (1983).

76. Newton, D.W., et al.: Lorazepam solubility in and sorption from I.V. admixture solutions. Am. J. Hosp. Pharm., *40*, 424, (1983).

77. Perentesis, G.P., et al.: Stability and visual compatibility of bretylium tosylate with selected large volume parenterals and additives. Am. J. Hosp. Pharm., *40*, 1010 (1983).

78. Nahata, M.C.: Stability of ceftriaxone sodium in intravenous solutions. Am. J. Hosp. Pharm., *40*, 2193 (1983).

79. Cheung, Y.W., et al.: Stability of cytarabine, methotrexate sodium and hydrocortisone sodium succinate admixtures. Am. J. Hosp. Pharm., *41*, 1802 (1984).

80. DasGupta, V., et al.: Stability of dobutamine HCl and verapamil HCl in 0.9% sodium chloride and 5% dextrose injections. Am. J. Hosp. Pharm., *41*, 616 (1984).

81. Hasegawa, G.R., et al.: Visual compatibility of amiodarone injection with other injectable drugs. Am. J. Hosp. Pharm., *41*, 1379 (1984).

82. Quebbeman, E.J., et al.: Stability of fluorouracil in plastic containers used for continuous infusion at home. Am. J. Hosp. Pharm., *41*, 1153 (1984).

83. Boehm, J.J., et al.: Shelf life of unrefrigerated succinylcholine chloride injection. Am. J. Hosp. Pharm., *41*, 300 (1984).

84. Walker, S.E., et al.: Stability of ranitidine HCl in total parenteral nutrient solution. Am. J. Hosp. Pharm., *42*, 590 (1985).

85. Quock, J.R., et al.: Stability of cytarabine in a parenteral nutrient solution. Am. J. Hosp. Pharm., *42*, 592 (1985).

86. Macias, J.M., et al.: Stability of morphine sulfate and meperidine HCl in a parenteral nutrient formulation. Am. J. Hosp. Pharm., *42*, 1087 (1985).

87. James, M.J., et al.: Stability of I.V. mixtures of aztreonam and ampicillin. Am. J. Hosp. Pharm., *42*, 1095 (1985).

88. Thompson, D.F., et al.: Compatibility of furosemide with aminoglycoside admixtures. Am. J. Hosp. Pharm., *42*, 116 (1985).

89. Mansur, J.M., et al.: Stability and cost analysis of clindamycin-gentamicin admixtures given every eight hours. Am. J. Hosp. Pharm., *42*, 332, (1985).

90. Quebbeman, E.J., et al.: Stability of mitomycin admixtures. Am. J. Hosp. Pharm., *42*, 1750 (1985).

91. James, M.J., et al.: Stability in intravenous admixtures of aztreonam and clindamycin phosphate. Am. J. Hosp. Pharm., *42*, 1984 (1985).

92. Nahata, M.C., et al.: Stability of tobramycin sulfate in admixtures with calcium gluconate. Am. J. Hosp. Pharm., *42*, 1987 (1985).

93. Wong, W.W., et al.: Stability of cefonicid sodium in infusion fluids. Am. J. Hosp. Pharm., *42*, 1980 (1985).

94. Boss, J.A., et al.: Stability of clindamycin phosphate and ceftizoxime sodium, cefoxitin sodium, cefamandole nafate, or cefazolin sodium in two intravenous solutions. Am. J. Hosp. Pharm., *42*, 2211 (1985).

95. Baptista, R.J., et al.: Stability of cimetidine HCl in a total nutrient admixture. Am. J. Hosp. Pharm., *42*, 2208 (1985).

96. Dandurand, K.R., et al.: Stability of dopamine hydrochloride exposed to blue-light phototherapy. Am. J. Hosp. Pharm., *42*, 595 (1985).

97. Concannon, J., et al.: Stability of aqueous solutions of amoxicillin sodium in the frozen and liquid states. Am. J. Hosp. Pharm., *43*, 3027 (1986).

98. Venkataramanan, R., et al.: Leaching of diethylhexyl phthalate from polyvinyl chloride bags into intravenous cyclosporin solution. Am. J. Hosp. Pharm., *43*, 2800 (1986).

99. Beijnen, J.H., et al.: Stability of intravenous admixtures of doxorubicin and vincristine. Am. J. Hosp. Pharm., 1986; *43*, 3022 (1986).

100. Yliruusi, J.K., et al.: Effect of flow rate and type of I.V. containers on adsorption of diazepam to I.V. administration systems. Am. J. Hosp. Pharm., *43*, 2795 (1986).

101. Stennett, D.J., et al.: Stability of levodopa in 5% dextrose injection at pH 5 or 6 Am. J. Hosp. Pharm., *43*, 1728 (1986).

102. Mehta, J., et al.: Stability of terbutaline sulfate admixtures stored in polyvinyl chloride bags. Am. J. Hosp. Pharm., *43*, 1760 (1986).
103. Riley, C.M., et al.: Interaction of aztreonam and nafcillin in intravenous admixtures. Am. J. Hosp. Pharm., *43*, (1986).
104. Nahata, M.C., et al.: Stability of phenobarbital sodium diluted in 0.9% sodium chloride injection. Am. J. Hosp. Pharm., *43*, 384 (1986).
105. Marble, D.A.: Stability of clindamycin phosphate with aztreonam, ceftazidime sodium, ceftriaxone sodium or pipercillin sodium in two intravenous solutions. Am. J. Hosp. Pharm., *43*, 1732 (1986).
106. Kuhn, R.J.: Stability of netilmicin sulfate in admixtures with calcium gluconate and aminophylline. Am. J. Hosp. Pharm., *43*, 1241 (1986).
107. Ptachcinski, R.J., et al.: Stability and availability of cyclosporin in 5% dextrose injection of 0.9% sodium chloride injection. Am. J. Hosp. Pharm., *43*, 94 (1986).
108. Tu, Y., et al.: Stability of papaverine hydrochloride and phentolamine mesylate in injectable mixtures. Am. J. Hosp. Pharm., *44*, 2524 (1982).
109. Visor, G.C., et al.: Stability of ganciclovir sodium in 5% dextrose or 0.9% sodium chloride injections. Am. J. Hosp. Pharm., *43*, 2810 (1986).
110. DeAbu, N.C., et al.: Stability of pentamidine isethionate in 5% dextrose and 0.9% sodium chloride injections. Am. J. Hosp. Pharm., *43*, 1486 (1986).
111. Nahata, M.C., et al.: Stability of gentamicin diluted in 0.9% sodium chloride injection in glass syringes. Hosp. Pharm., *22*, 1131 (1987).
112. Johnson, C.E., et al.: Compatibility of premixed theophylline and methylprednisoline sodium succinate intravenous admixtures. Am. J. Hosp. Pharm., *44*, 1620 (1987).
113. Nahata, M.C., et al.: Stability of vancomycin hydrochloride in various concentrations of dextrose injection. Am. J. Hosp. Pharm., *44*, 802 (1987).
114. Perry, M., et al.: Stability of penicillins in total parenteral nutrient solution Am. J. Hosp. Pharm., *44*, 1625 (1987).
115. Fitzgerald, K.A., et al.: Calcium and phosphate stability in neonatal parenteral nutrient solutions containing aminosyn PF. Am. J. Hosp. Pharm., *44*, 1396 (1987).
116. Nelson, R.W., et al.: Visual incompatibility of dacarbazine and heparin. Am. J. Hosp. Pharm., *44*,, 2028 (1987).
117. Raymond, G.C., et al.: Stability of procainamide hydrochloride in neutralized 5% dextrose injection. Am. J. Hosp. Pharm., *45*, 2513 (1988).
118. Riley, C.M.: Stability of milirone and digoxin, furosemide, procainamide hydrochloride, propanolol hydrochloride, quinidine gluconate, or verapamil hydrochloride in 5% dextrose injection. Am. J. Hosp. Pharm., *45*, 2079 (1988).
119. Behme, R.J., et al.: Incompatibility of ifosfamide with benzyl-alcohol preserved bacteriostatic water for injection. Am. J. Hosp. Pharm., *45*, 627 (1988).
120. Johnson, C.E., et al.: Compatibility of premixed theophylline and verapamil intravenous admixtures. Am. J. Hosp. Pharm., *45*, 609 (1988).
121. Thompson, D.F., et al.: Compatibility of verapamil hydrochloride with penicillin admixtures during simulated Y-site injection. Am. J. Hosp. Pharm., *45*, 142 (1988).
122. Collucci, R.D., et al.: Visual compatibility of labetalol hydrochloride injection with various injectable drugs during simulated Y-site injection. Am. J. Hosp. Pharm., *45*, 1357 (1988).
123. Karnatz, N.N., et al.: Stability of esmolol hydrochloride and sodium nitroprusside in intravenous admixtures. Am. J. Hosp. Pharm., *46*, 2057 (1989).
124. Chilvers, M.R., et al.: Visual compatibility of ranitidine hydrochloride with commonly used critical-care medications. Am. J. Hosp. Pharm., *46*, 2057 (1989).
125. Schaaf, L.J., et al.: Stability of esmolol hydrochloride in the presence of aminophylline, bretylium tosylate, heparin sodium and procainamide hydrochloride. Am. J. Hosp. Pharm., *47*, 1567 (1990).
126. Koberda, M., et al.: Stability of bleomycin sulfate reconstituted in 5% dextrose injection or 0.9% sodium chloride injection stored in glass vials or polyvinyl chloride containers. Am. J. Hosp. Pharm., *47*, 2578 (1990).
127. Stewart, J.T., et al.: Stability of ranitidine in intravenous admixtures stored frozen, refrigerated and at room temperature. Am. J. Hosp. Pharm., *47*, 2043 (1990).

128. Floy, B.J., et al.: Compatibility of ketorolac tromethamine injection with common infusion fluids and administration sets. Am. J. Hosp. Pharm., *47*, 1097 (1990).
129. Stewart, C.F., et al.: Compatibility of cisplatin and fluoroucil in 0.9% sodium chloride injection. Am. J. Hosp. Pharm., *47*, 1373 (1990).
130. Williams, M.F., et al.: In vitro evaluation of the stability of ranitidine hydrochloride in total parenteral nutrient mixtures. Am. J. Hosp. Pharm., *47*, 1574 (1990).
131. Wilson, T.D., et al.: Stability of milrinone and epinephrine, atropine sulfate, lidocaine hydrochloride or morphine sulfate injection. Am. J. Hosp. Pharm., *47*, 2504 (1990).
132. Thompson, D.F., et al.: Visual compatibility of enalaprilat with selected intravenous medications during simulated Y-site injection. Am. J. Hosp. Pharm., *47*, 2530 (1990).
133. Tripp, M.G., et al.: Stability of total nutrient admixtures in a dual-chamber flexible container. Am. J. Hosp. Pharm., *47*, 2496 (1990).
134. Wiest, D.B., et al.: Stability of amphotericin B in four concentrations of dextrose injection. Am. J. Hosp. Pharm., *48*, 2430 (1991).
135. Nahata, M.C., et al.: Stability of cefazolin sodium in peritoneal dialysis solutions. Am. J. Hosp. Pharm., *48*, 291 (1991).
136. Lee, D.K.T., et al.: Compatibility of cefoperazone sodium and furosemide in 5% dextrose injection. Am. J. Hosp. Pharm., *48*, 108 (1991).
137. Pugh, C.B., et al.: Visual compatibility of morphine sulfate and meperidine hydrochloride with other injectable drug during Y-site injection. Am. J. Hosp. Pharm., *48*, 123 (1991).
138. Holmes, S.E., et al.: Stability of miconazole in peritoneal dialysis fluid. Am. J. Hosp. Pharm., *48*, 286 (1991).
139. Lee, D.K.T., et al.: Compatibility of cefoperazone sodium and cimetidine hydrochloride in 5% dextrose injection. Am. J. Hosp. Pharm., *48*, 111 (1991).
140. Wade, C.S., et al.: Stability of ceftazidime and amino acids in parenteral nutrient solutions. Am. J. Hosp. Pharm., *48*, 1515 (1991).
141. Hatton, J., et al.: Stability of nizatidine in total nutrient admixtures. Am. J. Hosp. Pharm., *48*, 1507 (1991).
142. Gora, M.L., et al.: Stability of dobutamine hydrochloride in peritoneal dialysis solutions. Am. J. Hosp. Pharm., *48*, 1234 (1991).
143. Strom, J.G., et al.: Stability and compatibility of methylprednisolone sodium succinate and cimetidine hydrochloride in 5% dextrose injection. Am. J. Hosp. Pharm., *48*, 1237 (1991).
144. Riley, C.M., et al.: Stability of amrinone and digoxin, procainamide hydrochloride, propranolol hydrochloride, sodium bicarbonate, potassium chloride, or verapamil hydrochloride in intravenous admixtures. Am. J. Hosp. Pharm., *48*, 1245 (1991).
145. Lor, E., et al.: Visual compatibility of fluoconazole with commonly used injectible drugs during simulated Y-site administration. Am. J. Hosp. Pharm., *48*, 744 (1991).
146. Kintzel, P.E., et al.: Stability of amphotericin B in 5% dextrose injection at concentrations used for administration through a central venous line. Am. J. Hosp. Pharm., *48*, 283 (1991).
147. Lam, N.P., et al.: Stability of zidovudine in 5% dextrose injection and 0.9% sodium chloride injection. Am. J. Hosp. Pharm., *48*, 280 (1991).
148. Goodwin, S.D., et al.: Compatibility of ciprofloxacin injection with selected drugs and solutions. Am. J. Hosp. Pharm., *48*, 2166 (1991).
149. Ritchie, D.J., et al.: Activity of octreotide acetate in a total nutrient admixture. Am. J. Hosp. Pharm., *48*, 2172 (1991).
150. Anderson, P.M., et al.: Biological activity of recombinant interleukin-2 in intravenous admixtures containing antibiotic, morphine sulfate or total parenteral nutrient solution. Am. J. Hosp. Pharm., *49*, 608 (1992).
151. I.V. Additives and Pharmacy Technology of Sterile Products-1. Washington, D.C., American Society of Hospital Pharmacists, 1975.

152. Trissel, L.A., et al.: Parenteral Drug Information Guide. Washington, D.C., American Society of Hospital Pharmacists, 1974.
153. Trissel, L.A.: Handbook on Injectable Drugs. Washington, D.C., American Society of Hospital Pharmacists, 1992, Seventh Ed.
154. King, J.C.: Guide to Parenteral Admixtures. Berkeley, California, Cutter Laboratories.
155. Kirschenbaum, B.E., and Latiolais, C.J.: Injectable Medication: A Guide to Stability and Reconstitution. New York, McMahon Publishing Company, 1991.
156. Product brochure. Syracuse, N.Y., Bristol Laboratories.
157. Product brochure. Philadelphia, Pa., Wyeth Laboratories.
158. Savello, D., and Shangraw, R.: Stability of sodium ampicillin solutions in the frozen and liquid states. Am. J. Hosp. Pharm., 28, 754 (1971).
159. Shoup, L.K., and Thur, M.P.: The stability of frozen buffered penicillin G potassium injection. Hosp. Form. Mgt., 3, 38 (1968).
160. Boylan, J.C., Simmons, J.L., and Winely, C.L.: Stability of frozen solutions of sodium cephalothin and cephaloridine. Am. J. Hosp. Pharm., 29, 687 (1972).
161. Stolar, M.H., et al.: Effect of freezing on the stability of sodium methicillin injection. Am. J. Hosp. Pharm., 25, 32 (1968).
162. Carone, S.M., et al.: Stability of freezing solutions of cefazolin sodium. Am. J. Hosp. Pharm., 33, 639 (1976).
163. Parodi, J.F.: Stability of frozen antibiotic solutions in Viaflex infusion containers. Hosp. Pharm., 11, 178 (1976).
164. Granatek, A., and Kaplan, M.: Stability of frozen solutions of cephapirin sodium. Curr. Ther. Res., 16, 573 (1974).
165. Knecht, P.S., Eickholt, T.H., and Talley, J.R.: Activity of frozen solutions of cefazolin sodium packaged in glass and plastic disposable syringes. New Orleans, 33rd Annual Meeting American Society of Hospital Pharmacists, April 7, 1976.
166. Dinel, B.A., et al.: Comparative stability of antibiotic admixtures in minibags and minibottles. Drug. Intell. Clin. Pharm., 11, 226 (1977).
167. Dinel, B.A., et al.: Stability of antibiotic admixtures frozen in minibags. Drug Intell.Clin.Pharm., 11, 542 (1977).
168. Jurgens, R.W., et al.: Compatibility of amphotericin B with certain large volume parenterals. Am. J. Hosp. Pharm., 38, 377 (1981).
169. Moorhatch, P., et al.: Interactions between drugs and plastic I.V. fluid bags. Am. J. Hosp. Pharm., 31, 72 (1974).
170. Nation, R.L., et al.: Uptake of clonazepam by plastic I.V. infusion bags and administration sets. Am. J. Hosp. Pharm., 40, 1692 (1983).
171. Parker, W.A., et al.: Incompatibility of diazepam injection in plastic I.V. bags. Am. J. Hosp. Pharm., 36, 505 (1979).
172. Gardella, L.A., et al.: Intropin I.V. admixture compatibility: Part 1: Stability with common I.V. fluids. Am. J. Hosp. Pharm., 32, 575 (1975).
173. Mitchell, J.F., et al.: Heparin stability in 5% dextrose and 0.9% sodium chloride solution. Am. J. Hosp. Pharm., 33, 540 (1976).
174. Hirsch, J.I., et al.: Insulin adsorption to polyolefin infusion bottles and polyvinylchloride administration sets. Am. J. Hosp. Pharm., 38, 995 (1981).
175. Leach, J.K., et al.: Biological activity of dilute isoproterenol solution stored for long periods in plastic bags. Am. J. Hosp. Pharm., 34, 709 (1977).
176. Bergstrom, R.F., et al.: Stability of parenteral solutions of tobramycin sulfate. Am. J. Hosp. Pharm., 32, 887 (1975).
177. Chiou, W.L., et al.: Interaction between vitamin A and plastic I.V. fluid bags. JAMA, 223, 23 (1973).
178. Nedich, R.L.: Vitamin A absorption from plastic I.V. bags. JAMA, 224, 1531 (1973).
179. Tomecko, G.W., et al.: Stability of cefazolin sodium admixtures in plastic bags after thawing by microwave radiation. Hosp. Pharm., 37, 211 (1980).
180. Holmes, C.J., et al.: Activity of antibiotic admixtures subjected to different freeze-thaw treatments. Drug Intell. Clin. Pharm., 114, 353 (1980).
181. Smith, Kline & French, Letter on file, Nov. 25, 1983.

182. Eli Lilly Laboratories, Letter on file, Oct. 20, 1983.
183. Elliott, G.T., et al.: Stability of cimetidine hydrochloride in admixtures after microwave thawing. Am. J. Hosp. Pharm., *40*, 1002 (1983).
184. Hoechst-Roussel, personal communication.
185. Lederle Laboratories, Letter on file, Oct. 31, 1983.
186. Merck, Sharpe & Dohme, Letter on file, Oct. 28, 1983.
187. Holmes, C.J., et al.: Effect of freezing and microwave thawing on the stability of six antibiotic admixtures in plastic bags. Am. J. Hosp. Pharm., *39*, 104 (1982).
188. Ausman, R.K., et al.: Frozen storage and microwave thawing of parenteral nutrition solutions in plastic containers. Drug. Intell. Clin. Pharm., *15*, 440 (1981).
189. Cottrell, J.E., et al.: Intravenous nitroglycerin. Am. Heart J., *96*, 550 (1978).
190. Hill, N.S., et al.: Intravenous nitroglycerin. Chest, *79*, 69 (1981).
191. Derrida, J.P., et al.: Nitroglycerin infusion in acute myocardial infarction. N. Engl. J. Med., *297*, 336 (1977).
192. Baase, D.M., et al.: Nitroglycerin compatibility with intravenous fluid filters, containers and administration sets. Am. J. Hosp. Pharm., *37*, 201 (1980).
193. ECRI: Hazard: Nitroglycerin overinfusion with infusion devices through Tridil I.V. administration sets. Health Devices, *11*, 42 (1981).
194. ECRI: Nitroglycerin overinfusion hazard extended to Nitrostat I.V. administration sets. Health Devices, *11*, 71 (1981).
195. Signal. Newsletter, Am. Soc. Hosp. Pharm., Jan.–Feb., 1981.
196. Rock, M., et al.: Reducing I.V. nitroglycerin loss to an intravenous administration set by preliminary preparation. Am. J. I.V. Therapy Clin. Nutr., *9*, 37 (1982).
197. Raymond, G.G., et al.: Administration set purging for dosage adjustment in I.V. nitroglycerin therapy. NITA, *6*, 415 (1983).
198. Jacobi, J., et al.: Loss of nitroglycerin to pulmonary artery delivery systems. Am. J. Hosp. Pharm., *40*, 1980 (1983).
199. Tracy, T.S., et al.: Nitroglycerin delivery through a polyethylene-lined intravenous administration set. Am. J. Hosp. Pharm., *46*, 2031 (1989).
200. Hill, J.B.: Adsorption of insulin to glass. Proc. Pediatr. Soc., *102*, 75 (1959).
201. Wiseman, R., et al.: Prevention of insulin I adsorption to glass. Endocrinology, *68*, 354 (1961).
202. Hill, J.B.: The adsorption of I insulin to glass. Endocrinology, *65*, 515 (1959).
203. Weisenfeld, S., et al.: Adsorption of insulin to infusion bottles and tubing. Diabetes, *17*, 766 (1968).
204. Eli Lilly Laboratories to S. Turco. Letter on file, Temple University.
205. Petty, C., et al.: Insulin adsorption by glass infusion bottle, polyvinylchloride infusion containers and intravenous tubing. Anesthesiology, *40*, 400 (1974).
206. Weber, S.S., et al.: Insulin adsorption controversy. Drug Intell. Clin. Pharm., *10*, 232 (1976).
207. Peterson, L., et al.: Insulin adsorption on polyvinylchloride surfaces with implications for constant infusion therapy. Diabetes, *25*, 72 (1976).
208. Weber, S.S.: Availability of insulin from parenteral nutrient solutions. Am. J. Hosp. Pharm. *34*, 353 (1977).
209. Hirsch, J.I., et al.: Clinical significance of insulin adsorption by polyvinylchloride infusion systems. Am. J. Hosp. Pharm., *34*, 583 (1977).
210. Whalen, F.J., et al.: Availability of insulin from continuous low-dose insulin infusion. Am. J. Hosp. Pharm., *36*, 330 (1979).
211. Twardowski, Z.J., et al.: Insulin binding to plastic bags. Am. J. Hosp. Pharm., *40*, 575 (1983).
212. Twardowski, Z.J., et al.: Nature of insulin binding to plastic bags. Am. J. Hosp. Pharm., *40*, 579 (1983).
213. Kane, M., et al.: Binding of insulin to a continuous ambulatory peritoneal dialysis system. Am. J. Hosp. Pharm., *93*, 81 (1986).
214. Furberg, H., et al.: Effect of pretreatment with 0.9% sodium chloride or insulin solution or the delivery of insulin from an infusion system. Am. J. Hosp. Pharm., *43*, 2209 1986.
215. Talbot, E.M.: Dangers of adding insulin to intravenous infusion bags with fixed needle syringes. Br. Med. J., *289*, 678 (1984).

216. Dozier, N., et al.: Practical considerations in the preparation and administration of cancer chemotherapy. Am. J. I.V. Ther. Clin. Nutr., 9, 6 (1983).
217. LeRoy, M.L. et al.: Procedures for handling antineoplastic injections in comprehensive cancer centers. Am. J. Hosp. Pharm., 40, 601 (1983).
218. Provost, G.J.: Legal issues associated with the handling of cytotoxic drugs. Am. J. Hosp. Pharm., 41, 1115 (1984).
219. Stolar, M.H., et al.: Recommendations for handling cytotoxic drugs in hospitals. Am. J. Hosp. Pharm., 40, 1163 (1983).
220. Selevan S.G., et al.: A study of occupational exposure to antineoplastic drugs and fetal loss in nurses. N. Engl. J. Med. 313, 1178 (1985).
221. Falck, K., et al.: Mutagenicity in urine of nurses handling cytostatic drug. Lancet, 1, 1250 (1979).
222. Davis, M.R.: Guidelines for safe handling of cytotoxic drug in pharmacy departments of hospital wards. Hosp. Pharm., 16, 17 (1981).
223. ASHP technical assistance bulletin on handling cytotoxic drugs in hospitals. Am. J. Hosp. Pharm. 42, 131 (1985).
224. OSHA Work-practice guidelines for personnel dealing with cytotoxic (antineoplastic) drugs. Am. J. Hosp. Pharm. 43, 1193 (1986).
225. Gregoire, R.E., et al.: Handling antineoplastic drug admixtures at cancer centers: Practices and pharmacist attitudes. Am. J. Hosp. Pharm. 44, 1090 (1987).
226. Crudi, C.B.: A compounding dilemma. I've kept the drug sterile but have I contaminated myself. NITA, 3, 77 (1980).
227. Ladik, C.F., et al.: Precautionary measures in the preparation of antineoplastics. Am. J. Hosp., Pharm., 37, 1184 (1980).
228. Hoffman, D.M.: The handling of antineoplastic drugs in a major cancer center. Hosp. Pharm., 15, 302 (1980).
229. Tortorici, M.P.: Precautions followed by personnel involved with the preparation of parenteral antineoplastic medications. Hosp. Pharm., 15, 293 (1980).
230. Anderson, R.W., et al.: Risk of handling injectable antineoplastic agents. Am. J. Hosp. Pharm., 39, 1881 (1982).
231. Crudi, C.B., et al.: Possible occupational hazards associated with the preparation and administration of antineoplastic agents. NITA, 5, 264 (1982).
232. Zimmerman, P.F., et al.: Recommendations for the safe handling of injectable antineoplastic drug products. Am. J. Hosp. Pharm., 38, 1963 (1981).
233. Specialty Practice Committee on Parenteral Services: Guidelines For Safe Handling of Cytotoxic Drugs in Pharmacy Departments and Hospital Wards. Society of Hospital Pharmacists of Australia.
234. Stolar, M.H., et al.: Recommendations for handling cytotoxic drugs in hospitals. Am. J. Hosp. Pharm., 40, 1163 (1983).
235. Dozier, N., and Ballentine, R.: Practical considerations in the preparation and administration of cancer chemotherapy. Am. J. I.V. Ther. Clin. Nutr., 10, 6 (1983).
236. Hoffman, D.M.: Lack of urine mutagenicity of nurses administering pharmacy prepared doses of antineoplastic agents. Am. J. I.V. Ther. Clin. Nutr., 10, 28 (1983).
237. LeRoy, M.L., et al.: Procedures for handling antineoplastic injections in comprehensive cancer centers. Am. J. Hosp. Pharm., 40, 601, (1983).
238. Hennessy, K., et al.: Chemotherapy waste disposal: A safe and practical method. NITA, 5, 311 (1982).
239. Valanis, B., et al.: Use of protection by nurses during occupational handling of antineoplastic drugs. NITA, 8, 218 (1985).
240. American Society of Hospital Pharmacists: Technical assistance bulletin on handling cytotoxic drugs in hospitals. Am. J. Hosp. Pharm., 42, 131 (1985).
241. Council for Scientific Affairs: Guidelines for handling parenteral antineoplastics. JAMA, 253, 1590 (1985).
242. Stolar, M.H.: National survey of selected hospital pharmacy practices. Am. J. Hosp. Pharm., 33, 225 (1976).
243. Second Supplement to 1976 Edition of the Accreditation Manual for Hospitals, August, 1977.

244. NCC-LVP: Recommendations to pharmacists for solving problems with large-volume parenterals. Am. J. Hosp. Pharm., *33*, 231 (1976).

245. Mitchell, J.B.: Legal aspects of the I.V. admixture program. Apothecary, *7*, 13 (1975).

246. Burke, A.W.: Justifying an I.V. admixture program. I.V. additive review. Drug Intell. Clin. Pharm., *6*, 111 (1972).

247. Anderson, R.D.: A case for the I.V. admixture service—reducing patient risk. I.V. Top., *1*, 4 (1976).

248. Schmidt, S.: Procedure Guide for the Pharmacy Service. I.V. Additive Program. Department of Pharmacy, Kansas City College Osteopathic Medicine, 1974.

249. Garrison, T.: Planning an I.V. Admixture program. Pharmacy Services, Kansas City, MO.

250. Pang, F.: A Transition to Centralized I.V. Additive Service in a Private Hospital. Porter Memorial Hospital, Denver, CO.

251. Sherrin, R.P.: Sample Policies and Procedures for an I.V. Admixture Service. Riverside Methodist Hospital, Columbus, OH.

252. Shoup, L.K., and Godwin, N.H.: Implementation Guide—Centralized I.V. Admixture Program. Travenol Laboratories, 1977.

253. Hunt, M.L.: I.V. admixture training program for pharmacy personnel. Am. J. Hosp. Pharm., *31*, 467 (1974).

254. Hinshaw, W.R., and Wilken, L.O.: Training personnel for I.V. admixture programs. Am. J. Hosp. Pharm., *29*, 1025 (1972).

255. Muraida, R.M.: Pharmacy-nursing communications in an I.V. admixture program. Am. J. Hosp. Pharm., *32*, 889 (1975).

256. Lausier, M.: Computerized hospital information systems for an I.V. admixture service. Am. J. Hosp. Pharm., *34*, 976 (1977).

257. Souder, D.E., et al.: A computer-associated I.V. admixture system. Am. J. Hosp. Pharm., *30*, 1015 (1973).

258. Bergman, H.D.: Incompatibilities in large volume parenterals. Drug Intell. Clin. Pharm., *11*, 345 (1977).

259. NCC-LVP: Recommended methods for compounding I.V. admixtures in hospitals. Am. J. Hosp. Pharm., *32*, 261 (1975).

260. Steele, R.G., et al.: Rapid reconstitution and storage of certain I.V. antibiotics. Am. J. Hosp. Pharm., *30*, 1021 (1973).

261. Upton, J.H., Crouch, J.B., and Williams, H.M.: Mass reconstitution of neutral cephalothin sodium using tandem sequence filling. Am. J. Hosp. Pharm., *32*, 579 (1975).

262. Gouveia, W.A., Sceppa, J.M., and Janousek, J.P.: Experience with a 20-gm. Pharmacy Bulk Package of Keflin Neutral. Indianapolis, Indiana, Eli Lilly, 1974.

263. Hernandez, A.P., and Vanderveen, T.W.: Procedures for Reconstitution of Keflin Neutral. Indianapolis, Indiana, Eli Lilly, 1975.

264. Mueller, W.J.: Use of 20-gm. Ampoules of Keflin Neutral. Indianapolis, Indiana, Eli Lilly, 1975.

265. Van Der Linde, L.P., Campbell, R.K., and Jackson, E.: Guidelines for I.V. administration of drugs. Drug Intell. Clin. Pharm., *11*, 30 (1977).

266. Rapp, R.P., Grant, K., and Piecoro, J.J.: Guidelines for the administration of commonly used I.V. drugs. Drug Intell. Clin. Pharm., *10*, 206 (1976).

267. GIVP Manual. North Chicago, IL, Abbott Laboratories, 1979.

268. Food and Drug Administration, Rockville, MD: FDA Alert Letter, Nov. 29, 1990.

269. Crawford, S.Y., et al.: National Survey of Quality Assurance Activities for Pharmacy Prepared Sterile Products in Hospitals. Am. J. Hosp. Pharm., *48*, 2398 (1991).

270. Draft Guidelines on Quality Assurance for Pharmacy-Prepared Sterile Products. Am. J. Hosp. Pharm., *49*, 407 (1992).

271. The United States Pharmacopeia, 22nd rev. United States Pharmacopeia Convention, 1989, Rockville, MD.

272. Akers, M.J., et al.: Sterility testing of antimicrobial-containing injectable solutions prepared in the pharmacy. Am. J. Hosp. Pharm., *48*, 2414 (1991).

273. Murray, P.R., et al.: Sterility testing of a total nutrient admixture with a biphasic blood culture system. Am. J. Hosp. Pharm., 48, 2419 (1991).
274. Choy, F.N., et al.: Sterility-testing program for antibiotics and other intravenous admixtures. Am. J. Hosp. Pharm., 38, 453 (1982).
275. Condella, F., et al.: Evaluation of two sterility testing methods for intravenous admixtures. Hosp. Pharm. 15, 305 (1980).
276. Brier, K.L.: Evaluating aseptic techniques of pharmacy personnel. Am. J. Hosp. Pharm., 40, 400 (1983).
277. Morris, B.G., et al.: Quality-control plan for intravenous admixture programs. II: Validation of operator techniques. Am. J. Hosp. Pharm., 37, 668 (1980).
278. Dirks, I., et al.: Method for testing aseptic technique of intravenous admixture personnel. Am. J. Hosp. Pharm. 39, 457 (1982).

12

CHAPTER

Convenience Parenterals

Parenteral products are packaged in ampuls, vials, bottles, plastic bags, and disposable syringes (Figs. 12–1, 12–2, and 12–3). Although of long-continued use, the glass ampul has few advantages other than that of a unit package and therefore is designed for one-time use.

Ampuls

Injections packaged in ampuls are not required to contain an antimicrobial preservative; however, they frequently do, because the manufacturer sometimes uses the same product formula for the injection packaged in ampuls as is used for multiple-dose vials,* in which an antimicrobial preservative is required. In contrast to vials, ampuls do not provide dosage flexibility; sometimes a large number of ampuls must be opened to obtain the desired dose.

A great disadvantage of the glass ampuls is the contamination of the injection by glass particles when the container is opened.[1] In addition, the ampul is inconvenient to the user because the contents must be transferred to a syringe prior to administration. Originally, ampuls were opened by scoring the neck at the point of constriction with an ampul file to break off the top (Fig. 12–4). In larger ampuls in which the neck is not constricted, greater difficulty is encountered. The opening has been made easier by prescoring (T.C. Wheaton Co.) or inscribing the ampul neck with a circle of ceramic paint (Color-Break, Kimble). Baked onto the glass, the paint weakens the glass at the line of application and becomes the fracture point when pressure is applied to the sealed stem. Glass contamination of the solution still occurs, but ampul opening is easier.

---

*Injections for intracisternal, intraspinal, peridural, and large-volume injections are packaged for single use without preservatives.

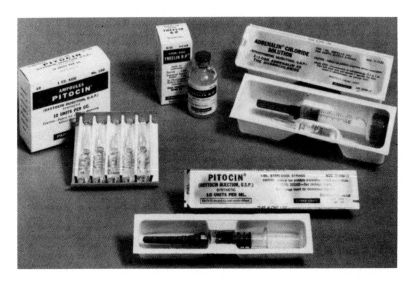

Figure 12–1. Parenteral packaging showing the ampul, vial, and disposable syringe. (Courtesy of Parke, Davis & Co., Detroit, MI.)

Vials

The availability of multiple-dose vials sealed with rubber closures permitted flexibility of dosage and reduced the unit cost per dose (Fig. 12–5). Several problems became apparent, however: increased possibility of microbial contamination with repeated withdrawals, coring and increased particulate contamination, possible error in dosage calculation, time required to withdraw the desired volume, and increased waste. These disadvantages tend to increase the ultimate patient cost per dose.

As discussed in Chapter 4, the use of rubber closures introduced the problem of coring, provided a source for particulate contamination, and afforded a packaging component capable of reacting with the solution and its additives to create physical and chemical difficulties. Several entries into a multiple-dose vial challenge the preservative system and increase the possibility of contaminating the containers. The likelihood of contaminating multiple-dose containers when the same syringe is used to enter two or more different products is apparent. The combination of two or more injections in the same syringe for a single administration is justified in some cases, as for preoperative medication, but the practice should be discouraged unless the compatibility of the agents is known.

To avoid some of the disadvantages of the ampul and multi-dose vial, single-dose vials have been used (Fig. 12–6). They eliminate the hazard of glass fragments and the disadvantages of multiple punctures and withdrawals.

In an effort to reduce manipulation and increase convenience, several manufacturers have produced some injections in vial containers designed for introducing their contents directly into intravenous fluid bottles. The closures of these containers are provided with rubber-covered plastic spikes that can be inserted directly into the intravenous bottle-stopper after removal of the

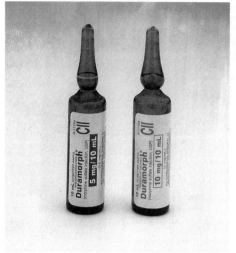

A

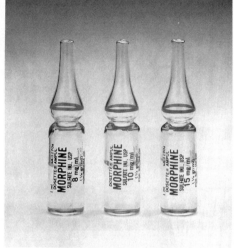

B

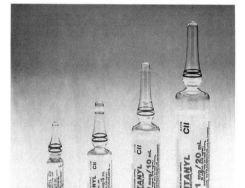

C

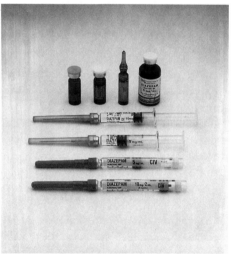

D

Figure 12–2. A–C, Dosette ampul vials. D, Ampuls and prefilled syringes. (Courtesy of Elkins-Sinn, Inc., Cherry Hill, NJ.)

spike's protective covering. The use of these convenience containers has been discussed in Chapter 8.

Double-chambered vials can be used to package a sterile powder with its vehicle. Known as the Mix-O-Vial (Upjohn), the bottom compartment of the container holds the sterile powder and is separated from the upper compartment holding the diluent by a rubber plug located at the constriction of the container (Fig. 12–7). The rubber closure sealing the container is twisted and pressure is applied to the top. The pressure on the solution in the upper compartment dislocates the plug and the diluent or vehicle flows into the

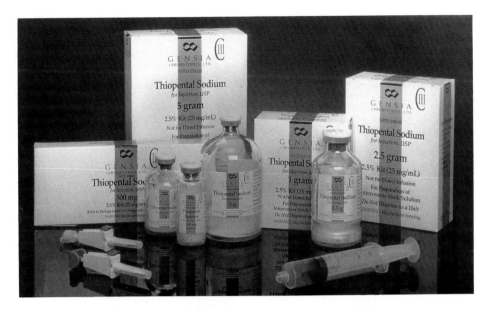

Figure 12–3. Assortment of small-volume parenterals (SVPs). (Courtesy of Gensia Laboratories Limited, Irvine, CA).

lower compartment, dissolving the sterile solid. When solution is complete, the contents may be removed in the usual manner with sterile syringe and needle (it is not necessary to inject air) or transferred by a transfer needle into an intravenous fluid. In the latter instance, the contents of the Mix-O-Vial are evacuated by the vacuum in the intravenous bottle. The container offers a convenient way to package a diluent with a drug that does not have sufficient stability in aqueous solution to be packaged as an injection, such as Solu-Cortef (Upjohn). It has also provided a means by which incompatible drugs are separated until time of administration. Eli Lilly and Company introduced the Redi Vial for the preparation of Kefzol for administration (Fig. 12–7B). In Bejectal (Abbott), the B complex and C vitamins are lyophilized as a sterile powder in the lower compartment and vitamin B_{12} is placed in the vehicle. The decomposition products of the former promote the decomposition of the latter even when combined in the dry state.

Prefilled Disposable Syringes

During World War II, the need for parenteral packaging that could be used immediately under emergency conditions became apparent. One approach led to the development of the Syrette. This unit consisted of a sealed flexible metal tube, not unlike an ophthalmic ointment tube, with the top designed to hold a needle. The sterility of the needle was protected by a glass sleeve that screwed onto the top of the tube holding the needle. Within the needle was a wire probe to be used to puncture the seal between the tube and the needle. For use, the glass sleeve was removed, the seal was punctured with the wire probe, the needle was inserted into the selected muscle, and the injection was expelled by applying pressure on the flexible metal tube. The

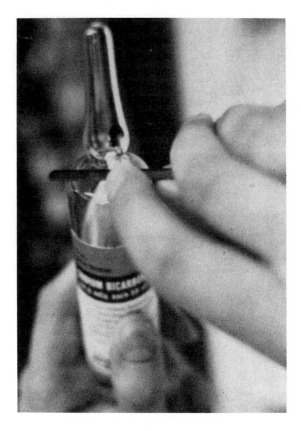

Figure 12–4. Opening large-volume ampul by scoring with ampul file.

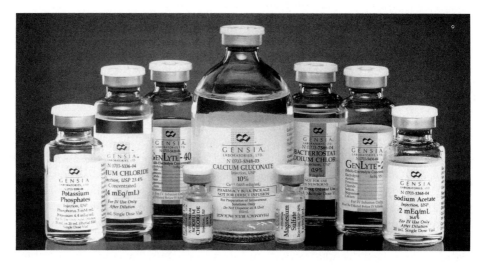

Figure 12–5. Small-volume parenteral vials. (Courtesy of Gensia Laboratories Limited, Irvine, CA.)

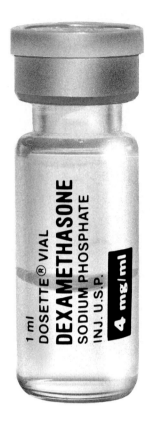

Figure 12–6.   Single-dose vial. (Courtesy of Elkins-Sinn, Inc., Cherry Hill, NJ.)

unit was developed for use with Morphine Sulfate Injection, but problems arising from sterility, injection-package compatibility, and leakage hindered its wider application.

Another early attempt at a convenient unit dose was the Ampin. This unit consisted of a glass ampul with its stem inserted in a piece of gum-rubber tubing holding a needle encased in a glass sleeve. To administer, the glass sleeve was removed and the needle was inserted into a muscle. The tip of the ampul in the tubing was broken, and the injection was allowed to flow into the tissues. The problems encountered led to abandonment of the Ampin.

It was also during this period that the Tubex (Wyeth)[2] system was originated. In the Tubex system, the injection is filled into a glass cartridge with needle attached and administered with a reusable stainless steel holder (Fig. 12–8). This was the first of many disposable systems using the prefilled cartridge or syringe. The syringe design has a 2-ml volume limitation. Prefilled syringe systems have proliferated as the result of their many advantages and an increased interest in unit-dose medication. The systems differ from the Tubex in two basic characteristics: the needle is not in contact with the medication prior to activation or use, and the cartridges are packaged as part of a disposable plastic holder ready for use.

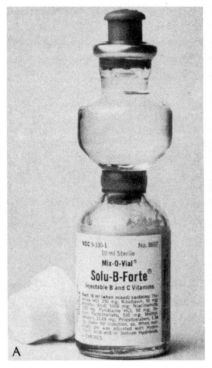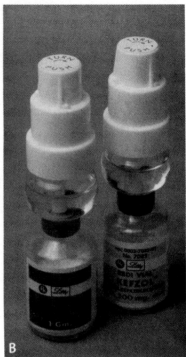

Figure 12–7. A, Double-chambered vial used to package sterile powder and vehicle separately. (Courtesy of Upjohn Company, Kalamazoo, MI.) B, Dual-compartment Redi Vial. (Courtesy of Eli Lilly and Co., Indianapolis, IN.)

Sterile prefilled disposable syringes are increasingly popular (Fig. 12–9). This form of convenience packaging offers several advantages: ease of administration, reduction of medication errors, and increased assurance of sterility. Good control of drugs, especially narcotics, can be achieved with these devices. The adequate labeling found on prefilled syringes saves nurses' time.

Several styles of prefilled disposable syringes are available. In most instances, the injection is packaged in a glass cartridge with the needle attached and is administered with a plastic or metal holder that may or may not be part of the original package (Fig. 12–9). The various syringes are listed in Table 12–1.

Prefilling Syringes

Many hospital pharmacists and medical practitioners prefer drugs packaged in prefilled syringes; however, some products have not been made available by the industry in this form. For these products, the hospital pharmacist must prefill syringes for use in the hospital. Components and equipment for prefilling syringes are available from several sources (Table 12–2). The procedure followed varies depending upon the source of the components.

Subdividing an injection packaged in an ampul or multiple-dose vial into individual syringes requires the same care and aseptic technique required in handling any other sterile product. The subdivision is preferably done in a

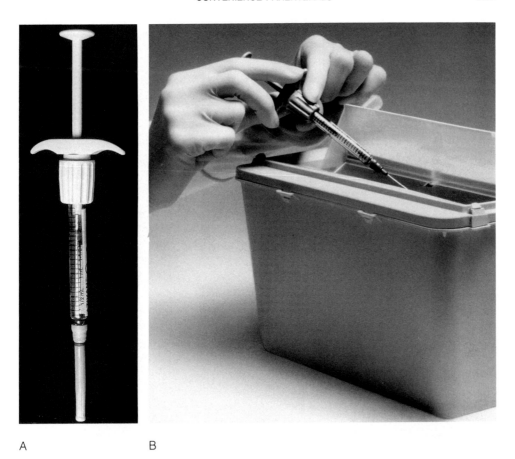

A   B

Figure 12–8. A, Tubex closed-injection system of prefilled cartridge. B, Disposal of used needles. (Courtesy of Wyeth-Ayerst Laboratories, Philadelphia, PA.)

laminar air-flow hood by trained personnel. To evaluate technique, the procedure can be followed using sterile trypticase soy broth as the product and incubating the filled syringes to demonstrate to personnel any instance of contamination.

After selecting a syringe system to be used and training the personnel to do the work, thought must be given to control—especially with respect to stability, sterility, and labeling. Removing an injection from its original container and subdividing it into disposable syringes create a new set of storage conditions for the injection. Both the volume of solution and the packaging materials to which it is exposed are now different. For these reasons, it cannot be assumed that an injection showing good stability in the original package will continue to exhibit good stability after subdivision. Therefore, it is prudent to place short expiration dates on prefilled syringes, usually 30 to 90 days. If stability data subsequently become available, the expiration date can be extended on future batches.

In removing a sterile solution from its original container and placing it into disposable syringes, the aseptic technique used in the procedure is the only assurance that sterility has been maintained. A sterility test on a number of

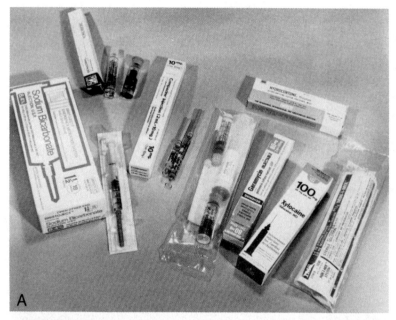

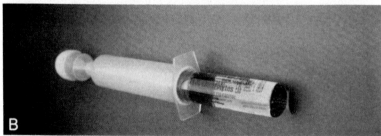

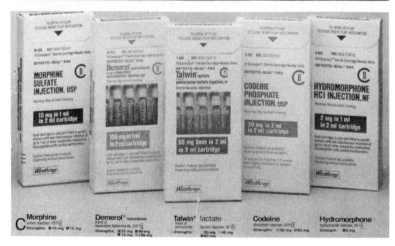

Figure 12–9. A, Various prefilled syringes. (Courtesy of Abbott Laboratories, North Chicago, IL.) B, Prefilled syringe. (Courtesy of Abbott Laboratories, North Chicago, IL.) C, Prefilled Capuject. (Courtesy of Winthrop Laboratories, New York, NY.) D, Capuject holder. (Courtesy of Winthrop Laboratories, New York, NY.) E, Heparin flush kit (Courtesy of Wyeth-Ayerst Laboratories, Philadelphia, PA.) F, Astra prefilled syringes. (Courtesy of Astra Pharmaceutical Products, Inc., Westborough, MA.)

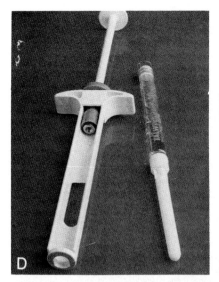

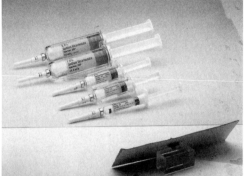

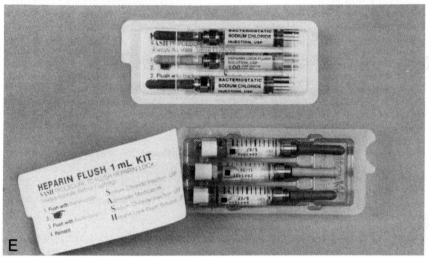

Figure 12–9. (*Continued*).

syringes selected at random from the batch will not necessarily assure that all the syringes in the batch are sterile. Therefore, the importance of aseptic technique in this procedure cannot be overemphasized. The consequences from a contaminated unit obtained in subdividing can be minimized by the immediate use of the unit. Prolonged storage of a contaminated unit may establish an incubation period that can be disastrous.

Hoar[3] described methods of extemporaneous syringe filling and studied the available methods and degree of contamination. McDonald et al.[4] and Stach[5] reported on various methods of prefilling syringes in the hospital pharmacy. Mantsch et al.[6] described a semi-automatic method using the FluiDose II for unit of use syringes. This study also compared the commonly available methods. A delivery system introduced by MPL offers syringes and syringe filling

Table 12-1. Prefilled Disposable Syringe Units

Manufacturer	System
Abbott Laboratories	Abboject*
American Critical Care	Rap-Add
LyphoMed	Bristoject
Eli Lilly & Co.	Hyporet[†]
E.R. Squibb & Sons	Unimatic[‡]
International Medication Systems (IMS)	Min-I-Jet, Flex-O-Jet, Add-A-Jet, Air-Way-Jet
Lederle Laboratories	Lederject
McNeil Pharmaceutical	(no trade name)
Merck Sharp & Dohme	(no trade name)
Merrell	M-N-L-Ject
Organon, Inc.	Redijects
Parke, Davis & Co.	Steri-Dose[†]
Pfizer Laboratories	Isoject[‡]
Roche Laboratories	Tel-E-Ject[†]
The Upjohn Co.	U-Ject[§]
Adria Laboratories	Stat-Pak[§]
Winthrop Laboratories	Carpuject[‖]
Wyeth Laboratories	Tubex[‖]

*The Abboject is a glass syringe with plastic component parts.
[†]The Hyporet, Tel-E-Ject, and Steri-Dose are completely assembled units. To use, the rubber needle sheath is removed and the injection is made.
[‡]The Isoject and Unimatic syringes also require activation prior to use. After activation the needle sheath covering is removed and used as the plunger.
[§]The U-Ject is an assembled unit that requires activation prior to use. Pressure applied on the plastic needle sheath pushes the needle through a rubber closure into the solution.
[‖]The Tubex and Carpuject systems are glass cartridges containing 1 or 2 ml of medication. The needle is attached to the cartridge and is covered by a rubber needle sheath. They must be placed in a holder for injection.

of hypodermic syringes (HyPod), nebulizer syringes (Nebuject), and oral pediatric syringes (Ped-Pod).

Few data exist for the justification of long-term storage of drugs in plastic syringes. Few studies have been done because of the various methods used to fill, package, and store syringes in addition to the variety of different plastic syringes manufactured and used. Variances in assay methods[7,8] have produced conflicting data on studies of the same drug. These difficulties make it ap-

Table 12-2. Methods for Prefilling Syringes

Becton-Dickinson method
Owens-Illinois method
Wyeth Tubex breech-fill method
Wyeth Tubex needle-fill method
Calibrated Cornwall syringe method
3-Way stop-disposable syringe method
Flui Dose II method (Mono-Med. Inc.)
MPL Solo Pak method (MPL-Solo Pak Div.)

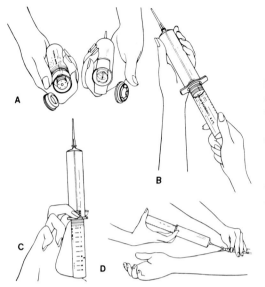

Figure 12–10. Abboject disposable syringe. A, Plastic caps are flipped from vial and injector. B, Vial is threaded into injector. The needle has penetrated the vial stopper and is in contact with the solution. C, Air has expelled. D, Medication is administered into injection site of intravenous fluid set. (Courtesy of Abbott Laboratories, North Chicago, IL.)

parent that those wishing to store drugs, particularly in plastic syringes, should back up storage times with individual stability studies.

Labelled prefilled disposable syringes have added a new dimension to parenteral therapy. They have increased safety and convenience while decreasing the work of personnel. They have helped in the accountability of drugs and aided in the implementation of new improved drug distribution systems. The lack of uniformity among the various systems is considered a disadvantage because it creates confusion for the user and makes it necessary to give in-service training for the use of these systems.

Packaging and Handling of CPR Drugs

The importance of packaging for parenteral drugs is amply demonstrated in the parenteral drugs used for cardiopulmonary resuscitation.

Drugs used in cardiopulmonary resuscitation (CPR) are supplied in ampuls, vials, pour bottles, and prefilled disposable syringes, but the prefilled disposable syringes are particularly useful when time and accuracy are of the utmost importance. Prefilled CPR syringes offer efficiency and speed in handling, proper labeling, and maintenance of sterility. Drugs may be ordered by milliliter, milligram, or ampul. Wherever possible, at least initial doses should be available in prefilled disposable syringes (PDS) as CPR drug stock on carts or in kits.

The systems known as Min-I-Jet and Add-A-Jet (International Medication Systems [IMS]), Bristoject (LyphoMed), and Abboject (Abbott Laboratories) contain a sterile prefilled glass vial of medication that fits into a plastic vial injector with a long, stainless steel needle shaft that punctures the rubber closure on the glass vial (Fig. 12–10). Emergency drugs such as sodium bicarbonate, epinephrine, calcium chloride, lidocaine, isoproterenol, metaraminol, and atropine are available in this type of prefilled syringe. Various concentrations and needle lengths are available for use as intravenous bolus or intracardiac injections. Certain medications are also supplied with a spike so that they can be used as intravenous solution additives. Astra Pharmaceuticals markets a 100-mg syringe for bolus injections of lidocaine as well as a special vial of lidocaine with transfer spike for use as an intravenous additive.

"Pre-op" Orders

In hospitals, the evening prior to operation, medications and food are commonly withheld from the patient. Bedtime sedations are administered and preoperative orders for medications to be administered before operation the following day are prescribed.

Commonly used pre-op orders are combinations of narcotics, anticholinergics, and barbiturates or phenothiazines. In an effort to avoid multiple injection, combinations of narcotics and anticholinergics are often prepared in the same syringe. Little information is available concerning the compatibility of multiple drugs in the same syringe. Usually, these injections are not stored for long periods; however, hospital pharmacists might want to package them in advance.

Drug Stability in Plastic Disposable Syringes

Selected prefilled manufacturer's disposable syringes have been available for several years. All current manufacturers' prefilled syringes are packaged in disposable glass (Type I U.S.P.); glass packaging is required for long-term stability. Often, the drug contacts the glass barrel, rubber closure, and stainless steel needle. Some manufacturers' prefilled syringes limit the contact of the drug with the glass barrel and rubber component parts; however, with this type of syringe, needle activation must be performed by the user prior to injection (e.g., Isoject).

Pharmacists have long seen a need to prepackage or prefill syringes; in many cases, because these syringes are not available commercially. Pharmacists prefill batch sizes in empty, disposable glass syringes. Many prefill glass and plastic syringes for extemporaneous use and sometimes for storage in a refrigerator or freezer. Many legitimate reasons exist to prepare and store drugs in syringes.

The introduction of mini-infusion (e.g., by Bard, Becton-Dickinson) has necessitated that drugs be placed in plastic syringes for use with these instruments.

Information concerning the stability of single drugs or combinations of drugs packaged in glass or plastic syringes has been scarce. Owing to the lack of data on drug stability in glass and, particularly, pharmacy-prepared prefilled plastic syringes, storage of drugs traditionally has been minimized. Many pharmacies use plastic prefilled syringes primarily for extemporaneous or immediate use. Although some pharmacists store drugs in prefilled plastic syringes, many then store the syringes in the freezer for future use. Methods and duration of storage of such frozen prefilled plastic syringes vary among hospital pharmacies; some maintaining their frozen supplies anywhere from 1 week to a full year.

An early report[12] described prefilling plastic syringes with insulin. Because diabetic patients may lose acuity of vision as their disease progresses, they become increasingly unable to prepare the drug themselves; thus, the long-term stability of prefilled insulin syringes is vital in diabetic therapy. Early reports by Lilly stated that NPH and Lente insulins could be stored in plastic Becton-Dickinson syringes for 5 to 7 days under refrigeration without altering potency. They also noted that "mixtures of Regular with NPH or Lente should be administered immediately."

A study of the stability of paraldehyde[13] in Jelco, Burron, and Monoject plastic syringes showed that the plastic syringe caused the paraldehyde to be chemically altered; therefore, it was not advisable to use plastic syringes with paraldehyde.

Levin et al.[9] studied several drugs in glass Tubex syringes for stability after a 3-month storage period. Most drugs retained their potency and physical appearance in this study.

Dietrich[10] prefilled preanesthetic medication combinations in glass Tubex syringes. Wyeth (now Wyeth-Ayerst) Laboratories confirmed the stability of meperidine-atropine combinations for up to 3 months under refrigeration.

Studies[14] of 5000 units of heparin in Becton-Dickinson plastic syringes revealed that heparin retained its stability for at least 4 weeks at room temperature.

Combinations of a preanesthetic mixture of hydroxyzine HCl and atropine sulfate were studied[11] for stability in Becton-Dickinson plastic syringes. No significant degradation was noted after 10 days of storage.

Weiner et al.[7] studied the stability of gentamicin sulfate for up to 90 days in both glass and plastic syringes. Storage in glass was deemed superior. Storage in plastic for 30 days resulted in an unacceptable (15%) loss of potency. The manufacturer of Garamycin (Schering) confirmed these results.[15]

Stanaszek et al.[16] studied the stability of hydroxyzine HCl, meperidine HCl, and atropine sulfate in glass and plastic syringes. The stability of these combinations was confirmed for up to 10 days in either type of syringe.

Kresel et al.[17] studied the stability of carbenicillin and oxacillin that had been frozen in glass and plastic syringes for up to 3 months. No instability was found in these drugs in either plastic or glass syringes.

Kleinberg et al.[18] studied the stability of frozen antibiotics stored in disposable hypodermic syringes. Their data suggest that cephalothin, cefazolin, cefamandole, and nafcillin, when frozen and stored at −20° C in Hy-Pod hypodermic syringes, may be used within 9 months of initial freezing.

Steitz et al.[19] studied the stability of tobramycin sulfate in plastic syringes. Storing tobramycin in plastic is not recommended by the manufacturer because of incompatibility with the plunger head of the syringe. This study showed that tobramycin sulfate in plastic syringes retained its stability for up to 2 months.

Jump et al.[20] studied the compatibility of nalbuphine HCl in combination with other preoperative medications in Tubex syringes. Diazepam and pentobarbital were not stable, although several other drugs were.

Sesin et al.[21] investigated the stability of 5-fluorouracil in plastic disposable syringes. 5-Fluorouracil was found to be stable for up to 7 days in plastic, Sherwood syringes.

Thiamine HCl, repackaged in disposable Glaspak, Styrex (plastic), or Hy-Pod (glass) syringes, was found to be stable for at least 84 days.[22]

A 7-day stability study of cytarabine in plastic and glass syringes showed acceptable limits of stability, although the authors maintained that repackaging in glass is optimal.[23]

Nafcillin sodium (Unipen) was found to be satisfactory in glass Tubex syringes when stored and frozen at −20° C for 3 months.[24]

Johnson et al.[25] confirmed the incompatibility of paraldehyde with plastic syringes.

Gaj et al.[26] studied the compatibility of doxorubicin HCl in combination with vinblastine sulfate when stored in Monoject plastic syringes. The authors noted 5-day stability.

Solutions of methotrexate sodium were found to be stable when stored in plastic syringes for up to 30 days.[27]

Combinations of chlorpromazine HCl, hydroxyzine HCl, and meperidine HCl, when stored at 4° C and 25° C in glass or plastic syringes, were found to be stable for 366 days.[28]

Combinations of meperidine HCl, promethazine HCl, and atropine sulfate were found to be stable in plastic syringes for at least 24 hours.[29]

Huey et al.[30] studied the contamination potential associated with plastic syringes. Three brands of plastic syringes were evaluated by subjecting them to in-use conditions and intentional microbial challenge. In 120 samples, no contamination was found. Plastic syringes apparently pose no additional contamination potential when compared with glass. Mitrano et al.,[31] in a study of frozen plastic syringes for use with a mini-infusor, found no compromise of sterility when using plastic syringes.

Azacitidine[32] stability was studied in Becton-Dickinson polypropylene plastic syringes. The drug was reconstituted in polypropylene syringes with ice-cold lactated Ringer's injection and then frozen at −20° C. Stability was achieved for 2 weeks. After thawing to room temperature, the syringes should be used within three hours. Speaker et al.[33] studied selected drugs for their stability and interaction with three different brands of plastic syringes: Becton-Dickinson, Sherwood, and Terumo Medical. The drugs studied included dexamethasone sodium phosphate, diatriazoate meglumine, diazepam, and nitroglycerin. Generally, drug interaction was minimal; however, lipophilic drugs had achieved a greater loss.

Pecosky et al.[34] compared the stability of calcitriol in several types of plastic tuberculin syringes. Calcitritol has greater affinity for *polyvinyl* chloride than for polypropylene.

Limited studies of the stability of drugs in plastic disposable syringes have been performed. Perhaps the time has come for a more complete evaluation of drug stability in plastic syringes. With pressure being applied on health care systems to reduce costs, and with the introduction of new I.V. drug delivery systems, it appears that such data will be needed for optimal pharmacy practice.

References

1. Turco, S.J., and Davis, N.M.: Glass particles in intravenous injections. N. Engl. J. Med., *287*, 1204 (1972).
2. Apat, J.A., and Elias, W.F.: Single dose disposable syringes—the Tubex system. Bull. Parenter. Drug Assoc., *19*, 61 (1965).
3. Hoar, M.E.: A study of methods involved in extemporaneous syringe filling and degree of contamination. Drug Intell. Clin. Pharm., *7*, 132 (1973).

4. McConald, D.E., Prisco, H.M., and Parente, R.J.: Prefilling syringes in the hospital pharmacy. Am. J. Hosp. Pharm., 29, 223 (1972).

5. Stach, P.E.: Method for the aseptic filling of unit dose syringes. Am. J. Hosp. Pharm., 31, 762 (1974).

6. Mantsch, M.E., Stach, P.E., and Sherrin, T.P.: FluiDose II—a semi-automatic method used in filling unit-of-use syringes. Drug Intell. Clin. Pharm., 10, 162 (1976).

7. Weiner, B., McNeely, D.J., Kluge, R.M., and Stewart, R.B.: Stability of gentamicin sulfate injection following unit dose repackaging. Am. J. Hosp. Pharm., 33, 1254 (1976).

8. Kresel, J.J., and Smith, A.L.: Stability of gentamicin in plastic syringes. Am. J. Hosp. Pharm., 34, 570 (1977).

9. Levin, H.J., Fieber, R.A., and Levi, R.S.: Stability data for Tubex filled by hospital pharmacists. Hosp. Pharm., 8, 310 (1973).

10. Dietrich, W.J.: Standardized preanesthetic medications in prefilled syringes. Am. J. Hosp. Pharm., 30, 805 (1973).

11. Beatrice, M.G., et al.: Psysico-chemical stability of a preanesthetic mixture of hydroxyzine hydrochloride and atropine sulfate. Am. J. Hosp. Pharm., 32, 1133 (1975).

12. Eli Lilly and Co. Letter, Dec. 20, 1972, on file, Temple University Hospital Pharmacy.

13. Elkins-Sinn, Inc., Cherry Hill, NJ. Study on file, Temple University Hospital Pharmacy.

14. Cohelfred Laboratory, Chicago, IL. Data on file, Temple University Hospital Pharmacy.

15. Chrai, S.S., et al.: Gentamicin sulfate injection repackaging in syringes. Letter. Am. J. Hosp. Pharm., 34, 920 (1977).

16. Stanaszek, et al.: Analysis of hydroxyzine HCl, meperidine HCl and atropine sulfate in glass and plastic syringes. Am. J. Hosp. Pharm., 35, 1087 (1978).

17. Kresel, J.J., et al.: Stability of carbenicillin and oxacillin frozen in syringes. Am. J. Hosp. Pharm., 35, 310 (1978).

18. Kleinberg, M., et al.: Stability of antibiotics frozen and stored in disposable hypodermic syringes. Am. J. Hosp. Pharm., 37, 1087 (1980).

19. Steitz, D.J., et al.: Stability of tobramycin sulfate in plastic syringes. Letter. Am. J. Hosp. Pharm., 37, 1614 (1980).

20. Jump, W.G., et al.: Compatibility of nalbuphine HCl with other pre-operative medications. Am. J. Hosp. Pharm., 39, 841 (1982).

21. Sesin, G.P., et al.: Stability study of 5-fluorouracil following repackaging in plastic disposable syringes and multidose vials. Am. J. I.V. Ther. Clin. Nutr., 8, 23 (1982).

22. Nolly, R.J., et al.: Stability of thiamine HCl repackaged in disposable syringes. Am. J. Hosp. Pharm., 39, 471 (1982).

23. Gannon, P.M., et al.: Stability of cytarabine following repackaging in plastic syringes and glass containers. Am. J. I.V. Ther. Clin. Nutr. 6, 11 (1983).

24. Wyeth Laboratories, Philadelphia, PA. Letter, May 12, 1983, on file, Temple University Hospital Pharmacy.

25. Johnson, C.E., et al.: Compatibility of paraldehyde with plastic syringes and needle hubs. Am. J. Hosp. Pharm., 41, 306 (1984).

26. Gaj, E., et al.: Compatibility of doxorubicin HCl and vinblastine sulfate. Am. J. I.V. Ther. Clin. Nutr., 5, 8 (1984).

27. Levay, I.D., et al.: Stability of refrigerated methotrexate sodium in a plastic syringe. I.V. Therapy News, January, 1985.

28. Conklin, C.A., et al.: Stability of an analgesic-sedative combination in glass and plastic single-dose syringes. Am. J. Hosp. Pharm., 42, 339 (1985).

29. Rhodes, R.S., et al.: Stability of meperidine HCl, promethazine HCl and atropine sulfate in plastic syringes. Am. J. Hosp. Pharm., 42, 112 (1985).

30. Huey, W.Y., et al.: Microbial contamination potential of sterile disposable plastic syringes. Am. J. Hosp. Pharm., 42, 102 (1985).

31. Mitrano, F.P., et al.: Microbial contamination potential of solutions in prefilled disposable syringes used with a syringe pump. Am. J. Hosp. Pharm., 43, 78 (1986).

32. Hartigh, J.D., et al.: Stability of Azacitidine in lactated Ringer's injection frozen in polypropylene syringes. Am. J. Hosp. Pharm., 46, 2500 (1989).
33. Speaker, T.J., et al.: A study of the interaction of selected drugs and plastic syringes. J. Parenter. Sci. Technol., 45, 212 (1991).
34. Pecosky, D.A., et al.: Stability and sorption of Calcitriol in plastic tuberculin syringes. Am. J. Hosp. Pharm., 49, 1463 (1992).

CHAPTER

Radiopharmaceuticals

Elaine D. Mackowiak

Nuclear pharmacy was recognized as the first specialty practice by the Board of Pharmaceutical Specialties in 1978. The Board defines nuclear pharmacy practice as "a patient oriented service that embodies the scientific knowledge and professional judgment required to improve and promote health through the assurance of the safe and efficacious use of radioactive drugs for diagnosis and therapy." Nuclear pharmacists are responsible for the procurement, storage, and dispensing of radiopharmaceuticals. Radiopharmaceuticals are drugs that contain radioactive atoms in their structure and are intended for human use for either diagnosis or treatment of diseases.

Because radiopharmaceuticals are drugs, they must meet the same criteria established by the FDA for other drugs before they are marketed. In addition to tests for chemical purity, sterility, pyrogenicity, efficacy, and safety, all radiopharmaceuticals must be tested for radiochemical purity to ensure that the radiation emitted by the drug is correct. The nuclear pharmacist routinely performs certain quality control procedures whenever radiopharmaceuticals are prepared or dispensed, which is in marked contrast with the handling of other types of pharmaceuticals. For example, each dose of radiopharmaceutical must be measured or assayed before it is dispensed. Nuclear pharmacists must follow guidelines of the Nuclear Regulatory Commission (N.R.C.), in addition to following federal and state regulations that pertain to the practice of pharmacy. If radiopharmaceuticals are to be transported from one facility to another, the appropriate regulations of the United States Department of Transportation must be followed.

Because special facilities are required for the preparation of radiopharmaceuticals, nuclear pharmacies have traditionally been located in departments of nuclear medicine within hospitals. Since the early 1980s, there has been a rapid growth of chains of centralized nuclear pharmacies separate from hospitals, primarily because of economic factors. These facilities are usually located in areas where they can serve a large number of hospitals. Nuclear Pharmacy Incorporated and Syncor International Corporation merged in August of 1985 under the name Syncor International Corporation, making it the largest nationwide chain of nuclear pharmacies, with over 100 service centers. In 1983, Mallinckrodt entered the nationwide market with its nuclear pharmacies, known as Diagnostic Imaging Services. In 1986, Summa Medical Corporation announced that it would enter the national radiopharmaceutical service network through the establishment of a subsidiary company, Summa Pharmacy Corporation, Inc. Since then, Summa was purchased by medi + physics, a division of Amersham. Smaller chains of centralized nuclear pharmacies exist in several regions and serve limited areas.

The majority of radiopharmaceuticals are intended for intravenous administration and nuclear pharmacists must use their expertise in aseptic technique in drug preparation. A vertical laminar flow hood is a necessity, and if radioiodine preparations are to be prepared, a fumehood equipped with special filters is needed. Because of the radioactive nature of these drugs, the nuclear pharmacists must become adept at manipulating syringes and vials that are in shields during the preparation and dispensing of radiopharmaceuticals.

Use of Radiopharmaceuticals

Radioactivity represents an unstable energy state within the nucleus of an atom. In an attempt to achieve a stable energy state, the excess energy is most often emitted in the form of alpha and beta particles, positrons which are also particles, or gamma rays—pure electromagnetic energy, or photon radiation. The usefulness of a radiopharmaceutical depends on both the type of radiation emitted and its energy.

An alpha particle possesses a double positive charge and has a mass of four atomic mass units. A beta particle has the same mass and charge as an electron. Neither of these particles is able to pass through the human body, which makes them useless as diagnostic agents when imaging of various organs is desired. Some radiopharmaceuticals that emit beta radiation are used for in vitro diagnostic studies or for therapeutic purposes. Positrons and gamma radiation are capable of penetrating through human tissue and are useful for both imaging studies and therapy.

Positrons are the antiparticles of beta particles. They have the same mass as beta particles, and the magnitude of their charge is the same but opposite in sign. Positrons immediately interact with electrons after they are emitted from the nucleus. The interaction occurs with such a great force that the mass of the positron and electron are converted to electromagnetic energy and two photons are created with an energy of 0.51 million electron volts. This conversion of mass to energy is called annihilation radiation.

Annihilation photons may be used in diagnostic imaging studies, but unfortunately the efficiency of the instrumentation currently used in nuclear medicine for their detection is rather poor. Some positron emitters being developed as radiopharmaceuticals have extremely short half-lives, for example, ^{13}N, ^{15}O, and ^{18}F have half-lives of 10 minutes, 124 seconds, and 112 minutes

Table 13–1. Radiopharmaceuticals Used for Therapy

Drug	Uses	Dose
Chromic Phosphate (^{32}P)	Irradiate pleural and peritoneal cavities	10–20 mCi
Sodium Phosphate Injection (^{32}P)	Polycythemia vera	1–12 mCi
Sodium Iodide (^{131}I)	Ablation of thyroid gland	5–200 mCi

respectively. The production of these short-lived radioisotopes is very expensive, as is the new instrumentation needed for scanning. Because of these factors, only a few sites are capable of performing positron studies.

When radionuclides, regardless of their nature, interact with any material, they cause ionization. The amount of ionization is related to the type and quantity of radiation present. In human tissue, the energy that the radionuclide transfers to tissue is referred to as the radiation absorbed dose or the rad, or as the gray if the International System of Units is used. This absorbed radiation is responsible for the biologic effects resulting from radiation.

Because alpha and beta particles penetrate through human tissue so poorly, all of the energy they lose through ionization is deposited in the tissues where they are concentrated. In certain malignant conditions, cell death may be the desired therapeutic goal and these particles may be useful. At the present time, there are no alpha-emitting radiopharmaceuticals; phosphorous-32, a beta-emitting radionuclide, is used in two radiopharmaceuticals. Table 13–1 lists the compounds of ^{32}P that are available for therapy.

Iodine-131, ^{131}I, emits both beta particles and gamma rays. When it is administered as Na^{131}I, it concentrates in the thyroid gland and causes necrosis of thyroid tissue due to the beta radiation. If the dose administered to the patient is greater than 30 millicuries, the patient must be hospitalized because the gamma rays from the ^{131}I make him a radiation hazard. The patient remains hospitalized until the quantity of ^{131}I present is less than 30 millicuries.

Milli Current research with monoclonal antibodies involves development of MCAs, which may be labeled with alpha- and beta-emitting radionuclides. These labeled antibodies will deliver the radionuclide to the targeted malignant cells, thereby reducing radiation dose to normal cells and tissues. If MCAs are labeled with gamma-emitting radionuclides, they can be used for diagnosis or therapy.

Cytogen's OncoScint, which is labeled with indium-111, is approved as a tumor imaging agent for selected groups of patients in the diagnosis of ovarian and colorectal cancer. Indium-111 emits gamma radiation. Myoscint, an ^{111}In-labeled MCA developed by Centocor, is in Phase III testing as a myocardial imaging agent. It will be used to evaluate the degree of necrosis in myocardial tissue in patients who have had myocardial infarcts.

Other radionuclides are also used to treat patients who have malignant diseases, but they are not considered radiopharmaceuticals. In teletherapy, cobalt-60, ^{60}Co, and cesium-137 (^{137}Cs), are used as external radiation sources. They are carefully shielded to deliver very large doses of radiation to precise tumor sites to kill malignant cells. Brachytherapy involves the implantation of radioactive sources in the patient by surgical procedures. These sources re-

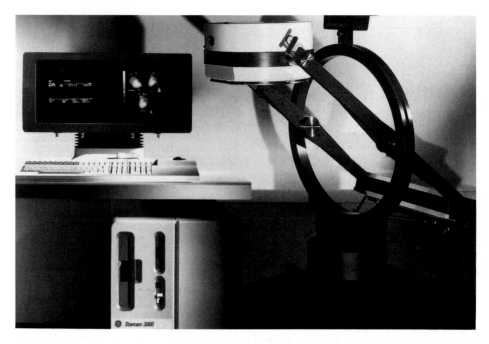

Figure 13–1. A general-use gamma camera, the Starcam 3000 XC/T, is also used for tomographic studies. A tomographic image provides a specific layer or "slice" in a specified region of the body to be viewed. (Courtesy of GE Medical Systems, King of Prussia, PA.)

main in the body for a limited time to deliver a specific radiation dose at the site where they are implanted. Then, they may be either removed surgically or allowed to remain in the body, where they undergo complete radioactive decay, like iridium-192. Both teletherapy and brachytherapy sources are used by the radiotherapy departments of hospitals.

An ideal diagnostic agent should have sufficient radiation energy to penetrate through the body after administration and be efficiently detected by the current instrumentation known as a gamma camera (Fig. 13–1), thus providing good quality images and producing as low a dose of radiation in the patient as possible. Gamma radiation, which is electromagnetic energy, readily penetrates through human tissue and is the form of radiation currently present in nearly all diagnostic radiopharmaceuticals. Technetium-99m, a gamma emitter, has an energy that is nearly ideal for current instrumentation. The degree of penetration of gamma radiation through tissue is directly related to its energy. In diagnostic procedures, the risk of significant biological harm from the radiation dose of radiopharmaceutical is extremely small, but, as with any drug, the benefit derived from the use of the drug must exceed the risk of its adverse effect.

Adverse effects from radiopharmaceuticals do occur, but are not due to the radioactivity. Like any parenteral drug, radiopharmaceuticals may cause hypotension, diaphoresis, and syncope. True allergic reactions are rare but do occur in those radiopharmaceuticals that contain serum albumin. Absorption, distribution, and excretion of radiopharmaceuticals may be affected by the concurrent administration of nonradioactive drugs that a patient may be taking. Nuclear pharmacists must be familiar with the increasing number of drug interactions that have been reported.

Unlike other drugs, radiopharmaceuticals do not produce a pharmacologic dose response. Rather than the mass or weight of drug administered, it is the radioactivity present in the drug that is responsible for its usefulness. The amount of radioactivity per unit of mass of drug is known as the specific activity. Radiopharmaceuticals in which all the atoms are radioactive are known as carrier-free drugs. High specific activity allows compounds, which have inherently toxic properties, to be used in patients because the mass of the drug present is so small. An example is thallium, as thallous chloride-201, a diagnostic agent widely used in cardiology.

Diagnostic radiopharmaceuticals are useful because they are a noninvasive means of determining physiologic functions or anatomic structure. Radioactivity in the drug molecule allows it to be monitored or followed as it circulates or concentrates in the body. It is the chemical or physical form of the drug, however, which determines its use as a diagnostic drug. For example, elemental iodine (I_2) is used as an antibacterial and antifungal agent, but potassium iodide and sodium iodide are used therapeutically as sources of iodide for the thyroid gland to synthesize thyroxine. If radioactive iodine-123 ($^{123}I_2$) is used, it will have antibacterial and antifungal properties. If radioactive sodium iodide-123 ($Na^{123}I$) is ingested, the iodide will be taken up by the thyroid gland and will be incorporated into the thyroxine. The distribution of $Na^{123}I$ in the thyroid permits it to be visualized by an appropriate detector so that its anatomic structure can be determined. Such a study is an imaging procedure or a scan. If the rate at which the $Na^{123}I$ is taken up by the thyroid is determined, the physiologic functioning of the gland may be evaluated.

The following mechanisms are responsible for most of the imaging studies currently performed.

Active Uptake or Active Transport. In this process, the organ accumulates the radiopharmaceutical by an active transport mechanism. If the organ is functioning normally, the distribution of radioactivity in the organ will be uniform. Abnormal results are obtained if there is an area of increased radioactivity or if there is an area devoid of radioactivity. Interpretation of the results depends on the organ being scanned and the radiopharmaceutical being used. The classic example of this type of study is thyroid scanning using radioactive iodine-123 as sodium iodide or radioactive sodium pertechnetate, $NaTcO_4$. If the patient has hyperthyroidism, the uptake of radionuclide will be exaggerated. The increased sites of radioactivity are referred to as "hot spots." Conversely, nonfunctioning thyroid tissue will not contain radio-activity and is known as a "cold spot," which may be either benign or malignant tissue requiring further evaluation.

Phagocytosis. Cells of the reticuloendothelial system (RES), the liver, spleen, and bone marrow, are responsible for the degradation of foreign materials of a certain size by phagocytosis. Sulfur colloid, containing particles from 0.1 to 1 μ, labeled with technetium-99m, is injected intravenously for imaging of the RES.

Capillary Blockade. Lung perfusion is evaluated by injecting radioactive particles 10 to 50 μ in size that have a diameter larger than that of the capillaries in the lung. After intravenous injection of radiolabeled albumin as either a macroaggregate or as microspheres, lung capillaries trap these particles. Distribution and intensity of radioactivity is directly related to regional perfusion. Note that, because very small quantities of drug are actually injected, no impairment in circulatory function occurs because of the small number of capillaries that are temporarily blocked by the process, except in patients who have pulmonary hypertension. The number of particles injected must be carefully controlled to prevent worsening of right-heart failure in this group of patients.

Compartment Localization. Injection of a radioactive tracer into a compartment, where it remains, allows evaluation of that compartment. For example, red blood cells labeled with technetium-99m are used for measuring the ejection fraction and wall motion of the heart.

Exchange Diffusion. The adherence of technetium-99m-labeled pyrophosphates or diphosphonates to the hydroxyapatite of bone by exchange diffusion permits visualization of the skeletal system.

In addition to imaging studies; radiopharmaceuticals may be used to evaluate physiologic processes in vitro. Many of these procedures involve the administration of a radiopharmaceutical by either mouth or intravenous injection, and the subsequent collection of some body fluid such as blood, urine, or feces for in vitro determination of the presence of radioactivity. Table 13–2 lists the imaging agents in current use and Table 13–3 lists radiopharmaceuticals used for routinely performed special studies.

Units of Radioactivity

Because radiopharmaceuticals are compounds whose atoms contain unstable nuclei, the unit of quantifying radioactivity describes the rate at which the nuclei decay. The curie (Ci) is the basic unit for quantifying radioactivity. One curie is defined as 3.7×10^{10} disintegrating atoms per second (dps). The dose of radiopharmaceutical is expressed in units of the curie, as either microcuries, μCi, or millicuries, mCi.

$$1 \text{ curie (Ci)} = 3.7 \times 10^{10} \text{ disintegrations per second (dps)}$$
$$1 \text{ millicurie (mCi)} = 3.7 \times 10^{7} \text{ dps}$$
$$1 \text{ microcurie (μCi)} = 3.7 \times 10^{4} \text{ dps}$$

In 1980, the scientific community adopted the System Internationale (SI) and the becquerel (Bq) became the new basic unit for quantifying radioactivity. One becquerel equals one disintegration per second.

$$1 \text{ becquerel (Bq)} = 1 \text{ dps,}$$

therefore

$$1 \text{ Ci} = 3.7 \times 10^{10} \text{ Bq or 37 gigabecquerels (GBq) (giga} = 10^{9})$$
$$1 \text{ mCi} = 3.7 \times 10^{7} \text{ Bq or 37 megabecquerels (MBq) (mega} = 10^{6})$$
$$1 \text{ μCi} = 3.7 \times 10^{4} \text{ Bq or 37 kilobecquerels (KBq) (kilo} = 10^{3})$$

Table 13–2. Radiopharmaceuticals Used as Imaging Agents

Organ Systems	Drug	Mechanism for Distribution
Cardiovascular System:		
Myocardial Imaging	^{201}Thallous chloride ^{82}Rubidium chloride	Analog for potassium that is extracted in proportion to myocardial blood flow; permits study of regional wall motion
	^{99m}Tc pyrophosphate	Combines with calcium released from mitochondrial cells in myocardium in infarcted cells
	^{99m}Tc sestamibi ^{99m}Tc teboroxime	Lipohilic drugs which penetrate into myocardial cells
Ventriculography	^{99m}Tc in vivo labeled red cells	Localization of red cells in blood compartment permits study of cardiac chambers and regional wall motion
Central Nervous System:		
Cerebral Anatomy	^{99m}Tc pertechnetate ^{99m}Tc gluceptate ^{99m}Tc DTPA (diethylene-triaminopentacetic acid)	Localizes in brain at sites where there is injury to blood brain barrier
Cerebral Blood Flow	^{99m}Tc pertechnetate ^{99m}Tc gluceptate ^{99m}Tc exametazine[†] ^{99m}Tc pentetate	Visualizes cerebral blood flow by localizing in blood compartment
	^{133}Xe gas ^{123}Iodoamphetamine*	Quantifies cerebral blood flow by determining rate of washout
Cerebrospinal Fluid	^{111}In pentetate	Localizes and follows flow of cerebrospinal fluid
Cerebral Metabolism	^{18}F deoxyglucose	Monitors glucose metabolism; used in diagnosis of epilepsy
Endocrine System:		
Adrenal Gland	^{131}I iodocholesterol ^{131}I iodomethyl-19-non-cholesterol	Cholesterol analog incorporated into adrenal corticosteroids
Thyroid	Na^{123}I, Na^{131}I	Active transport and organification
	^{99m}Tc pertechnetate	Active transport only
Gastrointestinal System:		
Gastrointestinal Bleeding	^{99m}Tc-labeled red blood cells ^{99m}Tc sulfur colloid ^{51}Cr-labeled red blood cells	Compartmental localization

Table 13–2.   *Continued*

Organ Systems	Drug	Mechanism for Distribution
Gastric Emptying	^{99m}Tc sulfur colloid ^{111}In pentetate ^{99m}Tc pentetate	Compartmental localization
Gastroesophageal Reflux	^{99m}Tc sulfur colloid ^{99m}Tc pentetate ^{111}In pentetate	Compartmental localization
Meckel's Diverticulum	^{99m}Tc pertechnetate	Active transport
Liver and Spleen Imaging	^{99m}Tc sulfur colloid ^{99m}Tc albumin colloid	Phagocytosis by reticuloendothelial cells
Spleen Image Only	^{51}Cr heat damaged autologous red blood cells ^{99m}Tc heat damaged autologous red blood cells	Spleen removal of damaged RBCs
Hepatobiliary Imaging	^{99m}Tc disofenin ^{99m}Tc mebrofenin ^{99m}Tc lidofenin	Active transport by polygonal cells in liver
Salivary Glands	^{99m}Tc pertechnetate	Active transport for evaluation of salivary flow
Genitourinary System: Cystography	^{99m}Tc pentetate ^{99m}Tc gluceptate	Compartmental localization
Diuretic Renography for Collecting System and Ureters	^{99m}Tc pentetate and furosemide	Clearance by glomerular filtration to evaluate mechanical obstruction (washout test)
Renal Function	^{99m}Tc pentetate ^{123}I or ^{131}I orthoiodohippurate ^{99m}Tc dimercaptosuccinic acid (DMSA) ^{99m}Tc mertiatide	Evaluation of glomerular filtration rate (renal clearance)
Renal Imaging	^{99m}Tc DMSA ^{99m}Tc gluceptate ^{99m}Tc mertiatide	Binds to renal tubules Binds to renal tubules
Renal Perfusion	^{99m}Tc pentetate ^{99m}Tc gluceptate	Compartmental localization
Testicular Imaging	^{99m}Tc pertechnetate	Compartmental localization
Pulmonary System: Perfusion	^{99m}Tc macroaggregates (MAA)	Capillary blockade
Ventilation	^{133}Xe gas ^{81m}Kr gas ^{99m}Tc pentetate aerosol	Diffusion in lungs proportional to regional ventilation
Skeletal System: Skeletal Imaging	^{99m}Tc medronate (MDP) ^{99m}Tc pyrophosphate (PYP) ^{99m}Tc oxidronate (HDP)	Chelation (binding) to hydroxyapatite

Table 13–2. *Continued*

Organ Systems	Drug	Mechanism for Distribution
Joint Imaging	^{99m}Tc pertechnetate ^{99m}Tc MDP	Accumulates at site of active synovitis
Miscellaneous Imaging: Inflammatory Processes	^{111}In oxine-labeled leukocytes ^{67}Ga citrate	Active uptake in abscesses and areas of active inflammation
Tumor Localization and Staging	^{67}Ga citrate	Active uptake in a variety of neoplasms
Thrombus Localization	^{125}I-labeled fibrinogen ^{111}In-labeled platelets	Incorporation into thrombus
Lacrimal System (Dacryocystography)	^{99m}Tc pertechnetate	Passive transport
Bone Marrow Imaging	^{99m}Tc sulfur colloid	Phagocytosis
Lymphatic Imaging	^{99m}Tc antimony sulfur colloid	Passive transport and phagocytosis

*Not currently available.
†Formerly known as ^{99m}Tc hexamethylenepropylene Amine Oxime (HM-PAQ).

Although the SI system has been officially adopted, the older terms still persist in current medical practice.

Since radioactive decay is a continuous process, the time the drug is to be administered must be known before the nuclear pharmacist can prepare the drug for dispensing. Radioactive decay is a first-order rate reaction, and the dose of the drug at any required time may be calculated from the following equation:

$$A = A_0 e^{-\lambda t}$$

where

A = Amount of radioactivity present at time t

A_0 = Amount of radioactivity present at time zero (t = 0)

λ = Decay constant

e = Base of the natural logarithm = 2.7183

Since the value of λ is expressed as the number of decaying nuclei per unit of time, it is not a convenient value to remember. It is much easier to use

Table 13–3. Radiopharmaceuticals Used for Special Studies

Drug	Usage
^{125}I or ^{131}I Human serum albumin (RISA)	Plasma volume
^{51}Cr Sodium chromate	Red blood cell volume Red blood cell survival time
^{57}Co cyanocobalamin (vitamin B$_{12}$)	Evaluate macrocytic anemias (Schilling test)

the term half-life, $T_{1/2}$. Half-life is the time required for one half of the original radioactive atoms to decay. From this definition, a relationship between λ and the above equation can be expressed as

$$A = A_0\, e^{\dfrac{-0.693\, t}{T_{1/2}}}$$

Each radioactive isotope of an element possesses its own decay rate, which cannot be altered. The following examples demonstrate the use of these formulas. At 6:00 AM, a vial of technetium, ^{99m}Tc, contained 20 mCi (740 MBq). What is the activity at 8:00 AM? $T_{1/2}$ for ^{99m}Tc is 6 hours.

$$A = 20 \text{ mCi (740 Mbq) } e^{-(0.693/6 \text{ hours}) \times 2 \text{ hours}}$$
$$A = 20 \text{ mCi (740 Mbq) } e^{-0.231}$$
$$A = 15.9 \text{ mCi (587.4 MBq)}$$

If a 15-mCi dose of ^{99m}Tc is needed at 9:00 AM, how much ^{99m}Tc must be dispensed at 6:00 AM?

$$15 \text{ mCi (555 Bq) } = A_0\, e^{-(0.693/6 \text{ hours}) \times 3 \text{ hours}}$$
$$A_0 = 15 \text{ mCi (555 Bq) } e^{0.3465}$$
$$= 21.2 \text{ mCi (745 Bq)}$$

Because radioactive·decay is constant, correction factors for decay may be calculated for predetermined elapsed times. These values are compiled in tabular form so that the pharmacist does not have to perform a calculation for each time period. The following is an example of such a table for ^{99m}Tc:

Elapsed time (Hr)	Correction factor (fraction remaining)
0	1.00
0.25	0.97
0.50	0.94
0.75	0.92
1.00	0.89
1.25	0.86
1.50	0.84
1.75	0.82
2.00	0.79

Each dose of radioactive drug must be assayed before dispensing by using a dose calibrator, as shown in Figure 13–2. A dose calibrator contains an air-filled chamber coupled to an electrometer that measures that amount of ionization produced by a radiopharmaceutical. The amount of ionization created in the chamber is directly proportional to the quantity of radiation emitted by the radiopharmaceutical. Each radiopharmaceutical emits radiation at a specific energy, and the dose calibrator has a series of calibrated buttons that may be set to detect the given energy of the radiopharmaceutical to be measured. When the appropriate button is selected, the dose calibrator's digital

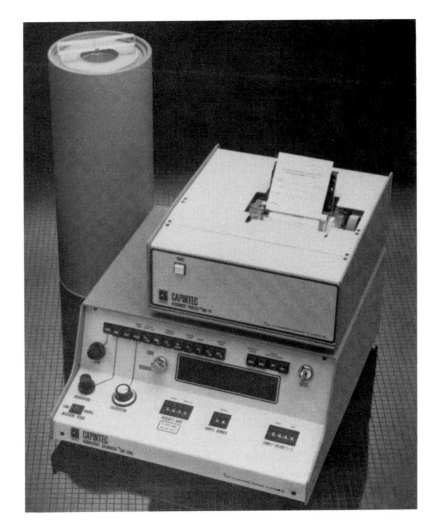

Figure 13–2. The model CRC-30BC dose calibrator features a computer and a permanent printout that can be used to record patient dose and to provide a table of precalibrated dose and volume of dose to be delivered. Results of molybdenum-99 assay required for quality control of radiopharmaceuticals may also be recorded. (Courtesy of Capintec, Inc., Ramsey, NJ.)

display indicates the dose in either mCi or μCi (or in becquerels). Once the radiopharmaceutical is prepared, both the total amount of radioactivity and the concentration, mCi/ml, will decrease as time elapses. This means that, to administer the same dose of radioactivity throughout the day, the volume of drug to be dispensed must be increased.

Example: The concentration of ^{99m}Tc is 20 mCi per 0.5 ml at 6:00 AM If 20 mCi are to be dispensed at 8:00 AM, what volume should be dispensed? At 8:00 AM the concentration of drug will be 15.9 mCi per 0.5 ml; therefore, 0.63 ml must be dispensed to provide the required dose of 20 mCi.

Each radiopharmaceutical has an expiration time or date that is determined by the radionuclide that is present in the drug.

Preparation of Radiopharmaceuticals

Radiopharmaceuticals are dispensed at the direction of a physician who has a license from the Nuclear Regulatory Commission. Radiopharmaceuticals are available in two basic forms:

1. The radiopharmaceutical is purchased from the manufacturer in its final form for dispensing by the pharmacist. The drug already contains radioactive atoms in its molecule; the nuclear pharmacist must calculate the appropriate amount of drug to be dispensed. Examples of this type of radiopharmaceutical are cyanocobalamin ^{57}Co capsules, sodium iodide ^{131}I capsules or liquid, and thallium chloride ^{201}Tl injection.

2. The majority of radiopharmaceuticals are obtained as kits. The manufacturer provides a chemical compound or drug that contains no radioactivity; this is known as an intermediate. The pharmacist compounds or makes the radiopharmaceutical at the time of dispensing, when an appropriate quantity of radionuclide is added to the intermediate chemical.

$$\text{Intermediate} + \text{Radionuclide} \rightarrow \text{Radiopharmaceutical}$$

Radioactive technetium-99m, ^{99m}Tc, is the radionuclide used in the preparation of most drugs sold as kits.

Some nuclear pharmacies are becoming involved in the labeling of cells that are used for diagnostic purposes. For example, blood is taken from a patient and the leukocytes are separated and are labeled or tagged using indium oxine, ^{111}In. The labeled cells are then injected back into the patient for studies to determine unknown sites of infection. Red cell labeling with ^{99m}Tc, in vivo or in vitro is used in several studies of the cardiovascular system.

Both the chemical and radiologic properties of ^{99m}Tc contribute to its usefulness for preparation. ^{99m}Tc is a transition metal, and it exists in several valence states. In the form of pertechnetate ion, TcO_4^-, it behaves as iodide and will be concentrated by the thyroid gland. If the thyroid is first blocked by the administration of potassium iodide, KI, or potassium perchlorate, $KClO_4$, to the patient, the pertechnetate will remain in circulation, which allows it to be used for other studies such as cardiac shunt detection and quantitative compartmental analyses of left and right heart function.

If technetium is in its reduced valence state, it can combine with the chemical intermediates to form compounds that are used in a large variety of studies, as can be seen in Table 13–2. The reduction of technetium is achieved by the use of stannous chloride during preparation of the radiopharmaceutical.

The desirable radiologic properties of ^{99m}Tc include a gamma ray that has an energy of 0.14 MeV (million electron volts), which is detected with good efficiency by the instrumentation currently available in nuclear medicine. It also gives relatively low radiation doses to patients because of its short half-life, 6.02 hours, and its gamma energy.

The 6-hour half-life means that the drug is too expensive to order directly from a pharmaceutical manufacturer because much of it would decay before it could be used. The problem of obtaining ^{99m}Tc at reasonable cost was solved when Powell Richards of Brookhaven National Laboratories described a generator system that provided for ^{99m}Tc to be easily separated and removed from molybdenum-99, ^{99}Mo, its parent compound.

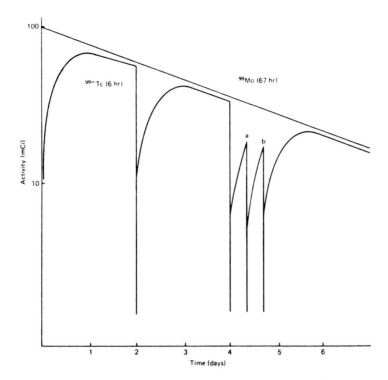

Figure 13–3. Typical curve demonstrating transient equilibrium in a ^{99}Mo/^{99m}Tc generator system. As ^{99}Mo decays, its activity decreases, while the activity of the ^{99m}Tc being formed starts to increase. The ^{99m}Tc activity increases until it reaches a maximum at about 23 hours. Whenever the generator is eluated on day 2 or day 4, the ^{99m}Tc activity falls to a minimum value, which is determined by the efficiency of the elution process itself. Points a and b on the curve indicate elution of ^{99m}Tc at intervals of 8 and 17 hours on day 4. (From Saha, G.B.: Fundamentals of Nuclear Pharmacy. New York, Springer-Verlag, 1979, p. 56.)

When ^{99}Mo, a readily available radionuclide, undergoes radioactive decay, it produces ^{99m}Tc. The amount of ^{99m}Tc produced will increase until it reaches maximum activity, which occurs in about 23 hours (Figure 13–3). At that point, the generator has reached transient equilibrium at which time the amount of ^{99m}Tc being produced is equal to the amount of ^{99}Mo present. In this generator system, the ^{99}Mo is absorbed on a column of alumina. If the alumina column is eluted with sterile normal saline, the ^{99m}Tc will be separated from the ^{99}Mo and eluted from the column. Because ^{99}Mo has a half-life of 67 hours, it will continue to produce enough ^{99m}Tc for several days' use. This generator system provides an economical source of ^{99m}Tc for the preparation of radiopharmaceuticals in nuclear pharmacy.

Figure 13–3 shows the relationship between the amount of ^{99m}Tc and the decay of ^{99}Mo over a period of several days. It must be noted that the maximum amount of ^{99m}Tc is available after 23-hour intervals, but that the actual quantity available each day decreases because of the ongoing decay of the ^{99}Mo.

Because the total activity of ^{99m}Tc decreases daily, the generator may be eluted with smaller volumes of normal saline to provide a product that will have approximately the same concentration of ^{99m}Tc/ml/day. For example, if a 1600-mCi ^{99m}Mo generator is eluted with 20 ml of sterile normal saline at the time of its calibration, and the efficiency of the elution process is 80%, 64 mCi/ml will be obtained (1600 mCi × 0.8/20 ml). If this generator is eluted 2 days later, only 1248 mCi of ^{99m}Tc would be on the column. Because elution of the column is only 80% efficient, the total amount of ^{99m}Tc available is 998 mCi. To obtain the same concentration of ^{99m}Tc, only 15.6 ml of sterile saline should be used for the elution. If this method of elution using decreasing volumes is not followed, the concentration of ^{99m}Tc/ml will decrease daily, resulting in a larger volume of radiopharmaceutical being dispensed to provide the same dose of radioactivity for the patient.

There are two types of technetium generator systems, wet and dry. Squibb and New England Nuclear produce a dry generator. In this system, the alumina column remains dry until the elution is done. A vial of sterile saline is attached to the system and a sterile evacuated vial of equal or greater volume is attached to the system to begin the elution. All the sterile saline is drawn through the generator into the evacuated vial.

The dry system allows more accurate control of the actual volume used in the elution process. The vial that collects the eluent must be shielded during this process at all times to reduce the radiation dose the pharmacist receives. Because radioactivity causes the formation of peroxides and free radicals in aqueous solution, the dry column system reduces this process and theoretically should result in a more trouble-free generator. The dry system reduces the possibility that the valence of the technetium will be changed during storage and elution. All elutions must be performed with a sterile saline solution that is free from bacteriostats and/or preservatives, to prevent any alteration of the valence state of technetium.

The second type of generator is a wet system produced by Mallinckrodt and Union Carbide. This system has an internal supply of sterile saline, and the alumina column is always saturated or wet. The volume of eluent used is determined by the volume of the sterile evacuated vial used during elution. Manufacturers generally provide evacuated vials to be used in their systems. Pharmacists must be thoroughly familiar with the generator system used in their nuclear pharmacy and should consult the manufacturer's package insert prior to use.

Two additional generator systems are used for diagnostic imaging procedures. The radionuclides produced in these systems have such short half-lives that the eluants from the stationary adsorption columns are administered directly to the patient without any preparation by the pharmacist.

Rubidium-82, ^{82}Rb, a positron emitter, has a half-life of 75 seconds. The parent radionuclide is strontium-82 (^{82}Sr), which is absorbed on a column of stannic oxide. The half-life of ^{82}Sr is 25 days. The shielded column is eluted at a rate of 50 ml per minute with a special infusion system containing Sterile Sodium Chloride Injection USP directly into the patient. ^{82}Rb behaves like potassium and is used as a cardiac perfusion agent.

Lung ventilation studies may be performed with krypton-81m, which has a half-life of 13 seconds. It is obtained from the decay of rubidium-81, which has a half-life of 4.6 hours. The ^{81}Rb is absorbed on a column of BioRad AG50 resin. The eluant is a stream of humidified oxygen which is inhaled by the patient from a device attached directly to the generator.

Quality Control

The manufacturer usually performs all the quality control tests necessary for nonradioactive drugs, but for radiopharmaceuticals, the nuclear pharmacist is responsible for performing some quality control analyses. Radiopharmaceuticals that are dispensed in the form in which they are obtained from the manufacturer are dispensed in the same manner as their nonradioactive counterparts, but all other radiopharmaceuticals must first be subjected to quality control examination by the nuclear pharmacist. Nuclear pharmacy emphasizes this role in its practice. Quality control must be performed in several areas.

1. Because all doses of radiopharmaceutical must be assayed to determine the quantity of radioactivity or dose of drug before dispensing, the dose calibrator itself, which is shown in Figure 13–2, must be calibrated on a daily basis. Because radionuclides with different energies are used in nuclear medicine, the appropriate energy to be measured is selected on the dose calibrator by depressing a push button that bears the chemical symbol of the radionuclide to be dispensed. Calibration of the dose calibrator must be performed daily when used with radionuclides that are traceable to the National Bureau of Standards. This is an NRC requirement and is known as the constancy test. NRC requests that other tests be performed during the year to ensure that the response of the instrument is linear with the dose and that the dose calibrator is accurate.

2. The eluent from the ^{99}Mo-^{99m}Tc generator must be analyzed for both molybdenum and aluminum breakthrough. The N.R.C. and U.S.P. limit the quantity of ^{99}Mo and aluminum permitted in the technetium eluent.

Measurement of ^{99m}Mo may be made with either the dose calibrator or a sodium iodide (thallium activated) scintillation detector. In a scintillation detector, the gamma radiation of the radiopharmaceutical produces light that is directly proportional to the quantity of gamma energy present. The scintillation detector converts the light signal into an electrical signal by means of a photomultiplier tube. This electrical signal may be displayed on a cathode ray tube (CRT) after being sorted by a pulse analyzer (Fig. 13–4). (Each radionuclide has its own characteristic spectrum due to the radiation it emits.) This process is referred to as gamma-ray spectroscopy. Once the scintillation detector is calibrated, the quantity of radioactivity present and the identification of its energy ensure the pharmacist of the radionuclide purity of the radiopharmaceutical.

3. During the elution process, it is possible that aluminum from the column may be released and may contaminate the eluent. The U.S.P. sets the limits for the amount of aluminum permitted in the eluent and requires that a colorimetric test be performed.

4. The radiochemical purity of a drug must also be established before it is dispensed. Radiopharmaceuticals that contain technetium-99m use it either as the free pertechnetate ion in $Na^{99m}TcO_4$ or as reduced technetium that is bound to the intermediate present in the kit. Although standard chemical techniques such as precipitation or solvent extraction may be used, paper and thin-layer

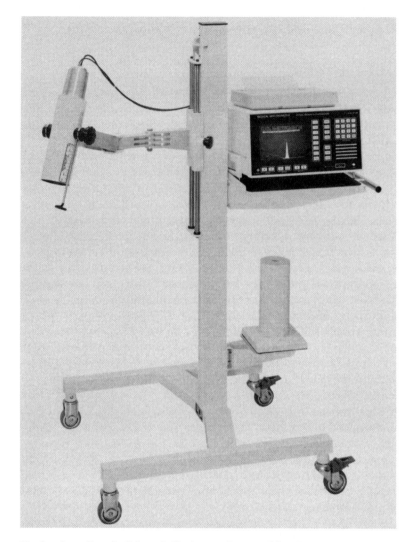

Figure 13–4. A sodium iodide scintillation probe used for thyroid studies is connected to a multichannel analyzer (MCA), which displays the energy spectrum of the gamma-emitting radiopharmaceutical used for the study. (Courtesy of Atomic Products Corporation, Center Moriches, NY.)

chromatography are the techniques most often used in determinations of radiochemical purity. For example, in an acetone solvent, free pertechnetate moves with the solvent front, whereas technetium that is bound remains at the point of origin. Determination of the amount of radioactivity at the origin and at the solvent front on the chromatogram is satisfactory for performing this U.S.P. test. Other solvent systems are also acceptable for use in performing this test.

Some newer radiopharmaceuticals have more stringent requirements to ensure quality. Because of stability problems, ^{99m}Tc exametazine (Ceretec) requires that quality control be performed immediately before use, and the package insert recommends that a combination of three different chromatographic tests be used. The radiopharmaceutical must be administered to the patient within 30 minutes after its formulation.

5. The majority of radiopharmaceuticals dispensed are intended for intravenous injection and undergo the same tests for sterility and pyrogenicity as used for other pharmaceuticals. Radiopharmaceuticals dispensed in the form supplied by the manufacturer require no further testing.

The ^{99}Mo-^{99m}Tc generator used in nuclear pharmacy is sterile and pyrogen-free when it is obtained from the manufacturer. All elutions of the generator are with Sodium Chloride for Injection, U.S.P. If aseptic procedures are followed, the ^{99m}Tc obtained by elution should also be sterile. This ^{99m}Tc is used then either directly as $Na^{99m}TcO_4$ for diagnostic studies or combined with the intermediate in the various kits. The chemicals in the kit are also sterile and pyrogen-free when purchased. If final sterilization must be performed in the nuclear pharmacy, membrane filters, such as Millipore, are used except when the drug to be dispensed is a colloid or particulate. All preparations should be prepared in a vertical laminar flow hood and should be tested for sterility, following the methods prescribed in U.S.P. XXII. Because both the fluid thioglycollate medium and the soybean-casein in digest medium require from 7 to 14 days for completion, the short half-lived radiopharmaceuticals would be decayed before testing could be completed. This means that sterility data are not available until after the radiopharmaceutical has been administered to the patient.

One test that is useful in evaluating sterility in radiopharmaceuticals with extremely short half-lives involves an in vitro test using carbon-14 labeled glucose. A trypticase soy broth culture medium that contains ^{14}C labeled glucose is incubated with the drug to be tested. Any microorganisms present in the sample will metabolize the labeled glucose, producing $^{14}CO_2$, which is detected by using an ionization chamber. An automated instrument available for performing this radioassay is the Bactec instrument. The test may be completed in less than 24 hours, which is an advantage for testing radiopharmaceuticals. Most kits prepared with ^{99m}Tc have a 6-hour expiration time.

6. As with sterility testing, pyrogenicity testing is usually performed after the radiopharmaceutical is dispensed. U.S.P. XXII describes the rabbit test for pyrogen testing, which is a rather long procedure. More recently, the limulus amebocyte lysate (LAL) has been used. This test may be performed in about 1 hour and is described in Chapter 3.

Safety

The nuclear pharmacist prepares drugs that contain high levels of radioactivity, and all available techniques to reduce radiation exposure must be employed. The pharmacist must wear disposable gloves and a laboratory coat to prevent direct contamination of skin and clothing. Three factors that determine the radiation dose received by the pharmacist are time, distance, and shielding.

Time. The longer it takes to prepare the radiopharmaceutical, the greater the radiation exposure to the pharmacist. To minimize the time that the pharmacist is exposed to radiation, all needed materials should be readied before

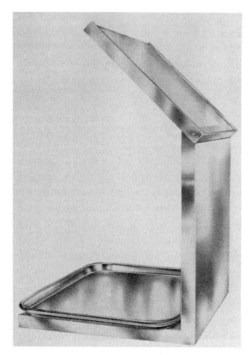

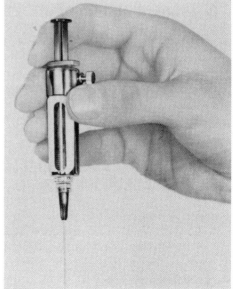

Figure 13–5. Shield used to provide protection to the head and body of workers who handle radionuclides that emit gamma radiation. (Courtesy of Atomic Products Corporation, Center Moriches, NY.)

Figure 13–6. Syringe shields are used to reduce radiation exposure to fingers and hands of nuclear pharmacists. (Courtesy of Atomic Products Corporation, Center Moriches, NY.)

the preparation of the radiopharmaceutical begins. The pharmacist must work quickly, but not with such haste that carelessness could become a factor. Before a procedure is to be performed for a first time, a "dry run" should be done; i.e., the complete procedure should be performed, using nonradioactive material.

Distance. Because gamma radiation exposure varies as the inverse square with its distance from the body, radioactive drugs should be stored and handled in such a way as to maximize the distance between the pharmacist and the source of radioactivity. Thus, working at arm's length provides a significant reduction of radiation exposure to the body of the pharmacist. For highly radioactive drugs, tongs or other remote handling devices should be used.

Shielding. Shielding is used to reduce radiation exposure. Lead bricks and lead shields are used for storing the ^{99m}Mo-^{99m}Tc generator. Lead shields are also used for vials containing radioactivity and for dispensing syringes containing radiopharmaceuticals. Lead glass shields, such as the one shown in Figure 13–5, are used to protect the pharmacist's body during the preparation of radiopharmaceuticals. To protect the hands while doses are being drawn, lead glass, lead acrylic, and tungsten syringe shields are available (Figure 13–6). These shields may reduce finger and hand exposure to ^{99m}Tc by as much as 150%.

If the procedures that have been outlined are followed during preparation, dispensing, and storage of radiopharmaceuticals, the pharmacist's radiation dose will be kept to a very low level. The risk of biologic effects to the nuclear pharmacist from this occupational exposure is very small and is acceptable by today's standards for radiation safety.

Biological Bibliography

Carey, J.E., Jr., Kline, R.C., and Keyes, J.W., Jr. (eds.): Manual of Nuclear Medicine Procedures. Boca Raton, FL, CRC Press, 1983.

Chilton, H.M., and Witcofabi, R.L.: Nuclear Pharmacy: An Introduction to the Clinical Application of Radiopharmaceuticals. Philadelphia, Lea & Febiger, 1986.

Hladik, W.B., III, Nigg, K.K., and Rhodes, B.A.: Drug induced changes in the biologic distribution of radiopharmaceuticals. Semin. Nucl. Med., 12:184 (1982).

Hladik, W.B., Saha, G.B., and Study, K.T.: Essentials of Nuclear Medicine Science. Baltimore, Williams & Wilkins, 1987.

Nuclear Pharmacy Practice Standards, Section on Nuclear Pharmacy. Academy of Pharmacy Practice, American Pharmaceutical Association. Washington, D.C. (1978).

Rhodes, B.A., and Croft, B.Y.: Basics of Radiopharmacy. St. Louis, C.V. Mosby, 1978.

Saha, G.: Fundamentals of Nuclear Pharmacy. 3rd Ed. New York, Springer-Verlag, 1992.

Srivastava, S.V., and Chervu, L.R.: Radionuclide labeled red blood cells: Current status and future prospects. Semin. Nucl. Med., 14:68 (1984).

CHAPTER

Devices

The federal Food, Drug, and Cosmetic Act defines the term "devices" as instruments, apparatus, and contrivances, including their components, parts, and accessories, intended (1) for use in the diagnosis, cure, mitigation, treatment, or prevention of disease in man or other animals; or (2) to affect the structure or any function of the body of man or other animals. In this chapter, the term "devices" is used for the equipment needed for the administration of parenteral drugs. These devices include syringes, cannulas, and final filtration mechanisms. Like parenteral dosage forms, these devices must be sterile, pyrogen-free, and free from particulate matter.

Syringes

Even after the recognition of the necessity to use sterile equipment for the parenteral administration of sterile solutions late in the nineteenth century, there was a lack of materials for making syringes suitable for steam sterilization. In 1896, an all-glass syringe with a cylindrical piston ground to fit a graduated glass barrel was invented by Karl Schneider, a mechanic of H. Wolfgang Luer of Paris. This syringe was able to withstand steam sterilization. The Luer syringe was the prototype of the present-day glass syringe. Soon afterward, an American patent was issued and subsequently sold to Becton, Dickinson and Company in 1898.

With the development of local anesthesia, there came a demand for a secure and easy method of removing and attaching the needle to the syringe. Several attempts were made and some of the approaches were successful. About 1925, the Luer-Lok syringe was developed by Col. F.S. Dickinson of Becton, Dickinson and Company. The Luer-Lok syringe has a thread inside the metal tip that engages the rim of the needle, and only a half-turn is needed to fasten securely or to remove the needle from the syringe.

Syringe tips have been categorized into four basic groups (Fig. 14–1):

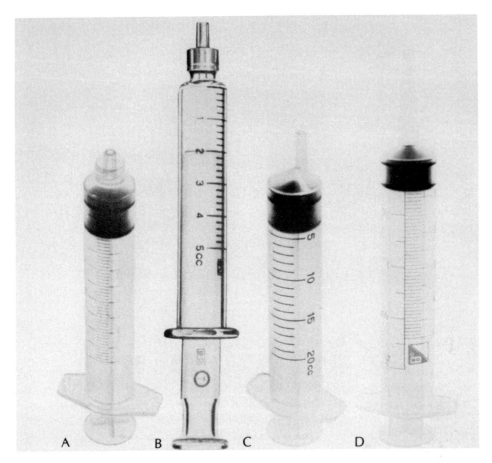

Figure 14–1. Syringe tips. A, Luer-Lok tip; B, Luer Slip tip; C, eccentric tip; D, catheter tip.

1. Luer-Lok Tip. This kind of tip is stronger than a regular tip. It is permanently attached to reinforce a heavy glass base on the syringe and is threaded to accept a Luer-Lok needle. Once attached, the needle is locked to the syringe until unlocked. It cannot pop off accidentally.
2. Luer Slip Tip. Luer Slip needles do not lock in place. They have the disadvantage of sometimes allowing the needle to pop off from the pressure of injection.
3. Eccentric Tip. This infrequently used tip is designed off-center for use when the needle is to be kept as nearly parallel to the field of injection as possible.
4. Catheter Tip. This is not used for injection, but when surgical tubing or a catheter is to be attached directly to the syringe. This type of syringe tip is commonly used for irrigation.

Types of Syringes

Syringes currently used can be classified according to their composition as glass reusable, glass disposable, and plastic disposable. Disposable syringes

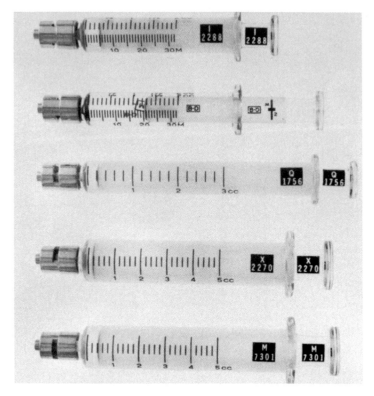

Figure 14–2. Reusable glass Luer-Lok syringes. (Courtesy of Becton, Dickinson and Co., Rutherford, NJ.)

are intended for one-time use only. It is standard practice to use disposable syringes for injection. In a few situations, disposable plastic syringes are reused, for example, for multiple injections into the same patient or in admixture programs when the same drug may be required during the day. This practice should be discouraged. The infection hazard from reusing disposable plastic syringes has been published.[1] The possibility of leaching and other drug interactions exists when drugs are stored in plastic syringes,[2] and the practice of such storing should be discouraged. One report[3] described experimental tissue culture death related to possible syringe extraction. A comparison of disposable syringe systems has been published.[4] The desirability of one over another depends on cost, product packaging, needle sharpness, ability to read dosage measurement, safety during and disposability after use, and individual preference.

Syringes are available in sizes from 1-ml to 60-ml capacity, and all share the design of a round plunger or piston within a barrel. For reusable syringes, the glass plunger is ground to fit a given barrel exactly, and for many syringes the parts cannot be interchanged. The needle affixed to the tip of the syringe barrel may be held in place by friction or locked in place, as is the Luer-Lok syringe (Fig. 14–2). In the latter instance, the needle is not dislodged by pressure from the plunger or by improper placement. The barrel of the syringe is graduated in milliliters; the larger the syringes, the larger are the

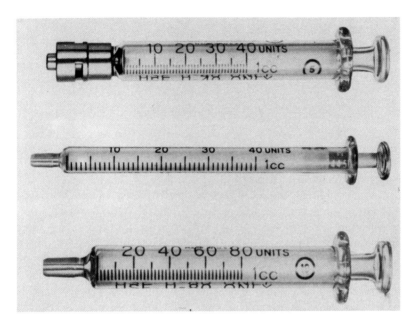

Figure 14–3. Insulin syringes. (Courtesy of Becton, Dickinson and Co., Rutherford, NJ.)

graduated increments. In the design of syringes for small volumes such as 1 ml, the barrel is long and slender to give greater accuracy in measuring volumes.

Insulin syringes are graduated in units of insulin (40 units, 40 and 80 units, 80 units, and 100 units per ml) (Fig. 14–3). Approximately 1,000,000 diabetics require daily insulin; it is estimated that 400,000,000 insulin injections are administered annually. About 75% of these injections are made with disposable syringes.[5] Three insulin strengths are available: U-40, U-80, and U-100. Separate syringes for each insulin strength are required. It is anticipated that in the future the U-100 insulin will replace the lower strengths currently available.

The two basic lengths of insulin syringes are long and short. The total volume is the same in both. The long type offers scale markings that are farther apart, allowing the scale to be read more easily. Syringes should not be used interchangeably.

U-100 syringes are available from a number of suppliers. In addition, several manufacturers have introduced low-dose insulin syringes—0.5 ml used for U-100 insulin and calibrated up to 50 units.* By reducing the capacity, the accuracy is increased, and for those diabetics using low doses this type of syringe is preferred. The Busher automatic injector[†] has been used as a semi-automatic method of injecting insulin, providing automatic insertion of the needle at the proper depth and angle. A pressure type of device that utilizes no needle is also available.[‡]

---

*Becton, Dickinson and Co., Rutherford, NJ; Sherwood Medical, St. Louis, MO.
†Becton, Dickinson and Co., Rutherford, NJ.
‡Medi-Jector-Daystrol Scientific, Inc., Minneapolis, MN.

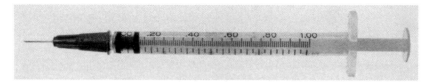

Figure 14–4. Plastic tuberculin syringe. (Courtesy of Becton, Dickinson and Co., Rutherford, NJ.)

Tuberculin syringes have capacities of 1 ml, and a volume of 0.05 ml can be measured with accuracy (Fig. 14–4).

Owing to the problems (such as serum hepatitis) associated with cleaning and resterilization of glass reusable syringes, along with breakage and high cost, glass reusable syringes have made way for disposable syringes (Fig. 14–5). Glass disposable syringes cost less than glass reusable ones, but more than those made from plastic. Compared with plastic syringes, glass disposable syringes have the advantage of possessing the handling and physical characteristics associated with glass. Injections stored in glass may present fewer compatibility problems than those stored in plastic. When injections must be stored, disposable glass syringes are preferred.

Plastic syringes are usually made from either polyethylene or polypropylene plastic and are available as sterile packaged items (Fig. 14–6). They are sterilized after packaging with either ethylene oxide or radiation. Syringes made

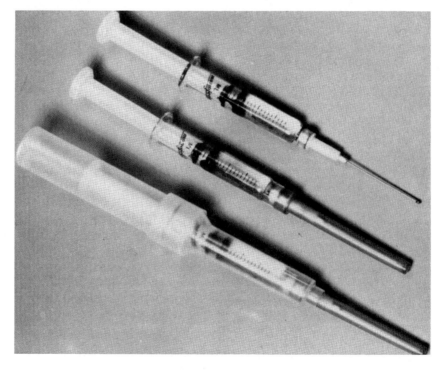

Figure 14–5. Disposable glass syringes. (Courtesy of Sherwood Corporation, St. Louis, MO.)

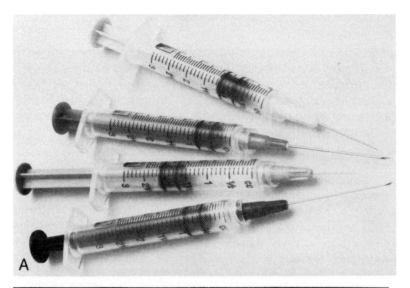

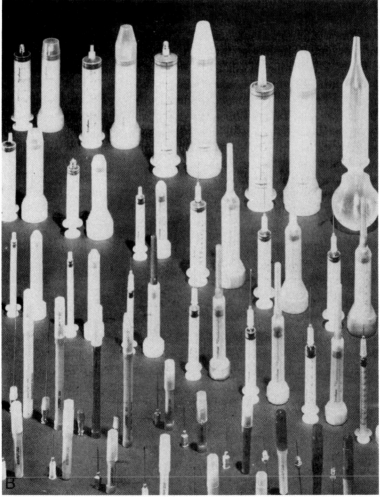

Figure 14–6. Disposable plastic syringes. (A, Courtesy of Becton, Dickinson and Co., Rutherford, NJ. B, Courtesy of Sherwood Corporation, St. Louis, MO.)

from polypropylene are stable to autoclaving, which is important in the preparation of surgical trays. Only polypropylene plastic syringes can be packed into these trays for resterilization in an autoclave. Prefilled syringes and the filling of prefilled disposable syringes are discussed in Chapter 12. Several companies manufacture plastic disposable syringes (American Hospital Supply; Becton, Dickinson and Co.; Sherwood Medical Industries).

Syringes and "Dead Space"

All syringes contain so-called dead space. The dead space refers to the space occupied by the needle bore and the space above the needle, the hub, and the space in the hub of the syringe. The dead space varies with the needle size and the manufacturer of the needle and syringe. It is of no consequence when preparing for a usual injection; the extra volume drawn into the syringe during aspiration remains in the syringe after injection. The syringe calibration takes the dead space into consideration. The syringe markings start above the syringe hub. Dead space becomes of some consequence when two drugs are drawn up into the same syringe, particularly if the dose is concentrated into a small volume of liquid.

The problem of dead space is particularly important when preparing insulin mixtures. Kochevar and Fry[5] made a significant contribution when they recognized the following:

> The problem that dead space volume presents when preparing insulin mixtures in the syringe is illustrated by the following example. Assume the "dead space" to be 8 insulin units of volume and the mixture to be prepared is 20 units of NPH Insulin and 10 units of Regular Insulin. The desired ratio of insulins in this example is 2:1 (NPH to Regular).
>
> When the 10 units of Regular Insulin are drawn into the syringe, 18 units are actually present in the syringe (measured volume plus "dead space" volume). When the 20 units of NPH Insulin are then drawn, the final mixture in the syringe is composed of 18 units of Regular Insulin and 20 units of NPH Insulin. The patient will receive a total of 30 units of insulin, but instead of the 20 units of NPH Insulin and 10 units of Regular Insulin (2:1), he will receive 15.8 units of NPH Insulin and 14.2 units of Regular Insulin (1.1:1). The error in the ratio of this particular example is considerable. As the total dose of insulins and the ratio of insulins vary, so will the error produced by the "dead space" volume. The error will also of course depend on the order of mixing of the insulins. If the order of mixing in the above example were reversed, the ratio would be greater than 2:1 (2.8:1).
>
> If the patient is currently stabilized on a particular dose, technique, and syringe system, there would seem to be little problem as long as he remains on that regimen. However, changing the total dose, ratio of insulins, mixing technique, and/or the syringe system may have considerable effect on maintaining an expected glycemic response.[5]

Four different brands of syringes were studied, and considerable dead space variance existed among brands. The FDA Drug Bulletin[6] noted this hazard, and manufacturers of insulin syringes are aware of the problem and are required to include a warning statement in the labeling of their products. Inaccurate dosage of insulin because of dead space variance was also noted by Shainfield[7] and by Rosenbloom.[8] Feingold[9] also confirmed dead space errors in plastic as well as in various brands of glass syringes.

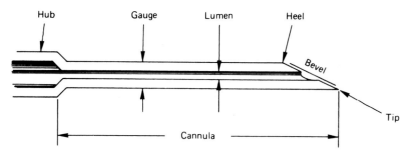

Figure 14–7. Diagram of a hollow, metal intravenous needle.

Cannulae

Hollow Needles

The device most frequently used for penetrating the skin is a hollow needle made from stainless steel composed of nickel, chromium, and iron. As shown in Figure 14–7, the needle consists of a hollow shaft enlarged at one end to form a hub by which it is attached to a syringe or an administration set. The other end of the needle is beveled, forming a tip to maximize ease of insertion and to reduce tissue trauma (Fig. 14–8A). Some needles are coated with silicone for lubrication and aid in penetration. Needle sizes are specified by the length of the cannula and the gauge. Needles range in length from $^3/_8$ to 6 in. The gauge of the needle refers to the outside diameter (O.D.) of the shaft and is based on the Birmingham wire standards (Fig. 14–8B). Hollow needles

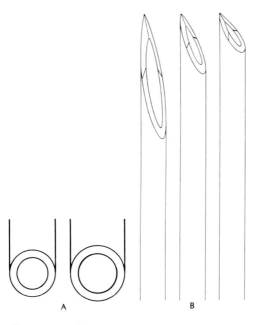

Figure 14–8. A, Needle gauges. B, Needle bevels. Left to right: regular, short, and intradermal.

are available in sizes from 13 to 27 gauge. A 13-gauge needle has an O.D. of 0.095 in., whereas the 27-gauge needle has an O.D. of 0.016 in.; thus, the larger the gauge of the needle, the smaller the diameter and the lumen.

Needles are available commercially designated as "thin-wall." As the name indicates, the wall of the needle is thinner than that of the conventional needle. It offers the advantage of a larger lumen for a given outside diameter. The larger-sized lumen allows fast flow rates, while the outside diameter is kept small. The three basic needle bevel designs are available as follows:

1. *Regular.* Most common design used. Particularly useful for I.M. and S.C. injections.
2. *Short bevel.* Useful for intravenous and intraspinal use where there is danger of penetrating the blood vessel wall.
3. *Intradermal.* Designed for intradermal administration.

In selecting a needle, the choice of length depends on the site of administration and the depth of penetration into the body, whereas the gauge depends on the viscosity of the fluid to be injected or withdrawn. Long, small-gauge (large-lumen) needles are preferred for venipuncture in adults and for intramuscular injections. For infants, penetration of small veins, and intradermal and subcutaneous injections, large-gauge (small-lumen) needles are used. A wide variety of needles (beyond common usage) is required for various special purposes: radiology, anesthesia, biopsy, cardiovascular and eye work, transfusion, blood collecting, hemorrhoidal and tonsil procedures, tracheotomy. The selection of needle size frequently depends on the clinician. A suggested needle selection, depending on the site of administration, as followed at Temple University Health Sciences Center is shown in Table 14–1.

In the past, needles were sharpened and sterilized for reuse. Currently most needles are considered disposable and are used only once.

Winged Needles

Originally used for pediatric and geriatric patients, the winged needle (scalp-vein; butterfly; Minicath; Venocut; scalp and small vein set; prn adapter; E-Z Set; Miniset; small vein administration set) is becoming increasingly popular for intravenous therapy. It consists of a stainless steel needle, two flexible wing-like projections mounted on the needle, a short length of flexible tubing, and a female adaptor that can accept any fluid administration set (Fig. 14–9). The wings are used to make the venipuncture and then are taped to the patient to keep the needle securely within the vein.

Winged needles are commonly used for intermittent heparin therapy. The proximal end contains a gum rubber plug that can be used as an injection site. Winged needles are $^3/_4$ in. long and 16 to 23 gauge.

Heparin Locks

A heparin lock is a scalp vein infusion set (needle attached to $3^1/_2$-in. plastic tubing) (Fig. 14–9A) capped by a resealable latex diaphragm. These sets are available from several companies. Originally used for pediatric and geriatric patients, heparin locks are becoming increasingly popular for a variety of other uses, such as the intermittent or continuous administration of fluids or drugs including heparin. The use of a heparin lock unit has the advantage of access to the vascular system, allows the patient more flexibility than hanging KVO

TABLE 14–1.   Needle Selection

Injection Site	Length Range (in.)	Gauge Range
Intradermal (intracutaneous)	$^1/_4$ to $^5/_8$	24 to 26
Subcutaneous (hypodermic)	$^1/_4$ to $^5/_8$	24 to 25
Intramuscular	1 to 2	19 to 22
Intravenous		
Metal needle	1 to 2	15 to 25
Winged needle	$^3/_4$ to 1 $^1/_2$	16 to 23
Plastic needle	3 to 5	15 to 21
Intracatheter	11 $^1/_2$	15 to 21
In-lying catheter	12, 36	14, 15
Hypodermoclysis		
Adult	2	19
Pediatric	1 to 1 $^1/_2$	20 to 22
Intraosseous		
Biopsy needle	4 $^1/_4$	10
Aspiration needle	2	16
Intra-articulate (intrasynovial)	1 to 3	19 to 22
Intraperitoneal	4 to 6	14
Intramyocardial	3 $^1/_2$	18 to 21
Intrathoracic	5 to 6	13
Intraspinal (intravertebral)		
Adult	3 to 5	20 to 22
Pediatric	1 to 1 $^1/_2$	25
Neonatal	$^1/_2$ to 1	27

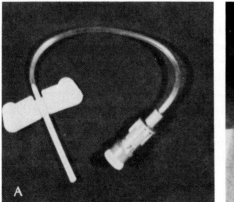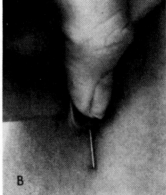

Figure 14–9.   Butterfly infusion set has dual-purpose wings molded onto needle cannula. During venipuncture, wings fold flat against patient's skin and serve as an anchor for taping (A). When wings are folded together, they can be used as a needle holder (B). Butterfly infusion sets are available in a variety of sizes and styles. Special-purpose sets are available for surgical, pediatric, geriatric, hemodialysis, and intermittent intravenous procedures. (Courtesy of Abbott Laboratories, North Chicago, IL.)

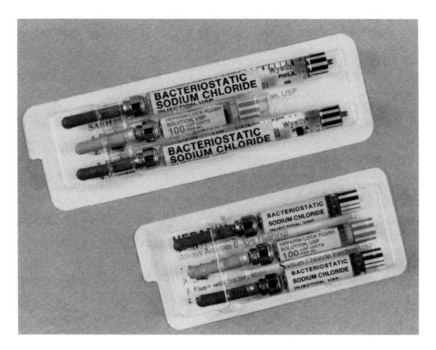

Figure 14–10. Heparin flush kit. (Courtesy of Wyeth Laboratories, Philadelphia, PA.)

I.V. fluid, allows reduction of volume of fluid administered from I.V. (this is particularly important with cardiac patients in whom fluid volumes must be kept limited), and eliminates KVO bottles. Locks can be used for collection of blood samples for glucose tolerance, kidney function, and other tests, thus eliminating the need for multiple punctures. Patients with locks can carry on drug administration outside the hospital environment. Some disadvantages to heparin locks include occlusion or blood clotting within the lock (needle bore or tubing); the possibility of speed shock or damage from a drug being rapidly introduced into the circulation; and the inadvertent push of drugs into the lock that should be diluted first. Some drugs are incompatible with the heparin that may be present in the lock and special techniques are required to prevent drug-heparin incompatibility. The use of large-bore needles should be avoided, because multiple punctures may damage the diaphragm.

When heparin locks are in place for intermittent therapy (and when heparin is not the drug being used for therapy), it is necessary to place a sufficient amount of diluted heparin (heparin-saline) solution in the lock to maintain the patency of the set.[10] Although no standard exists as to the concentration of this solution, only small amounts are needed. In one survey[11] of hospitals, concentrations of heparin varied from 0 to 1000 units of heparin per milliliter; most hospitals used 100 units/ml. A volume of approximately 0.2 to 0.4 ml is required to fill the cannula. A number of manufacturers have made available heparin solutions of 100 units/ml for use in these sets (Fig. 14–10). The incompatibilities of heparin have been reported.[12] Thomas[13] reported meperidine and heparin precipitation when heparin was used to maintain the patency of the lock; and other drug incompatibilities have been reported.[14] This means that, before each intermittent drug injection through the cannula, the lock must be flushed with 1 ml of sodium chloride injection to remove the heparin. The diluted heparin solution is then added.

Use of 1000 units/ml heparin solution has been reported to cause transient increase in the activated partial thromboplastin time.[15] This concentration should be avoided. A comparison by Hanson[16] of KVO versus heparin lock on the incidence of complications showed that overall complications were equal. Hanson et al.,[17] in a series of experimental and clinical studies followed by clinical observations and evaluation, showed that a concentration of 10 U.S.P. units of sodium heparin per milliliter of normal saline solution will maintain potency of heparin locks without affecting the clotting time, prothrombin time, or activated partial thromboplastin time. A procedure of flushing the heparin lock with 1 ml of the recommended heparin-saline solution following each intravenous injection of medication, or every 8 hours if medications are not given more frequently, is suggested.

Stern et al.[18] reported on the use of the lock to inject numerous antibiotics, digoxin, ethacrynic acid, and vitamin K without complications or incidents. Kimmel[19] used the lock to inject steroids, heparin, and antihemophilic factor without complications. Rucker and Harrison[20] described a procedure for the I.V. administration of antibiotics on an outpatient basis utilizing the heparin lock. Ferguson et al.[21] reported on the complications with heparin-lock needles. Their data suggest that heparin-lock needles be removed every 48 to 72 hours or at least every 4 days to lessen the risk of phlebitis. The proper techniques for insertion, care, and maintenance of heparin locks have been discussed by DeFina.[22] The use of heparin locks in neonates has also been reported.[23]

Wiltsee has described the use of the heparin needle to obtain difficult venipunctures.[24] Couchonnal et al.,[25] in a study of heparin locks, found a significant reduction in cases of phlebitis when the heparin lock was used with iodophor solution as a skin preparation. Several questions are asked frequently concerning heparin locks. How often should they be changed? Heparin-lock needles must be changed routinely every 72 hours, or sooner if evidence of phlebitis or bacteremia develops. How should the heparin lock be cleared? Heparin-lock flush solutions and saline solutions are used to keep the lock clot free and prevent heparin-drug incompatibilities.

The procedure is as follows:
1. Before administering medication, clear lock with Sodium Chloride Injection, U.S.P.
2. Administer medication.
3. Clear lock again with Sodium Chloride Injection, U.S.P.
4. Reinstill heparin-lock flush solution.

In recent years, the use of heparin flush solutions has been called into question.[26,27] At least five different studies[27-31] affirm that 0.9% sodium chloride injection is as effective as heparin for maintaining the patency of intermittent intravenous devices. Apparently this issue is not resolved; pharmaceutical manufacturers continue to sell large amounts of heparin lock kits for patency.

Volume Occupied by Central Venous Catheters and Implantable Vascular Access Devices

Several types of central venous catheters are used in hospitals and on an outpatient basis. They are used for a variety of parenteral medications, such as total parenteral nutrition solutions, cancer chemotherapy, long-term anti-biotic therapy, and blood components, as well as other medication. The length of time central venous catheters remain in place can vary from days to months and, in some few cases, years. When not in use, central catheters require heparinization (Heparin-Lock Flush Solution, U.S.P.) in order to maintain patency of the catheter lumen.

The amount of heparin required to maintain patency has not been standardized. Concentrations used have varied from no heparin to 1000 units/ml; the volume of heparinized saline has also varied considerably. An enlightening study[32] of four commonly used catheters (Hickman, Broviac, Centrasil, Intrasil) illustrated that the volume of heparinized solution that would be required to fill these catheters ranged from 0.2 ml (Centrasil) to a high of 1.90 ml (Hickman).

Newton et al.[33] studied the volume occupied in vascular access devices in order to determine the quantity of heparin necessary for a flush. The volume occupied by the extension set and the ports ranged from 0.21 ml to 1.18 ml. Although no standard for adequate flushing exists, the devices studied can aid the practitioners in formulating a reasonable judgment.

Practitioners should be aware that only small amounts of heparin are required to fill these catheters completely.

Indwelling Catheters

Fluids and drugs can be administered into veins by the use of plastic catheters, eliminating the need for multiple punctures during prolonged intravenous therapy. These catheters are made from materials such as polyvinyl chloride, Teflon, and polyethylene, and should be radiopaque to ensure that they will be visible on x-ray films. Accidental severance or loss of a part of the catheter necessitates its surgical removal. All catheters should be removed within 48 hours of insertion.

The choice of catheter depends on the length of time of the infusion, the purpose of the infusion, and the condition and availability of the veins. Three types of catheters are available:

1. Plain plastic catheter (in-lying catheter; cutdown catheter). This device consists of a variable length of plastic tubing (without needle) designed for insertion into a vein by surgical incision (cutdown). This type of catheter is usually reserved for emergency situations in which superficial veins are unavailable for percutaneous venipuncture (Fig. 14–11).

2. Catheter-over-needle or catheter-outside-needle (plastic needle; catheter mounted on a needle; Jelco; Angiocath; Abbocath-T; Medicut; Medicath). The catheter accompanies the needle into the vein during venipuncture. Once in the vein, the catheter hub is held in place, and the needle is removed and discarded; the plastic catheter remains in the vein (Fig. 14–12). The connection is then made with the administration set. The catheter-over-needle is used for routine percutaneous venipuncture of peripheral veins for intravenous infusion of solutions and drugs. Plastic stylets are available for insertion to maintain patency if intermittent infusion or injection is required.

3. Catheter-inside-needle (intracatheter; catheter inserted through needle; Venocath; Intracath; Intramedicut). This catheter consists of a stainless

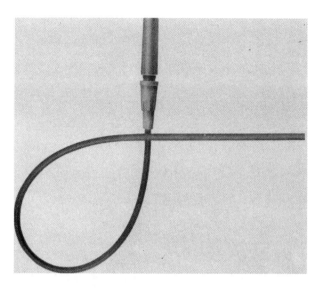

Figure 4–11. Plain plastic catheter.

steel needle with a length of plastic tubing lying inside its lumen (Fig. 14–13). After venipuncture is made, the plastic catheter is advanced the desired distance into the vein. After being withdrawn, the needle remains on the external portion of the device and is secured with tape to the patient. The catheter should never be withdrawn through the needle because there is danger of the needle point shearing the catheter; this could result in fragments migrating into the vein where they can cause emboli. This type of catheter is generally preferred to a surgical cutdown catheter.

Internal Methods Utilized To Achieve Intravascular Access

Implantable Devices: Implantable Ports*

Broviac and Hickman catheters have been used to achieve long-term venous access in various diseases. Although these catheters are widely used, they are associated with some morbidity, including fracture of catheters, entrance site infection, and catheter sepsis. Implantable catheters have been developed to overcome catheter complications and are designed to permit repeated access to the infusion site. For repeated I.V. fluid delivery, the system can be used repeatedly. The implantable catheter consists of implantable grade silicone tubing connected to a stainless steel port with a self-sealing septum that allows needle access (Fig. 14–14). The delivery catheter can be placed in a vein, cavity, artery, or CNS system. The system is accessed with a Huber point needle through the skin into the self-sealing silicone plug positioned in the center of the portal.

The specialized Huber point needle is designed with an angle level that reduces coring and permits easy entry. These implantable ports can be used

*Infuse-A-Port, Infusaid Corporation, Norwood, MA; Port-A-Cath: Pharmacia Laboratories, Piscataway, NJ.

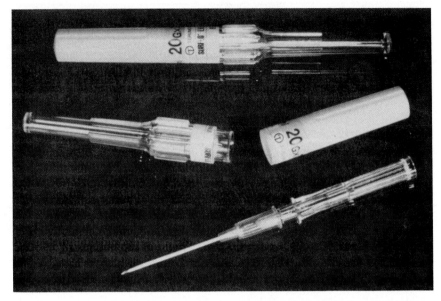

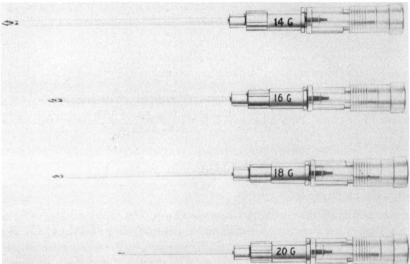

Figure 14–12. Catheter-over-needle. (Top, courtesy of Terumo Corporation, Piscataway, NJ. Bottom, courtesy of Abbott Laboratories, North Chicago, IL.)

for the injection of I.V. fluids, total parenteral nutrition, chemotherapy, antibiotics, and other drugs.

Some advantages of implantable devices include:

1. Need for a long-term access site to venous, arterial, and spinal systems.
2. Increased dependence on "nonhospital" treatment of chronic disease states.
3. Direct infusion on a target organ or tumor.
4. Decrease the infection rates seen with percutaneous catheters or repeated spinal taps.
5. Allow greater mobility for the patient (return to normal function).

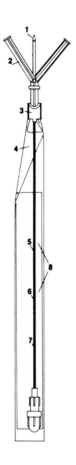

Figure 14–13. Flexible intravenous catheter-inside-needle (Venocath). This catheter is radiopaque so that its position in the vein is readily visible on x-ray films. A removable stainless steel stylet prevents the catheter from buckling while being threaded into the vein. After the needle is withdrawn from the vein, a folding guard shields the entire length of the needle. The assembly consists of (1) needle, (2) folding needle guard, (3) quick-release clip securing protective sleeve, (4) protective sleeve, (5) ultrasoft catheter tubing, (6) nonbuckling stainless steel stylet for easy catheter "threading," (7) full-length radiopaque stripe, and (8) 11 $\frac{1}{2}$-in. plastic catheter. (Courtesy of Abbott Laboratories, North Chicago, IL.)

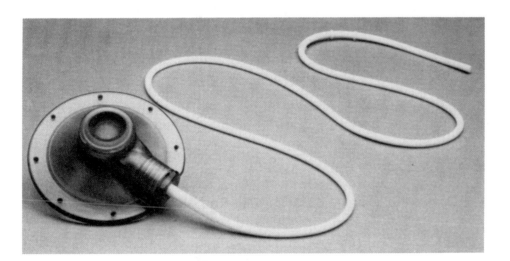

Figure 14–14.   Infuse-A-Port. (Courtesy of Infusaid Corporation, Norwood, MA.)

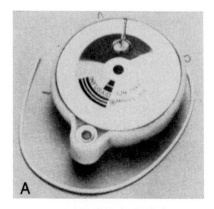

Figure 14–15. Photograph (A) and diagram (B) of Infusaid Model 400 Implantable Pump. (Courtesy of Infusaid Corporation, Norwood, MA.)

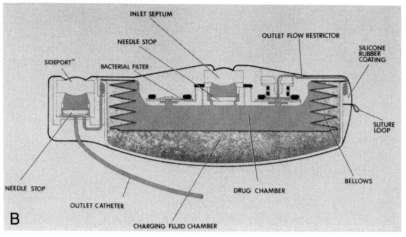

Implantable Devices: Implantable Pumps

Infusaid Implantable Pump*. The Infusaid Implantable Pump was approved for selected drug administration (Fig. 14–15). This pump is the size of a hockey puck and weighs approximately 6-1/2 oz. The construction is titanium, stainless steel, and polypropylene. The injection part is constructed of silicone rubber and has a usable life of at least 2000 punctures. Under normal use, this device has an 8 years plus life span.

The internal power supply uses freon in equilibrium between the gaseous and liquid states and is "recharged" with each refilling process. This supplies power for as long as the pump is needed. As the pump is refilled, it compresses the gas back into the liquid state, thus allowing a fresh supply of "energy" for the next cycle. The capacity of this pump is 50 ml, which can be administered over 14 days. The pump accuracy is stated as +3%. The cost of one model is approximately $4,000. This cost does not include the surgical implant procedure. The 14-day cycle cannot be altered to any degree.

Infusaid Model 400 Implantable Drug Delivery System*. The Infusaid Model 400 Implantable Drug Delivery System is designed for long-term therapy in

---

*Infusaid Corporation, Norwood, MA.

TABLE 14–2. Final Filtering Devices

Trade Name	Manufacturer	Type of Filter	Porosity (μ)
Final filter	Baxter Healthcare Laboratories	Membrane	0.5
In-line membrane filter	McGaw Laboratories	Membrane	0.45
RPM filter	McGaw Laboratories	Depth	5 (approx.)
Saif filter	Abbott Laboratories	Membrane	1
Saftiset I.V. filter	Cutter Laboratories	Membrane	1
Microporous final I.V. filter	Extracorporeal Medical	Membrane	0.45
Microporous final I.V. filter	Extracorporeal Medical	Membrane	0.22
Aspiration needle with filter	Sherwood Medical Industries, Inc.	Stainless steel	5
5-μ filter needle	Jelco Laboratories	Stainless steel	5
Filter straw	Burron Medical Products	Nylon	5
Ultipor	Pall Corporation	Membrane	0.22
IVEX-2	Abbott Laboratories	Membrane	0.22
MP-5	Baxter Healthcare Laboratories	Depth	5
Extension set	Baxter Healthcare Laboratories	Membrane	0.22
PMF	McGaw Laboratories	Depth	5
ACF	McGaw Laboratories	Membrane	0.22

ambulatory patients. The Model 400 with a 47 ml usable drug volume delivers a precise, continuous flow to a selected organ or site via a soft, non-traumatic, non-thrombogenic silicone rubber catheter. The Model 400 also features an auxiliary sideport septum, completely bypassing the pumping mechanism, for delivery of direct bolus injections to the target site. This allows the clinician to easily supplement the continuos infusion with additional drugs, objectively assess disease states, or monitor catheter location and drug perfusion with the use of radio-labeled microspheres.

Final Filtering Devices

Concern for the occurrence of particulate matter in large-volume parenteral solutions, whether it originated in the solutions, as the result of drug admixture incompatibilities, from manipulation of the solution, or from the administration set, led to the suggestion to produce intravenous administration sets with a suitable filter in the chamber to retard the passage of undesirable particles. In the design of devices that followed, the intravenous fluid or drug enters a chamber containing a membrane filter and passes through the filter prior to entering the vein. Devices are available with membrane filters having varying porosities (Table 14–2). In hyperalimentation therapy, the filters have shown value in preventing septicemia and in reducing phlebitis. Several manufacturers have designed relatively inexpensive depth-type filters for use in recovering drugs from vials and ampuls. Filter aspiration needle, 5-micron filter needle, filter straw, and RPM filter are examples. Filters having a porosity of 0.22 μ may require an infusion pump for satisfactory flow.

Final filters have several limitations. Administration of blood, emulsions, or suspensions through final filters is contraindicated. Air lock may be a problem for personnel not familiar with these devices. When wet, membranes with a porosity of 0.22 and 0.45 μ are impervious to air at normal pressures. Air in the system causes blockage. In order to prevent air lock, the filter housing must be completely purged of air prior to use. The more recently developed filters provide air eliminators that solve the problem of air blockage. Use of these devices requires additional training and may be confusing in the training period. Cost of administration of medication is increased. The single greatest advantage of final filter devices is their ability to reduce the infusion of particulate matter into the vascular system.[34,35]

Because endotoxin can pass freely through bacterial retaining filters, one of the concerns for the use of inline filters is the release of endotoxin produced by bacteria trapped on the filter.[36,37]

In a clinical setting, antibiotics are frequently administered along with the intravenous fluid. In such a case, the contaminating bacteria susceptible to the antibiotic probably would not have a chance to proliferate on the filter. Such contamination could occur, however, if antibiotics were administered subsequently to beginning I.V. administration. Because there is no way of telling during use whether the filters have been contaminated, subsequent administration of antibiotics increases the risk of endotoxin release. As a precaution, if antibiotics are to be initiated during intravenous fluid administration, the inline filter should be changed prior to beginning therapy. Also, if antibiotics are being administered through a medication chamber on a 12- to 24-hour basis, it is advisable to replace the filter every 24 hours. Continual administration of antibiotics during I.V. infusion lessens the risk of bacterial proliferation on the filter; and consequently, minimizes the risk of releasing pyrogenic substances.

Competitive Products

Filtration can be accomplished by either depth or screen type filters. Filters may be add-on, purchased separately from the administration set and added on at time of use; or inline, an integral component of the administration set. There may be air-eliminating venting of air to a reservoir in the unit, or an air-venting filter that vents air to the atmosphere. The first generation filters, which are still available, are non-air-eliminating or air-venting. A problem that has occurred with air-venting filters when they have been used with pumps (pressure) and one particular drug multivitamin infusion is weeping of the drug through the hydropholic (air-venting) membrane. Multivitamin infusion contains a surfactant (surface-tension reducing agent) that under the pressure of pumps allows the hydrophobic (non-wettable filter) to be wetted, with the resulting effect of weeping of the drug. Manufacturers have introduced high-pressure (HP) filters to solve this problem.

Drug Adsorption to Membrane Filters

Although considerable information is available concerning the clinical use of filters in entrapping particles and microorganisms, little information exists describing drug adsorption to the filter. Wyeth Laboratories conducted ampicillin assays on clinically used filters. Assay reports indicated no filter adsorption of ampicillin: "All solutions had identical and acceptable potency."[38]

A publication by Wagman et al.[39] described adsorption of considerable amounts of various antibiotics, including gentamicin, to various filter media; however, none of these filters media (cellulose powder, diatomaceous earth, and Seitz filter sheets) resembles the characteristics and qualities of clinical filters. Subsequent assays indicated that "little or no activity was removed by the membrane filter."[40]

Work done at the University of Kentucky[41] showed insignificant quantities of penicillin blocked by the filter. Assays of bleomycin sulfate (Blenoxane)[42] through a 0.45-μm membrane filter indicated insignificant adsorption.

Work done by Huber et al.[43] using 0.22-μm filters with amphotericin B (a colloidal suspension) indicated filter adsorption. These authors indicated that 0.22-μm filters were inappropriate for use with this product. At pH 5.6, only filters with pore sizes of 1.0 μm or greater showed acceptable results. In contrast, Piecoro et al.[44] studied filtration of amphotericin B infusions; their data showed that filtration through 0.85- and 0.45-μm filters did not reduce the in vitro antimicrobial activity, and filtration through 5-, 0.45-, and 0.22-μm filters did not alter the concentration of the drug, as shown spectrophotometrically.

No significant drug loss occurred[45] with prochlorperazine, dexamethasone, digoxin, hydrocortisone, lidocaine, or isoproterenol when filtered through a 0.45-μm filter. Stennet et al.[46] studied drug loss of cefazolin sodium (10 mg/ml) through a 0.22-μm filter and a 0.45-μm filter and found no drug loss.

Butler et al.[47] showed that the potency of drugs administered intravenously in small doses could be significantly reduced during inline filtration with a filter containing a cellulose ester membrane. Measurable reduction in potency occurred with digitoxin, insulin, mithramycin, and vincristine sulfate. No reduction in potency occurred with bleomycin sulfate, cyanocobalamin, ergonovine maleate, folic acid, heparin, levarterenol bitartrate, oxytocin, and vinblastine sulfate.

Goldberg et al.[48] also showed that insulin adsorption occurred with an inline membrane filter (McGaw 0.45-μm filter [V5545]). However, in a follow-up study by Wigert et al.,[49] using an Ultrapor membrane (Pall Corp.), no significant adsorption occurred and these authors concluded that the composition of the filter membrane affects adsorption.

Reports in the literature on a few filters and limited amounts of drugs indicate that drugs administered in low doses might present a problem with drug bonding to the filter. The reason that adsorption to the filter material is limited is that the filter material (substrate) surface area and weight relative to the drug are small, approximately 10 cm^2 and 50 to 60 mg, respectively. Therefore, if the drugs are in solution, removal of the drug occurs owing to the interaction of the drug and bonding sites on the filter substrate. For filter material substrates, the potential bonding sites are small, no more than 1 to 2% of the total weight of the filter.

Many clinically used filters are nitrate or acetate esters of cellulose. These compounds are polar and have residual hydroxyl groups that might become involved with drug adsorption interaction. Hydrophobic interactions between

TABLE 14–3. Drug Filterability—Summary of References

	Filterable Through Membrane Filter	Filtering Not Recommended
Amphotericin B[43]		X
Ampicillin[38]	X	
Bleomycin[47]	X	
Cefazolin[46]	X	
Cyanocobalamin[47]	X	
Dexamethasone[45]	X	
Digitoxin[47]		X
Digoxin[45]	X	
Ergonovine[47]	X	
Folic acid[47]	X	
Gentamicin[39,40]	X	
Heparin[47]	X	
Hydrocortisone[45]	X	
Insulin[43,47–49]		X
I.V.-Fat		X
Isoproterenol[45]	X	
Norepinephrine[45]	X	
Bitartrate[47]	X	
Lidocaine[45]	X	
Mithramycin[47]		X
Nitroglycerin[49]		X
Oxytocin[47]	X	
Penicillin[41]	X	
Prochlorperazine[45]	X	
Vinblastine[47]	X	
Vincristine[47]		X

the hydrocarbon portions of the drugs filtered and the linear cellulose molecules are also thought to be involved in drug adsorption. By treating the membrane with an agent capable of both hydrophilic and hydrophobic hydration, the polar groups as well as the linear cellulose moiety would be blocked and binding could be minimized. Proprietary treatment of the filter membranes reduces the binding capability of the membrane material.[50]

Product brochures (Millipore Corporation, Baxter Healthcare Laboratories) state "Minute quantities of drugs from intravenous solutions may adsorb to containers, administration sets and membrane filters. Therefore, supplemental dosages of 5 mg or less should be administered through the latex bulb with filter set slide clamp open."

Although the amount of current information suggests that little adsorption or absorption takes place with membrane filters, minute dosages of drugs 5 mg or less should not be filtered until sufficient data are available to confirm insignificant adsorption. Because of the controversy regarding the use of filters with amphotericin B, it is probably best to avoid any type of clinical filter with this antibiotic until this is resolved.

TABLE 14-4. Characteristics of Currently Available Blood Filters*

Filters	Type	Pore Size (Microns)	Material	Manufacturers Recommended # of Units (Whole Blood)	Priming Volume	Absolute Retention Rate (Diameter of Largest Particle Which Could Still Pass Through Filter)	Contraindications for Use	Unloading and Channeling of Particles	Contact Area of Blood and Filter Material
Microaggregate Blood Filters									
PALL SQ40S	Screen	40 μm	Polyester screen	10 units	20 ml	Retains particles greater than 40 μm	None known	No	Relatively small
BENTLEY Pff100	Depth	265 μm 60 μm 20 μm	Screen filter (2 layers of polyurethane foam)	5–10 units	80 ml	Cannot be determined	Not for use with fresh blood, platelet and platelet concentrates	Possible	Relatively large
SWANK 2010	Depth	20 μm	Dacron wool fiber	8 units	68 ml	Cannot be determined	Not for use during transfusion of platelet packs of fresh whole blood used as primary therapy for thrombocytopenia, platelet dysfunction or similar conditions	No	Relatively large
FENWAL 4C2423	Depth	20 μm	Non-woven polyester fibers	5–10 units	60 ml	Cannot be determined	Not for use with fresh blood. Filtration is not advised if specific replacement of platelets and WBCs desired	Possible	Relatively large

TABLE 14-4. Continued

Filters	Type	Pore Size (Microns)	Material	Manufacturers Recommended # of Units (Whole Blood)	Priming Volume	Absolute Retention Rate (Diameter of Largest Particle Which Could Still Pass Through Filter)	Contraindications for Use	Unloading and Channeling of Particles	Contact Area of Blood and Filter Material
HEMA™ 9131 or 9132	Combo Screen and Depth	Over 90 μm, 50–90 μm, 20 μm	Special proprietary composite (screen depth rolled around screen depth). Removes debris in multiple stages.	2–4 units	60 ml	Cannot be determined	Do not use when transfusing platelet packs, platelet concentrates or platelet-rich plasma	Possible	Relatively large
PEDIATRIC FILTER Fenwal 4C2428	Depth	20 μm	Non-woven polyester fiber	Up to 10 40 ml aliquots	8–9 ml	No information at this time	Not for use with platelets	No	No information at this time
Standard Blood Administration Sets									
FENWAL Straight Type Blood Recipient Set 4C2116	Clot screen	170 μm	Lexan plastic nylon mesh	1–2 units	8 ml	Retains particles Greater than 170 μm	None stated	Unclear	Relatively small
FENWAL 80-Micron Filter Sets 4C2431 or 4C2199	Double screen	200 μm, 80 μm	Polyester screen	4 units	30 ml	No information at this time	None stated	No	Relatively small

*As of June 1984.
Reprinted with permission, Intravenous Therapy News, *11*, 9, 1984. Roberta D. Schell, RN

Because of their large particle size, emulsions, such as Liposyn and Intra-lipid, should not be administered through filters. Pharmaceutical suspensions should never be filtered (e.g., fat emulsions, blood, sterile suspensions, insulin suspensions). Blood cannot be filtered through the usual membrane filters, and many of the blood components such as albumin are not readily filterable through the membrane filters. (See Table 14–3).

Blood Filters

The standard blood filter used in clinical practice is designed to remove all particulate matter larger than 170 μm. With the introduction of extracorporeal circulation and open heart surgery, cardiovascular surgeons have become concerned about debris present in stored blood. These microaggregates consist largely of platelets and fibrin in addition to fat. Some reports suggest that blood debris plays an important role in the pathogenesis of post-traumatic pulmonary insufficiency.[51–53] Studies have shown that organ function can also be impaired by microaggregates.[54,55] Others have shown that multiple pulmonary emboli occur after massive blood transfusion.[56,57] The conventional 170-μm nylon screen filter on blood administration sets has been found to be inadequate for removing microemboli. Also, it becomes clogged rapidly because of its limited area. In response to this need, new filters (Table 14–4) have been developed, with larger surface areas, which can remove microemboli smaller than 40 μm. These filters have the capability of high flow and permit at least 10 units of blood to be filtered through the same unit.

See Appendix 5 for I.V. Devices.

References

1. Blogg, C.E., Ramsay, M.A.E., and Jarvis, J.D.: Infection hazard from syringes. Br. J. Anaesth., 46, 260 (1974).
2. Turco, S.: Data on file, Temple University School of Pharmacy.
3. Garver, K.L., Marchese, S.L., and Boas, E.G.: Amniotic fluid-culture: Possible role of syringes. N. Engl. J. Med., Letters, 295, 286 (1976).
4. Frisk, A.P., and Jeffrey, L.P.: A comparison of disposable syringe systems. Apothecary, October 1974.
5. Kochevar, M., and Fry, L.K.: Insulin and dead space volume. Drug Intell. Clin. Pharm., 8, 33 (1974).
6. Dead space and insulin dosage errors. FDA Drug Bulletin, 5, 10 (1975).
7. Shainfield, F.J.: Errors in insulin doses due to the design of insulin syringes. Pediatrics, 56:302 (1975).
8. Rosenbloom, A.L.: Advances in commercial insulin preparations. Am. J. Dis. Child., 128, 631 (1974).
9. Feingold, A.: Volume of syringe-needle dead space. Am. J. Hosp. Pharm., Letters, 33, 756 (1976).
10. Thomas, R.B., and Salter, F.J.: Heparin locks: Their advantages and disadvantages. Hospital Formulary, 8, 536 (1975).
11. Deeb, E.N., and DiMattia, P.E.: How much heparin in the lock? Am. J. I.V. Ther., 3, 22 (1976).
12. Turco, S.J.: I.V. drug incompatibilities with heparin sodium. Am. J. I.V. Ther., 3, 16 (1976).
13. Thomas, R.: Meperidine HCl and heparin sodium precipitation. Hosp. Pharm., 9, 356 (1974).
14. King, J.G.: Guide to Parenteral Admixtures. Cutter Laboratories, Inc., 1978.
15. O'Neill, T.J., Tierney, L.M., and Provix, R.J.: Heparin lock-induced alterations in the activated partial thromboplastin time. JAMA, 227, 1297 (1974).

16. Hanson, R.L.: Heparin—lock or keep open I.V.? Am. J. Nurs., 76, 1102 (1976).
17. Hanson, R.L., Grant, A.M., and Majors, K.R.: Heparin-lock maintenance with ten units of sodium heparin in one milliliter of normal saline solution. Surg. Gynecol. Obstet., 142, 373 (1976).
18. Stern, R.C., Pittman, S., Doershuk, C.F., and Matthews, L.W.: Use of a heparin-lock in the intermittent administration of I.V. drugs. Clin. Pediatr., 11, 521 (1972).
19. Kimmel, R.: Keys to using the heparin-lock. Nursing, 3, 52 (1974).
20. Rucker, R.W., and Harrison, G.M.: Outpatient I.V. medications in the management of cystic fibrosis. Pediatrics, 54, 358 (1974).
21. Ferguson, R.L., Rosett, W., Hodges, G.R., and Barnes, W.S.: Complications with heparin-lock needles, a prospective evaluation. Ann. Intern. Med., 85, 583 (1976).
22. DeFina, E.: How we use heparin-locks. Am. J. I.V. Ther., 3, 27 (1976).
23. Signal. Am. Soc. Hosp. Pharm. Newsletter, 1, 10 (1977).
24. Wiltsee, I.G.: Obtaining difficult venipunctures via heparin well needle technique. Am. J. I.V. Ther., 13, 1 (1977).
25. Couchonnal, G.J., et al.: Complications with heparin-lock needles. JAMA, 242, 2098, (1979).
26. Cyganski, J.M., et al.: The case for the heparin flush. Am. J. Nurs., 796 (1987).
27. Dunn, D.L., et al.: The case for the saline flush. Am. J. Nurs., 798 (1987).
28. Epperson, E.L.: Efficacy of 0.9% sodium chloride injection with and without heparin for maintaining indwelling intermittent injection sites. Clin. Pharm., 3, 626 (1984).
29. Shearer, J.: Normal saline flush versus dilute heparin flush. NITA, 12, 425 (1987).
30. Hamilton, R.A., et al.: Heparin sodium versus 0.9% sodium chloride injection for maintaining patency of indwellings intermittent infusion devices. Clin. Pharm., 7, 439 (1988).
31. Lombardi, T.P., et al.: Efficacy of 0.9% sodium chloride injection with or without heparin sodium for maintaining patency of intravenous catheters in children. Am. J. Hosp. Pharm., 45, 2578 (1988).
32. Pituk, T.L., DeYoung, J.L., and Levin, H.J.: Volumes of selected central venous catheters. Implications for heparin flush use. NITA, 6, 98, (1983).
33. Newton, R., et al.: Volumes of implantable vascular access devices and heparin flush requirements. NITA, 8, 137 (1985).
34. Turco, S.J., and Davis, N.: A comparison of commercial final filtration devices. Hosp. Pharm., 8, 141 (1973).
35. Turco, S.J., and Davis, N.: Clinical significance of particulate matter: a review of the literature. Hosp. Pharm., 8, 137 (1973).
36. Rusmin, S., et al.: Consequences of microbial contamination during extended intravenous therapy using inline filters. Am. J. Hosp. Pharm., 32, 373 (1975).
37. Rusmin, S., et al.: Effects of antibiotics and osmotic change on the release of endotoxin by bacteria retained on intravenous inline filters. Am. J. Hosp. Pharm., 32, 378 (1975).
38. Wyeth Laboratories: Data on file, Temple University School of Pharmacy. July 27, 1975.
39. Wagman, G.H., et al.: Binding of aminoglycoside antibiotics to filtration materials. Antimicrob. Agents Chemother., 7, 316, (1975).
40. Schering Laboratories: Letter to S. Turco, on file, Temple University School of Pharmacy. Aug. 3, 1975.
41. Rusmin, S.W., et al.: Effect of in-line filtration on the potency of drugs administered intravenously. Am. J. Hosp. Pharm., 34, 1071 (1977).
42. Bristol Laboratories: Letter to S. Turco, on file, Temple University School of Pharmacy. Aug. 5, 1975.
43. Huber, R.C., et al.: In-line final filters for removing particles from amphotericin B infusions. Am. J. Hosp. Pharm., 32, 173 (1975).
44. Piecoro, J.J., et al.: Particulate matter in reconstituted amphotericin B and assay of filtered solutions of amphotericin B. Am. J. Hosp. Pharm., 32, 381 (1975).
45. Stiles, M., and Allen, L.V.: Retention of drugs during in-line filtration of parenteral solutions. Infusion, 3, 67 (1979).

46. Stennet, D.J., et al.: Effect of membrane filtration in 10 mg/ml cefazolin admixtures. Am. J. Hosp. Pharm., 36, 657 (1969).
47. Butler, L.D., et al.: Effect of in-line filtration on the potency of low dose drugs. Am. J. Hosp. Pharm., 37, 935, (1980).
48. Goldberg, N.J.: Insulin adsorption to an in-line membrane filter. N. Engl. J. Med., Letters, 298, 1480 (1978).
49. Wingert, T.D.: Insulin adsorption to an air-eliminating in-line filter. Am. J. Hosp. Pharm., 38, 382 (1981).
50. Reducing drug absorption on inline I.V. filters. Parenterals, 1(4), 5 (1983).
51. Reul, G.J., Beall, A.C., and Greenberg, S.D.: Protection of the pulmonary microvasculature by fine screen blood filtration. Chest 66, 4 (1974).
52. Reul, G.J., et al.: Prevention of post traumatic pulmonary insufficiency. Arch. Surg., 106, 386 (1973).
53. Cullen, D.J., and Ferrara, L.: Comparative evaluation of blood filters. Anesthesia, 41, 568 (1974).
54. Goldiner, P.L., and Howland, W.S.: Filter for prevention of microembolism during massive transfusion. Anesth. Anal., 51, 717 (1972).
55. Soeter, J.R., et al.: Comparison of filtering efficiency of four new in-line blood transfusion filters. Ann. Surg., 181, 114 (1975).
56. Marshall, B.E., et al.: Effects of Intercept micropore filtration of blood on microaggregates and other constituents. Anesthesia, 44, 525 (1976).
57. Connell, R.S., and Swank, R.L.: Pulmonary microembolism after blood transfusion. Ann. Surg., 177, 40 (1973).

Bibliography—Implantable Systems

1. Ecoff, E., et al.: Implantable infusion port. NITA, 12 406 (1983).
2. Fulks, K.D., and Kenady, D.E.: Techniques of chemotherapy delivery for cancer patients. Hosp. Formula, 22, 248 (1987).
3. Gyves, J., et al.: Totally implanted system for intravenous chemotherapy in patients with cancer. Am. J. Med., 73, 841 (1983).
4. Kwan, J.W.: Use of infusion devices for epidural or intrathecal administration of spinal opioids. Am. J. Hosp., 47, 18 (1990).
5. May, G.S., and Davis, C.: Percutaneous catheters and totally implantable access systems. J. Int. Nursing, 11, 97 (1988).
6. McGovern, B., et al.: A totally implantable venous access system for long term chemotherapy in children. J. Pediatr. Surg., 6, 725 (1985).
7. McIntyre, K.E., et al.: Early experience with an implantable reservoir for intravenous chemotherapy. Arizona Med., 42, 308 (1985).

Ophthalmic Preparations

Preparations for the eye may be solutions (eye drops or eyewashes), suspensions, or ointments. In special cases, ophthalmic injections are used. Ophthalmic preparations share with other sterile products the characteristics of sterility and freedom from particulate matter. With the exception of the limited number of ophthalmic injections, preparations for the eye are topical dosage forms used for their local effect, and hence it is not necessary that they be free from pyrogens. Because of their method of use and the drugs employed, ophthalmic preparations differ from parenterally administered agents in the substances added to enhance the activity and to maintain the stability and sterility of the products, as well as their packaging.

Requirements

Sterility is the most important requirement. Improperly prepared ophthalmic solutions can carry many organisms, the most dangerous of which is *Pseudomonas aeruginosa*. Eye infections from this organism have resulted in blindness; it is especially dangerous to instill nonsterile products in an eye when the cornea is abraded. Particulate matter can be irritating to the eyes, resulting in discomfort to the patient, and methods are available for its elimination.

Although the number of commercially prepared ophthalmic products available to the physician continues to increase, frequently the pharmacist (pharmacy service) is called upon to dispense an ophthalmic preparation of a composition unavailable on the market. In an evaluation of the sterility and concentration of 100 samples of 1% pilocarpine hydrochloride solutions prepared in pharmacies and companies throughout the United States, 52 of 66 solutions prepared by local pharmacists were contaminated with bacteria and/ or fungi, whereas only one of 34 samples prepared by pharmaceutical companies for interstate commerce and dispensed by local pharmacies was contaminated.[1] In the latter samples, the concentration of pilocarpine hydrochloride was also more uniform; those of locally prepared solutions varied greatly.

More recently,[2,3] eyesight loss and other ocular damage have occurred from ophthalmic products prepared by pharmacists. Pseudomonas organisms survied in autoclaved containers, with the resultant effect of infection and loss of vision. This incident prompted the FDA[4] to issue an alert letter to pharmacists describing the seriousness of products that require sterility.

Two recent cases of blindness and eye damage to many other people were reported by the FDA[5] from a commercially produced ophthalmic product as a result of eye pressure buildup. The event in Pittsburgh[2] prompted Reynolds[6] to publish guidelines for the preparation of sterile ophthalmic products.

With care and training, however, the pharmacist can extemporaneously prepare an ophthalmic solution that is satisfactory in all respects.

In the formulation of eye preparations, whether industrially or extemporaneously, consideration is given to a number of factors: the type of preparation and how it is to be used, the activity and stability of the drug involved, the adjustment of tonicity, the choice of the sterilization method, and the means by which the product is to be packaged.[7]

Tonicity

Tonicity refers to the osmotic pressure exerted by a solution from the solutes or dissolved solids present. Tear fluid and other body fluids exert an osmotic pressure equal to that of normal saline or 0.9% sodium chloride solution. A solution with a greater amount of solutes than tear fluid has a greater osmotic pressure and is called "hypertonic." Conversely, a solution with less solute has a lower osmotic pressure and is "hypotonic." The eye can tolerate solutions having tonicity values ranging from equivalents of 0.5% to 1.6% sodium chloride without great discomfort.

Tonicity of eyewashes assumes a greater importance than that of eye drops because of the volume of solution that is used. With eyewashes and the help of an eye cup, the eye is flooded with solution, thus overwhelming the ability of the tear fluid to adjust to any difference in tonicity. If the tonicity of the eyewash is not near that of the tear fluid, pain and irritation result.

In preparing ophthalmic solutions, the tonicity of a solution can be adjusted to that of lacrimal fluid by the addition of a suitable solute such as sodium chloride. If the osmotic pressure of the drug at the desired concentration exceeds that of the tear fluid, nothing can be done if the desired drug concentration is to be maintained, since the solution is hypertonic. For example, 10 and 30% solutions of sodium sulfacetamide are hypertonic, yet concentrations of less than 10% do not give the desired clinical effect. For hypotonic solutions, several methods are available for calculating the amount of sodium chloride to adjust the tonicity of an ophthalmic solution; one is the freezing point depression method.

Tear fluid, like other body fluids, contains sufficient solute to lower the freezing point of the solution 0.52° C. Likewise, 0.9% sodium chloride solution lowers the freezing point 0.52° C. The two solutions exerting the same osmotic pressure are isotonic.

Consider the eyewash solution containing 1% boric acid. From freezing point depression values found in the literature,[8,9] note that 1% boric acid lowers the freezing point 0.29° C. Therefore, sufficient sodium chloride must be added to make up the difference.

Tear fluid lowers freezing point . . . . 0.52° C
1% boric acid lowers freezing point . . . . 0.29° C
Sodium chloride to be added to lower freezing
point (f.p.). . . . . 0.23° C

If 0.9% sodium chloride lowers f.p. 0.52° C, then the amount required to lower it 0.23° C can be calculated by direct proportion.

$$\frac{0.52° \text{ C}}{0.9\%} = \frac{0.23° \text{ C}}{\text{X}}; \text{X} = 0.40\%$$

Thus, 0.40% sodium chloride will be added to 1% boric acid solution to make the solution isotonic with the lacrimal fluid.

If the ophthalmic solution contains more than one ingredient, the contribution of each must be calculated. The difference between the sum of freezing point depressions effected by each ingredient and 0.52° C indicates the amount that the calculated quantity of sodium chloride will contribute.

Among the drugs used in the eye are local anesthetics, anti-inflammatory, anti-infective, antihistamine, miotic, and mydriatic agents. Alkaloidal compounds such as the salts of homatropine, atropine, pilocarpine, and physostigmine make up the latter two classes. These alkaloidal materials are more active in their nondissociated form, liposoluble and readily absorbed by the cornea; however, to prepare satisfactory solutions, the water-soluble salts must be used. To achieve optimum activity and at the same time to obtain a satisfactory solution, the solutions are frequently buffered at pH 6.8. The nondissociated form is more readily available when drops of the alkaloidal solution are instilled in the eye, which has a pH of 7.4. In buffering solutions of alkaloidal salts near pH 7, there is a loss in the time during which the solution will be stable, the alkaloidal solutions being more stable at pH 3 to 5. This precludes the sterilization of the buffered solution with heat and indicates brief storage periods before use. Alkaloidal solutions are prepared commercially at a lower pH to improve the shelf-life of the product. It has been shown that the long-term stability problem inherent in formulating an ophthalmic solution of an alkaloidal salt at pH 6.8 can be solved by lyophilization. The lyophilized product can be stored for extended periods without degradation.[10] The eye will tolerate solutions having pH values over a wide range provided they are administered in small volumes.

A convenient method for buffering and adjusting the tonicity of an ophthalmic solution prepared extemporaneously is the Hammarlund and Pedersen-Bjergaard method, described in *U.S.P. XXI*. The method entails adding a sufficient volume of distilled water to a given amount of drug to make an isotonic solution of the drug. This isotonic solution is made to a final volume with an isotonic vehicle. Because both the drug solution and the vehicle are isotonic, the combination remains isotonic. Consider the following example.

℞

Homatropine hydrobromide	1%
M. Ft. collyr. isotonic	60 ml

The *U.S.P.* recommends that ophthalmic solutions of salts of homatropine be buffered at pH 6.8 and suggests a formula for a suitable isotonic phosphate buffer. From Table 15–1, note that 1 g of homatropine hydrobromide requires sufficient distilled water to give a final volume of 19 ml to obtain an isotonic solution.

In the given prescription, 600 mg of homatropine hydrobromide are needed; therefore, by direct proportion, it can be determined that 600 mg require sufficient volume of distilled water to give a final volume of 11.4 ml.

$$\frac{1000}{19} = \frac{600}{X}; X = 11.4 \text{ ml}$$

The prescription would be filled as follows:

℞

Homatropine hydrobromide	600 mg
Purified water to make	11.4 ml
(pH 6.8) Isotonic phosphate buffer qs ad	60 ml

When the drug does not require a buffer, as is the case with many anti-infective agents, local anesthetic agents, and antihistamines, a 1.9% boric acid solution serves as a suitable vehicle. To the isotonic solution of the drug, sufficient boric acid solution is added to bring the solution to volume, as shown in the following example.

℞

Tetracaine hydrochloride	0.5%
M. Ft. collyr. isotonic	30 ml

From Table 15–1, note that 1 g of tetracaine hydrochloride requires sufficient distilled water to give a final volume of 20 ml to obtain an isotonic solution.

In the above prescription, 150 mg of tetracaine hydrochloride are needed; therefore, by direct proportion, it can be determined that 150 mg require sufficient volume of distilled water to give a final volume of

$$\frac{1000}{20} = \frac{150}{X}; X = 3 \text{ ml}$$

The prescription would be filled as follows:

℞

Tetracaine hydrochloride	150 mg
Purified water to make	3 ml
Boric acid vehicle	qs ad 30 ml

In the example above in which a buffer is not used, the solution can also be adjusted to tonicity using sodium chloride by calculating the amount re-

TABLE 15–1.   Volumes of Water for Isotonicity*

Drug (1 g)	Volume of Isotonic Solution (ml)
Atropine Sulfate	14.3
Benoxinate Hydrochloride	20.0
Boric Acid	55.7
Butacaine Sulfate	22.3
Chloramphenicol Sodium Succinate	15.7
Chlorobutanol (hydrous)	26.7
Cocaine Hydrochloride	17.7
Colistimethate Sodium	16.7
Dibucaine Hydrochloride	14.3
Ephedrine Hydrochloride	33.3
Ephedrine Sulfate	25.7
Epinephrine Bitartrate	20.0
Epinephrine Hydrochloride	32.3
Eucatropine Hydrochloride	20.0
Fluorescein Sodium	34.3
Homatropine Hydrobromide	19.0
Homatropine Methylbromide	21.0
Neomycin Sulfate	12.3
Penicillin G Potassium	20.0
Phenacaine Hydrochloride	22.3
Phenylephrine Hydrochloride	35.7
Phenylethyl Alcohol	27.7
Physostigmine Salicylate	17.7
Physostigmine Sulfate	14.3
Pilocarpine Hydrochloride	26.7
Pilocarpine Nitrate	25.7
Piperocaine Hydrochloride	23.3
Polymyxin B Sulfate	10.0
Procaine Hydrochloride	23.3
Proparacaine Hydrochloride	16.7
Scopolamine Hydrobromide	13.3
Silver Nitrate	36.7
Sodium Bicarbonate	72.3
Sodium Biphosphate	44.3
Sodium Borate	46.7
Sodium Phosphate (dibasic, heptahydrate)	32.3
Streptomycin Sulfate	7.7
Sulfacetamide Sodium	25.7
Sulfadiazine Sodium	26.7
Sulfamerazine Sodium	25.7
Sulfathiazone Sodium	24.3
Tetracaine Hydrochloride	20.0
Tetracycline Hydrochloride	15.7
Zinc Sulfate	16.7

*The United States Pharmacopeia. XXII Revision. Easton, PA, Mack Publishing Company, 1990.

quired by any of the commonly used methods. The following procedure uses the freezing point depression method:

℞

Tetracaine hydrochloride	0.5%
Sodium chloride	—
Purified water	qs 30 ml

Tear fluid lowers freezing point .... 0.52° C

0.5% tetracaine hydrochloride lowers f.p. .... 0.06° C

Sodium chloride to be added to lower f.p. .... 0.46° C

If 0.9% sodium chloride lowers f.p. 0.52° C, then the amount required to lower it 0.46° C can be calculated by direct proportion.

$$\frac{0.52° \text{ C}}{0.9\%} = \frac{0.46° \text{ C}}{X}; X = 0.8\%$$

Thus, 0.8% sodium chloride will be added to 0.5% tetracaine hydrochloride solution to make the solution isotonic with lacrimal fluid

℞

Tetracaine hydrochloride	150 mg
Sodium chloride	240 mg
Purified water	qs ad 30 ml

Sterilization

Sterility is one of the important characteristics for ophthalmic solutions. Because the stability to heat of extemporaneously prepared ophthalmic solutions is frequently unknown, these solutions are best sterilized by microbiologic filtration. Disadvantages of this method of sterilization include not only the fact that it fails to remove viral contaminants but also that it places greater emphasis on the importance of aseptic technique involved in sterilization of the solution and its subsequent packaging. Sterile membrane filters, available as sterile plastic disposable units, offer a practical method of sterilizing small volumes (Swinnex and Millex, Millipore Corporation) (Fig. 15–1).[11,12] The solution to be sterilized is taken up in a clean but not necessarily sterile syringe. The sterile plastic holder containing a sterile membrane filter is fastened to the tip of the syringe, and the solution is expelled from the syringe through the sterile filter into a sterile container (Fig. 15–2). The plastic unit and filter are disposable. Sterilization of ophthalmic solutions by filtration also clarifies the solution by removing particulate matter. Some ophthalmic drugs in solution can be sterilized by autoclaving in the final container, provided the drug is stable. Because the stability of extemporaneously prepared ophthalmic solutions is frequently not known, filtration is the method of choice.

Preservation

Repeated use of an ophthalmic solution from the same container by a single individual, or the use of the solution from a common container for a number

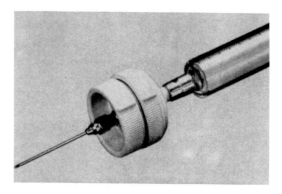

Figure 15–1. Disposabe filter unit (Swinnex). (Courtesy of Millipore Corporation, Bedford, MA.)

of individuals, increases the probability that microbial contaminants will be introduced into the solution. Serious infections can be transferred from person to person in this way. To prevent this, antimicrobial preservatives are included in all ophthalmic solutions with the exception of those packaged for one-time use, such as preparations used in ophthalmic surgical procedures.

In ophthalmic solutions, the contaminant causing the greatest concern is *Pseudomonas aeruginosa*. There is no preservative or combination of preservatives that can be guaranteed to be effective against all forms of *Pseudomonas*.[13] The most commonly used preservative is benzalkonium chloride (1:10,000); higher concentrations are irritating to the ocular tissues. Being a cationic drug, benzalkonium chloride is incompatible with anionic drugs as well as with nitrates and salicylates. Other preservatives are phenylmercuric acetate and nitrate (1:50,000), phenylethanol (1:200), and chlorobutanol (1:200). The latter is stable only near pH 5 to 6 and is used only with solutions in this pH range. The preservation requirements for any pharmaceutical system are unique for that system and depend not only on the drug and its concentration but also on the other additives and the type of packaging.[14] An increasing number of ophthalmologists prefer to use a nonpreserved solution because the patient has shown an allergic reaction to the commonly used preservatives. In this instance, it is better to prepare several 1- or 2-ml units so they can be discarded after initial use.

To increase the time during which the solution is in contact with the cornea, the viscosity of ophthalmic solutions can be increased by the addition of a suitable thickening agent such as one of the cellulose derivatives, methylcellulose, hydroxypropylcellulose, or polyvinyl alcohol. The *U.S.P.* suggests the use of 0.5% methylcellulose. Cellulose solutions cannot be filtered for sterilization; they must be autoclaved. When they are autoclaved, the cellulose derivative precipitates from solution because of decreased water solubility with increase in temperature, but clears upon cooling to room temperature. When a heat-labile drug is combined with a cellulose derivative, the components of the solution must be sterilized separately and then combined aseptically. The drug in solution is sterilized by filtration, and the cellulose derivative solution by autoclaving.

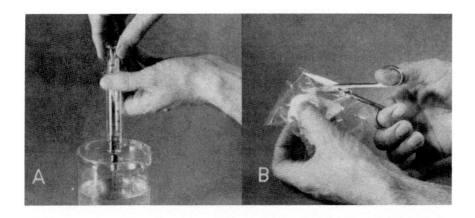

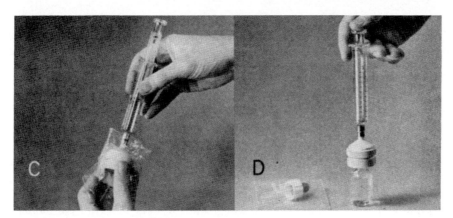

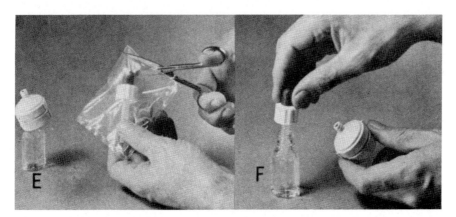

Figure 15–2. Operation of disposable filter unit (Swinnex). A, The syringe is filled with liquid to be filtered before attaching the Swinnex unit. B, The sealed plastic bag containing a sterilized unit is cut open with sterile scissors so that the female Luer end is accessible. C, The syringe containing the preparation is attached to the female end of the Swinnex unit while the unit is held through the bag. D, By applying pressure to the syringe plunger, the liquid passes through the filter and into the bottle. E, The sealed plastic bag containing a sterile eyedropper is then cut open with sterile scissors. F, The eyedropper is removed and placed in the bottle, replacing the Swinnex unit. (Courtesy of Millipore Corporation, Bedford, MA.)

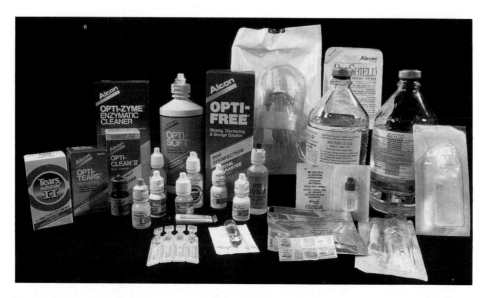

Figure 15–3. Ophthalmic preparations packaged in multiple- and single-dose containers. (Courtesy of Alcon Corporation, Fort Worth, TX.)

A newer approach to ophthalmic drug delivery is found in the form of membrane inserts (Ocusert, Alza). The ophthalmic insert is a device consisting of a drug-containing core surrounded by a flexible copolymer membrane through which the drug diffuses. The membrane, when placed under the eyelid, allows a drug such as pilocarpine to diffuse in therapeutic quantities over a 7-day period. The insert is situated and removed with a technique similar to that used for inserting and removing a soft contact lens.[15]

Another insert-type ophthalmic product is a small, rod-shaped, water-soluble solid consisting of 5 mg hydroxypropyl cellulose (Lacrisert, Merck Sharp & Dohme). It contains no other ingredients. The cellulose gum acts to stabilize and thicken the precorneal tear film and prolong the tear film breakup. It is indicated in patients with dry-eye syndromes.

Packaging

Ophthalmic solutions prepared extemporaneously are packaged either in polyethylene "droptainers" or in glass dropper bottles (Figs. 15–3 and 15–4). To maintain the sterility of the solutions, the containers must be sterile. The polyethylene containers are sterilized with ethylene oxide, whereas glass dropper assemblies can be suitably wrapped and autoclaved. Commercially prepared single-dose units with a volume of 0.3 ml or less are packaged in sterile polyethylene tubes and heat-sealed.

Ophthalmic Ointments

Ophthalmic ointments provide another means by which a drug can be held in contact with the eye and the surrounding tissues without being washed out by the tear fluid. The base for ophthalmic ointments is usually white pet-

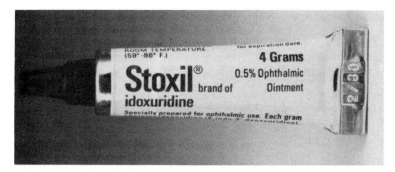

Figure 15–4. Sterile ophthalmic ointment. (Courtesy of SmithKline Beecham, Philadelphia, PA.)

rolatum, although in some cases water-soluble bases are desirable.[16] The drug, if not soluble, is dispersed throughout the base. In the preparation of sterile ophthalmic ointments, the base is sterilized by dry heat and combined aseptically with the sterile drug and sterile additives.[17,18] Antibiotics are usually isolated as sterile powders, whereas other chemicals must be sterilized with dry heat.

Cobalt-60 gamma radiation has been successfully used for the sterilization of ophthalmic ointments. Tetracycline hydrochloride (Achromycin) ophthalmic ointment and chlortetracycline hydrochloride (Aureomycin) ophthalmic ointment are the first pharmaceutical products for which radiation has been approved as the method of sterilization.[19] Radiation sterilization is a form of terminal sterilization, that is, sterilizing the product following packaging. In addition to meeting sterility requirements, ophthalmic ointments must also pass tests designed to limit the number and size of metal particles present. Originally, metal particles were found to be contaminants of the metal tubes in which the ointment was packaged.

Ophthalmic Suspensions

With the advent of steroids, aqueous suspensions were prepared for use in the eye because the water solubility of the steroids is too low for the desired concentration in solution. In preparing ophthalmic suspensions, the steroid in microfine form, the particles being in the range of 10 μm, is suspended in an aqueous vehicle. The vehicle is made isotonic with sodium chloride and includes a surfactant, thickening agent, and antimicrobial preservative. Because it is insoluble, the suspended sterile solid does not contribute to the tonicity of the vehicle. The steroid is either crystallized as sterile material or sterilized with dry heat. The vehicle is autoclaved, and the suspension is prepared by mixing aseptically prior to filling into the final package under aseptic conditions. For drugs not available as sterile ophthalmic suspensions, such as amphotericin B and nystatin, the injectable sterile suspension is frequently used to prepare a suitable ophthalmic suspension.

Instillation

When instilling ophthalmic solutions, the greatest danger is that of contamination. The preparations are more easily applied by someone other than the patient. The one administering the solution should wash his hands prior to instilling the drops. The patient is seated with his head tilted back, looking upward. The person instilling the solution pulls the patient's lower lid gently downward and drops the solution into the outer corner of the lower lid, taking care that the dropper or the tip of the plastic container does not become contaminated by touching the surface of the eye or the eyelashes.

In dispensing an ophthalmic preparation, it is the responsibility of the pharmacist to inform the patient concerning its use, to ensure that it will be properly handled and stored.

References

1. Macdonald, R., Jr., Keller, K.F., Bhatt, M.M., and Cox, H.B.: Sterility and concentration of pilocarpine solutions. Am. J. Ophthalmol., 68, 1099 (1962).
2. Associated Press: Pittsburgh woman loses eye to tainted drugs; 12 hurt. Baltimore Sun, Nov. 9:3A (1990).
3. Associated Press: Eye drops injuries prompt an F.D.A. warning. NY Times, Dec. 9:391 (1990).
4. FDA Alert Letter. Food and Drug Administration, Rockville, MD, Nov., 29 (1990).
5. Wall Street Journal: FDA suspects eye-care fluid blinded two. Oct. 21:B1 (1991).
6. Reynolds, L.A.: Guidelines for the preparation of sterile ophthalmic products. Am. J. Hosp. Pharm, 48, 2438 (1991).
7. The United States Pharmacopeia. XXI Revision. Mack Publishing Company, Easton, PA, 1985, p. 1338.
8. The Merck Index. 10th Ed. Rahway, NJ, Merck & Co., 1983, pp. Misc 47–Misc 49.
9. Siegel, F.P.: Tonicity, osmoticity, osmolality, and osmolarity. In Remington's Pharmaceutical Sciences. 17th Ed. Edited by A.R. Gennaro. Easton, PA, Mack Publishing Company, 1985, pp. 1465–1472.
10. Garrell, R.K., and King, R.E.: Stabilization of homatropine hydrobromide ophthalmic solution at pH 6.8 by lyophilization. J. Parenter. Sci. Tech., 36, 2 (1982).
11. Sterilization of Ophthalmic Solutions by Millipore Filtration. Application Report AR-1. Bedford, MA, Millipore Corporation, 1973.
12. Preparing Sterile, Particle-Free Fluids in the Hospital Pharmacy. Application Manual AM 303. Bedford, MA, Millipore Corporation, 1973.
13. Eriksen, S.P.: Preservation of ophthalmic, nasal, and otic products. Drug Cosmet. Industr., 107, 36 (1970).
14. Mullins, J.D.: Ophthalmic preparations. In Remington's Pharmaceutical Sciences. 17th Ed. Edited by A.R. Gennaro. Easton, PA, Mack, 1985, p. 1562.
15. Akers, M.J., Schoenwald, R.D., and McGinity, J.W.: Ophthalmic drug development. Drug Devel. Indust. Pharm., 3, 203 (1977).
16. Newton, D.W., Becker, C.H., and Torosian, G.: Physical and chemical characteristics of water-soluble semisolid, anhydrous bases for possible ophthalmic use. J. Pharm. Sci., 62, 1538 (1973).
17. Rosenberg, S.J.: Procedures important in the manufacture of ophthalmic preparations. Bull. Parenter. Drug Assoc., 24, 94 (1970).
18. O'Neill, J.L., Polli, G.P., and Fong, D.T.K.: Sterile ophthalmic ointments—pilot plant phase. Bull. Parenter. Drug Assoc., 27, 201 (1973).
19. Nash, R.A.: Radiosterilized tetracycline ophthalmic ointment. Bull. Parenter. Drug Assoc., 28, 181 (1974).

CHAPTER 16

Allergen Extracts

John D. Grabenstein

Allergen extracts comprise a unique pharmacopeia of more than 1000 distinct immunotherapeutic agents. The United States Food & Drug Administration (FDA) recognizes allergen extracts as useful in diagnosing allergic hypersensitivity and other allergic disorders. Of all allergen extracts licensed, approximately 60% are also efficacious in the treatment of certain allergic diseases, such as allergic rhinitis and asthma.[1-3] Most allergen-extract prescriptions are not compounded in laminar-flow hoods, most are inadequately labeled, and few are subjected to adequate quality control. Most facilities compounding allergen-extract prescriptions could use the help and consultation of a pharmacist.[4]

Allergic rhinitis affects an estimated 5 to 22% of the general population, ranking as the sixth most prevalent disease in the United States. An estimated 5 million Americans may be allergic to cat allergen. An estimated 1.4 million Americans per year receive some 35 million individual allergen injections, accounting for greater than $30 million in sales. Allergen extracts are probably the greatest single potential source of drug-induced anaphylaxis risk.[1,5-6]

In 1911, Noon[7] and Freeman[8] introduced the use of extracts of various plant pollens to treat allergic rhinitis ("hay fever"), beginning what was previously alluded to as hyposensitization or desensitization, but is now commonly known as immunotherapy. Allergen extracts are selective, parenteral immunostimulants that reduce allergic symptoms in 70% or more of properly treated pa-

---

The opinions or assertions contained herein are the private views of the author and are not to be construed as official or reflecting the views of the U.S. Department of the Army or the Department of Defense.

TABLE 16–1. Examples of FDA-Approved Allergen Extracts

Major Group	No. of FDA-Approved Extracts		Examples of Individual Allergen Extracts
	Diagnosis	Therapy	
Foods	289	0	Chicken egg albumin, casein, bovine alpha lactalbumin, beta lactoglobulin, almond (*Prunus amygdalus*), gum acacia (*Acacia senegal*), scallops (*Pecten irradians*)
Animals	32	32	Cat allergen-1; dog, horse, rat, guinea pig danders; chicken, duck, goose, pigeon feathers
Grasses	*	*	Kentucky blue (June; *Poa pratensis*), red top (*Agrostis alba*), perennial rye (*Lolium perenne*), Bermuda (*Cynodon dactylon*), meadow fescue (*Festuca eliatior*), velvet (*Holcus lanata*)
Insects	38	12	Fire ant (*Solenopsis invicta*), German cockroach, mite (*Dermatophagoides farinae*)
Molds	70	70	Genera (note: many individual species within each species): Alternaria, Aspergillus, Cladosporium, Fusarium, Monilia, Mucor, Helminthosporium, Penicillium, Phoma, Rhizopus, Saccharomyces, Tricophyton
Trees	*	*	White oak (*Quercus alba*), Arizona cypress (*Cupressus arizonica*), cottonwood (*Populus deltoides*), red maple (*Acer rubrum*), mountain cedar (*Juniperus sabinoides*), American elm (*Ulmus americanus*)
Weeds	*	*	Short ragweed (*Ambrosia elatior*), common sagebrush (*Artemisia tridentata*), saltbush (*Atriplex wrightii*), wingscale (*Atriplex canescens*), lambs quarters (*Chenopodium album*)
Other inhalants	23	5	House dust, cotton linters, gum arabic, gum karaya, green tobacco leaf, gum tragacanth, silk, castor bean

* = Total botanical pollens: 486 for both diagnosis and therapy.

tients.[1–3,9] In the United Kingdom, allergen extracts are called desensitizing vaccines.[10]

Allergen extracts result from the passage of an extracting fluid (or menstruum) through tree, grass, or weed pollen, animal pelts, feathers, foods, molds, or other airborne particles that elicit allergic symptoms when inhaled by hypersensitive patients. This process is not unlike the percolation of ground coffee beans, with the allergen extract analogous to the fluid we call coffee. Each allergen extract is a crude, complex mixture of many proteins, carbohydrates, and other components. Table 16–1 lists examples from each of the major groups of allergen extracts.[11–12]

FDA's Advisory Panel on Review of Allergenic Extracts confirmed the efficacy of allergen extracts in relieving symptoms of allergic asthma and allergic rhinitis,[1,9] often called type I hypersensitivities. Immunodiagnosis involves puncture ("prick") and/or intradermal application of individual dilute allergen extracts. Immunotherapy begins with minute, subcutaneous doses of one or several extracts individualized to the patient. Weak doses are administered once or twice weekly, escalating through a set of serial dilutions over the course of a few months to a maintenance dose every 2 to 4 weeks. The prescription for such a treatment formula is actually an intricate sterile-products order.

The FDA advisory panel divided allergen extracts into category I (safe, effective, and not misbranded) or category II (unsafe, ineffective, or misbranded). Two interim categories are also in use: category IIIA (not enough data available for final classification, yet interstate commerce may continue until final classification is made) and category IIIB (not recommended for continued licensure during the period of definitive testing).[1,9] Each extract received two distinct evaluations, one for use in diagnosis and one for use in immunotherapy. For example, cockroach extracts are listed in category I for diagnosis, but in category IIIB for therapy.

Immunoglobulin G (IgG, or "blocking antibody") specific to each allergen appears in human serum following injection of several doses of an extract.[2-3] This IgG is believed to compete for specific immunoglobulin E (IgE or "reagin") generated as the patient becomes hypersensitive to a specific environmental allergen. Bound to receptors on mast cells, the IgE produces allergic reactions on coupling with an antigen through the release of histamine and other mediators.. With allergen-extract immunotherapy, serum IgE levels decrease over time. Other responses have also been noted, but the complete mechanism of action has not been defined.

Allergen extracts also may be used in the diagnosis and treatment of veterinary allergy.[13] Dosage is the same for large and small animals as for human adults. Animals in which a large financial interest is invested, such as trained dogs, are the most likely candidates for such veterinary immunotherapy.

Several practices in allergy diagnosis and therapy have never been scientifically validated, yet persist among some clinicians. Unproven diagnostic and therapeutic techniques include subcutaneous and sublingual provocation testing, end-point neutralization therapy, Candidiasis hypersensitivity ("yeast overgrowth"), cytotoxic testing, Rinkel titration testing, total immune disorder syndrome, urine autoinjection, and others. Patients may anecdotally claim efficacy from these techniques, but these methods have not been shown to be efficacious in objective, blind studies.[14-16]

The Pharmacist's Role

The pharmacist, especially one who has experience in compounding intravenous admixtures, is uniquely qualified to supervise the compounding of allergen-extract prescriptions. The same compounding principles apply: maintenance of sterility, adequate documentation, potency validation, compounding-process validation, and various quality-control and quality-assurance analyses.[4,17-18] Clinical pharmacy opportunities also exist to enhance patient care and patient education.[19-22] Use of pharmacists to supervise the compounding of allergen-extract formulae improves the quality and reliability of these prescriptions and allows the allergy-immunology clinic staff more time for direct patient care and education. It is conceivable that entrepreneur pharmacists could contract with office-based allergists to compound allergen-extract prescriptions on a fee-for-service basis. Certainly all hospital-based allergen-extract compounding should receive a pharmacist's oversight.

References useful to the pharmacist compounding allergen extracts include review articles,[4,18,23] *Remington's Pharmaceutical Sciences*,[12] textbooks on botany (including U.S. Department of Agriculture publications), descriptive literature from manufacturers, and reports of the FDA Advisory Panel on Review of Allergen Extracts.[1,9]

Potency Measurement

Most allergen-extract products sold in the United States bear the proviso "No U.S. Standard of Potency." This caution is needed because the assays most widely used for allergen-extract concentrations [weight-to-volume extraction ratios (W/V) and protein nitrogen units (PNU)] have only a limited correlation to biologic and immunologic activity.

W/V extraction ratios indicate the relative quantities of pollen or other allergen extracted per given volume of extraction fluid. W/V ratios of 1/10 or 1/20 (i.e., 1 gram of source material per 10 or 20 ml of fluid) are most common. But these ratios are a process description that do not reflect the allergenicity of the resulting drug. The specific antigenic proteins extracted from the raw allergenic source material are not measured, nor is potency uniform from batch to batch.

PNU standardization measures the total protein content in a finished extract, by either the Kjeldahl or ninhydrin methods. Unfortunately, this assay measures protein without regard to the presence, absence, or consistency of specific antigenic character. The most common commercial products of this type contain 20,000 PNU/ml. House-mite and house-dust extracts usually contain 5000 PNU/ml.

Correlation between the W/V and PNU systems is incomplete and inconsistent. PNU assays for 1/10 W/V allergen-extract products generally range from 12,000 to 150,000 PNU/ml, depending on the allergen. Grass extracts typically exhibit PNU content at the top of this range, while the protein content of mold extracts tends toward the low end. W/V products of any given allergen routinely vary in their PNU content by as much as ±25% between batches.[2] House-dust extracts, because their source material is so poorly defined, exhibit the widest degree of variance.

Even pollens taken from the same field in successive years yield extracts of varying potency. If allergens were available in pure form, then mass alone would be sufficient standardization, as it is for most drugs. Unfortunately, the active ingredients of only a few allergen extracts have been identified, although much investigation is underway in this area. The new composite immunologic measurement system, allergy units (AU), increases qualitative and quantitative uniformity and lot-to-lot reproducibility. AU products are standardized by skin-test titration, corroborated with other in vitro techniques such as cross-radioimmunoelectrophoresis (CRIE) and the radioallergosorbent test (RAST).[24–29] The standardization of AU products is analogous to that of insulin, that is, standardization by biologic activity. FDA first licensed products with this form of standardization in 1983.

Any empiric comparison between the various standardization systems bears potential risks. Comparisons should be used only for general guidance; converting patients from one system of immunotherapy to another must be done cautiously. Allergens of different standardization types should not be combined.

The AU-standardization methods are not perfected. They attempt to measure the composite activity of a product with numerous independent components by use of a single potency value. Whether or not these assuredly potent extracts will actually increase the efficacy of immunotherapy is currently under study. Distinct biologic measurement systems have been developed for several major antigenic determinants, such as antigen E (AgE) for short ragweed, cat allergen-1 (CA-1), and others. For example, the antigen *Amb a* I (formerly called antigen E[30]) is a good barometer for predicting the relative presence of other companion antigenic determinants in a given lot of short-ragweed extract. But *Amb a* I alone is not sufficient to relieve allergic symptoms in most short ragweed-sensitive patients. A more complex mixture of allergens is required to treat most patients sensitive to this pollen.[3,31–32] Since 1972, short-ragweed extracts must contain not less than 135 AgE units/ml. The exact concentration must be printed on each vial label. AU-standardized cat extracts must contain 10 to 20 CA-1 units/ml.

The enhanced reproducibility of the AU-standardized products is expected to provide a marked improvement in the dose-response characteristics of these extracts. Regulatory authority for allergen extracts rests with the FDA Center for Biologics Evaluation and Research (CBER).[33–34] CBER regulations require that all new allergenic product-licensing requests include immunologic AU standardization.

Allergists commonly reject generic substitution of allergen-extract products because of the lack of potency uniformity between manufacturers and between lots of any single manufacturer. Cross-allergenicity between similar botanic groups, especially among the grasses, has been documented.[35–36] Additive effects of cross-reactive allergens may precipitate an adverse reaction.

Labeling

The concentration of allergen-extract prescriptions may be labeled on the basis of total allergen content (TAC) or according to the concentration of the greatest single allergen present in the formula (GSAP), according to prescriber preference. Because each specific allergen can be considered to interact with the human immune system independently, labeling on the basis of each allergen (GSAP) may be advisable. Caution should be exercised when allergen-extract prescriptions from both labeling systems are compounded or stored in the same location.

For example, a vial containing ten 1-ml portions of 1/10 W/V concentrates may be labeled 1/100 W/V (based on the concentration of the greatest allergen present) or 1/10 W/V (based on total extract present). Vials labeled 1/100 W/V under each of the two systems would actually vary from each other by a power of 10, a difference that is potentially fatal in exquisitely sensitive patients.

The nomenclature system for individual allergens is recommended by the International Union of Immunological Societies.[30] The system is based on the first three letters of the genus name, followed by the first letter of the species name, and then a Roman numeral. For example, antigen E of short ragweed [*Ambrosia artemisiifolia (elatior)*] is now called *Amb a I*.

Manufacture

Steps in allergen-extract manufacture include grinding, defatting, the actual extraction, preliminary filtration, dialysis, concentration, sterilization, and packaging. Good manufacturing practices (GMPs) on the industrial scale are important to the uniformity and reproducibility of allergen extracts.[11–12,33]

Source materials are ground or subdivided by other means to increase surface area and promote extraction of allergenic components. Ether or some other solvent is used to defat the source material; this step clarifies the product and removes any nonspecific irritants. Extraction itself is accomplished with buffered saline, Coca's solution, or some other menstruum for 16 to 72 hours with periodic agitation. The resultant fluid is coarsely filtered to remove the remnants of the source material. Some extracts are dialyzed to remove other irritants. Concentration by evaporation or dialysis may be employed if needed. At least one manufacturer precipitates proteins from the extract at this point with cold acetone (AP, acetone-precipitated, Hollister-Stier Laboratories, Spokane); the precipitable proteins are retained and returned to aqueous solution. Because allergen extracts are thermolabile, sterile filtration with a membrane filter, followed by packaging, concludes the manufacturing process. The manufacturers' quality-control program includes sterility testing and safety and toxicity testing in guinea pigs, rabbits, or mice. Expiration dates of 18 months for aqueous products and 36 months for glycerinated and freeze-dried extracts following release from manufacturer are common.

An extract's quality and potency are directly related to the quality of allergenic source materials from which it is derived. Pollens for extraction must be free of other contaminating pollens and may contain not more than 1% extraneous material. Freeze-dried products may contain not more than 1% residual moisture. Animal source materials may contain hair, dander, or epithelium.

Mold extracts are obtained from dried production cultures from which media has been removed. Source materials may contain mycelia, spores, or mold mats. MMP-process mold extracts (Hollister-Stier Laboratories, Spokane) contain nondialyzable mold metabolites.

Allergenic constituents of house dust consist primarily of human and animal (especially cat) dander, hair, foods, feathers, detergents, mold spores, fibers, dust mites (*Dermatophagoides farinae* and *pteronyssinus*), silk, pollens, and other inhalants. Nonspecific irritants and dyes may be removed during processing by dialysis.[1–2,33–34]

Cat allergen-1 standardized cat hair and dander extract is not directly interchangeable with cat allergen-1 standardized cat-pelt extracts or nonstandardized cat extracts. Standardized cat extracts prepared from cat hair and dander or the whole cat pelt are similar in content of cat allergen-1, the major allergen for cat-sensitive patients. Hair and dander extracts and pelt extracts, however, differ in their content of other allergenic molecules. Owing to the difference in quantity of the extraneous components in cat-pelt and cat hair and dander extracts, these extracts should not be interchanged during therapy. If patients are to be switched from one product to the other, the initial dose must be based on skin tests using the new extract.

Food extracts are licensed by the FDA for immunodiagnosis only. There is no convincing scientific evidence that food allergen extracts are safe and effective for immunotherapy. Food for extracts is defatted and dehydrated before extraction. Although most foods are extracted in aqueous buffered solution, some are extracted with a fluid containing sodium formaldehyde sulfoxylate 0.1%. Some food extracts are extremely potent, such as peanut extract.

Dosage Forms and Diluents

Several sterile dosage forms are marketed: solutions, suspensions, and lyophilized powders for reconstitution. The solutions may be either aqueous [commonly using 0.03% human serum albumin (HSA) as a protein preservative, 0.9% sodium chloride for tonicity, and 0.4% phenol as an antimicrobial agent] or glycerinated.[37–40] Solutions of 50% glycerin in sterile water for injection provide the highest degree of protein preservation, but glycerin injections may cause local irritation or sterile abscesses. Alum-precipitated suspensions of allergen extracts must be diluted with 0.9% sodium chloride and 0.4% phenol. Addition of HSA as a diluent to these products will disrupt the adsorbed, delayed-release character of the allergen-alum complex. Lyophilized extracts may be reconstituted with either 0.03% HSA with sodium chloride and phenol, or with 50% glycerin. All diluents must be sterile and non-pyrogenic.

Alum-precipitated products are available in two forms, Allpyral (Hollister-Stier Laboratories, Spokane) and Center-Al (Center Laboratories, Port Washington, NY), which are not interchangeable. They are prepared from aqueous extracts by formation of aluminum hydroxide precipitation complexes and standardized by PNU content. Each 0.5 ml dose may contain not more than 850 μg of aluminum. Additionally, Allpyral products are extracted with pyridine, which in certain cases has resulted in reduced biologic activity.[1] Both preparations should be resuspended before use.

Adsorption of the allergen onto the alum moiety slows the biologic release of the allergen, allowing faster dosage progression and fewer adverse reactions. Adverse reactions that do occur may be delayed in onset by one or more hours. Alum-precipitated suspensions of allergen extracts should be diluted with sodium chloride 0.9% with phenol 0.4% ("phenol-saline") only. Admixture of alum-precipitated allergen extracts with diluents containing HSA disrupts the prolonged-release character as the HSA competes with the alum for the allergen. Increased immediate bioavailability of the prescription results.

Stability of allergen extracts is shortest at low concentrations, because of protein adsorption to the walls of glass containers. Protein degradation and enzymatic autodigestion are other major factors. Stability is favored by low temperatures, although freezing may precipitate some proteins, especially those of high molecular weight.[24,37-39]

Diagnostic Testing

A unique formula for allergen-extract immunotherapy is prescribed for each patient, based on patient history and reactivity to skin test reagents. Allergen extracts for skin testing are in solution at weaker concentrations than those used for therapy. To diagnose hypersensitivity, patients may be tested with a series of injections of allergen extracts on their forearms and/or backs. Transcutaneous (puncture or "prick") and intradermal applications of extracts elicit an immediate-hypersensitivity reaction in sensitive patients consisting of induration ("wheal") and erythema ("flare") of varying magnitude. Intradermal (ID) tests tend to be more sensitive and reliable but more painful than prick or scratch tests. Because intradermal tests have more ready access to mast cells, weaker concentrations are used than for prick testing.[16,29,41-43]

Antihistamines suppress cutaneous reactions to extracts applied during skin testing for 48 to 72 hours.[2-3,44] Positive (histamine base 0.1 to 1 mg/ml) and negative (HSA or appropriate diluent) controls must also be applied to assure proper interpretation of test results. The viscous diluent glycerin retards the flow of a prick test reagent into neighboring reagents, but may increase the incidence of false-positive reactions. Single-component extracts are the optimal choice for testing because combining several extracts may reduce the independent concentrations to ineffective levels. Second, in the event of a positive reaction, the clinician would not know if the patient reacted to all or only some of the components.

After testing, individualized formulae for allergen-extract immunotherapy are prescribed for patients based on patient history and reactivity to the skin-test reagents. Multiple-allergen extracts are commonly combined into one to three separate solutions for therapy, depending on the number of extracts indicated and common seasonal exposure. Combinations of allergens should be limited so that each allergen is present at a therapeutic concentration. Typical concentration ranges for testing and for immunotherapy are listed in Table 16–2.[2-3,29] Several prescriptions may be written for a given patient to independently control therapy of distinct allergens and manage adverse reactions.

Compounding

Allergen extracts may be dispensed only on the order of a physician. A complete allergen-extract prescription specifies the allergen-extract components desired, their relative concentrations, demographic information on the patient, and a treatment schedule. Extract contents should be identified by both genus and species names to ensure uniformity when refill prescriptions are compounded.[18] For example, a prescription calling for oak extract should be clarified for the oak species desired, such as red oak (*Quercus rubra*), white oak (*Quercus alba*), or scrub oak (*Quercus dumosa*). Examples used by the U.S. Army allergen-extract pharmacy at Walter Reed Army Medical Center, Washington, DC, are shown in Figures 16–1 through 16–3.[18,45]

TABLE 16–2.   Diluents for Allergen Extracts

Dosage Form	Preferred Diluent	Comment
Alum precipitated allergen extracts (e.g., Allpyral, Center-Al)	0.9% NaCl with 0.4% phenol (use no other diluent)	Avoids disruption of adsorbed, delayed-release character
Allergen extracts in true solution (w/v, PNU, or AU systems)	0.03% human serum albumin with 0.9% NaCl and 0.4% phenol, or 50% glycerin	Protein preservative and antimicrobial properties
Lyophilized allergen extracts	0.03% human serum albumin with 0.9% NaCl and 0.4% phenol, or 50% glycerin	Protein preservative and antimicrobial properties
Hymenoptera venoms	0.03% human serum albumin with 0.9% NaCl and 0.4% phenol	Protein preservative and antimicrobial properties

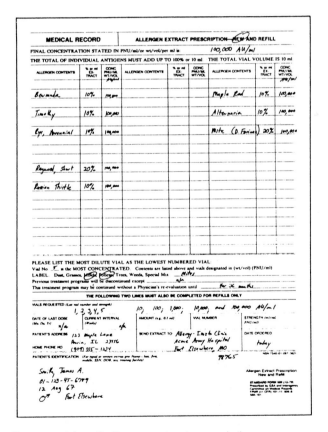

Figure 16–1.   Form used for all allergen-extract prescriptions.

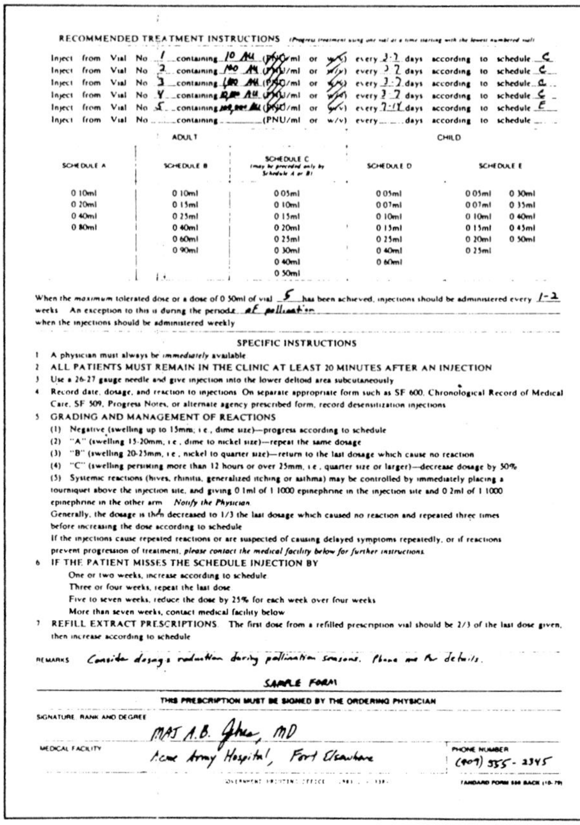

RECOMMENDED TREATMENT INSTRUCTIONS (Progress treatment using one vial at a time starting with the lowest numbered vial)

Inject from Vial No 1 containing 10 AU (PNU/ml or w/v) every 3-7 days according to schedule C
Inject from Vial No 2 containing 100 AU (PNU/ml or w/v) every 3-7 days according to schedule C
Inject from Vial No 3 containing 1,000 AU (PNU/ml or w/v) every 3-7 days according to schedule C
Inject from Vial No 4 containing 10,000 AU (PNU/ml or w/v) every 3-7 days according to schedule C
Inject from Vial No 5 containing 100,000 AU (PNU/ml or w/v) every 7-14 days according to schedule E
Inject from Vial No ___ containing ___ (PNU/ml or w/v) every ___ days according to schedule ___

ADULT			CHILD		
SCHEDULE A	SCHEDULE B	SCHEDULE C (may be preceded only by Schedule A or B)	SCHEDULE D	SCHEDULE E	
0 10ml	0 10ml	0 05ml	0 05ml	0 05ml	0 30ml
0 20ml	0 15ml	0 10ml	0 07ml	0 07ml	0 35ml
0 40ml	0 25ml	0 15ml	0 10ml	0 10ml	0 40ml
0 80ml	0 40ml	0 20ml	0 15ml	0 15ml	0 45ml
	0 60ml	0 25ml	0 25ml	0 20ml	0 50ml
	0 90ml	0 30ml	0 40ml	0 25ml	
		0 40ml	0 60ml		
		0 50ml			

When the *maximum* tolerated dose or a dose of 0 50ml of vial 5 has been achieved, injections should be administered every 1-2 weeks An exception to this is during the periods of pollination when the injections should be administered weekly

SPECIFIC INSTRUCTIONS

1 A physician must always be *immediately* available
2 ALL PATIENTS MUST REMAIN IN THE CLINIC AT LEAST 20 MINUTES AFTER AN INJECTION
3 Use a 26-27 gauge needle and give injection into the lower deltoid area subcutaneously
4 Record date, dosage, and reaction to injections On separate appropriate form such as SF 600, Chronological Record of Medical Care, SF 509, Progress Notes, or alternate agency prescribed form, record desensitization injections
5 GRADING AND MANAGEMENT OF REACTIONS
(1) Negative (swelling up to 15mm; i e., dime size)—progress according to schedule
(2) "A" (swelling 15-20mm, i e , dime to nickel size)—repeat the same dosage
(3) "B" (swelling 20-25mm, i e , nickel to quarter size)—return to the last dosage which cause no reaction
(4) "C" (swelling persisting more than 12 hours or over 25mm, i e , quarter size or larger)—decrease dosage by 50%
(5) Systemic reactions (hives, rhinitis, generalized itching or asthma) may be controlled by immediately placing a tourniquet above the injection site, and giving 0 1ml of 1 1000 epinephrine in the injection site and 0 2ml of 1 1000 epinephrine in the other arm *Notify the Physician*
Generally, the dosage is then decreased to 1/3 the last dosage which caused no reaction and repeated three times before increasing the dose according to schedule
If the injections cause repeated reactions or are suspected of causing delayed symptoms repeatedly, or if reactions prevent progression of treatment, *please contact the medical facility below for further instructions*
6 IF THE PATIENT MISSES THE SCHEDULE INJECTION BY
One or two weeks, increase according to schedule
Three or four weeks, repeat the last dose
Five to seven weeks, reduce the dose by 25% for each week over four weeks
More than seven weeks, contact medical facility below
7 REFILL EXTRACT PRESCRIPTIONS The first dose from a refilled prescription vial should be 2/3 of the last dose given, then increase according to schedule

REMARKS Consider dosage reduction during pollination seasons. Phone me for details.

SAMPLE FORM

THIS PRESCRIPTION MUST BE SIGNED BY THE ORDERING PHYSICIAN

SIGNATURE, RANK AND DEGREE MAJ A.B. [illegible], MD

MEDICAL FACILITY Acme Army Hospital, Fort Elsewhere

PHONE NUMBER (409) 555-2345

STANDARD FORM 5?? BACK (10-79)

Figure 16–2. Recommended treatment schedule completed on the reverse side of the prescription form.

Quality-control procedures during compounding emphasize (1) maintenance of sterility during manipulation of sterile components, needles, syringes, and containers, (2) confirmation of identity and volume of each allergen extract included, (3) accurate product labeling, and (4) complete compounding documentation, including manufacturer and lot number.

Because end-product testing of these complex mixtures is not possible and the consequences of a compounding error may include anaphylaxis or death, compounding pharmacists should emphasize error prevention. Double-check systems should be used at each compounding step to minimize transcription errors, inaccurate calculations or measurements, and transposition of vials or labels.[18] Inadvertently challenging a patient directly with a full-strength antigen may result in anaphylaxis or even death.

Patient profile cards should be maintained on all patients to provide a permanent record of immunotherapy prescribed and dispensed (Fig. 16–3). Additional space may be used to record concurrent medications, including nonprescription allergy medications.

Allergen-extract prescriptions, like all sterile products, should be compounded with aseptic technique in laminar air-flow hoods.[18,46–47] Separate needles and syringes should be used for each component to avoid cross-contamination

Smith, James A.   Allergy-Immunization Clinic
SSN: 01-123-45-6789   Acme Army-Community Hospital
Dependent/Son/Retired/US Army   Fort Elsewhere, MO 98765
Dr. (MAJ) Jones/today/Typist _____   Telephone: (202) 576-2185

Rx # 135791   Contains: 100,000 Allergenic Units/mL   Lot #:
Grasses: Bermuda .... 10%   1.0 mL _____
               Timothy .... 10%   1.0 mL _____
               Perennial Rye .... 10%   1.0 mL _____
Weeds: Ragweed, Short .... 20%   2.0 mL _____
               Russian Thistle .... 10%   1.0 mL _____
Trees: Maple, Red .... 10%   1.0 mL _____
Molds: Alternaria .... 10%   1.0 mL _____
House Dust Mite (*Dermatophagoides farinae*) .... 20%   2.0 mL _____
Dispense: Vials 1, 2, 3, 4, 5: 10; 100; 1,000; 10,000; and 100,000 AU/mL
Reviewer _____ Compounder _____ Checker _____ Packer _____ Date shipped _____

Refill: Rx # 201202   today   Vials #: 4 & 5: 10,000 and 100,000 AU/mL
Lots: ____;   ____;   ____;   ____;   ____;   ____;   ____;   ____.
Reviewer _____ Compounder _____ Checker _____ Packer _____ Date shipped ____

Figure 16–3. Patient profile card.

of stock containers with extraneous allergens. For a standard set of four 10-fold serial dilutions, the most concentrated vial is compounded first. Each dilution is then compounded by withdrawing a 1 ml aliquot and adding it to a 9 ml vial of suitable diluent. Prefilled 1.8, 4.5, and 9 ml vials are commercially available to facilitate compounding.

Extracts should be refrigerated, not frozen. Temperature recording graphs and alarms on refrigerators can help preclude catastrophic loss of inventory. Potency loss in stock containers as a result of repeated warming and cooling by chilling should be minimized during compounding sessions. Insulated trays at the side of the laminar flow hood are effective for this purpose. Allergenic prescriptions should be shipped by the most expeditious means (e.g., first class U.S. Mail or equivalent) to maximize stability. Because of the intricacies of compounding and the potency variation from one compounded prescription to the next, 12-month expiration dates for full-strength vials are frequently used. More dilute concentrations may be assigned shorter expiration dates.

Quality Assessment

End-product testing for identity of allergenic prescriptions is not feasible with current technology. Sterility testing is appropriate, using thioglycollate and soybean-casein media.[48] If samples are to be withdrawn with the same needle from a serial dilution set, samples should be drawn proceeding from the most dilute to the most concentrated vial. Pyrogen testing is not warranted. Protein assays, iso-electric focusing (IEF), radioallergosorbent test inhibition (RAST-I), and other assays are useful to validate potency and biologic activity of distinct allergen extracts prior to purchase or sequentially during storage.[18,49] Methods to monitor error rates and trends in compounding are described elsewhere.[18]

Patient Education

Patients should be involved in the management of allergic diseases. Avoidance of allergens is always the first method of management; environmental control is similarly important. Patients can be counseled on management and reporting of delayed adverse reactions, coincident use of non-prescription medications, and compliance with course of therapy.

Standard dosage schedules for diagnosis and therapy are included in Table 16–3 and Figure 16–2. Dosage reductions are frequently prescribed if the patient misses a scheduled injection, when therapy from a refill prescription is initiated, or during appropriate pollination seasons. Patients are advised not to double the dose to make up for a missed dose. Immunotherapy should be provided only in a setting where complete emergency equipment and personnel to treat anaphylaxis are immediately available. Anaphylaxis may occur without warning, usually within the first 30 minutes after an injection, even during the maintenance phase of therapy.[50–51] Routine use of antihistamines before allergen-extract injections may mask immediate hypersensitivity symptoms until a rapidly emerging anaphylactic episode erupts, and this use should be avoided.

Hymenoptera Venoms

Similar to allergen extracts are the purified, lyophilized venoms of the insect order *Hymenoptera* (honeybee, wasp, white-faced hornet, yellow hornet, and yellowjacket), licensed by FDA in 1978. At least 40 people die each year from anaphylaxis subsequent to stings from honey bees, wasps, or the vespids (the group of yellow jackets and hornets). Many other insect-related deaths are probably misattributed to heart attacks or other causes.[23,52–53]

Most venoms are harvested by physical dissection of the insects' venom sacs. In the case of the honeybee, the insect is stimulated electrically to sting; the extruded venom is then collected from a suitable receptacle. These products are assayed by mass of dried venom and standardized by hyaluronidase activity. The active ingredients include hyaluronidase, phospholipase A_2, acid phosphatase, and various peptides and vasoactive amines (such as histamine and dopamine). Specific stabilities for reconstituted venoms are provided by the manufacturers. Stability is shortest for dilute solutions (as low as 24 hours), but quite lengthy for the 100 μg/ml concentrate (as long as 12 months).[52,54–55]

The vespid venoms (white-faced hornet, yellow hornet, and yellowjacket) are significantly cross-antigenic. Wasp venom is slightly cross-reactive with the vespids. Honeybee venom is the most unique. The venom dose of an average insect sting is approximately 60 μg for honey bees, 2.4 μg for yellowjackets, 3.7 for hornets, and 10 mcg for wasps.[56] A standard maintenance dose is 1 ml of 100 μg/ml at 30-day intervals.

Although two manufacturers offer mixed-vespid formulations, such triple combinations should be used for therapy only; individual venoms should be used for diagnostic skin testing. An informal survey in mid-1985 among clients of the U.S. Army Allergen Extract Laboratory suggests that users consistently prefer the convenience of reconstituting starter kits over compounding proper dilutions manually.[23]

TABLE 16–3. Standard Concentrations and Dosages for Diagnosis and Therapy

Standardization System	Diagnostic Tests		Immunotherapy Dosage*†		Frequency	
	Prick	Intradermal	Initial	Maintenance	Initial	Maintenance
Immunometric	10,000–100,000 AU/ml	1–10 AU/ml	0.05 ml of 1–10 AU/ml	0.5 ml of 10,000 AU/ml	3–14 days	7–14 days
Weight/volume	1/100–1/10 W/V	1/1000–1/100 W/V	0.05 ml of 1/100,000 W/V	0.5 ml of 1/100 W/V	3–14 days	7–14 days
Protein nitrogen units	1000–2000 PNU/ml	100–200 PNU/ml	0.05 ml of 2 PNU/ml	0.5 ml of 2000 PNU/ml	3–14 days	7–14 days
Alum-precipitated extracts	Do not test with these products		0.1 ml of 100 PNU/ml	0.5 ml of 1000 PNU/ml	7–14 days	2–6 weeks
Hymenoptera venoms‡		0.1 ml of 0.001 to 1 µg/ml	0.02 ml of 0.01 µg/ml§	1 ml of 100 µg/ml	3–7 days‖	30 days

*Dosage is based on the concentration of the greatest single allergen present.
†Adult and pediatric doses are usually equivalent.
‡For safety, some clinicians administer one initial prick test at 0.1 µg/ml prior to intradermal tests.
§Usual initial dose is two 10-fold dilutions below first positive cutaneous reaction.
‖"Rush" immunotherapy under controlled conditions has also been effective.

Although purified venoms have completely replaced whole-body extracts (WBEs) for bees, wasps, and hornets, WBE are still employed for certain other *Hymenoptera* insects, including the imported fire ant (*Solenopsis invicta* and *Solenopsis richteri*). WBEs are prepared by macerating whole insects and then preparing an extract, a method similar to methods used for pollen extracts and other allergen extracts.[1] Fire-ant WBE contains at least 30 antigens, 5 of which may evoke IgE-mediated anaphylaxis, but antigen content varies from manufacturer to manufacturer. Despite some conflicting data, purified fire-ant venom appears to be no more effective than the corresponding whole-body extract, probably because these ants lack the enzymes that biodegrade venom protein in bee and vespid WBEs.[52,57–61]

Research Trends

Research currently focuses on purifying allergens, defining the allergenic determinants, and developing the evolving immunologic standardization systems. New immunologic methods, such as crossed radio-immunoelectrophoresis (CRIE), enzyme-linked immunosorbent assay (ELISA), and others will make further standardization feasible. Development of international reference preparations through the International Union of Immunological Societies (IUIS) is proceeding for *Alternaria* species, *Dermatophagoides pteronyssinus* mite, and others.

Research into various novel forms of allergen extracts has been under way for well over a decade. These studies aim to increase efficacy and decrease adverse effects associated with immunotherapy. None of these products has yet been licensed in the United States, although some are available in other countries.[62] Promising investigational forms of allergen extracts include formalin-treated allergens ("allergoids"), glutaraldehyde-treated allergens (i.e., polymerized allergens), and a polypeptide that mimics IgE.

Conclusion

Allergen extracts are safe and effective in the diagnosis and treatment of several allergic diseases. Immunodiagnostic reagents and immunotherapy prescriptions must be accurate, precise, and reproducible to serve the patient and to prevent adverse reactions. Sterile compounding procedures, patient profiles, and quality control tests of prospective batches of allergen extracts contribute to confidence in these prescription products.

Pharmacists can provide valuable input in the compounding of allergen-extract prescriptions on record keeping, aseptic technique, storage, and quality control. Entrepreneur pharmacists may contract with office-based allergists to compound allergen-extract formulae on a fee-for-service basis. All hospital-based allergen-extract compounding should receive a pharmacist's oversight. Use of pharmacists to compound allergen-extract formulae improves the quality and reliability of these prescriptions and allows the allergy-immunology clinic staff more time for direct patient care and education.

Clinical pharmacists in internal medicine, allergy, or pediatric settings should consider allergen extracts as diagnostic or therapeutic options in the management of allergic rhinitis, allergic asthma, and other disorders, especially in cases where pharmacotherapy has been inadequate. Pharmacists should take an active role in ensuring the optimal quality of diagnostic and therapeutic allergen extracts in their professional practices.

References

1. Food & Drug Administration: Biological products; allergenic products: Implementation of efficacy review. Fed. Reg., 50, 3082 (1985).
2. Baer, H., Anderson, M.C., and Turkeltaub, P.C.: Allergenic extracts. In Allergy: Principles and Practice. 3rd Ed. Edited by E. Middleton Jr., C.E. Reed, E.F. Ellis, N.F. Adkinson Jr., and J.W. Yunginger. St. Louis, C.V. Mosby, 1988, pp. 373–401.
3. Van Metre, T.E. Jr., and Adkinson, N.F., Jr.: Immunotherapy for aeroallergen disease. In Allergy: Principles and Practice. 3rd Ed. Edited by E. Middleton Jr., C.E. Reed, E.F. Ellis, N.F. Adkinson Jr., and J.W. Yunginger. St. Louis, C.V. Mosby, 1988, pp. 1327–44.
4. Grabenstein, J.D.: Allergen-extract compounding by pharmacists. Hosp. Pharm., 27, 148 and 165 (1992).
5. Grabenstein, J.D.: Comment on anaphylactic shock. Drug Intell. Clin. Pharm., 18, 646 (letter) (1984).
6. Naclerio, R.M.: Allergic rhinitis. N. Engl. J. Med., 325, 860 (1991).
7. Noon, L.: Prophylactic inoculation against hay fever. Lancet, i, 1572 (1911).
8. Freeman, J.: Further observations on the treatment of hay fever by hypodermic inoculations of pollen vaccine. Lancet, ii, 814 (1911).
9. Schaeffer, M., and Sisk, L.C.: Allergenic extracts: A review of their safety and efficacy. Ann. Allergy, 52, 2 (1984).
10. Committee on the Safety of Medicines: Desensitizing vaccines. Brit. Med. J., 293, 948 (1986).
11. Curtis, E.G.: Allergenic extracts. In Remington's Pharmaceutical Sciences. 15th Ed. Edited by A. Osol and J.E. Hoover. Easton, PA, Mack, 1975, pp. 1344.
12. Shough, H.R.: Allergenic extracts. In Remington's Pharmaceutical Sciences. 18th Ed. Edited by A.R. Gennaro. Easton, PA, Mack, 1990, pp. 1405–15.
13. Nesbit, G.H.: Canine allergic inhalant dermatitis: A review of 230 cases. J. Am. Vet. Med. Assoc., 172, 55 (1978).
14. Shapiro, G.G. and Anderson, J.A.: Controversial techniques in allergy. Pediatrics, 82, 935 (1988).
15. Selner, J.C., and Condemi, J.: Unproven diagnostic and therapeutic techniques for allergy. In Allergy: Principles & Practice. 3rd Ed. Edited by E. Middleton Jr., C.E. Reed, E.F. Ellis, N.F. Adkinson Jr., and J.W. Yunginger. St. Louis, C.V. Mosby, 1988, pp. 1571–97.
16. Council on Scientific Affairs: In vivo diagnostic testing and immunotherapy for allergy: Report I, Part II of the Allergy Panel. JAMA, 258, 1505 (1987).
17. Lawson, R.E.: Allergenic prescriptions: An expanded area of sterile compounding. Am. J. Hosp. Pharm., 20, 624 (1963).
18. Grabenstein, J.D.: Operation of an allergen-extract pharmacy. Am. J. Hosp. Pharm., 42, 1733 (1985).
19. Hunter, R.B., and Osterberger, D.J.: Role of the pharmacist in the allergy clinic. Am. J. Hosp. Pharm., 32, 392 (1975).
20. Grabenstein, J.D., Summers, R.J., and Renard, R.L.: A comprehensive allergen-extract monograph with advice for the patient. Ann. Allergy, 54, 185 (1985).
21. Owerbach, J., Winters, B., and Villella, W.: Pharmacist selection of allergy medication based on patient response to trial regimens. Am. J. Hosp. Pharm., 38, 856 (1981).
22. Tse, C.S.: Clinical pharmacy practice in an allergy clinic. Contemp. Pharm. Pract., 21, 20 (1978).
23. Grabenstein, J.D.: Immunotherapy for *Hymenoptera* insects: Bees, wasps, hornets, and fire ants. Hosp. Pharm., 27, in press.

24. Friesen, G.L., and Jones, R.M.: Standardized and partially purified allergen extracts: Concept and clinical evaluation of potency. Immunol. Allergy Pract., *6*, 163 (1984).

25. Turkeltaub, P.C., et al.: A standardized quantitative skin-test assay of allergen potency and stability: Studies of the allergen dose-response curve and effect of wheal, erythema and patient selection on assay results. J. Allergy Clin. Immunol., *70*, 343 (1982).

26. Yunginger, J.W.: Allergen standardization: 1984. J. Allergy Clin. Immunol., *73*, 316 (1984).

27. Reed, C.E., Yunginger, J.W., and Evans, R.: Quality assurance and standardization of allergy extracts in allergy practice. J. Allergy Clin. Immunol. *84*, 4 (1989).

28. Yunginger, J.W.: Standardization of allergen extracts. Ann. Allergy, *66*, 107 (1991).

29. Bousquet, J.: In vivo methods for study of allergy: Skin tests, techniques, and interpretation. *In* Allergy: Principles and Practice. 3rd Ed. Edited by E. Middleton Jr., C.E. Reed, E.F. Ellis, N.F. Adkinson Jr., and J.W. Yunginger. St. Louis, C.V. Mosby, 1988 pp. 419–36.

30. Marsh, D.G., et al.: Allergen nomenclature. J. Allergy Clin. Immunol., *80*, 639 (1987).

31. Norman, P.S., Winkenwerder, W.L., and Lichtenstein, L.M.: Immunotherapy of hayfever with ragweed Antigen E: Comparison with whole pollen extract and placebos. J. Allergy Clin. Immunol., *42*, 93 (1968).

32. Lichtenstein, L.M., Norman, P.S., and Winkenwerder, W.L.: A single year of immunotherapy for ragweed hayfever. Ann. Intern. Med., *75*, 663 (1971).

33. 21 CFR 210–211.

34. 21 CFR 680.1(a).

35. Weber, R.W., and Nelson, H.S. Pollen allergens and their interrelationships. Clin. Rev. Allergy, *3*, 291 (1985).

36. Leavengood, D.C., Renard, R.L., Martin, B.G., and Nelson, H.S.: Cross allergenicity among grasses determined by tissue threshold changes. J. Allergy Clin. Immunol., *76*, 789 (1985).

37. Nelson, H.S.: The effect of preservatives and dilution on the deterioration of Russian thistle (*Salsola pestifer*), a pollen extract. J. Allergy Clin. Immunol., *63*, 417 (1979).

38. Norman, P.S., and Marsh, D.G.: Human serum albumin and Tween 80 as stabilizers of allergen solutions. J. Allergy Clin. Immunol., *62*, 314 (1978).

39. Nelson, H.S.: Effect of preservatives and conditions of storage on the potency of allergen extracts. J. Allergy Clin. Immunol., *67*, 64 (1981).

40. Menardo, J.L., et al.: Effects of diluents on skin tests. Ann. Allergy, *51*, 535 (1983).

41. Nelson, H.S.: Diagnostic procedures in allergy: I. Allergy skin testing. Ann. Allergy, *51*, 411 (1983).

42. Bernstein, I.L. (Ed.): Proceedings of the task force on guidelines for standardizing old and new technologies used for the diagnosis and treatment of allergic diseases. J. Allergy Clin. Immunol., *82(Suppl)*, 487 (1988).

43. Council on Scientific Affairs: In vivo diagnostic testing and immunotherapy for allergy: Report I, Part I of the Allergy Panel. JAMA, *258*, 1363 (1987).

44. Grabenstein, J.D.: Drug interactions involving immunologic agents. II. immunodiagnostic and other immunologic drug interactions. DICP-Ann Pharmacother., *24*, 186 (1990).

45. Guilbert, T.V.: The feasibility of a common allergy extract preparation laboratory for the United States Army. Thesis, North Dakota State University, August 21, 1973.

46. Frieben, W.R.: Control of the aseptic processing environment. Am. J. Hosp. Pharm., *40*, 1928 (1983).

47. National Coordinating Committee for Large Volume Parenterals: Recommended guidelines for quality assurance in hospital centralized intravenous admixture services. Am. J. Hosp. Pharm., *37*, 645 (1980).

48. 21 CFR 610.12.

49. Grabenstein, J.D., Kosisky, S.E., and Summers, R.J.: Assessment of allergen-extract batches by sequential protein assay, iso-electric focusing (IEF) and RAST inhibition. Ann. Allergy, 55, 261 (1985).

50. Kaufman, C.R., Summers, R.J., and Renard, R.L.: Safety of immunotherapy (IT): A prospective study. Ann. Allergy, 52, 220 (1984).

51. American Academy of Allergy and Immunology: The waiting period after allergen skin testing and immunotherapy. J. Allergy Clin. Immunol., 85, 526 (1990).

52. Reisman, R.E.: Insect allergy. In Allergy: Principles and Practice. 3rd Ed. Edited by E. Middleton Jr., C.E. Reed, E.F. Ellis, N.F. Adkinson Jr., and J.W. Yunginger. St. Louis, C.V. Mosby, 1988, pp. 1345–64.

53. Lockey, R.F.: Immunotherapy for allergy to insect stings. N. Engl. J. Med. 323, 1627 (1990).

54. Product Information: Pharmalgen® Freeze-Dried Venom/Venom Protein Allergenic Extracts: Directions for Use. ALK America, Inc., Milford, CT, April 1987.

55. Product Information: Venomil™/Albay™ Hymenoptera Venoms. Hollister-Stier Laboratories, Spokane, WA. Revision code 355120-M09, undated.

56. Hoffman, D.R., and Jacobson, R.S.: Allergens in Hymenoptera venom. XII: How much protein is in a sting? Ann. Allergy, 52, 274 (1984).

57. Strom, G.B., Boswell, R.N., and Jacobs, R.L.: In vivo and in vitro comparison of fire ant venom and fire ant whole body extract. J. Allergy Clin. Immunol., 72, 46 (1983).

58. Paull, B.R., Coghlan, T.H., and Vinson, S.B.: Fire-ant venom hypersensitivity: I. Comparison of fire-ant venom and whole body extract in the diagnosis of fire-ant allergy. J. Allergy Clin. Immunol., 71, 448 (1983).

59. DeShazo, R.D., Butcher, B.T., and Banks, W.A.: Reactions to the stings of the imported fire ant. N. Engl. J. Med., 323, 462 (1990).

60. Stafford, C.T., et al.: Comparison of in vivo and in vitro tests in the diagnosis of imported fire-ant sting allergy. Ann. Allergy, 64, 368 (1990).

61. DeShazo, R.D., and O'Neil, C.: Treatment of allergy to fire-ant venom: The (allergy) doctor's dilemma. Ann. Allergy, 66, 1 (1991).

62. Grammer, L.C., and Shaughnessy, M.A.: Immunotherapy with modified allergens. Immunol. Allergy Clin. N. Am., 12, 95 (1992).

APPENDIX

Understanding Fluid Dynamics When Choosing IV Control Systems*

Stephen R. Ash and David J. Carr

Intravenous administration of fluids and medications has become standard practice in all hospitals. However, questions still arise concerning the optimal use of this therapy:

1. What causes the infusion rate to vary from minute to minute when using a gravity-flow system?
2. Do certain types of I.V. fluids necessitate use of a pump?
3. Can the accuracy of I.V. pumps be matched by I.V. controllers?
4. How effective are pressure alarms in detecting infiltration during pump infusion?

An I.V. administration system is essentially a hydraulic structure. A few simple principles of fluid dynamics are applicable to I.V. administration systems. A review of these principles is useful in understanding the problems of I.V. therapy and, consequently, in choosing the most effective method.

Pressure Gradient

The driving force of flow of a fluid through any device (tubing, clamp, filter, cannula, etc.) is termed the pressure gradient. This is the difference in the

*Reprinted with permission from Parenterals, Vol. 51, February/March 1987.
Edited for style consistency.

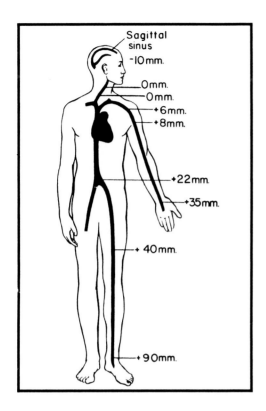

Figure A1–1. I.V. pressures, standing position.

pressure on a fluid before and after its flow through a device. Pressure is a familiar concept, but the units of measure may be confusing.

In medicine, the most common units of pressure are cm H_2O and mmHg. These units are derived from two measuring instruments—the water and mercury manometers. When using a manometer, such as in blood pressure measurement, a tube is attached that carries air under pressure. The air contacts fluid in a chamber at the bottom of the manometer. The mercury or water in the manometer rises until its height exerts a pressure equal to the air pressure. The height of the fluid column is then measured in cm H_2O. The conversion of cm H_2O to mmHg is simple. Because mercury is 13.6 times as heavy as water, the pressure of a 1 mm column of mercury equals that of a 13.6 mm or 1.36 cm column of water. These same units are used for measuring pressure in mechanical transducers.

The pressure generated by an I.V. container and length of tubing equals the vertical distance from the air inlet or the air-fluid interface of the solution container to the lowest part of the tubing. This distance is called the "hydrostatic pressure heap." For water, it equals the pressure created when fluid flow is at zero.

Obviously, raising or lowering the end of an I.V. changes the pressure at that point. Of course, the veins and arteries of the body also contain columns of fluid, in this case, blood. The weight of blood results in a higher pressure at the lower part of the body and at the end of any extremity, as shown in Figure A1–1. In measuring venous pressure, the pressure at a central point is taken as a reference. Central venous pressure is measured at the level of the right atrium. This point is approximately 10 cm down from the manubrium, whether the patient is in the supine or upright position. In measuring the pressure gradient of a gravity intravenous system, the same reference point may be used. In a gravity infusion system, the distance from the top of the I.V. fluid column (or to the air inlet of an I.V. container) to the right atrium is the pressure gradient driving the system.

Resistance

The second concept necessary for understanding flow in I.V. systems is resistance. Whether the term is used in politics, marketing, or psychology, resistance has a similar meaning. It indicates the amount of work necessary to accomplish a desired goal. When fluid flows through a tube or container, friction occurs between the moving fluid and the stationary walls of the container. This results in resistance to fluid flow. A large-diameter tube has a lower resistance than a smaller tube because the moving fluid is generally farther from the walls. With any tube or channel, the resistance is proportional to its length. A filter presents resistance to the flow of fluid because the flow channels are exceedingly small in diameter (0.2 to 0.45 μm, typically). However, the surface area of the filter can largely cancel this effect.

The higher the resistance in an I.V. system, the lower the flow at a given pressure. This relationship is expressed by the following:

$$\text{Resistance} = \frac{\text{pressure gradient}}{\text{flow rate}}$$

$$\text{Typical units:} = \frac{\text{cm } H_2O}{\text{ml/min}} \quad \text{or} \quad \frac{\text{mm Hg}}{\text{ml/min}}$$

The units indicate the rise in pressure to be expected from each ml/min increase in flow rate. When several flow elements are added successively in a line or series, the resistances are additive. Each extra component (such as a filter, clamp, length of tubing, or needle) adds to the total resistance. With a constant hydrostatic pressure head (as in gravity, infusion), increases in resistance diminish the flow rate.

With a pump, fluid volume is delivered at a constant rate. Each resistance results in a higher pressure in the fluid behind the resistance. If the resistance of a component of a flow system is known, measuring the pressure drop across the resistance allows the flow rate to be calculated. This is the basis of some flow meters. Conversely, if the flow rate is known and the pressure can be measured, the resistance of a system can be calculated (resistance = pressure divided by flow).

Resistance in a hydraulic system is generally independent of the flow rate. However, at high flow rates in small-diameter tubes, or when the diameter of a tube suddenly changes, flow may change from normal smooth "laminar" to "turbulent" (mixed) flow. Turbulent flow, however, is not a factor in the flow rates used in clinical settings in I.V. use, increasing the hydrostatic head pressure always increases the flow rate, although not necessarily linearly (Fig. A1–2).

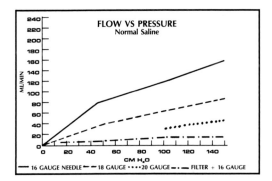

Figure A1–2. Flow rate (ml/min) versus hydrostatic pressure head (cmH₂O) for normal saline and various I.V. components.

Viscosity

In common terminology, viscosity denotes the thickness or thinness of a solution. Technically, it is a measurement of a solution's internal friction, as layers of fluid move relative to each other. The common unit of viscosity is centipoise (cp), which indicates relative thickness in comparison to water (1 cp). Solutions with high concentrations of solutes (such as 30% dextrose), and especially those with macromolecular solutes (such as albumin or dextran), have higher viscosities. Solutes generally have a greater effect on viscosity than on density. For example, 30% dextrose has a viscosity of 1.85 cp (1.85 times the viscosity of water), whereas its density is only approximately 1.10 times that of water.

Higher-viscosity solutions have higher resistance when passing through systems with small channels. Figure A1–3 indicates the flow of a 30% dextrose through an I.V. system using varying needle sizes. At the same pressure, and with the same needle or filter in line, the flow of 30% dextrose is lower than that of normal saline (Fig. A1–2).

Temperature also affects viscosity, especially in macromolecular solutions. The cooler the solution, the higher the viscosity. I.V. fluids and blood products are warmed to room temperature before infusion. Rooms vary in tem-

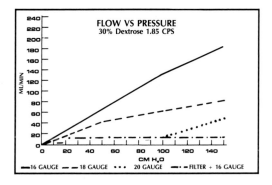

Figure A1–3. Flow rate (ml/min) versus hydrostatic pressure head (cmH₂O) for 30% dextrose and various I.V. components.

perature, though. Also, some I.V. fluids are prepared from frozen components and may be cool when delivered.

Drop Size

Most I.V. controllers and some pumps use drop-counting devices to measure the flow rate. This is done by positioning the drop to fall between a light and a light detector. Anyone who has operated a drop-counting controller knows that the user must first determine the type of solutes in the solution, and either enter this data into a volumetric rate-entry controller or manually adjust the drop rate in the drop-counting controller to yield the desired flow.[1] If the controller makes the conversion from drops/min to ml/hour, then it may be necessary to enter the volumetric accuracy required.

Several factors affect the size of drops that form at a small orifice. The most important is a fluid's tension—a force that develops at the interface between liquid and air. This tension is the reason why small volumes of water form round drops. When a drop is forming at an orifice, surface tension holds it to the orifice until the drop's weight causes it to fall. The speed of fluid flow also affects drop size, but this is not important in I.V. systems.

Several types of medications have "surfactant" properties. Surfactants are solutes that diminish the surface tension of fluids. Therefore, these substances markedly diminish the size of drops. An example is soluble B vitamins. Drop-counting devices must be adjusted whenever soluble B vitamins are in the solution. They must also be adjusted for solutions of widely varying density, such as those with high concentrations of dextrose or amino acid.

Compliance

The final concept needed to understand IV fluid flow is compliance, which describes both the size and the fullness of a container. It is expressed in terms of the volume change that causes a certain pressure alteration inside a particular container:

$$\text{Compliance} = \frac{\text{change in volume}}{\text{change in pressure}}$$

Typical units $= \text{ml/cmH}_2\text{O or ml/mmHg}$

The venous system is a highly compliant reservoir. When a liter of fluid is administered intravenously, the increase in venous pressure is only 4 or 5 mm Hg.[2] A greater amount of blood moves downward when the body remains sedentary. If a standing position is assumed, over 400 ml of blood shifts to the lower extremities. However, this transfer would be much greater if the compliance of the veins were not countered by muscular control of the diameter of the veins and the increase of venous tone by sympathetic activity.

The venous system is a low-resistance structure. Parallel vein channels exist in almost every part of the body, and the diameter of veins is large compared to that of arteries and arterioles, through which the blood loses about 90% of

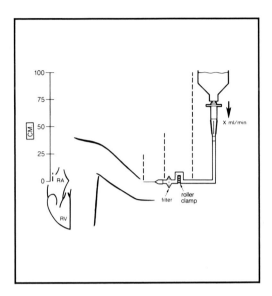

Figure A1–4.   Pressures in a gravity-control I.V. system with clamp, filter, and needle.

its pressure. The average pressure in peripheral veins is only 6 to 18 mmHg above that of the right atrium.[3-5] Although slight, this pressure is still sufficient to transport blood back to the heart at a rate equal to cardiac output.

The interstitial tissue that surrounds veins has also proven to be a mechanism of high compliance for blood flow. The pressure in the subcutaneous tissue is usually about 6 mm less than atmospheric pressure[3] representing a semivacuum condition. Only a small amount of free fluid is in interstitial tissue; it exists as a collagenous gel. Edema (the accumulation of free fluid) occurs only when venous pressure increases, when lymphatic vessels lose their ability to imbibe proteins and fluid, or when fluid is infused into the subcutaneous space by a needle. Once free fluid begins to accumulate, it collects easily. Guyton[3] has estimated that in a 70-kg person, over 70 l of fluid could be added to the interstitial space, with an increase in interstitial pressure of only 8 mmHg.

A Model of Intravenous Infusion

With this background, it is possible to construct a model for I.V. infusion. Pressures for this infusion are easier to calculate if the clamp, filter, and needle are all positioned at the level of the right atrium. Figure A1–4 indicates that expected pressures during gravity infusion with a 100-cm hydrostatic head. At usual I.V. infusion rates (<1 L/hr), there is only minimal pressure loss in the tubing. Therefore, the pressure exerted prior to the point where the clamp is placed equals the hydrostatic head of the I.V. fluid. The flow rate is determined primarily by the resistance of the clamp, filter, needle, and patient. Representative pressures at these respective locations are shown by dotted lines in the figure.

Infiltrating fluid into subcutaneous space may allow a significant amount of fluid to enter without a comparable increase in pressure. During infiltration, the pressures would still appear similar to those depicted in Figure A1–4.

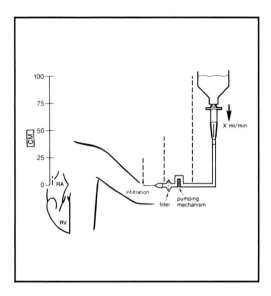

Figure A1–5. Pressures in an I.V. pump system with clamp, filter, and needle.

Figure A1–5 indicates the pressure changes that would occur during infusion of I.V. fluid with a pump. At the same time of flow rate as a gravity system (see Fig. A1–4), the pressures are the same at each point of the system. When the fluid's flow rate is the same, both gravity flow systems and pumps produce the same pressure in the system.

From this analysis, some commonly asked questions concerning I.V. infusion can be answered. Pressure monitors have been built into I.V. equipment to detect subcutaneous infiltration. It is not surprising that such monitors are often ineffective in detecting infiltration or blockage of the venous system. Gravity infusion systems have a significant variation in flow rate. This inconsistency results partially from "creeping" of the tubing in the clamp and the resulting change in resistance, and partially from changes caused by the position of the patient.

It is often thought that using an I.V. filter or high-viscosity fluid necessitates use of a volumetric pump.[6] This discussion indicates otherwise. As long as the hydrostatic pressure head is maintained at 100 cm H_2O and a drop-counting device accurately measures the flow rate, a gravity controller could deliver the desired flow rate. To determine the usefulness of gravity infusion systems, it would be helpful for filter manufacturers to indicate the resistance of their I.V. filter systems. Information on the viscosity of I.V. nutritional products would also be beneficial. Through a review of these data, it would be possible to determine whether gravity I.V. infusion would suffice or if a pump would be necessary.

In health care today, efficiency is as important as efficacy. The proper use of I.V. infusion devices provides an opportunity to improve both.

References

1. Turco, S.J.: Flow rate accuracy of a new volumetric controller. Am. J. I.V. Ther. Clin. Nutr., *10*, 18 (1983).

2. Brobeck, J.R. Jr. (Ed.): Physiological Basis of Medical Practice. 10th Ed. Baltimore, Williams and Wilkins, 1979, pp. 195–202.
3. Guyton, A.C. (Ed.): Human Physiology and Mechanisms of Disease. 3rd Ed. Philadelphia, W.B. Saunders, 1980.
4. Ganong, W.F. (Ed.): Review of Medical Physiology. Los Altos, C.A. Lange Medical Publishers, 1981, pp. 464–5.
5. Sheldo, C.A., Balik, E., Ohanalal, K., et al.: Peripheral postcapillary venous pressure—a new hemodynamic monitoring parameter. Surgery, 92, 663 (1981).
6. Kelly, W.N., and Christenson, L.A.: Selective patient criteria for the use of electronic infusion devices. Am. J. I.V. Ther. Clin. Nutr., 10, 18 (1983).

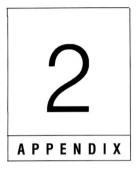

APPENDIX

Implantable and External Central Catheters*

Sandra L. Smith and Victoria E. Leach

The prolonged use of peripheral veins for parenteral nutrition, chemotherapy administration, infusion of intravenous fluids or blood products, and blood sampling usually causes pain, thrombosis, and psychologic distress. Indwelling peripheral catheters, called heparin locks or heparin wells, have long been used for intermittent administration of medications on a long-term basis, but have not eliminated the problems encountered in using peripheral veins for long-term therapy. The recent development of subcutaneously implanted systems has made a significant contribution to long-term venous infusion techniques. Increasing sophistication and improvement in the techniques employed to gain access to the circulatory system have resulted in the development of devices commonly referred to as indwelling catheters or vascular access devices (VADs).

In general, VADs can be classified into two categories: totally implanted devices and, the type often referred to as external catheters. The totally implanted system requires less home maintenance care, while the external-catheter type of VAD, since it exits the body, requires more intensive care and attention.

Before the selection of a VAD, several factors must be considered in order to determine the appropriate device to be used. The length and type of therapy may play a role in device selection. If therapy involves frequent blood

*Reprinted with permission from Parenterals, Vol. 52, April/May 1988.
Edited for style consistency.

sampling procedures or the administration of incomplete agents, a multilumen catheter may be preferable to a single-lumen catheter. Since the external-catheter VAD requires home management, patients should be assessed for their ability to comply with the required dressing changes and heparin or saline instillations. Finally, patient preference should be considered.

Placement

The insertion of totally and partially implanted VADs involves a surgical procedure. A centrally located superficial vein, usually the external jugular, cephalic or saphenous vein, is isolated through a small cutdown incision. For external-VAD placement, a separate proximal incision is made on the chest wall and the catheter is directed through a subcutaneous tunnel between the two incisions. The catheter is threaded into the superior vena cava just above the right atrium of the heart. The placement of implanted VADs involves inserting the catheter into the desired central vessel, then routing the catheter through a subcutaneous tunnel to the portal body site. The body of the port is then secured in a subcutaneous pocket over a bony prominence. Current research indicates that the distal end of the catheter should rest in the superior vena cava, well above the right atrium, to prevent catheter breakage and migration.[1]

External Catheters

External Long-term Catheters. The external-catheter type of VAD is made of medical-grade Silastic or silicone rubber. It is tunneled subcutaneously and has a Dacron sheath incorporated into the subcutaneous tunnel to enhance tissue ingrowth, preventing the progress of infection from the skin exit site to the venous entrance. The external end of the catheter has a Luer-lock connector to permit a tight junction with intravenous tubing and to allow secure capping of the catheter when it is not in use. Catheters are available in radiopaque or clear-with-radiopaque-stripe configurations, so that the placement can be confirmed fluoroscopically. External-catheter VADs are used for the administration of intravenous fluids, medications, blood products and parenteral nutrition, and for blood sampling.

A Silastic catheter was described in 1973 by Broviac et al.[2] This was the prototype of several of the external catheters currently in use. The Broviac, Hickman, Corcath, and Quinton catheters are similarly constructed, the major difference being lumen size. Dual- and triple-lumen catheters have been developed, in which a color coding system is used to identify the internal lumen size and corresponding external catheter. The dual-lumen model of the Quinton family of catheters, called the dual-lumen Raaf, provides two lumens of identical size in a single round or oval catheter. The design allows for 30% more fluid-carrying capacity than the Hickman or Corcath catheters. A Quinton triple-lumen catheter is also available. All require dressing changes and heparin instillation several times a week.

The Groshong catheter differs from the other external-catheter VADs in that it incorporates a three-position valve and a rounded, closed, radiopaque distal tip. Slight pressure opens the valve outward to allow for infusions, while

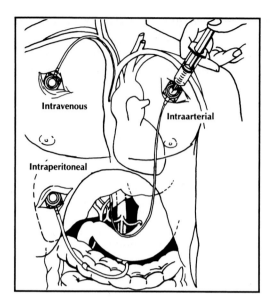

Figure A2–1. A variety of drugs and fluids may be delivered via the pathways shown, as well as intrathecally. Such catheters eliminate many problems associated with long-term therapy.

negative pressure, created by syringe aspiration, allows for blood withdrawal. This valve is thought to reduce greatly the potential for retrograde blood flow, air embolism, and catheter occlusion. The need for clamping is virtually eliminated. Maintenance with saline flushes is required once a week, whereas heparin flushes are recommended for the other external catheters. The Groshong catheter is currently available in the single-lumen design. Multilumen Groshong catheters will be introduced.

Complications from the use of external-catheter VADs include infection, site cellulitis, occlusions, dislodgement, and leakage. Care must be taken to prevent air from entering the catheter. Only nontraumatic clamps should be used to prevent damage to the catheter tubing. Recent versions of the Hickman, Broviac, and Corcath catheters have included a clamping device as part of the catheter and a reinforced clamping sleeve to prevent damage. Repair kits are available for external-catheter VADs if the external portion of the catheter is damaged.

Refer to Table I, Figure A2–2 for a comparison of the aforementioned catheters.

External Short-Term Catheters. Short-term multilumen central venous catheters have emerged from the need for devices suited to a number of applications in modern medicine: continuous or intermittent administration of fluids or medications, simultaneous administration of medications that are or may be incompatible, administration of blood products, parenteral nutrition, central venous monitoring, and blood sampling.

Many types of short-term venous catheters are manufactured. Their selection often depends on the insertion site to be used and the catheter with a 15-gauge internal lumen diameter and 22-inch length. A 7- to 9-inch-long centrally placed catheter of the same diameter is called the Centrasil. These devices are used primarily for chemotherapy administration, since their narrow diameter makes blood withdrawal difficult.

Multilumen central venous catheters generally have three separate and distinct lumens of various lengths running throughout the length of the catheter. The extensions (pigtails) are clear for easy observation of blood and infusions. An example of this type of catheter is the Arrow-Howes triple-lumen catheter. The recommended use of the individual lumens is outlined in Table II, Figure A2–2.

The Swan-Ganz catheter is another external short-term that is used almost exclusively in critical care settings. It is balloon-tipped and flow-directed, with several ports (pigtails) on the distal end. They are soft and pliable to allow the force of blood to propel them into the right ventricle and pulmonary artery. Multiple lumens are of benefit because of the numerous cardiac values obtained from patients. Dual-lumen Swan-Ganz catheters are designed to monitor pulmonary artery and pulmonary artery wedge pressures and to allow sampling of venous blood. The pulmonary artery lumen must be used with continuous heparinization flush solution under pressure to maintain patency.

Proper insertion is rarely difficult. The antecubital, femoral, internal jugular, or subclavian vein can be used as an insertion site. The last site is preferred because it allows for full arm movement with minimal tension place on the catheter. After venipuncture has been performed, a guide wire is passed into the vein using a dilator sheath. The dilator and wire are removed and the catheter is inserted through the sheath and placed in the vein.

Central venipuncture for the insertion of short-term external catheters has numerous clinical uses, but is associated with potential complications such as pneumothorax, arterial puncture, sepsis, and brachial plexus injury. The complications associated with the Swan-Ganz catheter insertion (dysrhythmia, local or endocardial infections, pulmonary artery perforations, balloon rupture, air embolism, pulmonary infarction and hemorrhage, and pneumothorax) have been reported. Once the catheter is in position, it is important to monitor the pulmonary artery pressure continuously to ensure that the catheter is not lodged in a wedge position—a complication that could cause pulmonary artery injury.

Implantable Devices

Implantable VADs or vascular access ports have become a welcome addition to the world of central lines. The use of these devices has escalated in the last five years and introduces an acceptable variance in choice. Ports are indicated in patients who require repeated venous access. The use of ports has decreased the time required for patients and families to care for the system, as they require maintenance flushing only once every three to four weeks. Decreased patient responsibility, improved self body-image, and freedom of activity are patient advantages. The nursing time required to care for these devices is decreased, since needle and dressing change need be done only about every seven days, when the port is in use. The system should not be placed in patients with a known infection or in those with inadequate tissue to support the device.

Several manufacturers produce implantable ports under such names as Midiport, Infuse-a-port, Microport, and Port-a-Cath, to name a few. The features of the ports vary, but the functional aspects of the ports remain similar. The

TABLE I

	Lumen size (ID)	Approx. Prime Vol.
Single-Lumen Catheters		
Broviac Pediatric	0.5mm	0.15ml
Broviac Pediatric	0.7mm	0.3ml
Broviac	1.0mm	0.7ml
Hickman	1.6mm	1.8ml
Quinton	0.75mm	0.9ml
Quinton	1.0mm	1.0ml
Quinton	1.5mm	2.0ml
Groshong	1.5mm	0.9ml
Groshong	1.3mm	0.7ml
Groshong	1.1mm	0.4ml
Groshong	0.7mm	0.13ml
Corcath	1.0mm	1.0ml
Corcath	1.5mm	2.0ml
Corcath Pediatric	0.71mm	0.14ml
Dual-Lumen Catheters		
Hickman Pediatric	0.7mm/1.3mm	0.5ml/1.0ml
Hickman	0.7mm/1.3mm	0.6ml/1.3ml
Leonard	1.3mm/1.3mm	1.3ml/1.3ml
Hickman	1.6mm/1.6mm	1.8ml/1.8ml
Raaf	1.0mm/1.0mm	1.2ml/1.2ml
Raaf	1.5mm/1.5mm	2.2ml/2.2ml
Raaf	1.9mm/1.9mm	2.7ml/2.7ml
Corcath	1.0mm/1.5mm	1.2ml/2.2ml
Triple-Lumen Catheters		
Hickman	1.0mm/1.0mm/1.5mm	0.7ml/0.7ml/1.6ml
Quinton	1.0mm/1.0mm/1.25mm	1.2ml/1.2ml/1.7ml

TABLE II

LUMEN	PROXIMAL	MIDDLE	DISTAL
Suggested lumen usage	Blood Sampling and General Access	TPN only or General Access	CVP Readings Blood Products General Access

Above references are to use of Arrow-Howes triple-lumen catheter.

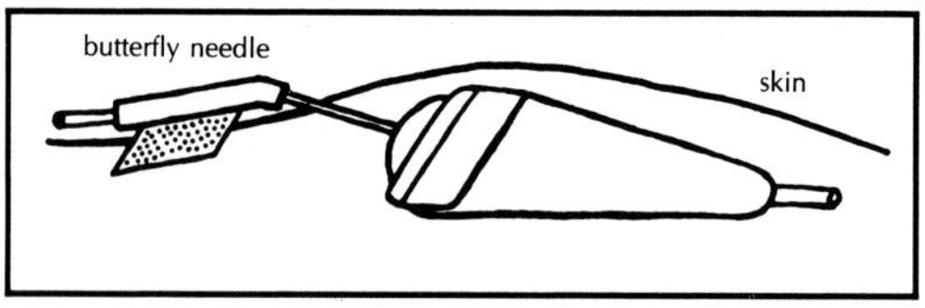

Figure A2–2. Norport-SP (skin-parallel) access port.

base of the port is constructed of metal or plastic, with the dome of the port consisting of a self-sealing system. Implantable vascular access ports are used primarily for entrance to the vascular system and require management as do other central venous lines (Fig. A2–2). However, implantable ports may also be used for other applications, such as the following:

1. Intraperitoneally, for the delivery of antineoplastic drugs or antibiotics to the abdominal cavity or for the removal of ascites or abdominal fluid;
2. Intrathecally, for the delivery of analgesics to the spinal area and for the administration of intrathecal antineoplastic drugs; and
3. Intraarterially, for the administration of antineoplastic agents through an artery or to remove fluid during body overload.

Until recently, the designs of the implanted ports have remained fairly similar. A newly introduced port with a design unlike those currently in use is the Norport-SP (Fig. A2–2). Unlike the other implanted vascular access ports, the Norport-SP (skin-parallel) is accessed with a straight Huber needle that is parallel to the skin rather than at a 90° angle. It was designed to facilitate longterm infusion via ambulatory infusion pumps, but is not limited to this application.

Initial postoperative complications form the insertion of implantable VADs include hematoma, accumulation of serous fluid at the surgical site, infection, respiratory distress, persistent pain, pneumothorax, and pleural effusion. Other complications include catheter blockage and migration, fibrin sleeve formation, needle dislodgement, infiltration, twiddler's syndrome[1] (catheter problems caused by patients who disturb the injection port), and air embolus.

Summary

The use of VADs provides an alternate method of accessing the vascular system. These devices have facilitated the implementation of treatment plans, provided greater patient comfort and self-image, and in some instances decreased the length of hospital stays. Those involved in caring for patients with VADs must be aware of the proper techniques for needling, dressing, and maintaining these devices, since improper care could result in complications and possibly fatal consequences for the patient. Health care professionals will continue to be challenged with the development of new designs and applications of these devices.

References

1. Gebarski, S., and Gebarski, K.: Chemotherapy port, twiddler's syndrome—A need for pre-injection radiotherapy. Cancer, 54, 38 (1984).
2. Broviac, J., Cole, J., and Scribner, B.: A silicone rubber atrial catheter for prolonged parenteral nutrition. Surg. Gynecol. Obstet., 136, 602 (1973).

Bibliography

1. Goodman, M., and Wickham, R.: Venous access devices: An overview. Oncology Nursing Forum, 11, 16 (1984).
2. Lokich, J., Bothe, A., Benotti, P., et al.: Complications and management of implanted venous access catheters. J. Clin. Oncol., 3, 10 (1985).
3. Moore, C., Erikson, K., Yanes, C., et al.: Nursing care and management of venous access ports. Oncology Nursing Forum, 13, 35 (1986).
4. Niemczura, J.: Rules to remember when caring for the patient with a Swan-Ganz catheter. Nursing, 15, 39 (1985).
5. Pituk, T., De Young, J., Levin, H., et al.: Volumes of selected central venous catheters. National Intravenous Therapy Association, 6, 97 (1983).
6. Ryan, L., and Gough, J.: Complications of central venous catheterization for total parenteral nutrition. National Intravenous Therapy Association, 7, 29 (1984).
7. Taylor, J., and Taylor, J.: Vascular access devices: Uses and aftercare. J. Emerg. Nurs., 13, 160 (1987).
8. Winters, V.: Implantable vascular access devices. Oncology Nursing Forum, 11, 25 (1984).

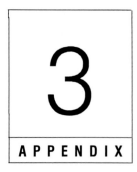

APPENDIX

Aseptic Techniques

In preparing and handling sterile dosage forms, the term "aseptic technique" refers to the ability of personnel to manipulate sterile preparations, sterile packaging components, and sterile administration devices in a way that excludes the introduction of viable microorganisms. As described in the text, the sources of contamination in aseptic handling of sterile materials are the area in which the procedures are done and the personnel involved. The cleaner the area, the less likelihood of introducing contaminants contributed by the environment. For this reason, laminar air flow, if properly utilized, provides optimum conditions for aseptic manipulations. These conditions include a well-lighted area and filtered air flowing at a velocity sufficient to maintain the critical working space free of viable material and particulate matter that can carry viable microorganisms.

Regardless of the cleanliness of the personnel involved, it is not practical to remove all microorganisms from the skin and hands to the point where they are sterile. Sterile gloves can be used and are recommended as a means of reducing the likelihood of contamination. Sterile gloves can give the operator a false sense of security, however, and the same precautions must be used with gloves as without them. In handling devices such as syringes, the hands must be placed only on those parts that will not come into contact with the sterile preparation. For example, the plunger of the syringe, which eventually will come into contact with the inner surface of the syringe barrel, should not be handled.

Viable material can be present on particulate matter constantly being shed by the operator and in the contribution made by his respiratory tract. The risk of contamination from the respiratory tract can be reduced by the use of masks. Personnel with colds should not be permitted to perform aseptic operations.

Prior to performing aseptic manipulations, the operator should make certain that the sterile materials, such as syringes, intravenous fluids, injections, and the like, are intact and protective wrappings have not been broken. Intravenous fluid bottles and other containers should be examined for cracks, imperfect closures, and particulate matter. With a proper attitude and an understanding of the reasons for the manipulations, the operator can become adept in aseptic techniques with practice.

Use of Syringes and Needles

Syringes and needles are used to directly inject a medicament into a body tissue and, in reconstitution and intravenous additive programs, to transfer medication from one container to another. Most syringes and needles are disposable, intended for one-time use only. When received, they are sterile and pyrogen-free and packaged to maintain these characteristics.

Syringes are available with or without needle attached; they are wrapped in paper or in a rigid plastic cover. Needles supplied separately are protected by an outer wrap of rigid or semirigid plastic. The needle shaft is protected by a rigid plastic needle sheath. The choice of the needle size depends on the tissue to be penetrated. For reconstitution of sterile solids, factors affecting the selection of needle size are viscosity, volume of liquid to be withdrawn, size of drug container, and nature of the rubber closure to be penetrated.

If two drugs are to be combined in the same syringe, special precautions must be taken. The two drugs must be compatible, and cross-container contamination must be prevented. If two different drug vials are penetrated, the needle must be aseptically changed after the first withdrawal.

Removal of Sterile Syringe from Package and Placement of Needle

1. Select a syringe of the size appropriate for the need.
2. Examine the integrity of the outer wrap; pin holes or breaks in the wrap render the syringe nonsterile.
3. With paper-wrapped syringes, peel sides apart and expose syringe. Avoid touching the plunger rod.
4. Select needle (if not attached) and examine the package for breaks.
5. Peel back needle wrapping and expose hub.
6. Aseptically remove plastic protective cap from syringe.
7. Attach needle to syringe with a twist, keeping needle sheath intact; avoid touching needle hub.
8. When ready to use, pull needle sheath straight off.
9. Perform transfer or injection.
10. Replace needle sheath.
11. When ready to discard, remove needle and place in designated disposal container. Some manufacturers provide destruction devices for needles.

Withdrawal of Contents of Ampuls

Glass ampuls are single-use containers that are sealed by fusion of the glass tips. Their capacities vary from 0.5 ml to 50 ml. A colored band, either blue or gold, around the constricted neck indicates that the ampul has been prescored to facilitate opening. The absence of a band indicates that the constricted neck must be filed prior to use; in which case, a file is pacakged with the ampul or small group of ampuls. The syringe for withdrawal is in an unwrapped, ready position for withdrawal with the needle sheath in place. The length of needle and size of syringe should be such that the contents of the ampul can be removed. Any air in the syringe is removed.

1. With the ampul in the upright position, tap it gently to release solution that may be trapped in the stem above the constricted neck. When ampules contain dry powders, as in the case of barbiturates, the diluent is injected into the ampul, solution is affected, and solution is then withdrawn back into the syringe.
2. Wipe neck of ampuls with an alcohol swab. Wrap swab around the neck of the ampul, thus avoiding cuts if the ampul breaks when being opened.
3. Using swab, thumb, and index finger on neck of ampul, and the thumb and the index finger of the other hand on the base of ampul, snap off neck (Fig. A3–1A). If ampul resists breaking, rotate ampul and repeat procedure. Inspect the opened ampul for glass particles.
4. Maintaining sterility, remove needle sheath. If air is present in syringe, remove it. Injection of air into ampul may cause overflow. Tilt ampul, submerge needle in solution, and avoid touching the bottom and outside rim of ampul with needle (Fig. A3–1B, C, D). Keeping the needle submerged will prevent air from being drawn into syringe.
5. Pull plunger back with thumb, using index finger for support, placing it on wing of the syringe (Fig. A3–1E). For larger ampuls, grasp the ampul and syringe base with one hand and pull the plunger back with the thumb and index finger of the other hand (Fig. A3–1F). Discard any unused solution.
6. Hold syringe with needle upward, tap syringe gently to allow air bubbles to surface, remove air bubbles if any, and eject slowly to remove air in needle.
7. Read volume of solution by aligning rubber end of plunger rod with calibration markings on barrel of syringe (Fig. A3–1G).
8. Replace needle sheath.

Withdrawal of Contents from Vials

Vials are molded glass containers holding sterile solutions, dry-filled powders, or lyophilized drugs. Vials are sealed with rubber closures secured by aluminum bands. Vials may be for single or multiple use; this determines the type of aluminum seal placed on the vials. Some vials have a plastic disk dustcover attached to the aluminum seal, removable at time of use. If the vial is for single use only, the aluminum band will be completely removable and will expose the entire rubber closure. For single-dose vials, the rubber closure is removed and solution is withdrawn directly with syringe and needle. For multiple-dose vials, only the target area of the closure is exposed.

The syringe for withdrawal is in an unwrapped, ready position with the needle sheath in place. The length of needle and size of syringe should be such that vial contents can be removed. Ideally, the smallest-gauge needle should be used to minimize coring.

1. Remove dustcover, if present, and aluminum tab over target area and discard. Cleanse the exposed rubber surface with an alcohol swab. Avoid

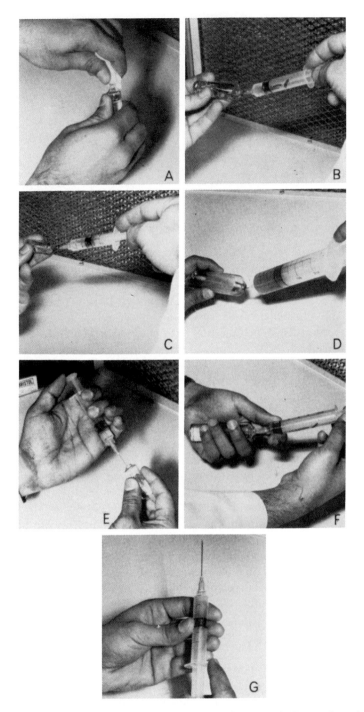

Figure A3–1. Procedure for withdrawing contents of ampul. *A,* Snap off neck of ampul; *B, C,* and *D,* tilt ampul and submerge needle in injection; *E,* pull plunger back with thumb; *F,* use thumb and index finger to pull plunger back on large syringes; *G,* determine volume with calibrations on syringe barrel.

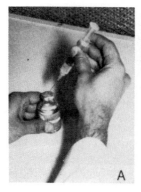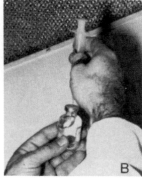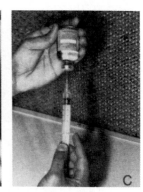

Figure A3–2. Procedure for withdrawing contents of vial. *A,* and *B,* Method of penetrating rubber closure to minimize coring; *C,* withdrawing injection from vial.

excess alcohol and lint as they may be carried with the needle into the vial.

2. Remove needle sheath from syringe and calibrate plunger rod to the volume of solution desired. A volume of air equal to the volume of solution needed must be injected into the vial in order to equalize pressure differential.

3. Penetrate the rubber closure with the needle, its beveled edge up, at an angle of approximately 60°. As the closure is penetrated, but before complete penetration, elevate the needle to a verticle position (90°). This technique minimizes coring (Fig. A3–2A, B).

4. Invert vial and inject air from syringe into vial; avoid bubbling air through solution (Fig. A3–2C).

5. Holding the vial with one hand and the needle and syringe with the other, draw the solution into syringe, keeping the needle submerged to avoid entrance of air into syringe. Withdraw a slightly larger volume of solution than is needed.

6. Withdraw the needle from the vial, the syringe and needle held upward, and tap the syringe gently to allow air bubbles to surface. Remove air bubbles, if any, and eject solution slowly to remove air from needle.

7. Read volume of solution by aligning rubber end of plunger with calibration markings on barrel of syringe.

8. Replace needle sheath.

Reconstitution of Sterile Solids

If a drug is in the form of a sterile solid, either a dry-filled or a lyophilized powder, the proper diluent is added to the container and solution is effected. The procedure described previously can be used for adding the diluent and withdrawing the solution. The most common diluents are Sterile Water for Injection, Bacteriostatic Water for Injection, and Sodium Chloride Injection. For some products such as Librium Injection, special sterile diluents are supplied with the drug. The diluent and the volume necessary for reconstitution are specified in the package brochure. When large amounts of diluent must be added for reconstitution, as for cephalothin sodium (Keflin), 4 g, a sterile needle placed into the container will facilitate venting.

Procedure for Plate Counts

Plate counts provide a means for determining the degree of contamination found in the environment or in a sterile filling area. Contamination rarely is absent completely. Plate counts indicate sudden or unexpected increases in contamination and the contaminants, if identified, can indicate the source. The record of plate counts over a period of time indicates the normal degree of contamination for a facility. Any excessive deviation from normal counts indicates a possible problem. For example, the movement of large pieces of equipment, repair of air conditioners, maintenance work within air ducts, and the like can upset the normal environment. A break in aseptic techniques or an illness of an operator can also increase the count. Routine cleaning procedures can be monitored by this method.

Agar plates are prepared according to the directions found on the container of the nutrient medium. The dehydrated material is placed in solution, poured onto Petri plates, covered, and autoclaved. If stored prior to use, the plates are kept in the refrigerator. Sterile disposable agar plates are available (Falcon Plastics). On the day of the count, the plates are dispersed throughout the area to be monitored and uncovered. They are placed approximately 5 feet apart and exposed for 10 to 20 minutes. During exposure, personnel remain out of the area. Exposure time and location are maintained as constants in order to compare counts made on different days.

After exposure, the plates are incubated in an inverted position for 1 week at 32° C. Following incubation, the number of colonies on each plate is counted and recorded. If reusable plates have been used, they are sterilized and washed for future use. The plate count may be done once a day or several times during the week.

Evaluation of Aseptic Filling Technique

Frequently, it is desirable to evaluate individual techniques in aseptic manipulations. The procedures help personnel to gain confidence in themselves and assure their supervisors that they can carry out aseptic procedures satisfactorily. One procedure consists of subdividing sterile culture medium such as soybean casein digest medium or trypticase soy broth into sterile containers under the same conditions used in aseptic manipulations for parenteral products. Incubation of the filled containers will show any contaminant introduced by personnel. Sterile agar plates placed strategically around the area while the filling is done will help the operator evaluate his technique and perhaps interpret the result. A procedure that can be used for evaluating the manipulations in subdividing sterile culture medium into vials within a laminar air flow hood is as follows:

1. Prepare and sterilize six agar plates.
2. Wash and sterilize 25 vials and rubber closures.
3. Prepare a quantity of soybean digest medium or trypticase soy broth and sterilize either in the autoclave or by membrane filtration.

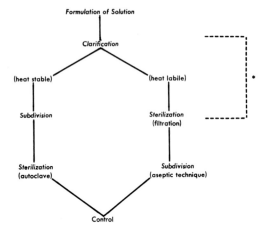

Figure A3–3. Sterilization method for parenteral product.

* May be combined as one step.

4. Disinfect the laminar air flow hood.
5. Place the sterile agar plate within the hood in positions strategic to the manipulations to follow.
6. Using a sterile Cornwall syringe (see Fig. 5–12), subdivide the sterile nutrient broth into the vials and seal.
7. Incubate the vials and plates for 1 week at 32° C.
8. After 1 week's incubation, note the number of contaminated vials, if any.
9. Note the presence of any colonies growing on the plates.

Suggested Procedural Approach for Extemporaneous Preparations

The factors to be considered in the preparation of a parenteral product are the added substances required, the sterilization method (Fig. A3–3), packaging components, dosage requirements, stability, and possible toxicity. Additives are kept to a minimum and used in the lowest effective concentration.

The ideal container permits one-time use only, thus eliminating multiple violations and possible microbiologic and cross-contamination. Additionally, a one-time use package obviates the necessity for an antimicrobial agent. Known vehicles and additives should be used. Vehicles other than water for injection should be used in minimal amounts. Preferably, parenterals should be packaged in clear containers so that the contents can be viewed. Light-sensitive drugs can be protected by an outer wrapping.

The pharmacist may be requested to prepare a small number of units extemporaneously, or he may be preparing a large routine batch. He may have prior experience in preparation, or the product may be new to him. The approach taken on a new request starts with questioning the prescribing physician. Is the product for animal or human use? Will it be administered in large volume or small volume? By what route will it be given? Is the dose proper? Is it needed immediately or will there be time for testing? Does the request have the proper authorization? The answers to these questions may dictate the method of preparation and other criteria. The literature is re-

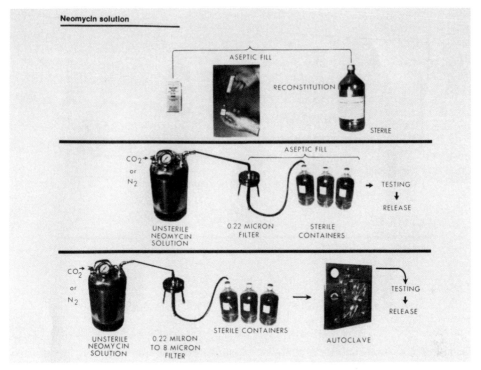

Figure A3–4. Flow chart for preparation of sterile, pyrogen-free neomycin irrigation solution. Top panel shows Method 1; center. Method 2; bottom, Method 3. (From Turco, S.J.: Preparing sterile neomycin sulfate solution. Hosp. Pharm., 7, 146 (1972).)

viewed to determine the product's use, dose, and stability. Once the pharmacist has ascertained the rationale for the product, he may proceed in its preparation.

Consideration must be given to expiration dating; the shortest possible dating is best.

Labeling must be clear and must indicate whether the drug is restricted to a particular patient.

A pharmacy release form may be necessary for signature by the prescribing physician if adequate time for testing is not available. This procedure will make the physician aware of this factor.

Any portion of the prepared product remaining after use should be returned to the pharmacy and destroyed.

Sterile Neomycin Sulfate Solution*

Neomycin sulfate is illustrative of a sterile product that may be prepared in a variety of ways. Although its solutions are frequently required in hospitals, sterile neomycin sulfate solutions are not available commercially and must be prepared by the pharmacist. The following methods describe the several approaches to preparation (Figs. A3–4 and A3–5). The methods can be

---

*Turco, S.J.: Preparing sterile neomycin sulfate solution. Hosp. Pharm., 7, 146 (1972).

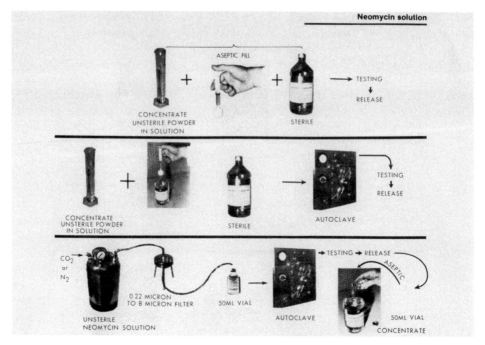

Figure A3–5.   Flow chart for preparation of sterile, pyrogen-free neomycin irrigation solution. Top panel shows Method 4; center, Method 5; bottom, Method 6. (From Turco, S.J.: Preparing Sterile neomycin sulfate solution. Hosp. Pharm., 7, 146 (1972).)

applied also to other sterile solutions that must be prepared extemporaneously by the hospital pharmacist.

Method 1. This method requires a commerical source of Sterile Water for Injection in a pour container, sterile neomycin sulfate, and a sterile disposable syringe. The neomycin sulfate is aseptically reconstituted, drawn into the syringe, and added to the Sterile Water for Injection. This rapid method has the advantage of requiring no special equipment; filtration and autoclaving times are avoided. Customarily, 1000 ml of a 1% solution are prescribed, thereby requiring the reconstitution of 20 0.5-g vials of neomycin sulfate. The 5-g vials are no longer available.

Method 2. This method utilizes sterilization by membrane filter. Nonsterile neomycin sulfate powder in solution is filtered and collected in sterile containers. Sterility testing and assays for potency are usually done. This method is used for batch-sized lots. When done properly, this technique results in a sterile, pyrogen-free clear solution. Disadvantages include the aseptic technique required and the additional equipment necessary. Since the entire solution must be filtered, a large volume of solution must be filtered, as compared with some of the other methods.

Method 3. This method is similar to Method 2 except that the solution is sterilized terminally by autoclaving. The filtration step in reality becomes a clarification step. Even though the final step utilizes terminal sterilization, good practice dictates that the procedure be conducted as if an aseptic fill were being done. Autoclaving will neither destroy pyrogens nor remove particulate matter. The solution prepared by this procedure is discolored as compared with that prepared by Method 2.

Method 4. This method uses nonsterile neomycin sulfate powder. The desired concentrate is prepared in Water for Injection or Sterile Water for Injection. The appropriate volume of nonsterile concentrate is drawn into a syringe and filtered through a 25-mm Swinnex or Millex filter containing a 0.22-membrane. The filtrate is syringed into a sterile container holding the sterile vehicle. This procedure is carried out using aseptic technique. It is similar to Method 1, but unlike in Method 1, the neomycin sulfate concentrate must be sterilized by filtration through a sterile membrane filter.

Method 5. In this method, the final product is autoclaved; otherwise the procedure is the same as that in Method 4. The filtration step becomes a clarification step. If this procedure is used for the preparation of multiple containers, it becomes necessary to place a prefilter in the Swinnex unit to minimize clogging of the membrane. Like the solution prepared by Method 3, this solution is discolored.

Method 6. This method is much the same as Method 3 except that the concentrated product is placed in vials for future use. At time of use, it is added aseptically to the diluent. A detailed description of this method is given to illustrate the procedure and the equipment required. This procedure can be adapted for other chemicals.

Day prior to preparation:

1. One hundred 50-ml vials are washed, packed in inverted position in covered containers, and placed in the hot-air oven for at least 4 hours at 170° C to render them sterile and pyrogen-free. When an oven is not available, vials can be washed with Water for Injection or Sterile Water for Injection and autoclaved at 121° C for 20 minutes. In the latter instance, the vials should be suitably wrapped for autoclaving.
2. A membrane filter having a porosity of 0.22 μ is placed in a 90-mm stainless steel filter holder; prior to use, the filter holder is washed with Water for Injection. A coarse prefilter is placed above the membrane filter to reduce clogging. If the final product is to be sterilized terminally in the autoclave, a filter with a larger porosity rating can be used for clarification. Both ends of the filter holder are wrapped in kraft paper or muslin, then autoclaved for 20 to 30 minutes.
3. The Tygon or rubber tubing to be used with the sterilization unit is washed well with Water for Injection or Sterile Water for Injection and autoclaved for 20 minutes.
4. Glass containers to be used for the preparation and collection of the sterile filtrate are washed with Water for Injection, covered with aluminum foil, and placed in the hot-air oven for 4 hours at 170° C to render them sterile and pyrogen-free.
5. A Cornwall syringe or other pipetting unit to be used in subdividing the sterile solution into sterile vials is assembled, adjusted to deliver a volume of 50.5 ml, washed well with Water for Injection, wrapped, and autoclaved for 20 minutes.
6. Control sheets are prepared and labels printed.

Day of preparation:

1. The laminar air flow hood is wiped down with disinfectant solution and the blower is turned on.
2. One hundred rubber closures are rinsed well with Water for Injection and drained; this is repeated several times. The closures are immersed in Water for Injection in a covered container, autoclaved for 20 minutes, then removed to laminar air flow hood.
3. The following materials are arranged within the hood:
   Wrapped sterile filter holder with sterile membrane in place
   Tygon tubing for pressure tank
   Sterile receiving flask
   Sterile Cornwall syringe adjusted to deliver 50.5 ml
   Covered container with sterile pyrogen-free vials
   Sterile cylindrical 100-ml graduate to check delivery
   Sterile gloves and a sterile pair of forceps for application of rubber closures
4. The solution is prepared as follows:
   Formula

% Concentration	% Ingredient	g/5000 ml
10	Neomycin sulfate	500.0
0.1	Sodium bisulfite	5.0
qs	Water for Injection qs	5000.0 ml

   Procedure:
   Place 500 g of neomycin sulfate in previously sterilized beaker, add several liters of Water for Injection by stirring to dissolve the chemical. Dissolve the sodium bisulfite and make up the solution to a volume of 5000 ml with Water for Injection.
5. Clarification and sterilization of solution:
   Rinse a stainless steel pressure tank with Water for Injection, drain well, and add the solution prepared as directed above.
   Remove the wrapping from the membrane filter holder within the hood and assemble the setup. Tighten the bolts on the 90-mm stainless steel filter holder and connect holder to the pressure tank with the sterile Tygon tubing. Using an inert gas such as compressed nitrogen, apply pressure to the tank and force the solution through the sterilizing membrane into the sterile receiving container.
6. Subdivision of the solution:
   Put on the sterile gloves, open the wrapped Cornwall syringe, and place the sinker of the syringe within the sterile solution. Check the delivery volume of the syringe; if satisfactory, fill into sterile vials.
   The second operator, using sterile forceps, applies sterile rubber closures to the vials as they are filled. After the entire batch is filled, aluminum seals are applied and sealed with a hand crimper.
7. Autoclaving.
8. Testing.

Problems

Calculations Involving Milliequivalents

1. How many grams of sodium bicarbonate are needed to provide 40 mEq of bicarbonate ion? The mEq weight of sodium bicarbonate is 0.084.

    Answer: 3.36 g

2. How many milliequivalents of potassium are in a 20,000,000-unit vial of potassium penicillin G? One milligram of potassium penicillin G equals 1595 units; the atomic weight of potassium is 39; the molecular weight of potassium penicillin G is 372; and the mEq weight of potassium is 0.039.

    Answer: 33.6 mEq

3. In preparing a solution containing calcium chloride U.S.P., what weight of chemical is needed if each 10 ml are to contain 50 mEq calcium chloride? The mEq weight of calcium chloride U.S.P. is 0.0735.

    Answer: 3.7 g per 10 ml

4. How many milliequivalents of magnesium ion are present in an ampul containing 10 ml Magnesium Sulfate Injection U.S.P.? Magnesium Sulfate Injection contains 50% $MgSO_4 \cdot 7H_2O$. The mEq weight of magnesium sulfate hexahydrate is 0.123.

    Answer: 40 mEq

5. How many milliequivalents of calcium ion are present in an ampul containing 10 ml Calcium Gluconate Injection U.S.P.? This injection contains 10% wt/vol calcium gluconate. The mEq weight of calcium gluconate is 0.215.

    Answer: 4.6 mEq

6. How many milliequivalents of potassium ion are present in 1000 ml of a solution containing 5.968 g of potassium chloride? The molecular weight of potassium chloride is 74.6.

    Answer: 80 mEq

Calculations in Intravenous Preparations

1. The pharmacy receives a physician's order for one day's supply of TPN solutions (two containers), each containing additives. The original computer-generated order is shown in Figure A3–6. Figure A3–7 is a pre-printed, non-computer-generated TPN order; the markings are pharmacist notes. The procedure and techniques followed in the filling of this order vary depending on the intravenous system used and the packaging of the additives available for use. For this hopsital, the standard composition (order A–6) of the basic solution is as follows (order #542):

Amino Acid (A.A.) 8.5%	500 cc
Dextrose Injection (D50)	500 cc
Sodium Chloride Injection	60 mEq
Sodium Acetate Injection	10 mEq
Potassium Chloride Injection	60 mEq
Potassium Phosphate Injection	18 mM

```
                                    PHCE
113-89-97-0-1170 07/27/91   08:15 AM
                          5WEST   511A
ENTERED BY:                  MD
ORDER TYPE:


  TPN...CENTRAL LINE START, BOTTLE
AA8.5% 500CC + D50 500CC
NACL 60MEQ
NA ACETATE 10MEQ
KCL 60MEQ
K PHOS 18MM
MAG SULF 16MEQ
CA GLUC 10MEQ
```

```
    MULTIVITAMINS 10ML
    FOLIC ACID 1MG
    TRACE ELEMENTS 3ML
    RATE
    85CC/HR
    X1 BAG
      ORDER #: 542.
    EXPIRES:_____
    PREPARED BY:_____
    -*-
```

Figure A3–6. Computer generated physican's order for TPN.

```
                                    PHCE
  113-89-97-0-1170 07/27/91   08:15 AM
                           5WEST   511A
    ENTERED BY:              MD
    ORDER TYPE:


      TPN...CENTRAL LINE BOTTLE #2,
    AA8.5% 500CC + D50 500CC
    NACL 60MEQ
    NA ACETATE 10MEQ
    KCL 60MEQ
    K PHOS 18MM
    MAG SULF 16MEQ
    CA GLUC 10MEQ
```

```
    RATE
    85CC/HR
    X1 BAG
      ORDER #: 543.
    EXPIRES:_____
    PREPARED BY:_____
    -*-
```

Magnesium Sulfate Injection	16 mEq
Calcium Gluconate Injection	10 mEq
Multivitamins	10 ml
Folic Acid Injection	1 mg
Trace Elements	3 ml

Procedure for preparing TPN
   The AA and Dextrose are combined.
The following additives are added:

Sodium Chloride Injection (100 mEq/40 ml)	24 ml
Sodium Acetate Injection (2 mEq/ml)	5 ml
Potassium Chloride Injection (20 mEq/ml)	30 ml
Potassium phosphate Injection (2 mM/ml)	9 ml
Magnesium Sulfate Injection (4 mEq/ml)	4 ml

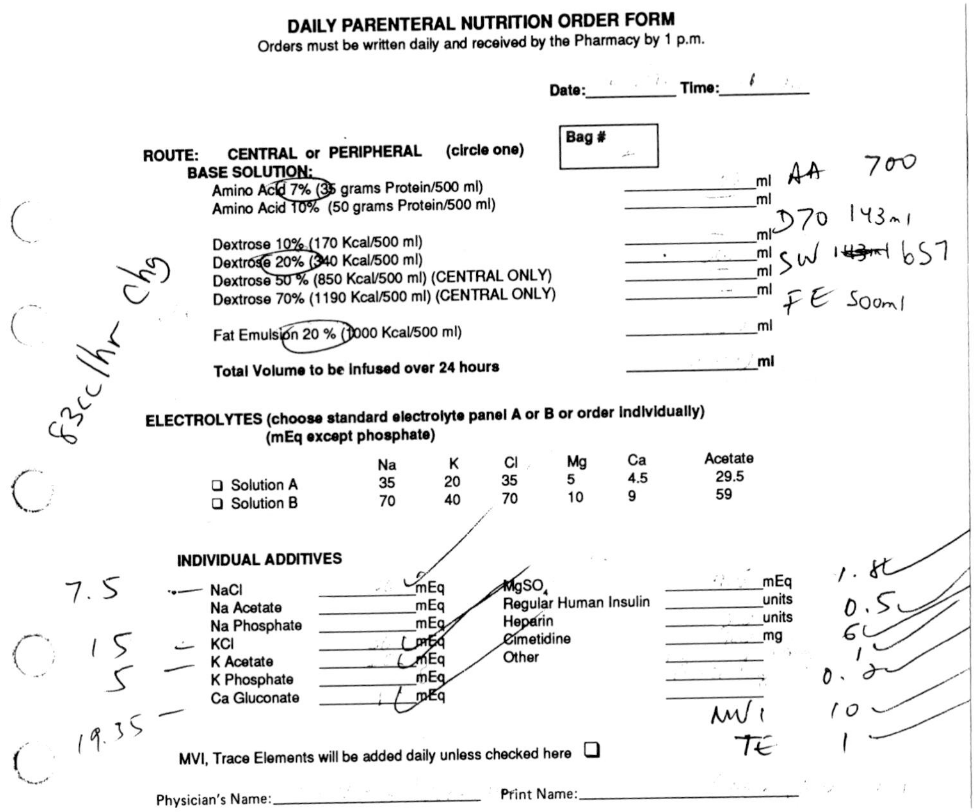

DAILY PARENTERAL NUTRITION ORDER FORM

Orders must be written daily and received by the Pharmacy by 1 p.m.

Date:_____ Time:_____

Bag #

ROUTE: CENTRAL or PERIPHERAL   (circle one)
BASE SOLUTION:
Amino Acid 7% (35 grams Protein/500 ml)   _____ml AA 700
Amino Acid 10% (50 grams Protein/500 ml)   _____ml

Dextrose 10% (170 Kcal/500 ml)   _____ml D70 143 ml
Dextrose 20% (340 Kcal/500 ml)   _____ml SW 113 657
Dextrose 50 % (850 Kcal/500 ml) (CENTRAL ONLY)   _____ml
Dextrose 70% (1190 Kcal/500 ml) (CENTRAL ONLY)   _____ml FE 500ml

Fat Emulsion 20 % (1000 Kcal/500 ml)   _____ml

Total Volume to be Infused over 24 hours   _____ml

ELECTROLYTES (choose standard electrolyte panel A or B or order individually)
(mEq except phosphate)

	Na	K	Cl	Mg	Ca	Acetate
☐ Solution A	35	20	35	5	4.5	29.5
☐ Solution B	70	40	70	10	9	59

INDIVIDUAL ADDITIVES

NaCl _____ mEq	MgSO₄ _____ mEq
Na Acetate _____ mEq	Regular Human Insulin _____ units
Na Phosphate _____ mEq	Heparin _____ units
KCl _____ mEq	Cimetidine _____ mg
K Acetate _____ mEq	Other
K Phosphate _____ mEq	
Ca Gluconate _____ mEq	

7.5
15
5
19.35

1.8
0.5
6
0.2
10

MVI
TE

MVI, Trace Elements will be added daily unless checked here ☐

Physician's Name:_____   Print Name:_____

83cc/hr chg

Figure A3–7.   Preprinted noncomputerized TPN order.

Calcium Gluconate Injection (4 mEq/10 ml)	25 ml
Multivitamins	10 ml
Folic Acid Injection (1 mg/ml)	1 ml
Trace Elements	3 ml

Container #2 (order 543) for this patient is similar; however, the second container does not contain the multivitamins, folic acid, or trace elemnts because adequate daily doses are present in the first container (order #542).

After the admixtures are prepared, they are capped, labeled, and inspected.

  a. What infusion rate is required at 85 mL/hr
      Administration set delivery rate—10 drops/mL
      Volume to be administerd 1000 mL—113 mL = 1113 mL plus additives

$$85cc/hr = \frac{85}{60 \text{ min}} = 14 \text{ drops/minute}$$

  b. Approximately what quantities of dextrose and amino acid is this patient receiving the first 8 hours?

      4.25% AA/Liter = 85 mL × 4.25% = 3.61 g

25% Dextrose/Liter = 85 × 25% = 21.2 g

c. How many calories are presented by the dextrose?

21.2 g × 3.4 Cal/gram = 72 Calories

d. Order #542 contains 10 mEq calcium gluconate. The ampul describes that container as 10 mL, 10% solution. How many mEq Calcium Gluconate are contained in one ampul?

mEq weight of calcium gluconate is 0.215

$$mEq = \frac{Wtg}{mEq\ Wt} = \frac{1}{0.215}$$

mEq = 4.65 mEq/lg ampul

Diagnosis: Rule Out Myocardial Infarction

Allergies: Penicillin

Container 1

Start I.V. with 5% dextrose containing 0.45%

- Sodium Chloride Injection
- Add 20 mEq Potassium Chloride
- Add 8 mEq Magnesium Sulfate
- Run I.V. 40 ml/hour

Container 2

- Add Lidocaine 1 g to 500 ml 5% Dextrose Injection
- Run I.V. 2 kg/min
- Patient weighs 68 kg

Container 3

- Add 10,000 units of Heparin to 500 ml of 0.45% (1/2 normal)
- Sodium Chloride Injection
- Run at 800 units/hour

2. The pharmacy receives the request for 250 ml of an infusion solution containing 15% dextrose and 0.2% sodium chloride. This is not commercially available and has to be prepared extemporaneously.

Available to the pharmacist are the following:

50% Dextrose Injection U.S.P.—50-ml vial
Sodium Chloride Ion-O-Trate—100 mEq or 5.84 g/40 ml
Sterile Water for Injection

Procedure:

Dextrose required:

250 ml × 15% = 37.5 g = 75 ml of 50% Dextrose Injection

Sodium chloride required:

250 ml × 0.2% = 0.5 g = 3.5 ml of Ion-O-Trate

Volume of solutions: 78.5 ml

From a 250-ml container of Sterile Water for Injection, remove and discard 78.5 ml of the water.

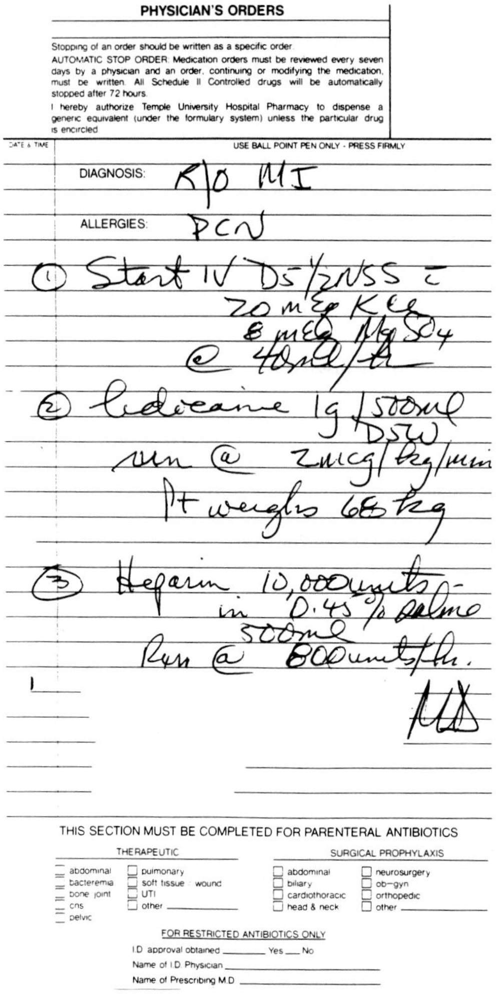
PHYSICIAN'S ORDERS

Stopping of an order should be written as a specific order.
AUTOMATIC STOP ORDER: Medication orders must be reviewed every seven days by a physician and an order, continuing or modifying the medication, must be written. All Schedule II Controlled drugs will be automatically stopped after 72 hours.
I hereby authorize Temple University Hospital Pharmacy to dispense a generic equivalent (under the formulary system) unless the particular drug is encircled.

DATE & TIME — USE BALL POINT PEN ONLY - PRESS FIRMLY

DIAGNOSIS: R/O MI

ALLERGIES: PCN

(1) Start IV D5 1/2NSS c̄
20 mEq KCl
8 mEq MgSO4
@ 40ml/hr

(2) Lidocaine 1g/500ml
D5W
run @ 2mcg/kg/min
Pt weighs 68 kg

(3) Heparin 10,000 units
in D.45% saline
500ml
Run @ 800units/hr.

THIS SECTION MUST BE COMPLETED FOR PARENTERAL ANTIBIOTICS

THERAPEUTIC: abdominal, bacteremia, bone joint, cns, pelvic, pulmonary, soft tissue wound, UTI, other ______

SURGICAL PROPHYLAXIS: abdominal, biliary, cardiothoracic, head & neck, neurosurgery, ob–gyn, orthopedic, other ______

FOR RESTRICTED ANTIBIOTICS ONLY
I.D. approval obtained ______ Yes ___ No
Name of I.D. Physician ______
Name of Prescribing M.D. ______

Figure A3–8. A somewhat typical I.V. order for drug additives.

Add 75 ml of 50% Dextrose Injection and 3.5 ml of the Sodium Chloride Ion-O-Trate; total volume of solution, 250 ml.

Seal with additive cap, label, and inspect.

3. A physician's order is received for 50 ml of 5% Dextrose Injection containing 40 mg of gentamicin. The directions indicate that it is to be infused over a 60-minute period. What is the labeled rate?

A volume control set such as the Buretrol (Baxter) is used; this set delivers 60 drops/ml.

$$\frac{50 \text{ ml}}{60 \text{ min}} = 0.83 \text{ ml/min}$$

$$0.83 \text{ ml/min} \times 60 \text{ drops/ml} = 50 \text{ drops/min}$$

4. The pharmacy is requested to prepare an admixture containing isoproterenol, 2 mg, in 500 ml of 5% Dextrose Injection. Available are 5-ml
ampuls of Isoproterenol Hydrochloride Injection, 1:5000.

    a. How much of the additive is to be added?
       A 5-ml ampul of 1:5000 solution (0.2 mg/ml) contains 1 mg of
       isoproterenol hydrochloride. Therefore, the contents of 2 5-ml
       ampuls are to be added.
    b. The directions indicate that 4 μg are to be infused per minute.
       If a Baxter administration set is used, how many drops should be
       given per minute?

       Administration set delivery rate is 10 drops/ml
       Concentration of solution is 2000 μg/500 ml or 4 μg/ml
       Requested rate is 4 μg/min

       Therefore, 1 ml/min or 10 drops/min.

5. The pharmacy is requested to prepare a 1,000,000-unit dose of potassium
penicillin G in 1 ml. Available to the pharmacy is Potassium Penicillin
G (Squibb) in a vial containing 20,000,000 units. Reconstitution information on the vial indicates that when 31.6 ml of Sterile Water for Injection are added, the resulting solution (40 ml) contains 500,000 units
per ml.

From the information given, it is concluded that the antibiotic powder
occupies a volume of 8.4 ml (40 ml − 31.6 = 8.4 ml). Therefore, to
reconstitute the antibiotic to give the concentration of 1,000,000 units/
ml, a total volume of 20 ml is required. The difference between 20 ml
and 8.4 ml is the volume of Sterile Water for Injection to be added to
the vial to give the desired concentration.

The Parenteral Prescription

Physicians' orders for intravenous admixtures are also called parenteral prescriptions. Several prescriptions are reproduced in this section as they were
written. In many instances, they can be prepared by several methods, depending on the intravenous solution system used in the hospital and the type
of packaging of the additives available. Common to all methods of preparation
are aseptic technique, accuracy, and the area in which they are prepared, the
laminar air flow hood. For the prescriptions given below, a method of preparation is indicated in which the Baxter solution system is used.

1.   ℞   1000 ml 5 D/W with 40 mEq KCl + Vits

          Run at 100 ml/hr

Remove aluminum seal from 5% Dextrose in Water container and swab
closure with alcohol. Remove rubber protective sleeve from Potassium
Chloride Incert containing 40 mEq of KCl and place in administration
set opening of intravenous container, allowing the vacuum to draw the
solution into intravenous container. Remove empty Incert container.

Remove rubber protective sleeve from Vi-Cert, place in administration set opening of intravenous container, invert container with Vi-Cert in place, and pump Vi-Cert container to pull intravenous fluid into it. Tap the additive container until solution is effected.

Turn intravenous fluid container with Vi-Cert attached back to an upright position and empty the reconstituted vitamin solution from the Vi-Cert container into the intravenous fluid.

Remove additive container and place sterile additive cap on intravenous fluid container. Label, and check label, intravenous order, empty containers, and clarity of the admixture.

2.   ℞   1000 ml 1/2 NS   100 mg Solu-Cortef

         Run in over 8 hours

Remove aluminum seal from liter bottle of 0.45% Sodium Chloride Injection and swab closure with alcohol. Reconstitute Solu-Cortef packaged in Mix-O-Vial container.

Using sterile syringe and needle or sterile double-ended transfer needle, transfer the contents of the Solu-Cortef container to the 0.5 N saline injection, penetrating the intravenous fluid container through the opening in the closure for the administration set. Place sterile additive cap on container.

Label, and check label, intravenous order, empty container, and clarity of the admixture.

3.   ℞   Penicillin G 10 million units with 1000 ml 5 D/W

         Run in 8 hours

Remove aluminum seal from liter container of 5% Dextrose Injection and swab closure with alcohol. Remove aluminum center seal from 10-million-unit vial of Potassium Penicillin G (Squibb) and swab with alcohol.

Take up 15.5 ml of Sterile Water for Injection into a sterile 20-ml plastic syringe. Loosen the antibiotic powder by shaking the vial; inject the diluent while holding the vial horizontally and rotating. Withdraw needle and replace needle sheath. Shake vial and examine the reconstituted solution for clarity.

Using the same sterile syringe and needle, withdraw 20 ml of the antibiotic solution and add to the Dextrose Injection. Place sterile additive cap on container.

Label, and check label, intravenous order, empty container, and clarity of the admixture. Use solution within 24 hours.

4.   ℞   Edecrin 300 mg in 150 ml 5 D/W

         Over one (1) hour

Remove aluminum seal from 150-ml container of 5% Dextrose Injection and swab closure with alcohol. Using sterile 50-ml plastic syringe, withdraw 50 ml of the dextrose solution.

Remove seal from 3 100-mg vials of Edecrin, swab closures, and place 50 ml of 5% Dextrose Injection into each of the 3 vials. When the Edecrin is in solution, remove 50 ml of the solution from each of the 3 vials and inject into the intravenous container. Place sterile additive cap on container.

Label, and check label, intravenous order, empty containers, and clarity of admixture.

5.   R̥   Garamycin 80 mg I.V. NSS 100 ml

       Infuse one (1) hour

Remove aluminum seal from 100-ml container of Sodium Chloride injection and swab closure with alcohol.

Remove aluminum seal from vial of Garamycin, 80 mg/2 ml, and swab closure with alcohol. Using a sterile 2-ml plastic syringe, remove 2 ml and inject into container of sodium chloride solution. Place sterile additive cap on container.

Label, and check label, intravenous order, empty container, and clarity of admixture.

6.   R̥   Keflin 2 g I.V.

       Buretrol q 6 hr × 4

Remove aluminum seal from 2 4-g Keflin containers and swab closures with alcohol. Using a sterile 20-ml syringe, add 40 ml of Sterile Water for Injection to each of the 2 containers. The concentration in the vials is 1 g/10 ml.

Into each of 4 sterile 20-ml syringes, withdraw 20 ml of the Keflin injection. Replace the sterile needle sheaths.

Label with concentration and expiration date, check label, I.V. order, empty containers, and clarity of admixture. The contents of each 20-ml syringe, 2 g Keflin, will be placed in a volume control device (Buretrol, Baxter). The already hanging I.V. fluid will be used to dilute the solution to 100 ml.

7.   R̥   Methicillin 1 g q 6 h

       500 ml 5 D/W

Remove aluminum seal from 5000-ml container of 5% Dextrose Injection and swab closure with alcohol.

Remove aluminum seal from vial of Methicillin containing 1 g, swab closure with alcohol, and inject 1.5 ml Sterile Water for Injection.

Withdraw 2 ml of the antibiotic injection and inject into dextrose solution. Place sterile additive cap on container.

Label, check label, I.V. order, empty container, and clarity of admixture.

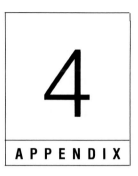

APPENDIX

Hazards Associated with Parenteral Therapy

Scope of Parenteral Therapy

According to one study,[1] it is estimated that, in the United States, an average of 7.5 medications is administered to each hospital patient every day, 30% in the form of injections. Another study[2] indicates that 39% of hospital patients received daily injections. It is believed that 25% of hospitalized patients are receiving I.V. therapy. Ten million patients receive intravenous therapy annually, accounting for 300 million I.V. containers per year. Over 800 million disposable syringes are used annually. Total injections in hospitals are well over the billion mark and account for 30% of the hospitals' drug budget. Hospital admissions continue to increase; in 1972 there were 33 million admissions, accounting for 442 million inpatient days;[3] in 1982, hospital admissions amounted to 40 million. As hospital admissions increase, so will the number of injections administered. Parenteral therapy is in increasing demand. Because of the requirements and nature of injectables, they are the most difficult to prepare and administer. The consequences of error are most severe. There is a tendency to associate the hazards of parenteral therapy with microbiologic contamination, and certainly the severity of contamination would justify this thinking. Many other hazards and problems with parenterals also exist, however, some subtle enough to escape the imagination.

Industry Expectations

In addition to the desired attributes of pharmaceuticals, such as clarity, stability, quality, and proper packaging, parenteral products require three additional qualities. They must be sterile, free of pyrogens, and free of particulate matter. These qualities are imparted during the manufacturing phases.

The user assumes, and rightfully so, that they are present in the product. From recent past history, however, this may not always be the case.

User Expectations

One would expect that, once the products arrive at the place of use, the user maintains the qualities imparted during the manufacturing processes. In addition, one would expect knowledgeable personnel to utilize the products in an acceptable environment. User-associated errors and problems are difficult to document; however, from a number of reports there is no question that they exist.

Institutional Hazards

These hazards are associated primarily with economic problems. The institution where parenteral drugs are used must provide sufficient, knowledgeable personnel, adequate space, and environmental support. We know also that this is not always the case. In a summary of medication errors of over 9400 individual reports over a 1-year period, it was shown that 24% of the errors were medication errors; I.V. errors accounted for 14% of the total incident reports.[4]

Psychologic Problems Associated With Injections

The emotional and psychologic aspects of parenteral therapy must be considered to achieve the goal of rational drug therapy. The reader is referred to Chapter 6.

Personnel Administering Parenteral Drugs

The personnel administering parenteral drugs must be adequate in number, knowledgeable, and well trained. Proper documentation and quality control in-house are imperative. It was the unanimous opinion of the National Coordinating Committee on Large Volume Parenterals (NCCLVP)[5] that there is a gross lack of knowledge in this area and that a major educational effort should be directed to all who in any way come in contact with large-volume parenterals. A study by Kaminski and Stolar[6] of 86 hospitals in 24 states and two Canadian provinces showed significant discrepancies between actual practice versus recommended practice, and an unacceptably high incidence of avoidable complications. The Joint Commission on Accreditation of Hospitals states that the hospital pharmacy should be responsible for the admixture of parenteral products when feasible; however, the NCCLVP found in a nationwide study that this was a responsibility of the diploma nurse in 92% of the hospitals surveyed.[7]

According to Anderson,[8] there is little or no surveillance of the system currently in vogue on most nursing units. Effective bacteriologic monitoring of techniques, components, or finished products of parenterals is almost unheard of in most hospitals.

Pain

Pain upon injection is common but difficult to document. One study in the *British Journal of Anaesthesia* involving 336 patients showed that 6% of patients had pain 24 hours after injection and 39% developed hematoma 24 hours

TABLE A4–1.   Degree of Infusion Phlebitis[12]

Scale No.	Description
0	None present
1	Tenderness without erythema
2	Tenderness with redness around the site of injection
3	Pain on touching, erythematous streak forming, no induration
4	Pain on touching, erythematous streak above injection site, vein hard and tender

after injection. The intramuscular complications from the drug ticarcillin showed that, of 206 patients, 16.5% (34) had side effects; 14% had pain at the injection site.*

Infusion Phlebitis

The term phlebitis, thrombophlebitis, phlebothrombosis, postinfusion phlebitis, infusion thrombophlebitis, venous thrombosis, and thrombophlebitis of superficial veins have all been used to describe a situation that can develop from intravenous infusion. A number of other factors may cause this disease, including obesity, acceleration of clotting, myocardial infarction, operation, anemia, shock, dehydration, venous stasis, pregnancy, and use of oral contraceptive drugs.[9,10]

The term *phlebitis* indicates inflammation of the vein. A thrombus is a clot in a blood vessel. Any injury that damages the endothelial cells of the venous wall can cause platelets to adhere and form a clot. The term thrombophlebitis is used to denote a twofold injury; thrombus formation plus inflammation. Apparently, these terms are used interchangeably by authors.

Infusion phlebitis is considered by some to be a major source of morbidity and patient discomfort in hospitals.

Clinical Signs and Incidence

An early sign of infusion phlebitis is tenderness above the insertion site of the cannula. Within hours, the vein becomes reddened, warm, and painful, with edema and stiffness. In the latent stages, the vein appears as a palpable, tender red cord.

In the clinical evaluation and determination of infusion phlebitis, various scales or ratings are used to define the clinical parameters. For example, Table A4–1 is a scale that was used in a study to define quantitatively the degree or extent of the disease.

Infusion phlebitis, a relatively minor complication, usually lasts for less than a week, although in some cases it may last for months.[11,12] Even minor cases, however, can induce fever, predispose to sepsis,[13,14] complicate the clinical picture, cause patient discomfort, and possibly lengthen hospital stay. The pathogenesis of infusion phlebitis, which remains unclear, is currently being investigated aggressively.

---

*Product information. Bristol, Tenn., Beecham Laboratories, 1976.

TABLE A4–2. Factors Implicated in Causing Phlebitis Associated with I.V. Drug Infusion

Type of cannula (plastic vs. needle)
Duration of therapy
Infection
Chemically irritating drugs
pH infusion fluid
Age, sex
Tonicity (osmolality)
Location of I.V. site
Decreased blood flow
Particulate matter

In 1970 Thomas et al.,[15] in a study of more than 1000 patients receiving postoperative infusin, observed complications in 69% of cases; 30% of the complications were phlebitis.

According to some reports, postinfusion phlebitis is responsible for 50% of hospital morbidity; it is seen in 25% of patients receiving intravenous infusion. The reported incidence of phlebitis traced to intravenous infusion of dextrose-containing solutions ranged from 15 to 24%.[16–18] Phlebitis reported to be caused by cephalothin infusion has ranged up to 50%.[19]

Some reports in the literature are confusing and conflicting. The parameters of measurement vary with the investigators. Diagnosis is not definitive; there are variations in the biologic model. Cases may be undiagnosed, unreported, or misdiagnosed. Some diseases can cause phlebitis, and intravenous infusion administration techniques may be a factor. Diagnoses made by various investigators used within a single study tend to complicate analysis of this disease.

Thomas et al.[15] noted the lack of a satisfactory clinical description of the types of complications, their severity, onset, and time course. If meaningful comparisons are to be made of the incidence and morbidity, a standard classification is required.

Causes of Infusion Phlebitis

The causes of infusion phlebitis are classified as (1) infection, (2) physical (trauma), and (3) chemical. A number of factors have been implicated in causing infusion phlebitis associated with intravenous drug administration. These are listed in Table A4–2.

Type of Cannula Used. In a study of polyethylene and Silastic catheters, Welch et al.[20] found that polyethylene catheters produced marked thrombosis within 10 days, whereas Silastic catheters maintained normal venous tissue.

The chemical composition of plastic I.V. catheters has been implicated as a source of irritation to some patients' veins. It has also been shown that the longer the catheter is left in place, the greater is the risk of infusion phlebitis. Mechanical trauma to the vessel occurs with venipuncture and cannula movement. Trauma to the vessel causes destruction of the platelets and release of thromboplastin. Adhesion of platelets to the cannula tip occurs with the formation of a clot. Blood flow is reduced, and stasis occurs with the clot, which increases in size.

Scalp vein and hollow needles do not stay in place as well as catheters; thus at times physicians prefer to use catheters. Plastic catheters are most often used in seriously ill patients. In several studies, the incidence of infusion phlebitis is compared with the type of cannula used. Collins et al.[21] reported the incidence of thrombophlebitis to be 39% with polyethylene catheters. Thomas et al.[15] found that overall venous complications were $2^{1}/_{2}$ times more common with plastic cannulae than with steel needles. More specifically, plastic cannulae caused 3 times more cases of phlebitis.

In studying venous complications associated with catheters, Thomas compared four types of catheters (plastic, polyvinylchloride (PVC), tetrafluoroethylene (TFE), and fluoroethylenepropylene (FEP)). Catheters made of FEP produced a significantly lower incidence of venous complications. Other studies[22-24] have shown that scalp vein needles produce a lower incidence of phlebitis and complications than did catheters.

Experts[25] conclude that steel cannulae are preferred over plastic catheters and that a lower rate of phlebitis is seen with steel needles. The chemical composition of plastic I.V. catheters may be a source of irritation to some patients. Therefore, the longer the I.V. catheter is left in place, the greater will be the risk of phlebitis. I.V. catheters should be changed routinely every 48 to 72 hours except where clinical circumstances dictate otherwise.

Duration of Therapy. Hussey[26] suggests that the frequent occurrence of thrombophlebitis is the result of long-term maintenance of needles or catheters.

The duration of infusion will most often dictate the type of cannula used. Generally, with infusions of short duration (1 to 3 days), steel needles are selected. Short plastic needles (catheter-over-needle type) may be used for longer infusions (3 to 5 days). Longer catheters, such as those used in parenteral nutrition, are used for therapy of long duration.

Several studies have shown that the degree of infusion phlebitis increased with the length of time the catheter was in place. One study[27] showed that the incidence of thrombophlebitis varied from 9% when the catheter was in place less than 24 hours to 58% when catheterization lasted longer than 24 hours. A similar study showed rates from 0.9% for less than 12 hours to 37% over 24 hours,[19] and up to 50% incidence in I.V. fluid therapy with cannulization up to 72 hours. Bolton-Carter[16] showed that, when the duration of infusion was under 8 hours, the incidence of phlebitis decreased from 52% to 5%.

Infection. Evidence indicates that phlebitis and other complications may cause a predisposition to catheter colonization,[13] although another study has shown that, with a 47% incidence of phlebitis (135 patients), only 9.7% had positive cultures. This author concluded that infection was not a cause of phlebitis.[27]

In a study of catheter contamination versus the incidence of phlebitis, Davidson[28] concluded that, although catheter contamination is often implicated as a contributing factor of local phlebitis, it is not the sole cause of phlebitis and a search for other causes is necessary. Welch et al.[20] also indicated a secondary role for bacteria in the development of phlebitis.

Chemical Irritation of Drugs. Many drugs induce infusion phlebitis by exerting an irritant effect on the vein: cephalothin, tetracycline, potassium chloride, penicillin, amphotericin B, and vancomycin are but a few.[14] The incidence of thrombophlebitis in one report on lidocaine was 50% versus 8.4% in the control.[29] The concentration and rate of drug administration also are factors in vein irritation. Several reports have recommended the use of such drugs as heparin, sodium bicarbonate, and steroids in the infusion to reduce the potential for phlebitis.[11,23,29–31]

Daniell,[31] in a double-blind study of 151 patients, noted that the addition of 1000 units of heparin to each liter of infusion fluid reduced the frequency of thrombophlebitis at infusion sites.

Schafermeyer[32] suggested that use of 500 units of heparin and 1 mg of hydrocortisone per liter of infusion containing cephalothin, gentamicin, kanamycin, or potassium salts will decrease phlebitis and increase longevity of cannulization.

Anderson et al.[33] reported that the median duration of venoclysis, which would produce thrombophlebitis, was 3.3 days. For infusions containing 1300 units of heparin per liter, the median was raised to 8.6 days.

Henney et al.[34] studied the thrombophlebitis potential of intravenous cytotoxic agents. In this study, 33% of all intravenously administered anticancer drugs were associated with the development of thrombophlebitis. Brand variation of the same drug has been associated with phlebitis. In one hopsital, a venous irritation problem was solved by changing one brand of nafcillin to another.[35]

Post-Infusion Phlebitis (PIP). This occurred in 17% of the patients receiving cephapirin or cefamandole. Of the patients receiving cefoxitin, 60% developed PIP.[36]

pH of Infusion Fluids. Several reports have associated the acidity of dextrose solutions with infusion phlebitis; one as early as 1952.[37–40] In one report,[41] the author notes the physician's surprise that 5% dextrose in water has an acid pH in the range of 4.4 to 4.6. These authors suggested that, if the pH had been printed on the bottle label, physicians would have been much more hesitant to use the product and would have realized earlier that this is one of the main causes of phlebitis developing after dextrose infusion.

It should be emphasized that nearly all intravenous infusion solutions are acidic. The *U.S.P.* allows pH range for Water for Injection from 5 to 7. The *U.S.P.* range for Dextrose Injection is 3.5 to 6.5. This pH range is necessary to ensure stability during sterilization and storage of commercially prepared solutions.

Dextrose solutions with a pH greater than 6 are not produced commercially because of caramelization. After autoclaving, these dextrose solutions range in pH from 3.5 to 5.5. Heat-producing breakdown products, which are acidic, glucuronic acid and 5-hydroxymethylfuraldehyde, account for the major portion of this acidity. At an alkaline pH, more breakdown products occur. However, for a short period of time (24 to 48 hours), dextrose can be buffered to a physiologic pH before administration without a significant degradation.[42,43]

Bolton-Carter et al.[17] in 1952 reported negative results with the buffering of I.V. dextrose. In response, Page et al.[37] reported a definite decrease in thrombophlebitis associated with buffering dextrose solutions and suggested that Bolton-Carter's negative results may have been caused by the irritant effects of the rubber administration sets. Page suggested control of all other factors and stated, "Only then can we be reasonably certain that correction of the acidity of glucose solutions affects the incidence of thrombophlebitis."

In 1960, Vere et al.[44] studied cold-sterilized and heat-sterilized dextrose solutions and their relationship to phlebitis. They found that autoclaved solutions are more acid and associated with a significantly higher incidence of thrombophlebitis (75%) than are solutions sterilized by filtration and with pH near neutrality (36%).

Elfving et al.[40] stated, "We regard it as clearly proven that the incidence of thrombophlebitis after infusion of 10% invert sugar can be reduced by bringing the pH of the infusion fluid close to neutral."

Fonkalsrud et al.[11] compared commercially available solutions and hospital-produced 5% dextrose and water, which was buffered. A threefold decrease in phlebitis resulted in buffered solutions. They concluded that pH of dextrose solutions is a major factor in causing phlebitis.

In another study, Fonkalsrud et al.[18] examined sections of canine vein after infusion with 5% dextrose solution and found severe endothelial injury, inflammation of the vein wall, and intraluminal thrombosis. Comparable sections of vein infused with buffered 5% dextrose solution showed little if any change.

Fonkalsrud et al.[18] studied 156 patients given unbuffered and buffered solutions, and unbuffered solutions containing heparin and hydrocortisone. The patients receiving unbuffered solutions had twice the incidence of phlebitis as did those receiving buffered solutions. The unbuffered heparin and hydrocortisone group also showed similar reduction in phlebitis.

Lebowitz et al.[39] studied the pH and total titratable acidity of intravenous infusion solutions. They showed that commercial infusion solutions have a low pH and considerable variations in acid content. It was stated that two manufacturers made pH adjustments prior to sterilization, and one manufacturer used lactic acid for pH adjustment for selected fluids.

Tse[45] suggested that acid intravenous infusion solutions have no significant buffer capacity and are easily buffered by the blood, and that phlebitis caused by acidity of such solutions is related to size of cannulae used. If a large-bore cannula is used in a small vein, blood flow is reduced around the cannula. The reduced blood flow is not enough to buffer the solution. Tse advises the use of large veins and small cannulae to achieve adequate blood flow.

In response to Lebowitz et al., Ansel[46] reported on the large buffering capacity of blood: that the presence of blood in proportions as small as 1:500 resulted in immediate buffering of acid solutions toward the pH of blood (7.4) and that the usual intravenous drip solution would rapidly be buffered by blood.

Moster,[47] reporting on the pH of drugs and blood, mixed various acid drugs with blood and showed that acid drugs, on coming into contact with the highly buffered blood, have no effect. Osmolality of intravenous infusion solutions is more important than pH.

Lipman[12] found no statistically significant difference between the incidence or severity of phlebitis caused by buffered versus unbuffered cephalothin.

Relationship of Age and Sex to Incidence of Phlebitis. In a study of 191 patients, Fonkalsrud et al.[11] have shown that men and women are equally susceptible to phlebitis. In the same study, younger patients (20 to 40 years)

were particularly susceptible to phlebitis. Thomas, however, found no difference in age groups.[15]

Other Factors. The osmolality of the infusion has been associated with
phlebitis. Hyperosmolar solutions (over 320 mOsm) are usually administered
via a large vein to minimize vein irritation.[38,45]

The arm is the preferred site for routine short-term intravenous infusion
therapy in adults. Catheterization of veins in the legs appears to be associated
with a considerably greater risk of thrombophlebitis and sepsis.[14,25]

Central venous catheters inserted in the arm and fed directly into the superior vena cava appear to cause less phlebitis than shorter catheters.[14]

There may be a relationship between particulate matter and phlebitis.[48] In
a study of 100 operative patients after operation, a 0.45-μ membrane filter
was found to dramatically minimize acute phlebitis and thrombophlebitis. A
comparison of the incidence of phlebitis in patients having infusion solutions
that were filtered and those not receiving filtered solutions showed a highly
significant decrease in frequency in the group using the filter. In the group
receiving nonfiltered solutions, phlebitis in 22 of 49, whereas only 1 of 51
developed phlebitis in the filter group. Work is continuing in this area. Recorded current phlebitis rates range from 11 to 70%. Hospitals having I.V.
teams report lesser rates.[49]

In one study[50] of over 7000 infusions, the I.V. team reduced the phlebitis
rate to below 4.5%. This study suggests that the person who performs the
venipuncture can cause a large percentage of occurrences of infusion phlebitis.

Conclusions

A review of the literature on infusion phlebitis indicates some confusion
about cause and prevention. Some of this confusion is the result of the many
factors associated with infusion phlebitis. The complexity of drug therapy and
treatment of ill patients adds to the confusion. In day-to-day hospital practice,
there is lack of concern by many medical personnel about infusion phlebitis,
since this disease is relatively unimportant in the total care of the severely ill
patient.

Abstracted conclusions by Maki and co-workers[14] concerning infusion phlebitis are as follows:

1. Anatomic location of cannulization. Lower extremities are more vulner-
    able to phlebitis.
2. Position of cannula tip. Central venous catheters inserted in the arm and
    fed directly into the superior vena cava appear to cause less phlebitis
    than shorter catheters.
3. Duration of cannulization. The incidence of phlebitis increases the longer
    catheters are left in place.
4. Type of cannula. Steel needles cause phlebitis less often than plastic
    catheters. This is because of small bore, ease of insertion, and nonthrom-
    bogenic surface.
    Several uncontrolled clinical trials have led investigators to conclude that
    siliconized catheters are less thrombogenic than polyethylene catheters.
    Heparin bonding reduced thrombogenesis and fluoroethylenepropylene
    caused virtually no phlebitis in a comparable study.

5. Cannula size and length. Catheters with large diameters may inflict greater damage on the vessel wall.

6. Type of infusion solution. Acidic solutions such as dextrose in water, especially if hypertonic, are likely to cause phlebitis.

7. I.V. medications. Antibiotics, cytotoxic drugs, electrolyte solutions, and anesthetic agents irritate the vascular endothelium.

8. pH infusion fluids. Several investigators have shown that neutralization of acidic infusion fluids with bicarbonate reduces the frequency of infusion-associated phlebitis. This has the disadvantages of additional manipulation and preparation of solution. Also, neutralization may broaden the spectrum of microbiologic proliferation. The addition of heparin and hydrocortisone are not definitive in reducing phlebitis.

9. Infusion-associated sepsis. The data indicate that patients with catheter-associated phlebitis may have increased risk of associated septicemia.

Infiltration and Intra-Arterial Injections

Infiltration or inadvertent intra-arterial injection of some drugs can cause severe necrosis resulting in tissue damage, gangrene, and ultimate loss of limbs. Alexander[51] reported on the occurrence of pedal gangrene in a patient receiving dopamine infusion of 10 μg/kg/min for 2 days. Gangrene has also been reported following dopamine infusion of 1.5 μg/kg/min.[52] The manufacturer recommends that dopamine be infused in a large vein to guard against the possibility of extravasation into tissue at the infusion site. Another report[53] describes gangrene in the feet and fingers of a patient receiving dopamine by infusion. Boltax et al.,[54] who also saw gangrene in one patient, advised the use of indwelling venous catheters for dopamine infusions. Inadvertent intra-arterially injected promethazine required amputation of the arm.[55] Inadvertent intra-arterial injection of haloperidol 10 mg and promethazine 50 mg required amputation of hand and forearm.[56] One estimate establishes infiltration rates as occurring in 25% of hospitalized patients receiving I.V. injections.

Gas gangrene following the intramuscular injection of adrenalin was first reported in 1946.[57] In 1960,[58] three cases caused by intramuscular injection of adrenalin-in-oil were reported, resulting in two deaths. Harvey and Purneil[59] described a fatal case of gas gangrene due to intramuscular injection of adrenalin-in-oil, suggesting that such injections be avoided.

The area of injection (buttocks) and the constriction caused by adrenalin promotes anaerobic infections such as *Cl. welchii*. Van Hook[60] reported a death caused by intramuscular injection of epinephrine-in-oil in the buttocks. Van Hook suggests 15-minute skin preparation with iodine compresses if epinephrine must be given intramuscularly.

Diffuse tissue damage following accidental intra-arterial injection of barbiturates or tranquilizers has been reported.[61–63] Other reports have described the hazards of the intra-arterial injection of barbiturates,[64] pentazocine,[65] and propoxyphene.[66]

Accidental injection of vincristine has occurred.[67,68] Accidental injection of vincristine into the spine has been reported.[63,69] Confusion between a heparin flush cartridge and a vaccine cartridge caused the inadvertent intravenous administration of influenza vaccine.[70] Although mechlorethamine is administered intravenously, accidental intramuscular injections have been reported.[71]

Numerous reports have been published of accidental extravasation associated with parenterals. This is particularly harmful in the extravasation of oncolytics and amine-type drugs.[72-77] Drug extravasation in venous access ports has also been reported.[78] Extravasation of drugs causes more severe problems in children.[79,80]

Particulate Matter and Filters

In the past two decades, considerable attention has been focused on particulate matter in parenteral solutions. The presence of particles in a wide variety of liquids and solids has been reported. Methods have been developed and are continuing to be developed for its analysis. Limited studies concerning its significance have been reported. Techniques and methods have been designed to minimize the presence of foreign materials. Various types of contaminants have been defined. Standards for the limits of particulate matter have been established in the U.S.P. for LVPs. Although some will question its clinical significance, few will deny its presence. With all the elucidation, discussion, and written clarification, however, the solution to the problem of particulate matter continues to elude us. Apparently, this evasiveness is the result of a number of factors, one of which is the complex nature of drugs and the component materials used to package drugs. Additionally, a need exists for better methods of analysis and techniques for the elimination of particulate matter. The generation of particulate matter in the clinical environment is not appreciated by many who function in this area of activity. A better understanding of particulate matter for the practitioner will go a long way toward solution of the problem.

Nature of Particulate Matter

Particulate matter encompasses many different materials and with increasing knowledge this list continues to grow. Identifications of cotton, glass, rubber, plastic, asbestos, tissue, insect fragments, ants, undissolved drugs, mold, fungi, bacteria, lint, hair, metal, and other debris have been made. Still other identified materials include polyvinylchloride, drug precipitates, undissolved chemicals, emulsion globules of diethylheptathalate (DEHP), sulfur, paraffin, zinc and other heavy metals, and metal fragments. Some materials remain to be identified. The theoretical possibilities for particulation would include any environmental material. The presence of particulate matter in parenteral drugs is partially the result of human activity, and until such time as this factor is controlled, the problem will persist. The fault cannot be laid to one group of individuals or activity; the cause is broad and cannot be narrowed to a specific contributor. Some of the particles found in infusions are listed in Table A4–3.

Factors that Contribute to Particulate Matter

Drug production and the environment in which drugs are produced are contributory factors to the presence of particulate matter. Tremendous efforts have been made by the pharmaceutical industry to better control the per-

TABLE A4–3.   Nature of Particles Found in Infusions

Garvan and Gunner (1963)	Millipore (1974)	Draftz and Graf (1974)	
Particles of 1-μ diameter	Colloidal particles	Pigments	
Black rubber particles up to	Metal	Filters	From
100 μ	Asbestos	Lacquer	rubber
Crystals	Cotton	flakes	bungs
Fibers	Dust	Maize starch	
Brown rust particles	Lint	Mica flakes	
Starch		Paper fibers	
Diatoms		Aluminum shavings	
Fungi		Polythene shavings	

sonnel and the environment of drug production. Drug packaging also makes a significant contribution; the generation of particulates from the contact of drugs with plastic, glass, and rubber components offers no simple solution. Drug manufacturers have devoted considerable effort to improve washing methods for glassware and equipment used to manufacture drugs. Better filtration techniques have been used. Employee training has been implemented. Particle analysis laboratories have been established in many pharmaceutical companies.

In preparation of drugs for use and ultimate administration to the patient, medical personnel make significant contributions toward the problem of particulate matter. Even with ideal techniques, needle coring, drug incompatibility, and glass from breaking ampuls add to the problem. Improper storage time and temperature are frequently factors in the hospital environment. The mixing and addition of complex drugs are frequent occurrences. In the administration of drugs to patients, all these add to the problem.

Occurrence of Particulate Matter

Particulate matter has been reported in a variety of products, infusion fluids, irrigating fluids, small-volume parenterals, dry-filled and lyophilized drugs, ophthalmic drugs, banked blood, dialysis solutions, hyperalimentation solutions, perfusion fluids, and various types of medical equipment.

Outlook and Improvements

Industrial improvements have occurred through better technology in the manufacturing and processing of drugs. Improved washing and filtration methods are employed. Improved air handling systems and environmental controls have been instituted. Establishment of standards for parenterals has made the state of the art more scientific. In the clinical setting, controlled admixture preparations and the use of filters have reduced particulation; above all, health care personnel have a better understanding of the problem of particulate matter. It is to be hoped that increased diligence, industrially and clinically, will upgrade the state of the art.

Clinical Significance of Particulate Matter

A review of the pertinent literature relating to the clinical significance of particulate matter up to 1973 was reported by Turco and Davis.[81] This 1973 review discusses 47 clinical reports concerning particulate matter and refers to an additional 45 reports. In the years that have elapsed since, relatively few new *clinical studies* have appeared in the literature.

In a study[82] conducted by the Pharmaceutical Manufacturers Association (PMA), an attempt was made to "define particulate matter in intravenously administered drugs and solutions." In this study, hundreds of rats were injected intravenously with varying quantities and sizes of *inert* polystyrene spheres. Necropsies were performed at varying periods of time from 1 hour to 28 days. Of 18 rats injected with 8×10^6 particles/kg at the 40-μ size, 13 developed labored respiration after injection and died within 3 to 5 minutes. One rat injected at the 4-μ size level with 4×10^5 particle/kg died within 3 minutes after injection. All the other rats injected with polystyrene particles or control vehicle were normal. Blood studies, organ weights, and pathologic criteria were eventually found to be normal in all animals. At the 4-μ size, particles were observed in the lung, liver, and spleen of test animals. With 10-μ particles, the lung was the principal site of deposition, although particles were found in the heart, liver, spleen, kidney, brain, and pancreas. The authors concluded that the "results of this study clearly demonstrate that nonreactive particles administered intravenously over a broad size range and up to dosages that produced death were without clinical or tissue toxicity." They further suggested the tremendous margin of safety that exists for drugs and parenteral solutions that contain low levels of nonreactive particulate material. In the discussions of this paper, attention was drawn to the fact that the conclusion drawn was not valid because of the artificial material studied. Duma,[83] reviewing the particulate matter problem,[84] noted that if infusion of glass, rubber, and starch is distasteful, then infusion of asbestos must certainly be unpalatable and unacceptable. An assessment of asbestos and its harmful effects has been made by Haley.[85]

Katz et al.[86,87] reported on visible glass generated from the breaking of glass ampuls of local anesthetic agents for epidural and caudal use. Speculating on possible granuloma formation and foreign body reaction that these injected particles might cause, these authors strongly recommended the use of small-bore needles, suitable filters, or filter aspiration needles to prevent these complications.

Lyon et al.[88] injected particulate matter containing dextran into several groups of animals, noting that there were definite histologic differences between the control and experimental groups, and suggested the particulate matter present in those samples of dextran studied contributed to granuloma formation. The histologic picture resulted in a diffuse perivascular granuloma formation in the lungs.

Furgang[89] explored the possibility that neurologic sequelae of regional anesthesia may in part be the result of injury and inflammation to neural tissue caused by glass fragments generated during the opening of ampuls.

Evidence was presented[90] in favor of adopting a micropore filtration and working techniques for bubble oxygenator prior to open heart surgery. Vast amounts of particulates had been found in bubble oxygenators used in the institution where the study was made. The authors noted that the incidence of postoperative neurologic deficits decreased after the incorporation of this technique. This publication is significant in that it illustrates that particulate contamination is also a consideration to be reckoned with in medical equipment.

In a study[91] of 173 patients undergoing cardiac catheterization and/or surgery, 14 (8%) had fiber emboli in routine autopsy sections. Fibers occurred in the pulmonary, renal, cerebral, and mesenteric arteries. The embolized fiber often resulted in narrowing or occlusion of the involved vessel. This study associated three cases of infarction with embolic fibers. The fibers were believed to be shed from cotton, gauze, sponges, gowns, and drapes and introduced into drug solutions. The authors concluded that particulate matter is a hazard and all steps to prevent its inadvertent administration should be considered.

Vidt[92] suggests that consideration be given to the routine use of in-line filters to prevent the infusion of particulate matter and microbial contamination.

Purkiss[93] injected cellular fibers into 40 mice; an additional 10 served as saline controls. In all dosed mice, lung sections contained granulomas. None of the lung sections taken from control mice showed granulomas.

The association between the introduction of foreign material during chronic peritoneal dialysis and peritonitis was first suggested by Zerefos et al.[94] Lasker,[95] observing considerable peritonitis with chronic peritoneal dialysis, designed a study[96] to determine whether peritoneal dialysis solutions containing particulate matter would cause a reaction. This study additionally attempted to determine whether reactions could be prevented by filtering the solution before its entry into the peritoneal cavity. Groups of mice were injected with filtered and unfiltered solutions. A high percentage of the injected animals showed particulate matter in the peritoneal membranes associated with an inflammatory reaction. This was prevented by final filtration of the solutions through 0.22- and 0.45-μ filters. The recommendation from this study was that chronic peritoneal dialysis be performed through a final filter.

Studies Involving the Analysis of Particulate Matter

Mead,[97] in a macroscopic analysis of over 81,000 I.V. infusion fluids, rejected 9122 (11.2%) because of the presence of visible particulate matter. Masuda et al.[98] studied the particulate content of various lyophilized, sterile, bulk-filled, and stable solutions of antibiotics. Of particular interest in this study was the comparison of carbenicillin manufactured by two different companies. One product contained a fivefold increase in particles attributed to the method of manufacture. The observation that lyophilized carbenicillin produced a less particulated product was also confirmed by Jeffrey et al.[99] Additional confirmations were made by Turco et al.[100-103] Particulate matter in diphenylhydantoin has been reported.[104,105] The implication of glass fragments being injected in considerable amounts was illustrated with furosemide.[106,107] Thousands of glass particles are generated with the breaking of large numbers of containers.

Of particular interest to pharmacists was the microscopic review[99] of over 19,000 containers of various antibiotics, which resulted in a rejection rate of 19.2%. Williams et al.[108] reported on the particulate contamination of I.V. fluids, administration sets, and cannulae. A comparative analysis of particulates in various manufactured ampules was reported on by Somerville et al.[109] Whitlow[110] studied the effects of particle generation of polyvinylchloride and glass containers. It was established from this study that significant numbers of particles can be generated in polyvinylchloride bags by the handling and dropping of these containers. The authors suggest that transport and storage conditions of plastic containers play a significant role in particle contamination of intravenous fluids.

In a comparative analysis[111] of particulate matter in spray-dried and lyophilized carbenicillin, it was shown that spray-dried carbenicillin can produce a material of low particulate contamination.

Mead[112] in a follow-up study of large-volume parenterals, examined over 33,000 solutions macroscopically and rejected 5400 units (16.2%). Of one batch of Ringer's Injection, 76% was particulated. Intravenous administration sets[113] have been studied for particulate matter and have been shown to contain varying amounts depending on the complexity of the set. A correlation exists[114] between the quantity of particulate matter and the amount of unfiltered drug solution added to the large-volume parenteral containers. Differences in storage and handling had an influence on the initial quantity of particles found in plastic bags. Levinson et al.[115] compared particles in I.V. solutions in glass and plastic. These results showed that particles found in glass and in plastic containers bore distinct differences. A study[116] of particulate matter in six commonly used I.V. solutions, evaluating five different methods of analyses, showed that the method of analysis gave varying particle counts.

In a study[117] of insoluble residues from various antibiotics, it appeared that the particulates were product-related rather than process-related, and that subtle degeneration of the product occurs. Schroeder and DeLuca,[118] studying various intravenous fluids, showed that of those solutions studied, none exceeded the *U.S.P. XIX* standard for particulate matter; however, particle counts increased as a function of additives, particularly antibiotic additives. In one study of cephalothin (Keflin) and cephapirin (Cefadyl),[119] it was shown that considerable differences in particulate counts can be found with different antibiotics because of differences in the manufacturing processes. These differences can also vary with the date of manufacture. In comparisons of particulate counts made when studying lyophilized antibiotics, these differences become less obvious.[120] The addition of additives to a parenteral nutrition base produces a significant increase in the concentration of particles.[121]

Although various methods for the detection of particulate matter have been reported in the literature by Ho,[122] Turco et al.,[123] Thomas et al.,[124] and Vidt,[125] none is without disadvantages. Newer methods are being developed.[126]

Phlebitis, Particulate Matter, and Filtration

Infusion phlebitis has been adequately reviewed in the literature along with the various causes and associations of this disease.[127] Various causes apparently lead to infusion phlebitis. An interesting study[128] published in 1972 was first to illustrate the possible relationship between particulate matter and infusion phlebitis. In this non-blind study of 100 postoperative patients, the effectiveness of a 0.45-μ filter was found to dramatically minimize acute phlebitis and thrombophlebitis. An analysis of the incidence of phlebitis in those patients who received filtered intravenous solutions showed a significant reduction in phlebitis. Only 1 of 51 patients receiving filtered drugs developed phlebitis, compared with 22 of 49 in the nonfiltered group. However, a study by Collin et al.[129] showed no effect in the reduction of infusion phlebitis with the use of in-line filters. In another study[130] of in-line filtration and the occurrence of phlebitis, no significant difference in the incidence of phlebitis in patients using the in-line final filter and those not using it was found. In a repeated double-blind study[131] of 146 patients using a 0.45-μ filter, a significant reduction in phlebitis was seen when in-line filters were used (25% phlebitis in filter group versus 62% in nonfiltered group).

There have been isolated clinical observations[132] that the use of filters reduces or eliminates phlebitis. In a study[133] utilizing a 5-μ filter, the incidence of phlebitis was significantly lower in patients receiving filtered intravenous solutions. Of 25 patients in the nonfiltered group, 14 developed phlebitis compared with 2 of 24 in the filtered group. Maddox et al.[134] in a study of cephalothin-induced phlebitis concluded that postinfusion phlebitis following cephalothin administration can be reduced by the concomitant addition of heparin and hydrocortisone or by the use of 0.22-μ in-line final filters.

In a study at Yale-New Haven Hospital[135] utilizing a 5-μ filter, no significant difference was found between the incidence or severity of infusion phlebitis associated with filtered and nonfiltered infusion. This group recommends that the use of 5-μ filters for the prevention of infusion phlebitis be discouraged.

In-line Filters and Contamination

Wilmore and Dudrick,[136] in an attempt to minimize microbial contamination during parenteral hyperalimentation, reported on the use of in-line filters. Of the more than 250 membrane filters studied during the period of evaluation, 7 positive bacterial cultures were obtained from the proximal surfaces. No systemic signs of bacteremia, septicemia, or phlebitis were observed. Seventeen filters became obstructed during use. On 14 occasions, microprecipitates resulted from drug incompatibility that occluded the membrane pores. Two filters developed air locks; one filter became obstructed from the inadvertent administration of blood proximal to the filter surface. The authors commented that the filters were accepted by patients and nurses and added no difficulties to the administration of intravenous fluids. They stated that "Use of the in-line final filter ensures sterile delivery of parenteral fluid, reducing the complications of infection and increasing patient safety during long-term I.V. therapy."

Myers[137] studied flow rates and microbial contamination of intravenous fluids. Of 43 filters, 6 showed bacterial contamination. Myers concluded that bacteria can be introduced inadvertently into intravenous fluids during administration and use of in-line filters could prevent this.

Butler et al.[138] studied the effective use of 0.45-μ and 0.22-μ filters in removing mycelial contamination in hyperalimentation solutions. Their results illustrated that the 0.45-μ filter was as effective in removing mycelial growth as was the 0.22-μ filter. Miller and Grogan,[139] in a study of 20 infants receiving intravenous nutrition, cultured 361 infusion systems. The infusion systems were attached to in-line bacterial filters. A 29.1% contamination rate was found. Multiple cultures at different points within the system indicated that the filters were effective in trapping and confining microorganisms in both forward and reverse directions. Collin et al.,[140] in a clinical study of 0.45-μ in-line filters, found no significant reduction in thrombophlebitis or in bacterial contamination of the cannulae. This group thought the filters to be inconvenient because of reduced flow rates and frequent filter blockage. Bunker et al.[141] used 0.5-μ filters for drugs used to test renal clearance. These authors concluded that the use of micropore filters was a justifiable addition in I.V. administration. Sarles et al.[142] were able to demonstrate a significant reduction in clinical peritonitis when filters were utilized. Of 140 dialyses, 34% produced positive cultures. These authors concluded that filters used in peritoneal dialysis drastically reduce the incidence of positive dialysis cultures and clinical peritonitis. Freeman et al.,[143] in a study of 105 medical and surgical patients, studied Millipore filters in 28 patients, none of whom had central venous nutritional sepsis, whereas 6 of 77 patients in whom filters were not used had central venous nutritional sepsis. Patients with filters required twice as many manipulations of the line as did those without filters because of the tendency of the filters to reduce flow rates.

Huber and Riffkin[144] studied various pore size filters to remove particles from amphotericin B solutions. These authors concluded that filters of not less than 1.0-μ porosity could be used to filter amphotericin B. All filters with 0.22-μ pores removed amphotericin B from solution and were, therefore, inappropriate for use with this product. In contrast to this study, Piecoro et al.[145] showed that filtration through 0.85- and 0.45-μ filters did not reduce the in vitro antimicrobial activity of amphotericin B, nor did filtration through 5-, 0.45-, and 0.22-μ filters alter the concentration of this drug, as shown spectrophotometrically.

The Medical Letter,[146] commenting on filters, concluded that "Final filters with a pore size of 0.45 μ or less remove particles and most bacteria and fungi from I.V. fluids. Atlhough these filters may reduce the incidence of phlebitis at the site of the cannula there is no evidence that they prevent infection or shorten the time of hospitalization, and they are expensive." Tenney and Dixon[147] in 1974 concluded that, although micropore filters for use in total parenteral nutrition (TPN) and other infusion therapy have theoretical advantages, insufficient data exist to recommend their use. Newman et al.,[148] in a study of 72 I.V. fluids using in-line filters, found 27% of the filters contaminated and concluded that their use was a positive means of trapping microorganisms and particles. Miller and Grogan,[149] in a follow-up study of in-line filters with intravenous nutritional solutions, concluded that single filters were effective in trapping organisms. Of more than 4800 cultures, 7.5% were positive. Serial in-line filters offered an advantage over a single filter. An evaluation[150] of an air-venting in-line filter in a 53-patient trial showed that this new, larger-surfaced filter was easy to use and gained the acceptance of nurses, pharmacists, and physicians.

Holland[151] suggests that micropore filters prevent air emboli and trap microprecipitates and other debris, and recommends the use of bacterial in-line filters for TPN solutions.

Meeker et al.[152] suggest in-line filters be used to prevent the infusion of particulate matter and microorganisms and air for intra-arterial infusions. In addition, in the event of set disruption, the filter will prevent bleeding via red cells clogging the membrane.

Rapp et al.[153] evaluated the 5-μ stainless steel filter as an in-line filter or prefilter. As a protective prefilter, the 5-μ filter device in combination with a 0.45-μ filter provided more uniform flow rates when additives were employed.

In a study assessing the relationship of contamination and infusion phlebitis, Rusmin et al.[154] found 11% of 146 I.V. solutions contaminated. This study also showed the absence of a strong correlation between infusion phlebitis and positive cultures, supporting the concept that particulate matter is a major cause of infusion phlebitis.

Filter Adsorption

Although considerable information is available concerning the clinical use of filters in entrapping particles and microorganisms, little information exists describing drug adsorption to the filter. An inquiry was received from a nurse[155] who questioned the use of filters for ampicillin; she was concerned about drug adsorption onto the filter. This prompted Wyeth Laboratories to conduct ampicillin assays, using the techniques used by this nurse. Assay reports indicated no filter adsorption of ampicillin; "all solutions had identical and acceptable potency."[156]

A publication by Wagman et al.[157] described adsorption of considerable amounts of various antibiotics including gentamicin to various filter media. However, none of these filter media (cellulose powder, diatomaceous earth, and Seitz filter sheets) resembles the current characteristics and qualities of clinical filters. Subsequent assays requested of these authors indicated that "little or no activity was removed by the membrane filter."[158]

Work done at the University of Kentucky[159] showed insignificant quantites of penicillin blocked by the filter. Assays of bleomycin (Blenoxane)[160] through a 0.45-μ membrane filter indicated insignificant adsorption.

Work done by Huber et al.[161] using 0.22-μ filters with amphotericin B indicated filter adsorption. These authors indicated that 0.22-μ filters were inappropriate for use with this product. At pH 5.6, only filters with pore sizes of 1.0 μ or greater showed acceptable results. In contrast to this, Piecoro et al.[162] studied filtration of amphotericin B infusions; their data showed that filtration through 0.85- and 0.45-μ filters did not reduce the in vitro antimicrobial activity, and filtration through 5-, 0.45-, and 0.22-μ filters did not alter the concentration of the drug, as shown spectrophotometrically.[98] Product brochures[162] state, "Minute quantities of drugs from intravenous solutions may adsorb to containers, administration sets, and membrane filters. Therefore, supplemental dosages of 5 mg or less should be administered through the latex bulb with filter set slide clamp open." Bacterial endotoxin retention by in-line intravenous filters has been studied by Baumgartner et al.[163] Of the filters tested, only one, composed of Poisidyne Nylon 66, was able to retain *Escherichia coli* endotoxin for 96 hours. Endotoxin retention requires further study.

Although the small amount of current information suggests that little adsorption or absorption takes place with membrane filters, minute dosages of drugs 5 mg or less should not be filtered until sufficient data are available to confirm insignificant adsorption. In the case of amphotericin B, because of the current controversy, it is probably best to avoid any type of clinical filter until this can be clarified. One might argue that we should not be concerned about adsorption of drugs to membrane filters considering that millions of pieces of pharmaceuticals are sterilized in the United States by membrane filtration. One cannot make a valid comparison, however, because industrial-sized batches render filter adsorption insignificant.

Catheter Complications

The use of tapered, plastic catheters inserted over a needle was first reported in the 1950s. I.V. catheter complications are many and varied.

Malposition of central venous pressure catheters has been reported.[164] This is a frequent occurrence, believed to happen in 25% to 38% of cases. In one study[165] of 73 central venous catheters thought to be correctly positioned, only 64% were in an acceptable position radiologically.

Several instances[166,167] of heart wall perforation by central venous catheters used in the administration of I.V. fluids have been reported. Fatal air embolism during insertion of central venous pressure (CVP) monitoring equipment was first described by Levinsky.[168] Venous air embolism is considered a dramatic complication of parenteral fluid therapy. It is probably necessary to inject a total of over 200 ml at a rate of 70 to 100 ml/sec to produce sudden death.[169] Air emboli via subclavian catheters have been described by Johnson et al.,[170] Lucas,[171] and others.[172,173] The risk of thrombosis and infection with indwelling radial-artery catheters has been studied.[174] Cortical blindness caused by subclavian vein catheterization has been reported.[175] Dinley[176] published on venous reactions related to in-dwelling plastic cannulae. Thromboembolic complications with Swan-Ganz catheters have been investigated.[177] A number of publications direct attention to the potential complications of breaking catheters.[178,179] Several accounts deal with catheter sepsis[180–187] in addition to other complications.[188–194] An extensive evaluation of catheter placement units has been published.[195] Diagnosis and management of catheter-related infections have been reviewed by Raad.[196]

Preservative Toxicity

Generally, preservatives used in reasonable amounts, like those contained in parenterals, are relatively nontoxic. Reports of toxicity as a result of misuse of formulated products have appeared in the literature, however. Toxic symptoms have been observed from the absorption of sodium bisulfite used to preserve peritoneal dialysis solutions.[197] Cronk[198] called attention to the potential dangers of phenol in glucagon dilution, noting that, for each milligram of glucagon, 0.2 g of phenol is injected. Clinical application of glucagon for myocardial contractile failure requires larger doses than those customarily used. Spodick et al.[199] commented on the undesirability of phenol. Schmidt et al.[200] reported on the sudden appearance of cardiac arrhythmia after dexamethasone injection. These authors speculated that the toxic effects may be due to the preservatives in dexamethasone. It has been suggested that sodium benzoate used as a solubilizer or buffer preservative in diazepam (Valium) injection and caffeine sodium benzoate injection is a potent bilirubin-albumin uncoupler, resulting in the development of kernicterus in infants.[201] Mizutan[202] reported on the high incidence of delayed hypersensitivity reactions associated with thimerosal. The possibility of bronchial irritation due to paraben-containing drugs used in inhalation therapy has been reported.[203] Concern has been focused also on paraben allergenicity. Nagel et al.[204] describe paraben-provoked bronchospasm and pruritus caused by intravenously injected paraben-preserved hydrocortisone. Sharer et al.[205] noted cardiovascular and respiratory depressant effects with large doses of diazepam. The major effects were attributed to the propylene glycol diluent. Chlorobutanol-caused eye irritation has been reported.[206] Eye irritation from procaine hydrochloride preserved with benzyl alcohol has been reported.[207] Preservatives present in parenteral products also possess the potential for diagnostic error[208] when the bacteriostatic-preserved product may be used for diagnostic testing.

The neurotoxicity of Bacteriostatic Water has been reported.[209] Benzyl alcohol present as a preservative in some multiple dose vials of bacteriostatic sodium chloride or Bacteriostatic Water for Injection has caused fatal toxic syndrome in premature infants. Two different medical centers reported the deaths. Benzyl alcohol has also been associated with hypersensitivity reactions. Several pharmaceutical manufacturers* are now producing preservative-free products in an effort to reduce the allergic response and/or toxicity of preservatives.

Extemporaneously compounded preservative-free injections provided by the pharmacist require special quality assurance procedures.[211]

Rubber Closure Compatibility and Stability

Interaction between preservatives (phenol, cresol, thiomersalate, chlorcresol, benzyl alcohol) and rubber closures have been reported, including rubber closure plastic interaction.[212] An extensive study by Lachman et al.[213] examining those factors that affect antibacterial preservative agents in solutions of rubber-stoppered containers showed that vials have a greater loss of preservative content than do ampuls. Vials stored in an inverted position have a greater loss of preservatives; natural rubber stoppers exert the least effect on preservative content. Interaction of rubber closures is not limited to parenteral products, as illustrated by a report of incompatibility with acetylcysteine packaged in syringes used for inhalation therapy.[214] Leaching of zinc and other heavy metals from rubber closures has been noted.[215,216] Liberation of hydrogen sulfide in large-volume parenterals has been reported.[217,218] Interaction between preservatives (sodium formaldehyde, sulfoxylate) and rubber components with the liberation of sulfur crystals has been responsible for the recall of meperidine.[219]

Labeling

Labeling[220] of parenteral containers is sometimes difficult to read and often can be read only with the best of lighting conditions and vision. Manufacturers have a number of problems associated with labeling. The small surface area available for the label, together with the desire to minimize the size of the label so that the user can inspect the contents, aggravates the situation.

---

*PF, Elkins-Sinn, Incorporated, Cherry Hill, NJ, and MPF, Astra Pharmaceutical Products, Incorporated.

Additionally, government requirements tend to fill up labels. In some cases, labeling is inconsistent, confusing, and inadequate,[221] and often leads to medication errors. Frequent causes of errors include (1) similarity of containers of different drugs, (2) indistinct labeling, (3) failure to read labels, and (4) confusing labeling.

Cases of administration of 50% dextrose in water instead of 5% D/W and Lasix in place of Neo-Synephrine, and mixups between morphine and oxytocin, edrophonium and curare, clindamycin (Cleocin) and Sterile Water for Injection have been reported.[222,223] Misunderstanding of labeling[224] such as "For I.V. Use" has resulted in direct I.V. push instead of proper dilution. Manufacturers' logos often take precedence over the drug name. The use of unnecessary decimal points and zeroes can lead to errors. For example, 100.0 can easily be mistaken for 1000; the zero after the decimal point is unnecessary and hazardous. Often the letters U.S.P. are too large. Many ampuls are difficult to read[225] and easily confused. Often, paper labels become unglued. Many multiple-dose containers tell the user to discard contents after initial use.[221]

Alyea[225] suggested that unsatisfactory labeling of ampuls can be solved by ceramic background with superimposed letters. Davis[226] also commented on the excellent ceramic labeling of ampuls. A publication concerning the labeling of LVPs by the NCCLVP presents the committee's view on labeling with specific recommendations.[227]

Energy and Time Required for Cold Large-Volume Intravenous Solutions to Reach Room Temperature

The only apparent research describing the effects of temperature upon the body when large-volume intravenous fluids are infused relates to the administration of blood. Bank blood is stored under refrigeration at 4° C. During handling, and by the time it is given to the patient, it has warmed up to some extent but is rarely administered at a temperature above 8 to 10° C. The incidence of cardiac arrest increases with the speed of blood administration. Patients who receive large amounts of cold bank blood become hypothermic. Hypothermia produces a depressed effect on the body. The first organ to become affected is the heart, which fails during cooling. Boylan and Howland[228] in 1962 described the detrimental effects of the transfusion of cold blood.

MacLean and Van Tyn[229] measured esophageal temperatures as low as 29° C when large quantities of blood were administered; they noted ventricular fibrillation as a complication. Boylan and Howland[230] measured the association of cardiac arrest and the temperature of cold infused blood. They found that, when 3000 ml of blood were administered at a rate of 50 to 100 ml per minute, 12 cardiac arrests occurred among 55 patients. Transfusions in excess of 6000 ml, at a rate greater than 100 ml per minute, caused cardiac arrest in 9 of 11 patients. The same workers, using a similar group of 40 patients, administered 3000 ml of warmed blood at a rate of 50 ml per minute. Only one cardiac arrest was observed in the 40 patients.

Tacchi[234] reported that the average time for refrigerated bank blood to reach the patient required 20 to 30 minutes, and there is little warming of the blood before its rapid infusion at this low temperature.

The clinical observations of VanderVeer[232] indicated that when the infusion rate is less than 10 ml per minute there is no problem because the blood can be warmed before it reaches the heart. With rapid administration rates, 50 to 100 ml per minute, however, cold blood can cause irreversible shock or cardiac arrest.

The infusion of cold intravenous admixture solutions would appear to present a different clinical situation from that which exists with blood. Flow rates are considerably slower than those used to administer blood; however, the biologic effects of refrigerated I.V. solutions have yet to be measured.

Carlson[233] pointed out that a horse in severe shock might require 36 L of 5% dextrose in water; the calories present in 2 l of this solution would be utilized to raise the temperature of the fluid from 25 to 37° C. These comments concerning energy loss in fluid therapy prompted us to look further into the energy requirements expended to heat cold intravenous fluid to room temperature. It is not uncommon for infusion fluids containing additives, especially parenteral nutritional solutions, to be refrigerated after preparation and prior to use.

A similar situation exists when intravenous fluids are administered at a temperature below that of body temperature. Energy must be expended to heat the fluid to body temperature. This constitutes an energy loss.

The calorie is equal to the amount of heat required to raise the temperature of 1 g water 1° C (the particular degree between 14.5 and 15.5° C). One thousand calories are equal to one kilocalorie (kcal).

One thousand calories (1 kcal) are required to raise the temperature of 1000 ml of 5% dextrose in water 1° C. To raise the temperature of 1000 ml of 5% dextrose in water from 2 to 37° C (35 degrees increase) requires approximately 35,000 calories (35 kcal). Each gram of dextrose U.S.P. is equivalent to 3.4 kcal. The 50 g of dextrose U.S.P. in 1000 ml of 5% dextrose in water contains 170 kcal; thus 35 of the 170 kcal present in 1 L of 5% dextrose in water would be dissipated in raising the temperature 35° C. This represents approximately 20% of the total calories present.

Turco,[234,235] studying the effects of time on cold (refrigerated) I.V. solutions, showed that when a refrigerated I.V. fluid is hung, the fluid entering the vein approaches room temperature within 10 minutes. To wait for a refrigerated fluid to approximate room temperature before allowing the solution to run seems futile considering that this rise in temperature, which requires over 4 hours, can be achieved in less than 10 minutes when the bottle is hung. More recently, this study was again confirmed by Stiles et al.[236]

Miscellaneous Hazards

Cracked Containers

The 1971 issue of Clin-Alert reported a 22-year-old mother who died of septicemia 20 hours after receiving a dextrose injection from a cracked, contaminated container.[237] Although the user is warned to examine the container for clarity and vacuum, cracked containers have been associated with real hazards. If they are used undetected, death can result. It has also been shown that microorganisms can exist in a container at counts of up to 10^6/ml without visible evidence of their presence.[238]

Multidose Use of Single-Dose Containers

Stolar suggests that multiple-dose vials not be used and that single-dose packages be used wherever possible.[239] Sterility and use patterns of multiple-dose vials showed that 4/1000 became contaminated during use.[240]

A frequent consideration of multidose vials is the time they may be stored after initial entry. A excellent review was presented by Moi et al.[241] A number of factors must be considered to achieve a sound judgmental answer; number of penetrations, effectiveness of the bacteriostatic agent, aseptic technique utilized, and storage environment. If storage labeling, and dating guidelines are followed, these authors recommend a 30-day storage of multiple dose vials after initial entry.

It is not uncommon in hospitals to observe containers formulated and manufactured for one-time use being used as multiple-dose containers. This is especially true with vials of Sterile Water for Injection. On occasion, a nurse, in an effort to conserve on cost, will remove a portion of a dose from an ampul, cover the ampul with adhesive tape or gauze, and administer the remaining portion at a later time. Solutions for irrigation, although marked for one-time use, are continually used for multiple doses, often in the operating room and for several patients. It is hoped that the parenteral drug industry can design a container that will circumvent this procedure.

Additions to Plastic Infusion Containers

Reports have described harm (phlebitis) to patients from improperly mixed additives, particularly potassium chloride added to plastic containers. Studies have shown that concentrated quantities of potassium chloride are infused when the container is not mixed properly.[242]

Other Dangers

Deteriorated and outdated parenterals pose a problem, especially with biologicals. Storage in hospitals is often inadequate; refrigeration space is often minimal. Storage and rotation of I.V. fluids are sometimes inadequate. Some hospital administrations tend to fail to recognize the importance of proper storage.

One article describes the entrance of an ant through the plastic airway of an I.V. container.[243] Medical personnel were alerted by the patient, who noticed a black object in the hanging I.V. bottle. Similar ant breaks have been described in medical literature.[244,245]

There are other hazards associated with physical, chemical, and therapeutic incompatibilities, including drug interactions that affect patient safety.

Administration of parenterals by the wrong route is not uncommon. This can be quite hazardous. For example, bethanecol (Urecholine) is given S.C. If given I.M. or I.V., overstimulation of the cholinergic system may occur, leading to arrhythmia and even cardiac arrest. Parenteral suspensions are never to be given I.V. NPH insulin, procaine penicillin, and insoluble steroids, and other agents have been documented as having been given I.V. inadvertently. Overfilling of drug containers by the manufacturer may lead to clinical problems of overdosage. In the case of one company, containers labeled "750 mg," when assayed, were found to contain from 1080 to 1152 mg.[246]

The use of the wrong diluent to dissolve a drug may cause instability, precipitation, and side effects. It is not difficult in a clinical situation for this to occur. Errors in parenteral medication are continually occurring.[247]

Deaths have occurred from the intravenous administration of vitamin E to neonates.[248] A medication error that was the cause of death in two children resulted from cisplatin overdose.[249] Glutaraldehyde in an operating room used to preserve tissue was accidentally injected into the spine to replace spinal fluid.[250] Numerous hazards from catheters have been reported. Separation of subclavian central venous catheters as a result of faulty manufacture has been reported.[251,252] Death from massive air emboli has occurred from the use of infusion pumps.[253] Defective I. V. pumps have caused paralysis as a result of infusion of air.[254] Death has also been known to occur from pump failure that resulted in drug overdose.[255]

There has been considerable publicity concerning errors with potassium chloride injection. Recent deaths[256] have occurred when vascular access catheters were flushed with potassium chloride injection that was mistaken for diluted heparin injection.

Device and equipment dead space can present delivery of an inaccurate dose of drug. Syringe dead space is a well-known problem associated with syringes and has been discussed elsewhere. Dead space can also become a hazard with other types of equipment and cannulae. In one study, between 10 and 30% of a 1-ml IV dose remained in the cannulae. It has been suggested that all cannulae be flushed after drug administration and flushed with the drug solution before insertion.[257]

It is difficult to assess the incidence of misuse, overuse, and abuse of parenteral drugs in the clinical setting; however, by being aware of the potential for hazards, the clinician can be on guard against tragedy.

Contamination

Contamination of Product

Between July 1, 1965, and November 10, 1975, large-volume manufacturers had 608 recalls of large-volume parenteral products. These recalls involved over 43 million distributed containers, and most of the recalls were associated with product contamination.[247] Fifty-four deaths and 410 injuries were associated with these products. The factual number of injuries is impossible to evaluate. Between January 1, 1970, and November 10, 1975, 17 recalls involving biologic large-volume parenterals (e.g., albumin) were issued because of contamination.[247] Six deaths and 11 injuries were associated with these products. In all probability, manufacturing problems constitute only a small percentage of morbidity and mortality caused by I.V. contamination. Studies reported by the Centers for Disease Control[258] and others[259] show rates of nosocomial (hospital acquired) infections to range from 1% to 15% and the mean rate to be 5%.

According to Duma and Latta,[260] the manufacturer has no way to guarantee the sterility of large-volume parenterals. Quality control sampling schemes are not designed to detect low-level contamination because of the small sample size tested. Duma also speculated that hospital pharmacists who subject their compounding to periodic, randomized sampling are also performing an exercise of questionable value, thus engendering a false sense of security. In 1969, one company alone recalled 900,000 containers with possible hairline cracks[247] that could result in contamination. In 1970, 9 deaths and over 400 cases of septicemia resulted from improperly sterilized commercially manufactured I.V. fluids.[261] In 1971 and 1972, 8 cases of bacteremia and 6 deaths resulted from improperly sterilized hospital-manufactured I.V. fluids.[262] In March, 1972,[263] 5 deaths were reported in Plymouth, England, of patients receiving 5% D/W manufactured and contaminated by a British company. In March, 1973, 5 patients developed septicemias related to intrinsically contaminated I.V. fluids.[264] Several other large-volume solution recalls have taken place.[265] A recall of millions of containers of small-volume parenteral products such as amines, anesthetics, and analgesics has taken place because of questionable sterility.[266]

In-Use Contamination of Infusion Fluids

Studies have shown that sterile solutions can easily become contaminated during use. Miller and Latiolais, in an evaluation of admixture systems containers for closed systems, found contamination rate with an air vent to be 8.4%; with the formerly used open system, 16.2%; and with the plastic bag system (not the one in use today), 17.7%.[267] Letcher et al. studied contamination rate of I.V. admixtures prepared in plastic containers and solution sets. They reported rates of contamination of 4.9% and 5.5%.[268] Studies at the Hospital of the University of Pennsylvania of over 1000 units of parenteral nutritional solutions, prepared by the pharmacy, showed rates of contamination to be 4 to 10%, depending on the efficiency of the laminar flow hood and the technique of the preparer; with excellent technique, the rate can be as low as 1%.[269] Deeb and Natsios cultured 85 in-use bottles of conventional I.V. fluids and found contamination rates of 38% for hyperalimentation and 3.8% for I.V. fluids.[270] Two C.D.C. studies have shown in-use contamination rates of 10% and 6.8% of two different I.V. fluid systems.[271,272] The rate of sepsis in total parenteral nutrition has ranged from zero to 27%.[273] In one report, a retrospective study of 33 cases of fungal septicemia showed that 22 patients developed infection, and fungal infection was the primary cause of death in 15 patients. In the same hospital, a prospective study revealed that 13 of 49 patients (27%) developed septicemia while receiving parenteral nutrition.[274] In a C.D.C. survey of 31 hospitals treating 2000 patients, the associated septicemia rate was 7%. Most investigators have found that fungi are responsible for a large portion of septicemias. The C.D.C. study showed 54% of the septicemias to be fungal.[275]

Many factors can cause in-use contamination of parenterals, and drug additives are a potential source. One study of contamination showed that, of 101 fluids samples, 61 had additives and 40 had no additives. Of the 61 with additives, 34 (55.7%) were contaminated; whereas of the 40 without additives, only 5 (12.5%) were contaminated.[276] The pharmacy control admixture program can be a potential source of contamination, as evidenced by a recent outbreak.[277]

Contamination of parenterals in use is a serious complication that deserves further study by the reader. An excellent in-depth study of microbiologic hazards of infusion therapy has been detailed by Maki.[278,279] The growth potential of fluids has been reviewed by Guynn et al.[280] Programs for monitoring and surveillance have been established.[281,282] Excellent guidelines for prevention and contamination are available.[275,281,282]

References

1. Highlights of a Study on Single Unit Drug Dispensing. Owens-Illinois, Toledo, 1968.
2. Turco, S.J.: Percentage of injections. Am. J. I.V. Ther., 4,50 (1977).
3. Oddis, J.A.: Address to the Annual Meeting of the Federal Wholesale Druggists Association, White Sulphur Springs, West Virginia, Sept. 17, 1973.
4. Anon: Forum. Harvard Med., 1(I), June, July, 1980.
5. NCC-LVP recommended methods for compounding intravenous admixtures in hospitals. Am. J. Hosp. Pharm., 32, 261 (1975).
6. Kaminski, M.F., Jr., and Stolar, M.: Parenteral hyperalimentation—A quality of care survey and review. Am. J. Hosp. Pharm., 31, 228 (1974).
7. Zellmer, W.A.: Editorial. Solving problems associated with large volume parenterals. Am. J. Hosp. Pharm., 32, 255 (1975).
8. Anderson, R.D.: A case for the intravenous admixture service—reducing patient risk. I.V. Top., 2, 4 (1976).
9. Current Diagnosis and Treatment. Los Altos, Calif., Lange Medical Publications, 1973.
10. Harrison's Principles of Internal Medicine, 6th ed., New York, McGraw Hill Book Co., 1970.
11. Fonkalsrud, E.W.: Effect of pH in glucose infusions on development of thrombophlebitis. J. Surg. Res., 8, 539 (1968).
12. Lipman, A.G.: Effect of buffering on the incidence and severity of cephalothin-induced phlebitis. Am. J. Hosp. Pharm., 31, 266 (1974).
13. Fuchs, P.C.: Indwelling intravenous polyethylene catheters. JAMA, 216, 1447 (1971).
14. Maki, D.G., et al.: Infection control in intravenous therapy. Ann. Intern. Med., 79, 867 (1973).
15. Thomas, E.T., et al.: Postinfusion phlebitis. Anesth. Analg., 49, 150 (1970).
16. Bolton-Carter, J.F.: Reduction of infusion thrombophlebitis by limiting duration of IV infusion. Lancet, 2, 20 (1951).
17. Bolton-Carter, J.F., et al.: Thrombophlebitis following intravenous infusions. Lancet, 2, 660 (1952).
18. Fonkalsrud, E.W., et al.: Prophylaxis against postinfusion phlebitis. Surg. Gynecol. Obstet., 133, 253 (1971).
19. Bogen, J.E.: Local complications in 167 patients with indwelling venous catheters. Surg. Gynecol. Obstet., 110, 112 (1960).
20. Welch, G.W. et al.: The role of catheter composition in the development of thrombophlebitis. Surg. Gynecol. Obstet., 138, 421 (1974).
21. Collins, R.B., et al.: Risk of local and systemic infection with polyethylene I.V. catheters. N. Engl. J. Med., 279, 340 (1968).
22. Crossley, K., and Matsen, J.M.: The scalp vein needle. JAMA, 220, 985 (1972).
23. Curry, J.T. et al.: Reduction of thrombophlebitis associated with indwelling catheters. J. Oral Surg., 31, 636, 1973.
24. Peter, G., et al.: Local infection and bacteremia from scalp vein needles and polyethylene catheters in children. J. Pediatr., 80, 78 (1972).
25. Control of infection from IV infusion. Med. Lett., 15, 26 (1973).

26. Hussey, H.H.: Iatrogenic nonsuppurative infected thrombophlebitis. JAMA, *235*, 535 (1976).

27. Cheney, F.W., et al.: Phlebitis from plastic IV catheters. Anesthesiology, *25*, 650 (1964).

28. Davidson, B.D.: Intravenous Catheter Contamination and Phlebitis. Presentation American Society Hospital Pharmacists, Midyear Clinical Meeting, Anaheim, Calif., Dec. 7, 1976.

29. Nordell, K., et al.: Thrombophlebitis following intravenous lignocaine infusion. Acta Med. Scand., *192*, 263 (1972).

30. Langdon, D.E., et al.: Thrombophlebitis with diazepam used IV. JAMA, *223*, 184 (1973).

31. Daniell, H.W.: Heparin in the prevention of infusion phlebitis. JAMA, *226*, 1317 (1973).

32. Schafermeyer, R.W.: Prevention of phlebitis. JAMA, *228*, 695 (1974).

33. Anderson, L.H., et al.: Venous catheterization for continuous parenteral fluid therapy: Use of heparin in delaying thrombophlebitis. J. Lab. Clin. Med., *38*, 585 (1951).

34. Henney, J.E., et al.: Thrombophlebitis potential of intravenous cytotoxic agents. Drug Intell. Clin. Pharm., *11*, 266 (1977).

35. McFadden, D.B.: Venous irritation from the use of nafcillin sodium 2 g I.V. minibag product. Am. J. Hosp. Pharm., *47*, 2655 (1990).

36. Baciewicz, A.M., et al.: Postinfusion phlebitis associated with selected cephalosporins. Am. J. I.V. Ther. Clin. Nutr., *9*, 9 (1982).

37. Page, B.H., et al.: Thrombophlebitis following IV infusions. Lancet, *2*, 788 (1952).

38. Horvitz, A., et al.: An experimental study of phlebitis following venoclysis with glucose and amino acid solutions. J. Lab. Clin. Med., *28*, 842 (1973).

39. Lebowitz, M.H., et al.: The pH and acidity of IV solutions. JAMA, *215*, 1937 (1971).

40. Elfving, G., et al.: Effect of pH on the incidence of infusion thrombophlebitis. Lancet, *1*, 953 (1966).

41. Clemetson, A.B., et al.: Strange effects of dextrose 5% water. N. Engl. J. Med., *280*, 332 (1969).

42. Osol-Farrar-Pratt: The Dispensatory of the United States. 25th Ed. Philadelphia, J.B. Lippincott Co., 1969.

43. Wolfrom, M.L., Schuetz, R.D., and Cavalieri, L.F.: Chemical interactions of amino compounds and sugars: III. The conversion of D-glucose to 5-(hydroxymethyl)-2-fural-dehyde. J. Am. Chem. Soc., *70*, 514, 1948.

44. Vere, D.W.: Venous thrombosis during dextrose infusion. Lancet, *2*, 627 (1960).

45. Tse, R.L.: pH of infusion fluids: A predisposing factor in thrombophlebitis. JAMA, *215*, 642 (1971).

46. Ansel, H.C.: Change in pH of infusion solutions upon mixing with blood. JAMA, *218*, 1052 (1971).

47. Moster, J.W.: The pH and osmolality of intravenously used drugs. JAMA, *216*, 1483 (1971).

48. Ryan, P.B., et al.: In-line filtration—A method of minimizing contamination in intravenous therapy. Bull. Parenter. Drug Assoc., *27*, 1 (1973).

49. NITA Update 6, Dec., 1985.

50. Costentino, F.: Personnel induced infusion phlebitis. Bull. Parenter. Drug Assoc., *31*, 288 (1977).

51. Alexander, C.S.: Pedal gangrene associated with the use of dopamine. N. Engl. J. Med., *293*, 591 (1975).

52. Collins, G.E.: Drug Information Bulletin, University of Alabama, 1976.

53. Julka, N.K., and Ndra, J.R.: Gangrene aggravation after use of dopamine. JAMA, *235*, 2812 (1976).

54. Boltax, R.S., Dineen, J.P., and Scarpa, F.J.: Gangrene resulting from infiltrated dopamine solution. N. Engl. J. Med., *296*, 823 (1976).

55. Clin-Alert 70, April 29, 1977.

56. Clin-Alert 70, April 29, 1977.

57. Cooper, E.V.: Gas-gangrene following injections of adrenalin. Lancet, *1*, 459 (1946).
58. Marshall, V., and Sims, P.: Gas gangrene after the injection of adrenalin-in-oil, with a report of three cases. Med. J. Aust., *2*, 653 (1960).
59. Harvey, P.W., and Purneil, G.V.: Fatal case of gas gangrene associated with intramuscular injections. Br. Med. J., *1*, 744 (1968).
60. Van Hook, R.: Gas gangrene after intramuscular injection of epinephrine: report of fatal case. Ann. Intern Med., *83*, 669 (1975).
61. Clin-Alert, 10, June 27, 1969.
62. Clin-Alert, 10, June 27, 1969.
63. Clin-Alert, 272, Dec. 17, 1971.
64. Lane, M.F.: Intra-arterial secobarbital. N. Engl. J. Med., *228*, 164 (1973).
65. Lindell, T.D., Porter, S.M., and Langston, C.: Intra-arterial injections of oral medication. N. Engl. J. Med., *287*, 1132 (1972).
66. Pearlman, H.S.: Intra-arterial injection of propoxyphene into brachial artery. JAMA *214*, 2055 (1970).
67. Solimando, D.A., et al.: Prevention of accidental administration of vincristine sulfate. Hosp. Pharm., *17*, 540 (1982).
68. ASHP Newsletter, April, 1985.
69. Dyke, R.W.: Treatment of inadvertent thecal injection of vincristine. N. Engl. J. Med., *18*, 1270 (1989).
70. Van Voris, L.P., et al.: Inadvertent intravenous administration of trivalent influenza vaccine. JAMA, *245*, 2422 (1981).
71. Owen, O.E., et al.: Accidental intramuscular injection of mechlorethamine. Cancer, *45*, 2225 (1980).
72. Reilly, J.J., et al.: Clinical course and management of accidental adriamycin extravasation. Cancer, *40*, 2053 (1977).
73. Clin-Alert *44*, March 17, 1978.
74. Olson, C., et al.: Amphotericin B extravasation. NITA, *8*, 299 (1985).
75. Cox, R.F.: Managing skin damage induced by doxorubicin HCl and daunorubicin HCl. Am. J. Hosp. Pharm., *41*, 2410 (1984).
76. Moore, R.A., et al.: Nafcillin necrosis. NITA, *7*, 61 (1984).
77. Faehnrich, J.: Extravasation. NITA, *7*, 49 (1984).
78. Reed, W.P., Newman, K.A., Applefeld, M.M., and Sutton, F.J.: Drug extravasation as a complication of venous access ports. Ann. Intern. Med., *102*(6), 788 (1985).
79. Brown, A.S., et al.: Skin necrosis from extravasation of intravenous fluids in children. Plastic Recon. Surg., *64*, 145 (1979).
80. Yosowitz, P., et al.: Peripheral intravenous infiltration necrosis. Ann. Surg., *182*, 553 (1975).
81. Turco, S., and Davis, N.: Clinical significance of particulate matter: a review of the literature. Hosp. Pharm., *8*, 137 (1973).
82. Giesler, R.M.: The biological effects of polystyrene latex particles administered intravenously to rats, a collaborative study. Bull. Parenter. Drug Assoc, *27*, 101 (1973).
83. Duma, R.J.: Particulate matter of particular interest. Ann. Intern. Med., *78*, 146 (1973).
84. Nicholson, W.J., et al.: Asbetos contamination of parenteral drugs. Science, *177*, 171 (1972).
85. Haley, T.J.: Asbestosis: a reassessment of the overall problem. J. Pharm. Sci., *64*, 1435 (1975).
86. Katz, H., et al.: Glass particle contamination of color-break ampuls. Anesthesiology, *39*, 354 (1972).
87. Katz, H., et al.: Glass particle contamination of solutions. JAMA, *229*, 1169 (1974).
88. Lyon, T.C., et al.: Particulate contamination of dextran for intravenous use: an in vitro and in vivo study. Milit. Med., *139*, 466 (1974).
89. Furgang, F.A.: (Correspondence) Glass particles in ampuls. Anesthesiology, *41*, 525 (1974).
90. Reed, C.C.: Particulate matter in bubble oxygenators. J. Thorac. Cardiovasc. Surg., *68*, 971 (1974).

 91. Dimmick, J.E.: Fiber embolization—a hazard of cardiac surgery and catheterization. N. Engl. J. Med., 292, 685 (1975).
 92. Vidt, D.G.: Use and abuse of intravenous solutions. JAMA, 232, 533 (1975).
 93. Purkiss, R.: Effects and distribution of intravenously administered cellulose particles in mice. J. Pharm. Pharmacol., 27, 290 (1975).
 94. Zerefos, N., et al.: Dialysis Ascites. A New Syndrome? 5th International Conference Nephrology, Mexico City, 1972.
 95. Lasker, N.: Personal communication.
 96. Lasker, N., et al.: Peritoneal reactions to particulate matter in peritoneal dialysis solutions. Trans. Am. Soc. Artif. Intern. Organs, 21, 324 (1975).
 97. Mead, W.B.: Particles in intravenous fluids. N. Engl. J. Med., 2, 1152 (1972).
 98. Masuda, J.Y., et al.: Particulate matter in commercial antibiotic injectable products. Am. J. Hosp. Pharm., 30, 72 (1973).
 99. Jeffrey, L.P., et al.: Quality Control—An Essential Tool in Particulate Contamination. Northeastern New York Society of Hospital Pharmacists, Albany, May 24, 1973.
100. Turco, S.J., et al.: Particulate contamination of carbenicillin products. (Letters) Am. J. Hosp. Pharm., 30, 770 (1973).
101. Turco, S.J., et al.: Particulate matter in Ancef and Kefzol. Am. J. Hosp. Pharm., 31, 222 (1974).
102. Turco, S.J., et al.: Particulate matter in lyophilized Kefzol. Am. J. Hosp. Pharm., 31, 772 (1974).
103. Turco, S.J., et al.: Particulate matter in carbenicillin. Hosp. Pharm., 11, 12 (1976).
104. Jeffrey, L.P., et al.: Glass particles in reconstituted sodium diphenylhydantoin injection. (Letters) Am. J. Hosp. Pharm., 28, 932 (1971).
105. Turco, S.J., et al.: Particulate contamination in sodium diphenylhydantoin injection. Am. J. Hosp. Pharm., 29, 186 (1972).
106. Turco, S.J., et al.: Glass particles in I.V. injections. N. Engl. J. Med., 287, 1204 (1972).
107. Turco, S.J., et al.: Preventing the injection of glass particles with furosemide. Hosp. Pharm., 7, 423 (1972).
108. Williams, A., et al.: Particulate contamination in I.V. fluids, administration sets and cannulae. Pharm. J., 211, 190 (1973).
109. Somerville, T.G.: Particulate contamination in ampoules: A comparative study. Pharm. J., 211, 128 (1973).
110. Whitlow, T.E.: Generation of particulate matter in large-volume parenteral containers. J. Pharm. Sci., 63, 1610 (1974).
111. Masuda, J.Y., et al.: Particulate contamination of spray-dried and lyophilized injectable carbenicillin. Am. J. Hosp. Pharm., 318, 189 (1974).
112. Mead, W.B., Particulate matter in I.V. solutions. N. Engl. J. Med., 292, 1355 (1975).
113. Harrison, M.M., et al.: Intravenous administration sets. Br. J. Anaesth., 46, 59 (1974).
114. Stokes, T.F.: Particulate contamination and stability of three additives in 0.9% sodium chloride injection in plastic and glass large-volume containers. Am. J. Hosp. Pharm., 32, 821 (1975).
115. Levinson, R.S., et al.: Detection of particles in intravenous fluids using scanning electron microscope. Am. J. Hosp. Pharm., 32, 1137 (1975).
116. Blanchard, J., et al.: Comparison methods for detection of particulate matter in large-volume parenterals. Am. J. Hosp. Pharm., 33, 144 (1976).
117. Rebagay, T., et al.: Residues in antibiotic preparations, scanning electron microscopic studies of surface topography. Am. J. Hosp. Pharm., 33, 433 (1976).
118. Schroeder, H.G., and DeLuca, P.P.: Particulate matter assessment of a clinical investigation of filtration and infusion phlebitis. Am. J. Hosp. Pharm., 33, 543 (1976).
119. Turco, S.J., et al.: A comparison of particulate matter in Keflin and Cefadyl. Hosp. Pharm., 11, 480 (1976).
120. Turco, S.J., et al.: A comparison of features of Kefzol and Ancef. Hosp. Pharm., 11, 482 (1976).

121. Fox, R.L., et al.: Particulate matter concentration in parenteral nutrition solutions. Am. J. I.V. Ther. Clin. Nutr. 9, 15 (1982).

122. Ho, N.: Particulate matter in parenteral solutions. Drug Intell., 1, 7 (1967).

123. Turco, S.J., et al.: Clinical significance of particulate matter. Hosp. Pharm., 8, 137 (1973).

124. Thomas, W.H., et al.: Particles in intravenous solutions: a review. N. Z. Med. J., 80, 170 (1974).

125. Vidt, G.D.: Use and abuse of intravenous solutions. JAMA, 232, 533 (1975).

126. Winding, O., et al.: Methods for determination and element analyses of particulate contamination in injectable solutions. Am. J. Hosp. Pharm., 33, 1154 (1976).

127. Turco, S.J.: Infusison phlebitis. Hosp. Pharm., 9, 422 (1974).

128. Ryan, P.B., et al.: In-line final filtration—a method of minimizing contamination in intravenous therapy. Bull. Parenter. Drug. Assoc., 27, 1 (1973).

129. Collin, J., et al.: Effect of a Millipore filter on complications of intravenous infusions: a prospective clinical trial. Br. Med. J., 4, 456 (1973).

130. Swift, R.G., et al.: The effect of in-line filtration on occurrence of phlebitis. Drug Intell. Clin. Pharm., 9, 76 (1975).

131. DeLuca, P.P., et al.: Filtration and infusion phlebitis: a double-blind prospective clinical study. Am. J. Hosp. Pharm., 32, 1001 (1975).

132. Lewis, J.: Value of filtering ampuls. Drug Intell. Clin. Pharm., 10, 293 (1976).

133. Evans, W.E., et al.: Double-blind evaluation of 5-μm final filtration to reduce postinfusion phlebitis. Am. J. Hosp. Pharm., 33, 1163 (1976).

134. Maddox, R.R., et al.: Double-blind study to investigate methods to prevent cephalothin induced phlebitis. Am. J. Hosp. Pharm., 34, 29 (1977).

135. Decker, E.L.: A study of the effect of in-line filtration on the incidence and severity of cephalothin induced infusion phlebitis. Unpublished data, Yale-New Haven Hospital.

136. Wilmore, D.W., and Dudrick, S.J.: An in-line filter for intravenous solutions. Arch. Surg., 99, 462 (1969).

137. Myers, J.A.: Millipore infusion filter unit: interim report of clinical trial. Pharm. J., 208, 547 (1972).

138. Butler, T.H., et al.: A comparative evaluation of the relative flow rates and the protective capabilities of the 0.22 and the 0.45 micron Millipore filters in preventing mycelial contamination in the course of hyperalimentation therapy in humans, a preliminary study. Drug. Intell. Clin. Pharm., 7, 317 (1973).

139. Miller, R.C., and Grogan, J.B.: Incidence and source of contamination of intravenous nutritional infusion systems. J. Pediatr. Surg., 8, 185 (1973).

140. Collin, J., et al.: Effect of a Millipore filter on complications of intravenous infusions: a prospective clinical trial. Br. Med. J., 24, 456 (1973).

141. Bunker, R., et al.: The use of micropore filters in the administration of intravenous fluids. Minn. Med., 57, 325 (1974).

142. Sarles, H.E., et al.: Peritoneal Dialysis Utilizing a Millipore Filter. Presented at Southeastern Dialysis and Transplantation Association Ninth Annual Meeting, Charleston, S.C. August 17, 1974.

143. Freeman, J.B., et al.: Preponderance of gram-positive infections during parenteral alimentation. Surg. Gynecol. Obstet., 139, 905 (1974).

144. Huber, R.C., and Riffkin, C.: In-line final filters for removing particles from amphotericin B infusions. Am J. Hosp. Pharm., 32, 173 (1975).

145. Piecoro, J.J., et al.: Particulate matter in reconstituted amphotericin B and assay of filtered solutions of amphotericin B. Am. J. Hosp. Pharm., 32, 381 (1975).

146. Med. Lett., 17, 35 (1975).

147. Tenney, J.H., and Dixon, R.E.: What risk of candidiasis from micropore filters in intravenous hyperalimentation? JAMA, 229, 467 (1974).

148. Newman, M.S., et al.: Microbial and particulate contamination during prolonged use of I.V. infusion sets. J. Hosp. Pharm., 33, 95 (1975).

149. Miller, R.C., and Grogan, J.B.: Efficacy of in-line bacterial filters in reducing contamination of intravenous nutritional solutions. Am. J. Surg., 130, 585 (1975).

150. Rapp, R., et al.: Evaluation of prototype air-venting in-line intravenous filter set. Am. J. Hosp. Pharm., 32, 1253 (1975).

151. Holland, R.R.: Filter system for intravenous alimentation. N. Engl. J. Med., 289, 487 (1973).
152. Meeker, W.R., et al.: Membrane filters—additional safety for intra-arterial infusions. Arch. Surg., 111, 201 (1975).
153. Rapp, R.P., et al.: Evaluation of 5-μm stainless steel filter as an intravenous in-line filter or prefilter. Am. J. Hosp. Pharm., 33, 352 (1976).
154. Rusmin, S., et al.: Microbial assessment of a clinical evaluation on filtration and infusion phlebitis. Bull. Parenter. Drug. Assoc., 31, 1 (1977).
155. Letter on file, Temple University School of Pharmacy.
156. Wyeth Laboratories: Data on file, Temple University School of Pharmacy.
157. Wagman, G.H., et al.: Binding of aminoglycoside antibiotics to filtration materials. Antimicrob. Agents. Chemother., 7, 316 (1975).
158. Schering Laboratories to Turco, S.: Letter on file, Temple University School of Pharmacy.
159. Abbott Laboratories to Turco, S.: Letter on file, Temple University School of Pharmacy.
160. Bristol Laboratories to Turco, S.: Letter on file, Temple University School of Pharmacy.
161. Huber, R.C., et al.: In-line filters for removing particles from amphotericin B infusions. Am. J. Hosp. Pharm., 32, 173 (1975).
162. Piecoro, J.J., et al.: Particulate matter in reconstituted amphotericin B and assay of filtered solutions of amphotericin B. Am. J. Hosp. Pharm., 32, 381 (1975).
163. Baumgartner, T.G., et al.: Bacterial endotoxin retention by inline intravenous filters. Am. J. Hosp. Pharm., 43, 681 (1986).
164. Royal, H.D., Shields, J.B., and Donati, R.M.: Misplacement of central venous pressure catheters and unilateral pulmonary edema. Arch. Intern. Med., 135, 1502 (1975).
165. Johnston, A.O.B., and Clark, R.B.: Malpositioning of central venous catheters. Lancet, 2, 1395 (1972).
166. Lamberth, J.J.: Catheter perforation of heart wall. N. Engl. J. Med., 291, 679 (1974).
167. Bell, J.A.: Malpositioning of central venous catheters. Lancet, 1, 105 (1973).
168. Levinsky, W.J.: Fatal air embolism during insertion of CVP monitoring apparatus. JAMA, 209, 1721 (1969).
169. Ordway, C.B.: Air embolus via cup catheter without positive pressure. Ann. Surg., 179, 479 (1974).
170. Johnson, C.L., et al.: Subclavian venipuncture: preventable complications. Report of two cases. Mayo Clin. Proc., 45, 712 (1970).
171. Lucas, C.F.: Air embolus via subclavian catheter. N. Engl. J. Med., 281 966 (1969).
172. Jose, M.: Fatal air embolism via subclavian vein. N. Engl. J. Med., 282, 688 (1970).
173. Richardson, J.D.: Intravenous catheter emboli. Am. J. Surg., 128, 722 (1974).
174. Gardner, R.M., et al.: Percutaneous indwelling radial-artery catheters for monitoring cardiovascular function. N. Engl. J. Meds., 290, 1227 (1974).
175. Clin-Alert, April 15, 1977.
176. Dinley, R.J.: Venous reactions related to in-dwelling plastic cannulae: a prospective clinical trial. Curr. Med. Res., 3, 607 (1976).
177. Goodman, D.J.: Thromboembolic complications with the in-dwelling tipped pulmonary arterial catheter. N. Engl. J. Med., 291, 777 (1974).
178. Soni, J., et al.: Nonsurgical removal of polyethylene catheter from the right cardiac cavities. Chest, 57, 398 (1970).
179. Bennett, P.J.: Use of intravenous plastic catheters. Br. Med. J., 2, 1252 (1963).
180. Udwadia, T.E., et al.: Accidental loss of plastic tube into venous system. Br. Med. J., 2, 1251 (1963).
181. Ayers, W.B.: Fatal intracardiac embolization from in-dwelling intravenous polyethylene catheter. Arch. Surg., 75, 259 (1957).
182. Collin, J., et al.: Infusion thrombophlebitis and infection with various cannulas. Lancet, 2, 150 (1975).

183. Ryan, J.A., et al.: Catheter complications in total parenteral nutrition. N. Engl. J. Med., *290*, 757 (1974).
184. Smith, J.A.: A clinical and microbiological study of venous catheterization. Can. Med. Assoc. J., *109*, 115 (1973).
185. Freeman, R., et al.: Analysis of results of catheter tip cultures in open-heart surgery patients. Thorax, *30*, 26 (1975).
186. Pace, N.L., et al.: Indwelling pulmonary artery catheters. JAMA, *233*, 893 (1975).
187. Greene, J.F., et al.: Septic endocarditis and indwelling pulmonary artery catheters. JAMA, *233*, 891 (1975).
188. Meguip, V., et al.: Hazards of long term venous catheterization. Lancet, *1*, 369 (1973).
189. Sayege, T.M., et al.: Hazards of intravenous cannulae. Lancet, *2*, 601 (1972).
190. Clin-Alert, Jan. 16, 1973.
191. Clin-Alert, Sept. 22, 1972.
192. Turke, H.: Intramedullary vs. intra-arterial infusion. N. Engl. J. Med., *293*, 309 (1975).
193. Hoshal, V.L.: The subclavian catheter. N. Engl. J. Med., *281*, 1425 (1969).
194. Walters, M.B., et al.: Complications with percutaneous central venous catheters. JAMA, *220*, 1455 (1972).
195. CVP measurement. Health Dev., *5*, 251 (1976).
196. Raad, I.I.: Vascular catheter-related Infections: Diagnosis and Management. J. New Dev. Clin. Med., *9*, 27 (1992).
197. Halaby, S.F., et al.: Absorption of sodium bisulfite from peritoneal dialysis solutions. J. Pharm. Sci., *54*, 52 (1965).
198. Cronk, J.D.: Phenol with glucagon in cardiotherapy. N. Engl. J. Med., *284*, 219 (1971).
199. Spodick, D.H., et al.: Phenol in glucagon diluent. N. Engl. J. Med., *284*, 500 (1974).
200. Schmidt, G.B., et al.: Sudden appearance of cardiac arrhythmias after dexamethasone. JAMA *221*, 1402 (1972).
201. Land, M.F.: Drug induced morbidity. Hosp. Form. Mgt., Oct. (1974).
202. Mizutan, H.: Hypersensitivity to thimerosal. N. Engl. J. Med., *289*, 1424 (1972).
203. Possibility of toxicity when inhaling parabens. Drug Ther., *5*, 158 (1975).
204. Nagel, J.E., et al.: Paraben allergy. JAMA, *237*, 1594 (1977).
205. Sharer, L., et al.: Intravenous administration of diazepam. Arch. Neurol., *24*, 169 (1971).
206. Personal communications, Temple University Hospital, 1977.
207. ASHP Newsletter 9, Sept., 1976.
208. Rein, M.F., et al.: Bacterial killing by bacteriostatic saline solutions—potential for diagnostic error. N. Engl. J. Med., *289*, 794 (1973).
209. Feasby, T.E., Hahn, A.F., and Gilbert, J.J.: Neurotoxicity of bacteriostatic water. Correspondence. N. Engl. J. Med., *308*, 966 (1983).
210. Anon: Letter, Department of Health & Human Services, F.D.A., May 28, 1982.
211. Levchuk, J.W.: Sterility of extemporaneously compounded preservative-free injections. Am. J. Hosp. Pharm., *48*, 71 (1991).
212. Coates, D.: Interaction between preservatives, plastics and rubber. Mfg. Chem. Aero News, Dec. (1973).
213. Lachman, L., et al.: Stability of antibacterial preservatives in parenteral solutions. J. Pharm. Sci., *51*, 224 (1962).
214. Subra, R.: Reactions of acetylcysteine with rubber. Am. J. Hosp. Pharm., *33*, 117 (1976).
215. APHA Newsletter, *15*, July 17, 1976.
216. Jetton, M.M., et al.: Trace element contamination of intravenous solutions. Arch. Dermatol., *136*, 782 (1976).
217. Abbott Laboratories to Turco, S.: Letter on file, Temple University.
218. Department Health, Education and Welfare to Turco, S.: Letter on file, Temple University.
219. Wyeth Laboratories: Meperidine recall. June 1976.

220. Parenter. Drug Assoc. Newsletter 8, March 1976.
221. Turco, S.J.: Hazards associated with parenteral therapy. Bull. Parenter. Drug. Assoc., *28*, 197 (1974).
222. Wang, B.C., et al.: Beware of misleading appearance of ampules and vials. Unpublished data.
223. Cohen, M.: Medication errors column. Hosp. Pharm., Monthly Reports, 1975–77.
224. Eli Lilly and Co. to Turco, S.: Letter on file, Temple University School of Pharmacy.
225. Alyea, J.O.: Labeling drug ampules. Anesthesiology, *39*, 358 (1973).
226. Davis, N.M.: (Editorial) What are you doing about poor labeling of injectables. Hosp. Pharm., *11*, 3 (1976).
227. NCC-LVP: Recommendations for labeling of large volume parenterals. Am. J. Hosp. Pharm., *34*, 495 (1978).
228. Boylan, C.P., and Howland, W.S.: Problems related to massive blood replacement. Anesth. Analg., *41*, 497 (1962).
229. MacLean, L.D., and Van Tyn, A.: Ventricular fibrillation. JAMA, *175*, 471 (1961).
230. Boylan, C.P., and Howland, W.S.: Cardiac arrest and temperature of bank blood. JAMA, *183*, 144 (1963).
231. Tacchi, D.: (Letter) Warming emergency blood-transfusions. Lancet, *1*, 782 (1967).
232. VanderVeer, J.B.: (Letter) Warming emergency and blood transfusions. Lancet, *1*, 1163 (1967).
233. Carlson, G.P.: Energy loss in fluid therapy. N. Engl. J. Med., *285*, 1328 (1971).
234. Turco, S.J., and Davis, N.M.: Temperature and energy changes of I.V. solutions. N. Engl. J. Med., *289*, 922 (1973).
235. Turco, S.J.: Temperature and energy changes of I.V. solutions. Hosp. Pharm., *12*, 584 (1977).
236. Stiles, M.L., et al.: Temperature of refrigerated I.V. fluids and admixtures during infusion. Am. J. Hosp. Pharm., *46*, 977 (1989).
237. Clin-alert, No. 117, 1971.
238. Maki, D.G.: Infection control in intravenous therapy. Ann. Intern. Med., *79*, 867 (1973).
239. Stolar, M.H.: Questions and Answers. Multidose vials. Am. J. Hosp. Pharm., *37*, 185 (1980).
240. Bawden, J.C., et al.: Sterility and use patterns of multiple-dose vials. Am. J. Hosp. Pharm., *39*, 294 (1982).
241. Moi, S., et al.: Time limit on multidose vials after initial entry. Hosp. Pharm., *26*, 805 (1991).
242. William, R.H.P.: Potassium overdosage: a potential hazard of nonrigid parenteral fluid containers. Br. Med. J., *1*, 714 (1973).
243. Rupp, C.A., and Forni, P.: Formic I.V. therapy. N. Engl. J. Med., *286*, 894 (1972).
244. Beatson, S.H.: Pharaoh's ants enter giving sets. Lancet, *1*, 606 (1973).
245. Cartwright, R.Y., et al.: Pharoah's ants. Lancet, *2*, 1455 (1973).
246. Smith, R.C.: No more overfill in cefuroxime sodium vials. Am. J. Hosp. Pharm., *43*, 2154 (1986).
247. Report of the Comptroller General of the United States: Recalls of Large-Volume Parenterals (MSD-76-67). March 12, 1976.
248. ASHP Newsletter, May 1984.
249. ASHP Newsletter, July 1981.
250. ASHP Newsletter, April, 1985.
251. Health Devices, November, 1983.
252. Sprague, D.H., and Sarwar, H.: Catheter embolization due to faulty bonding of catheter shaft to hub. Clinical Reports. Edited by B.R. Brown, Jr. Anesthesiology, *49*, 285 (1978).
253. Abernathy, C.M., and Dickinson, T.C.: Massive air emboli from intravenous infusion pump: etiology and prevention. Am. J. Surg., *137*, 274 (1979).
254. NITA Update, *4*, October, 1983.

255. NITA Update 5, February, 1984.

256. Macfie, A.G.: Equipment deadspace and drug administration. Anaesthesiology, 45, 145 (1990).

257. Cohen, M.R.: Potassium chloride injection mix-up. Am. J. Hosp. Pharm., 47, 2457 (1990).

258. Nosocomial Bacteremia Associated with I.V. Fluid Therapy. USA Morbid. Mortal. Wkly Rep. March 6, 1971.

259. Moore, W.L.: Nosocomial infections: an overview. Am. J. Hosp. Pharm., 31, 823 (1974).

260. Duma, R.J., and Latta, T.: What have we done—the hazards of intravenous therapy. N. Engl. J. Med., 294, 1178 (1976).

261. Nosocomial Bacteremias Associated With Intravenous Fluid Therapy. USA Morbid. Mortal. Wkly. Rep., Special Supplement. March 6, 1971.

262. Phillips, I., Eykyn, S., and Lasker, N.: Outbreak of hospital infections caused by contaminated autoclaved fluids. Lancet, 1, 1258 (1972).

263. Contaminated infusion fluids committee blames Evans medical management. Pharm. J., 209, 255 (1972).

264. Septicemias associated with contaminated I.V. fluids. Morbid. Mortal. Wkly. Rep., 22, 99 (1973).

265. Gold Sheet 9, July 1975.

266. Winthrop Laboratories: Urgent drug recall letter. June 30, 1976.

267. Miller, W.A., et al.: A comparative evaluation of compounding costs; and contamination rates of I.V. admixture systems. Drug Intell. Clin. Pharm., 5, 50 (1971).

268. Letcher, K., et al.: In-use contamination of intravenous solutions in flexible plastic containers. Am. J. Hosp. Pharm., 29, 673 (1972).

269. Hak, L.J.: Contamination incidence in I.V. solutions with additives. Annual Meeting of American Society Hospital Pharmacists, March 31, 1971.

270. Deeb, E.N., and Natsios, G.A.: Contamination of intravenous fluids by bacteria and fungi during preparation and administration. Am. J. Hosp. Pharm., 28, 764 (1971).

271. Maki, D.G., et al.: Nosocomial septicemia subsequent to contaminated I.V. fluids. Annual Meeting American Society Microbiology, May 5, 1971.

272. Maki, D.G., et al.: The infection hazard posed by contaminated I.V. infusion fluids. In Clinical and Laboratory Aspects of Bacteremia. Springfield, IL, Charles C Thomas, 1973.

273. Maki, D.G., et al.: Infection control in intravenous therapy. Ann. Intern. Med., 79, 867 (1971).

274. Curry, C.R., and Quie, P.G.: Fungal septicemia in patients receiving parenteral hyperalimentation. N. Engl. J. Med., 285, 1221 (1971).

275. Maki, D.G., et al.: Infection control in intravenous therapy. Ann. Intern. Med., 79, 867 (1973).

276. Arcy, P.F., and Woodside, W.: Drug additives: a potential source of bacterial contamination of infusion fluids. Lancet, 2, 96 (1973).

277. Primary Bacteria—Illinois. USA Morbid. Mortal. Wkly Rep. 25, 110 (1976).

278. Maki, D.G.: Preventing infusion-related infections. Drug. Ther., Hosp. Ed., 1, 37 (1977).

279. Microbiological Hazards of Infusion Therapy. Proceedings International Symposium. University Sussex, England, March 1976, 1966.

280. Guynn, J.B., Poretz, D.M., and Duma, R.J.: Growth of various bacteria in a variety of I.V. fluids. Am. J. Hosp. Pharm., 30, 321 (1973).

281. Hanson, A.L., and Shelley, R.M.: Monitoring contamination levels of in-use I.V. solutions using total sample techniques. Am. J. Hosp. Pharm., 31, 733 (1974).

282. Ravin, R.R., et al.: Program for bacterial surveillance of I.V. admixtures. Am. J. Hosp. Pharm., 31, 340 (1974).

283. McGowan, J.E.: Six guidelines for reducing infections associated with I.V. therapy. Am. Surg., 41, 713 (1976).

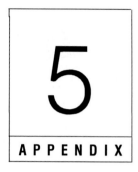

APPENDIX

Parenterals Derived
From Biotechnology

In 1982, Genentech/Lilly received approval to market the first recombinant DNA parenteral, Human Insulin. Since that time considerable research has gone into the production of clinically useful biotechnologic (biotech) parenterals. Recombinant DNA processes are illustrated in Figure A5–1. The types of products developed thus far* include:

• Immunomodulating Agents
    (Colony Stimulating Factor, CSF)

• Anticancer Agents
    (Interleukins)

• Antiviral Agents
    (Interferons)

• Hormones
    (Human Growth Hormone, Insulin)

• Vaccines
    (Hepatitis B, H. Flu)

• Antithrombotic Agents
    (Tissue Plasmenogen Activator, tPa)

• Diagnostics
    (Monoclonal Antibodies)

*Pharmaceutical Manufacturers Association
Biotechnology Medicines 1991 Survey Report
1100 15th Street, N.W.
Washington, DC 20005

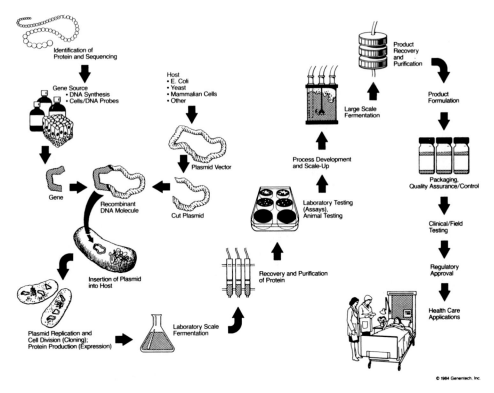

Figure A5-1. Recombinant DNA Product Development

Materials undergoing clinical study include anti-inflammatory agents, tissue repair agents, and vaccines for AIDS, cancer, and other diseases. Drugs produced from biotechnology will present new challenges for the pharmacist both in formulation and dispensing. Biotech drugs are more active on a weight basis and usually require a lower level dosage. Dosage errors become more critical. Most biotech drugs have limited stability and will require special methods of administration and storage. In the future, many will no doubt require specialized delivery systems for administration.

Thus far, 14 biotech drugs have been approved for clinical use (Table A5–1). Twenty-one are in Phase III clinical studies awaiting approval. Over 130 are in various phases of development (Table A5–2).

The Center for Biologics Evaluation and Review (CBER) has over 3200 Investigational New Drug Applications (IND) under review.

As a result of the stability sensitivities of proteins, the 14 biotech pharmaceuticals currently available are all manufactured as parenterals. Many are available as lyophilized parenterals (Table A5–3). Most have limited shelf-life after reconstitution (Table A5–4). All are supplied in low dosage, which attests to their potency (Table A5–5).

TABLE A5-1. Approved Drugs/Vaccines

Product Name	Company	Indication	U.S. Development Status
Actimmune®† interferon gamma-1b	Genentech* (S. San Francisco, CA)	management of chronic granulomatous disease	approved December 1990
Activase® alteplase, recombinant	Genentech* (S. San Francisco, CA)	acute myocardial infarction	approved November 1987
		acute pulmonary embolism	approved June 1990
Alferon®N† interferon alfa-n3 (injection)	Interferon Sciences (New Brunswick, NJ)	genital warts	approved October 1989
Engerix-B® hepatitis B vaccine (recombinant)	SmithKline Beecham* (Philadelphia, PA)	hepatitis B	approved September 1989
EPOGEN® epoetin alfa	Amgen* (Thousand Oaks, CA)	treatment of anemia associated with chronic renal failure, including patients on dialysis and not on dialysis, and anemia in Retrovir®-treated HIV-infected patients	approved June 1989
PROCRIT®† epoetin alfa	Ortho Biotech* (Raritan, NJ)	treatment of anemia associated with chronic renal failure, including patients on dialysis and not on dialysis, and anemia in Retrovir®-treated HIV-infected patients	approved December 1990

[PROCRIT was approved for marketing under Amgen's epoetin alfa PLA. Amgen manufactures the product for Ortho Biotech.] Under an agreement between the two companies, Amgen licensed to Ortho Pharmaceutical the U.S. rights to epoetin alfa for indications for human use excluding dialysis and diagnostics.

†Addition since 1990 survey. *PMA Member Company **PMA Research Affiliate

Product	Company (location)	Indication	Status
Humatrope® somatropin (rDNA origin) for injection	Eli-Lilly* (Indianapolis, IN)	human growth hormone deficiency in children	approved March 1987
Humulin® human insulin (recombinant DNA origin)	Eli Lilly* (Indianapolis, IN)	diabetes	approved October 1982
Intron A® interferon alfa-2b (recombinant)	Schering-Plough* (Madison, NJ)	hairy cell leukemia	approved June 1986
		genital warts	approved June 1988
		AIDS-related Kaposi's sarcoma	approved November 1988
		non-A, non-B hepatitis	approved February 1991
Leukine™† sargramostim (GM-CSF)	Immunex* (Seattle, WA)	autologous bone marrow transplantation	approved March 1991
Prokine™† sargramostim (GM-CSF)	Hoechst-Roussel* (Somerville, NJ)	autologous bone marrow transplantation	approved March 1991

[Prokine was approved for marketing under Immunex's sargramostim PLA. Immunex manufactures the product for Hoechst-Roussel.]

TABLE A5–1. *Continued*

Product Name	Company	Indication	U.S. Development Status
Neupogen®† filgrastim (rG–CSF)	Amgen* (Thousand Oaks, CA)	chemotherapy-induced neutropenia	approved February 1991
ORTHOCLONE OKT®3 muromonab-CD3	Ortho Biotech* (Raritan, NJ)	reversal of acute kidney transplant rejection	approved June 1986
Protropin® somatrem for injection	Genentech* (S. San Francisco, CA)	human growth hormone deficiency in children	approved October 1985
RECOMBIVAX HB® hepatitis B vaccine (recombinant), MSD	Merck* (Rahway, NJ)	hepatitis B prevention	approved July 1986
Roferon®-A interferon alfa-2a, recombinant/Roche	Hoffmann-La Roche* (Nutley, NJ)	hairy cell leukemia	approved June 1986
		AIDS-related Kaposi's sarcoma	approved November 1988

TABLE A5–2. Biotechnology Medicines In Development

Clotting Factors

Product Name	Company	Indication	U.S. Development Status
KoGENate	Cutter Biological,* Miles Inc.* (Berkeley, CA)	hemophilia	application submitted
Mono-IX† factor IX	Rhone-Poulenc Rorer* (Fort Washington, PA)	prophylaxis and replacement treatment of hemorrhagic complications of hemophilia B	application submitted
NovoSeven† recombinant factor VIIa	Novo Nordisk (Princeton, NJ)	treatment of hemophilia A&B with and without antibodies against factors VIII/IX	Phase II
RECOMBINATE™ anti-hemophilic factor (recombinant)	Genetics Institute** (Cambridge, MA) Baxter Healthcare (Deerfield, IL)	hemophilia	Phase II/III

Colony Stimulating Factors

Product Name	Company	Indication	U.S. Development Status
granulocyte/macrophage colony stimulating factor	Amgen* (Thousand Oaks, CA)	adjuvant to chemotherapy	Phase I/II
Leucomax® granulocyte/macrophage colony stimulating factor	Sandoz* (E. Hanover, NJ) Schering-Plough* (Madison, NJ) Genetics Institute** (Cambridge, MA)	treatment of low blood cell counts	application submitted

TABLE A5–2. Continued

Colony Stimulating Factors (continued)

Product Name	Company	Indication	U.S. Development Status
Leukine™ sargramostim (GM-CSF)	Immunex* (Seattle, WA)	allogeneic bone marrow transplants, adjuvant to chemotherapy	Phase III
		.... adjuvant to AIDS therapy	Phase II
Macrolin™ macrophage colony stimulating factor	Cetus** (Emeryville, CA)	cancer, fungal disease	Phase I
macrophage colony stimulating factor	Genetics Institute** (Cambridge, MA)	cancer, hematologic neoplasms, bone marrow transplants	Phase I
Neupogen® filgrastim (rG-CSF)	Amgen* (Thousand Oaks, CA)	AIDS leukemia, aplastic anemia	application submitted
Prokine™ sargramostim (GM-CSF)	Hoechst-Roussel* (Somerville, NJ)	neutropenia to secondary chemotherapy	Phase III

Dismutases

Product Name	Company	Indication	U.S. Development Status
superoxide dismutase	Bio-Technology General (New York, NY)	oxygen toxicity in premature infants	Phase I/II

Erythropoietins

Product Name	Company	Indication	U.S. Development Status
Marogen Sterile Powder / epoetin beta	Genetics Institute** (Cambridge, MA) Chugai-Upjohn (Rosemont, IL)	anemia secondary to kidney disease	application submitted
		autologous transfusion, substitute for transfusion	Phase II/III
PROCRIT® epoetin alfa	Ortho Biotech* (Raritan, NJ)	treatment of anemia associated with cancer and cancer chemotherapy	application submitted
		prevention of anemia associated with surgical blood loss, autologous blood donation adjuvant	Phase III

Growth Factors

Product Name	Company	Indication	U.S. Development Status
epidermal growth factor[†]	Chiron Ophthalmics** (Irvine, CA)	corneal and cataract surgeries	Phase III
epidermal growth factor	Chiron** (Emeryville, CA) Ethicon* (Somerville, NJ)	wound healing, skin ulcers	Phase II
fibroblast growth factor	California Biotechnology** (Mountain View, CA)	chronic soft tissue ulcers	Phase II
human recombinant basic fibroblast growth factor	Synergen (Boulder, CO)	venous stasis, diabetic leg and foot ulcers	Phase III

TABLE A5-2. *Continued*

Growth Factors (continued)

Product Name	Company	Indication	U.S. Development Status
insulin-like growth factor (IGF-1)	Genentech* (S. San Francisco, CA)	nutritional support/metabolism	Phase II
		type II diabetes	Phase I
insulin-like growth factor I	Chiron** (Emeryville, CA) CIBA-GEIGY* (Summit, NJ)	type II diabetes	Phase II
insulin-like growth factor I†	Kabi Pharmacia* (Piscataway, NJ)		Phase I
platelet-derived growth factor† (PDGF)	Amgen* (Thousand Oaks, CA)	chronic dermal ulcers	Phase I/II
platelet-derived growth factor† (PDGF)	Chiron** (Emeryville, CA) Ethicon* (Somerville, NJ)	skin ulcers	Phase II
platelet-derived growth factor† (PDGF)	ZymoGenetics (Seattle, WA)	diabetic ulcers	Phase I

Human Growth Hormones

Product Name	Company	Indication	U.S. Development Status
BioTropin human growth hormone	Bio-Technology General (New York, NY)	human growth deficiency in children	application submitted
		hip fractures in elderly, cancer, AIDS	Phase I
Norditropin somatropin (rDNA origin) for injection	Novo Nordisk (Princeton, NJ)	treatment of growth failure in children due to inadequate growth hormone secretion	application submitted
Protropin® somatrem for injection	Genentech* (S. San Francisco, CA)	chronic renal insufficiency	application submitted
		Turner's syndrome	Phase III
		burns (pediatric only)	Phase III
Saizen® somatropin (rDNA origin) for injection	Serono Laboratories (Norwell, MA)	long-term treatment of growth failure due to inadequate secretion of normal endogenous growth hormone	application submitted

Interferons

Product Name	Company	Indication	U.S. Development Status
Actimmune® interferon gamma-1b	Genentech* (S. San Francisco, CA)	small-cell lung cancer, atopic dermatitis	Phase III
		trauma-related infections, renal cell carcinoma	Phase II
		asthma and allergies	Phase I

TABLE A5–2. Continued

Interferons (continued)

Product Name	Company	Indication	U.S. Development Status
Alferon® LDO[†] interferon alfa-n3	Interferon Sciences (New Brunswick, NJ)	ARC, AIDS	Phase I/II
Betaseron® interferon beta	Berlex Laboratories* (Wayne, NJ)	multiple sclerosis	Phase III
		cancer	Phase I/II
Immuneron® interferon gamma	Biogen** (Cambridge, MA)	rheumatoid arthritis	Phase II/III
		venereal warts	Phase II
interferon consensus	Amgen* (Thousand Oaks, CA)	cancer, infectious disease	Phase II/III
interferon gamma	Amgen* (Thousand Oaks, CA)	cancer, infectious disease	Phase II
Intron A® interferon alfa-2b	Schering-Plough* (Madison, NJ)	superficial bladder cancer; basal cell carcinoma; chronic hepatitis B, delta hepatitis	application submitted
		acute hepatitis B, delta hepatitis; chronic myelogenous leukemia	Phase III
		HIV in combination w/Retrovir®	Phase I
R-FRONE®[†] recombinant interferon beta	Serono Laboratories (Norwell, MA)	treatment of malignant diseases unresponsive to standard therapies	Phase I

Product Name	Company	Indication	U.S. Development Status
Roferon®-A interferon alfa-2a, recombinant/Roche	Hoffmann-La Roche* (Nutley, NJ)	colorectal cancer in combination w/ 5-flourouracil	Phase II
		chronic and acute hepatitis B, non-A, non-B hepatitis; chronic myelogenous leukemia; HIV positive, ARC, AIDS, in combination w/Retrovir®	in clinical trials

Interleukins

Product Name	Company	Indication	U.S. Development Status
PEG interleukin-2	Cetus** (Emeryville, CA)	AIDS, in combination w/Retrovir®	Phase I
Proleukin aldesleukin (interleukin-2)	Cetus** (Emeryville, CA)	renal cell carcinoma	application submitted
		cancer	Phase II/III
		Kaposi's sarcoma, in combination w/ Retrovir®	Phase I
recombinant human interleukin-1 alpha†	Immunex* (Seattle, WA)	prevention of chemotherapy- or radiotherapy-induced bone marrow suppression, cancer immunotherapy	Phase I/II
recombinant human interleukin-1 beta†	Immunex* (Seattle, WA) Syntex* (Palo Alto, CA)	prevention of chemotherapy- or radiotherapy-induced bone marrow suppression, treatment of melanoma, cancer immunotherapy	Phase I/II
	Immunex* (Seattle, WA)	wound healing	Phase II

TABLE A5-2. Continued

Interleukins (continued)

Product Name	Company	Indication	U.S. Development Status
recombinant human interleukin-2	Amgen* (Thousand Oaks, CA)	cancer immunotherapy	Phase III
recombinant human interleukin-2	Hoffmann-La Roche* (Nutley, NJ) Immunex* (Seattle, WA)	cancer immunotherapy, in combination w/Roferon®-A	in clinical trials
recombinant human interleukin-3	Hoechst-Roussel* (Somerville, NJ) Immunex* (Seattle, WA)	bone marrow failure, platelet deficiencies, autologous bone marrow transplantation, adjuvant to chemotherapy	Phase I/II
		peripheral stem cell transplant	Phase I
recombinant human interleukin-4	Schering-Plough* (Madison, NJ)	treatment of immunodeficient diseases, cancer therapy, vaccine adjuvant and immunization	Phase I/II
recombinant human interleukin-4	Sterling Drug* (New York, NY) Immunex* (Seattle, WA)	cancer immunomodulator	Phase II

Monoclonal Antibodies

Product Name	Company	Indication	U.S. Development Status
anti-EGF receptor antibody† (RG-83852)	Rhone-Poulenc Rorer* (Fort Washington, PA)	adjunct for solid tumor treatment	Phase I

anti-epidermal growth factor[†] (EMD 55 900)	EM Industries (Hawthorne, NY)	treatment of malignant glioma	Phase II
anti-IL-2 receptor MAb	Immunex* (Seattle, WA)	prevention of graft vs. host disease in bone marrow transplants	Phase I/II
Anti-Leu-2 MAb	Becton-Dickinson (Mountain View, CA)	prevention of graft vs. host disease	Phase II
anti-LPS MAb	Cetus** (Emeryville, CA)	sepsis	Phase III
anti-pseudomonas MAb	Cutter Biological,* Miles Inc.* (Berkeley, CA)	pseudomonas infections	Phase I
anti-tumor necrosis factor	Chiron** (Emeryville, CA)	septic shock	Phase III
anti-tumor necrosis factor	Cutter Biological,* Miles Inc.* (Berkeley, CA)	clinical sepsis	Phase II/III
BI-RR-1[†]	Boehringer Ingelheim* (Ridgefield, CT)	prophylactic renal transplantation	Phase II
Capiscint[†]	Centocor (Malvern, PA)	atherosclerotic plaque imaging agent	Phase II
Centara[†] chimeric anti-CD4 antibody	Centocor (Malvern, PA)	rheumatoid arthritis, multiple sclerosis	Phase II
CenTNF[†] chimeric anti-TNF antibody	Centocor (Malvern, PA)	treatment of bacterial infections	Phase I

TABLE A5-2. *Continued*

Monoclonal Antibodies (continued)

Product Name	Company	Indication	U.S. Development Status
Centorex 7E3 MAb	Centocor (Malvern, PA)	anti-platelet prevention of blood clots	Phase II
Centoxin HA-1A MAb	Centocor (Malvern, PA)	sepsis and septic shock	application submitted
chimeric L6	Bristol-Myers Squibb/ Oncogen* (New York, NY)	breast, colon, lung and ovarian cancers	Phase I/II
E5™ MAb	Pfizer* (New York, NY) Xoma (Berkeley, CA)	gram-negative sepsis	application submitted
Fibriscint[†] anti-fibrin antibody	Centocor (Malvern, PA)	blood clot imaging agent	Phase III
GNI-250 MAb	Genetics Institute** (Cambridge, MA)	colorectal cancer	Phase I
HER-2 antibody[†]	Genentech* (S. San Francisco, CA)	breast, ovarian cancers	Phase I
human MAb (TI-23) to cytomegalovirus[†]	Cutter Biological,* Miles Inc.* (Berkeley, CA)	treatment of acute CMV disease in organ transplant (immunosuppressed) patients	Phase I
immunotoxin[†] (4197X-RA)	Houston Biotechnology (The Woodlands, TX)	prevention of secondary cataract	Phase I

ImmuRAID-CEA technetium 99m-FAb' fragment (colorectal)	Immunomedics (Warren, NJ)	extent of disease staging of colorectal cancer	application submitted
ImmuRAID-CEA[†] technetium-99m-FAb' fragment (lung)	Immunomedics (Warren, NJ)	extent of disease staging of lung cancer	Phase I
ImmuRAID-CEA[†] technetium-99m-FAb' fragment (breast)	Immunomedics (Warren, NJ)	extent of disease staging of breast cancer	Phase I
ImmuRAID-LL2[†] technetium-99m-FAb' fragment (lymphoma)	Immunomedics (Warren, NJ)	extent of disease staging of lymphoma	Phase I
ImmuRAID-MN3[†] technetium-99m-FAb' fragment (infectious disease)	Immunomedics (Warren, NJ)	diagnosis of fever of unknown origin	Phase I
ImmuRAIT-CEA iodine 131-intact IgG (colorectal)	Immunomedics (Warren, NJ)	treatment of colorectal cancer	Phase I
ImmuRAIT-LL2[†] iodine 131-intact IgG (lymphoma)	Immunomedics (Warren, NJ)	treatment of lymphoma	Phase I
LYM-1	Techniclone International (Tustin, CA)	lymphoma	Phase II
MAb	Lederle* (Wayne, NJ)	B-cell lymphoma, breast, colon and lung cancers	Phase I

TABLE A5–2. *Continued*

Monoclonal Antibodies (continued)

Product Name	Company	Indication	U.S. Development Status
MAb-L6	Bristol-Myers Squibb/Oncogen* (New York, NY)	breast, colon, lung and ovarian cancers	Phase II
murine MAb (IMelpgI) anti-idiotype against murine MAb to melanoma-associated antigen	IDEC Pharmaceuticals (Mountain View, CA)	malignant melanoma	Phase I
murine MAb (IMelpg2) anti-idiotype of melanoma associated antigen, 3A[†]	IDEC Pharmaceuticals (Mountain View, CA)	malignant melanoma	Phase I
murine monoclonal antibodies to human B-cell lymphomas (anti-idiotypes)	IDEC Pharmaceuticals (Mountain View, CA)	B-cell lymphoma	Phase III
Myoscint[†] mifarmonab	Centocor (Malvern, PA)	cardiac imaging agent	application submitted
ONCOLYSIN B anti-B4-blocked ricin	ImmunoGen** (Cambridge, MA)	IV treatment of B-cell leukemias and lymphomas	Phase II
		ex vivo treatment of autologous bone marrow and subsequent reinfusion in patients with acute myelogenous leukemia (AML)	Phase I/II

ONCOLYSIN M anti-My9-blocked ricin	ImmunoGen** (Cambridge, MA)	IV treatment of myeloid leukemias	Phase I/II
	ImmunoGen** (Cambridge, MA)	ex vivo treatment of autologous bone marrow and subsequent reinfusion in patients with acute myelogenous leukemia (AML)	Phase I/II
ONCOLYSIN S[†] N901-blocked ricin	ImmunoGen** (Cambridge, MA)	IV treatment of small cell lung cancer	Phase I/II
OncoRAD® GI103[†] CYT-103-Y-90	CYTOGEN** (Princeton, NJ) Sterling Drug* (New York, NY)	targeted radiotherapy for gastrointestinal malignancies	Phase II
OncoRAD® OV103 CYT-103-Y-90	CYTOGEN** (Princeton, NJ) Sterling Drug* (New York, NY)	targeted radiotherapy for ovarian cancer	Phase II
OncoScint® CR103 celocolab	CYTOGEN** (Princeton, NJ)	detection, staging and follow-up of colorectal cancer	application submitted
OncoScint® CR372[†] CYT-372-In-111	CYTOGEN** (Princeton, NJ)	detection, staging and follow-up of colorectal cancer	Phase I
OncoScint® OV103 celogovab	CYTOGEN** (Princeton, NJ)	detection, staging and follow-up of ovarian adenocarcinoma	application submitted
OncoScint® PR356 CYT-356-In-111	CYTOGEN** (Princeton, NJ)	detection, staging and follow-up of prostate adenocarcinoma	Phase II
ORTHOCLONE OKT®3 muromonab-CD3	Ortho Biotech* (Raritan, NJ)	reversal of heart and liver transplant rejection, renal prophylaxis	application submitted

TABLE A5–2. *Continued*

Monoclonal Antibodies (continued)

Product Name	Company	Indication	U.S. Development Status
ORTHOCLONE OKT4A[†]	Ortho Biotech* (Raritan, NJ)	prevention of organ transplant rejection	Phase I
ORTHOZYME® CD5+ muromonab CD5-RTA	Ortho Biotech* (Raritan, NJ)	treatment of graft vs. host disease	application submitted
		solid organ transplant rejection, type I diabetes	Phase I
pancarcinoma Re-186 MAb	NeoRx (Seattle, WA)	breast, colon, lung, ovarian, pancreatic and prostate cancers	Phase I
Panorex 17-1A MAb	Centocor (Malvern, PA)	colorectal cancer	Phase II
TNT	Techniclone International (Tustin, CA)	solid tumors	Phase I
XomaZyme®-791 MAb	Xoma (Berkeley, CA)	colorectal cancer	Phase I
XomaZyme®-CD5 Plus anti-CD5 MAb-ricin	Xoma (Berkeley, CA)	rheumatoid arthritis	Phase III
		type I diabetes, cutaneous T-cell lymphoma, inflammatory bowel disease	Phase I/II
XomaZyme®-CD7 Plus 4MRTA	Xoma (Berkeley, CA)	T-cell malignancies	Phase I
XomaZyme®-Mel MAb	Xoma (Berkeley, CA)	melanoma	Phase II

Recombinant Soluble CD4s (rCD4)

Product Name	Company	Indication	U.S. Development Status
CD4-IgG	Genentech* (S. San Francisco, CA)	maternal/fetal AIDS virus transfer	Phase I
rsCD4	Biogen** (Cambridge, MA)	ARC, AIDS	Phase II

Tissue Plasminogen Activators

Product Name	Company	Indication	U.S. Development Status
Activase®† alteplase, recombinant (tissue-plasminogen activator)	Genentech* (S. San Francisco, CA)	peripheral arterial occlusion	application submitted
		unstable angina	Phase III
		ischemic stroke	Phase III
tissue-plasminogen activator	Genetics Institute** (Cambridge, MA)	acute myocardial infarction, acute stroke, deep vein thrombosis, pulmonary embolism	Phase III

Tumor Necrosis Factors

Product Name	Company	Indication	U.S. Development Status
tumor necrosis factor	Biogen** (Cambridge, MA) Knoll Pharmaceuticals* (Whippany, NJ)	cancer	Phase II
tumor necrosis factor	Genentech* (S. San Francisco, CA)	cancer	Phase II

TABLE A5–2. *Continued*

Product Name	Company	Indication	U.S. Development Status
Vaccines			
AIDS vaccine[†] (r-gp-160)	Immuno AG (Vienna, Austria) National Institutes of Health (Bethesda, MD)	AIDS	Phase I
BMY-35047	Bristol-Myers Squibb/ Oncogen[*] (New York, NY)	melanoma	Phase I
gp120[†]	Genentech[*] (S. San Francisco, CA)	AIDS prophylaxis and treatment	Phase I
hepatitis B vaccine	Amgen[*] (Thousand Oaks, CA)	hepatitis B	Phase III
herpes vaccines	Chiron[**] (Emeryville, CA) CIBA-GEIGY (Basle, Switzerland)	herpes simplex 2, genital herpes	1 in Phase II 1 in Phase I
HIV immunotherapeutic vaccine[†] (RG 83894)	Immune Response Corporation (Carlsbad, CA) Rhone-Poulenc Rorer[*] (Fort Washington, PA)	treatment of asymptomatic HIV-infected patients	Phase II/III
HIV vaccines[†] (gp 120)	Chiron[**] (Emeryville, CA) CIBA-GEIGY (Basle, Switzerland)	AIDS	2 in Phase I

Product Name	Company	Indication	U.S. Development Status
malaria vaccines	SmithKline Beecham* (Philadelphia, PA) Walter Reed Army Institute of Research (Washington, DC)	malaria	3 in Phase II 2 in Phase I
Melacine™† melanoma vaccine	Ribi ImmunoChem Research (Hamilton, MT)	treatment of stage III/IV melanoma	Phase II as a therapeutic
VaxSyn® HIV-1 (gp160)	MicroGeneSys** (Meriden, CT)	AIDS	Phase II as a vaccine
		AIDS	Phase II as a therapeutic
VaxSyn® HIV-1† (rp24)	MicroGeneSys** (Meriden, CT)	AIDS	Phase I as a therapeutic

Others

Product Name	Company	Indication	U.S. Development Status
Antril™† anakinra (interleukin-1 receptor antagonist)	Synergen (Boulder, CO)	AML, CML, inflammatory bowel disease, rheumatoid arthritis, sepsis, septic shock	Phase II
Auriculin atrial natriuretic peptide	California Biotechnology** (Mountain View, CA)	heart and kidney failure	Phase II
DNase†	Genentech* (S. San Francisco, CA)	cystic fibrosis	Phase II
		chronic bronchitis	Phase I

TABLE A5–2. Continued

Others (continued)

Product Name	Company	Indication	U.S. Development Status
ImmTher[†] disaccharide tripeptide glycerol dipalmitoyl (macrophage activator)	ImmunoTherapeutics (Moorhead, MN)	metastatic colorectal cancer to the liver	Phase II
Imuvert ribosome and vesicles	Cell Technology (Boulder, CO)	brain cancer and other tumors	Phase II
MPL™[†] monophosphoryl lipid A	Ribi ImmunoChem Research (Hamilton, MT)	prevention or amelioration of gram-negative septic shock	Phase I
relaxin	Genentech* (S. San Francisco, CA)	cervical ripening to facilitate childbirth in women experiencing certain complications	Phase II
retroviral vector with tumor necrosis factor gene[†]	National Cancer Institute (Bethesda, MD) Cetus** (Emeryville, CA)	melanoma	Phase I
SLPI[†] secretory leukocyte protease inhibitor	Synergen (Boulder, CO)	cystic fibrosis, genetic emphysema	Phase II

The content of this chart has been obtained through government and industry sources based on the latest information. Chart current as of August 2, 1991. The information may not be comprehensive. For more specific information about a particular product, contact the individual company directly. For general information, contact the Pharmaceutical Manufacturers Association at (202)835-3463. *(If you are not receiving the biotechnology chart regularly but would like to, please send your request in writing to Editor, "Biotechnology Medicines in Development," Communications Division, Pharmaceutical Manufacturers Association, 1100 15th Street, NW, Washington, DC 20005.)*

Provided as a Public Service by the Pharmaceutical Manufacturers Association.

Copyright © 1991 by the Pharmaceutical Manufacturers Association. Permission to reprint is awarded if proper credit is given.

TABLE A5–3. Product Stability

	Physical Form	Shelf-life
Humulin	Liquid solution	2 years at 2–8° C
Protropin	Lyophilized powder	2 years at 2–8° C
Humatrope		
Roferon-A	Lyophilized powder	3 years at 2–8° C
Intron A	Lyophilized powder	2 years at 2–8° C
Activase	Lyophilized powder	2 years at 2–30° C
Recombivax-HB	Liquid solution	
Engerix-B	Liquid solution	
Orthoclone	Liquid solution	1 year at 2–8° C
Epogen	Liquid solution	

TABLE A5–4. Stability after Reconstitution (Lyophilized Products)

Roferon-A	1 month at 2–8° C
Intron A	1 month at 2–8° C
Humatrope	14 days at 2–8° C
Protropin	7 days at 2–8° C
Activase	8 hours at 2–30° C

TABLE A5–5. Recombinant Protein Drugs

	Vial Strength
Humulin	1000 units
Protropin	5 mg
Humatrope	5 mg
Roferon-A	3, 18 million units solution
	3, 18 million units lypho
Intron A	3, 5, 10, 25, 50 million units
Activase	20, 50 mg
Recombivax HB	5, 10 µg
Engerix-B	20 µg
Orthoclone OKT3	5 µg
Epogen	2, 4, 10,000 units

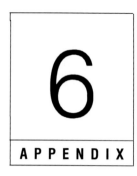

APPENDIX

Buyer's Guides

PUMPS AND CONTROLLERS

Mobile Pumps

Block Medical, Inc.

Address: 5957 Landau Court, Carlsbad, CA 92008
Instrument name/model: Venfuse V001000
Instrument cost: $3895 **Set cost:** $16.35
Flow/rate range: 0.1–300 ml/hr
Accuracy: ±6% **Net weight:** 1 lb
Power requirements: 2 9V vatteries, AC power or rechargeable battery pack
System alarms: occlusion, air in line, low battery, low reservoir, end of program, door open, malfunction, others
Miscellaneous comments: Delivers in 4 therapy modes; has exclusive remote monitoring capabilities; uses bar code programming

Burron Medical, Inc.

Address: 824 12th Ave, Bethlehem, PA 18018
Instrument name/model: Ambulatory Drug Delivery System—ADD-100/ADD-200/ADD-002
Instrument cost: Not supplied **Set cost:** Not supplied
Flow/rate range: 100 ml/hr (ADD-100); 200 ml/hr (ADD-200); 2 ml/hr (ADD-002)

Abstracted with permission from Pharmacy Practice News, July 1992

McMahon Publishing Co.
8th Annual Buyer's Guide to
Pumps and Controllers

Accuracy: ±10%–15%   **Net weight:** 3 oz
Power requirements: None
System alarms: None
Miscellaneous comments: Burron's ADD Pump Syustem provides an accu-
rate flow through the entire life of the pump, a visible and measurable fluid
reservoir, and the safety and convenience of propylene material

I-Flow Corporation

Address: 2532 White Road, Irvine, CA 92714
Instrument name/model: VIVUS 400 and 4000/2
Instrument cost: $3995 (2 channel), $4995 (4 channel)   **Set cost:** $14.90
Flow/rate range: 0.1–200 ml/per channel
Accuracy: ±10%   **Net weight:** 32 oz (2 channel);   35 oz (4 channel)
Power requirements: AC: 1A; also operates on 5 AA batteries
System alarms: Occlusion, low/dead battery, stop, empty, malfunction
Miscellaneous comments: The VIVUS 4000 System is the first multiple-chan-
nel remote-controlled ambulatory infusion system available

Ivion Corporation

Address: 2400 Industrial Lane, Broomfield, CO 80020
Instrument name/model: MedFusion WalkMed 440 PIC
Instrument cost: $3095   **Set cost:** Not supplied
Flow/rate range: 0.1–30.0 ml/hr, in 0.1-ml increments
Accuracy: ±5%   **Net weight:** 12.75 oz, with battery
Power requirements: 9V alkaline transistor battery
System alarms: Occlusion, under-delivery, over-delivery, system malfunc-
tion, bar open, depleted battery
Miscellaneous comments: Includes all features of WalkMed 410C, 4201/C
and 430 PCA. Distributed by Ivion Corporation, a wholly owned subsidiary
of Medex, Inc.

Ivion Corporation

Address: 2400 Industrial Lane, Broomfield, CO 80020
Instrument name/model: MedFusion WalkMed 410 C
Instrument cost: $2095   **Set cost:** $10.50–$12.50
Flow/rate range: 0.1–30.0 ml/hr, in 0.1-ml increments
Accuracy: ±5%   **Net weight:** 12.75 oz, with battery
Power requirements: 9V alkaline transistor battery
System alarms: Occlusion, under-delivery, over-delivery, system malfunc-
tion, bar open, depleted battery
Miscellaneous comments: Continuous delivery, including chelating agents and
chemotherapy; multiple applications, including epidural. Distributed by Ivion
Corporation, a wholly owned subsidiary of Medex, Inc.

Ivion Corporation

Address: 2400 Industrial Lane, Broomfield, CO 80020
Instrument name/model: MedFusion WalkMed 430 PCA
Instrument cost: $2695   **Set cost:** Not supplied
Flow/rate range: 0.1–30.0 ml/hr, in 0.1-ml increments

Accuracy: ±5% **Net weight:** 12.75 oz, with battery
Power requirements: 9V alkaline transistor battery
System alarms: Occlusion, under-delivery, over-delivery, system malfunction, bar open, depleted battery
Miscellaneous comments: PCA and continuous programming; PCA options and basal and/or bolus and remote bolus button; software and hardware lockouts available. Distributed by Ivion Corporation, a wholly owned subsidiary of Medex, Inc.

Ivion Corporation

Address: 2400 Industrial Lane, Broomfield, CO 80020
Instrument name/model: MedFusion WalkMed 420 PCA
Instrument cost: $2695 **Set cost:** $10.50–$12.50
Flow/rate range: 0.1–30.0 ml/hr, in 0.1-ml increments
Accuracy: ±5% **Net weight:** 12.75 oz, with battery
Power requirements: 9V alkaline transistor battery
System alarms: Occlusion, under-delivery, over-delivery, system malfunction, bar open, depleted battery
Miscellaneous comments: Intermittent and continuous programming; dose delivery with programmable time, for antibiotics and other scheduled drugs. Distributed by Ivion Corporation, a wholly owned subsidiary of Medex, Inc.

Ivion Corporation

Address: 2400 Industrial Lane, Broomfield, CO 80020
Instrument name/model: Intelliject Multi-Channel Infusion Pump
Instrument cost: $2940 **Set cost:** Not supplied
Flow/rate range: Adjustable 1–40.54 ml/hr
Accuracy: ±5% **Net weight:** 3.4 lb
Power requirements: 2 9V alkaline transistor battery
System alarms: Low battery, excessive back pressure, syringe empty, syringe not in place, door open, electronic fault, machine logic error
Miscellaneous comments: Programmable 4-channel operation for automated multiple or single-drug infusions, including automatic flushing, locking, and disconnect

Medical Technology Products, Inc.

Address: 107 Woodbury Road, Huntington, NY 11743
Instrument name/model: MTP 1001 and 1001A
Instrument cost: $1975 **Set cost:** $4.35
Flow/rate range: Model 1001: 0.1–499.9 ml/hr (volume 1–999 ml); Model 1001A: 1–499 ml/hr (volume 1–999 ml)
Accuracy: ±3% **Net weight:** 14.5 lb
Power requirements: AC: 110–115V available; DC: 12V adapter, battery life: 10 hr
System alarms: Air, occlusion, low battery, infusion complete (KVO), tamper alarm, call back alarm
Miscellaneous comments: Detachable power cord for patient mobility; carrying case available

Pharmacia Deltec

Address: 1265 Grey Fox Road, St. Paul, MN 55112
Instrument name/model: CADD-1 Ambulatory Infusion Pump, Model 5100 HFX
Instrument cost: $2595 **Set cost:** $14.25
Flow/rate range: 0–299 ml/24 hr or 90 ml/hr in fixed high flow mode
Accuracy: ±6% **Net weight:** 15 oz
Power requirements: 9V alkaline or lithium battery
System alarms: Power-up fault, pump in stop mode, low battery, depleted battery, low reservoir volume, programmed volume depleted, high pressure, system error
Miscellaneous comments: Designed for continuous IV chemotherapy

Pharmacia Deltec

Address: 1265 Grey Fox Road, St. Paul, MN 55112
Instrument name/model: CADD-TPN Ambulatory Infusion Pump, Model 5700
Instrument cost: $3595 (pump only); $3995 (pump, powerpack, backpack)
Set cost: $22
Flow/rate range: 10–400 ml/hr (using power pack; 10–2500 ml/hr (using 9V battery); KVO rate: 5 ml/hr
Accuracy: ±8% **Net weight:** 13 oz
Power requirements: 9V alkaline or lithium battery; rechargeable power pack; AC adapter
System alarms: Low reservoir volume, programmed volume depleted, infusion period completed, low battery, invalid rate, high pressure, others
Miscellaneous comments: Continuous delivery and continuous delivery with tapering for total parenteral nutrition therapy

Pharmacia Deltec

Address: 1265 Grey Fox Road, St. Paul, MN 55112
Instrument name/model: CADD-PLUS Ambulatory Infusion Pump, Model 5400
Instrument cost: $3395 **Set cost:** $14.25
Flow/rate range: 0–75ml/24 hr
Accuracy: ±6% **Net weight:** 15 oz
Power requirements: 9V alkaline or lithium battery
System alarms: Power-up fault, pump in stop mode, low battery, depleted battery, low reservoir volume, programmed volume depleted, high pressure, system error
Miscellaneous comments: Designed for intermittent or continuous I.V. antibiotic therapy; remote reservoir adapter and other accessories available

PCA Pumps

Abbott Laboratories

Address: One Abbott Park Road, Department 993, Building AP30, Abbott Park, IL 60064
Instrument name/model: Abbott Pain Management Provider

Instrument cost: $3795 **Set cost:** Not supplied
Flow/rate range: 1–25 ml/hr in epidural mode, or equivalent in mg or μg
Accuracy: ±5% fluid delivery **Net weight:** Approx. 2 lb
Power requirements: 2 9V batteries, AC power converter
System alarms: End of infusion, internal malfunction, low battery, occlusion, air in line, call back alert, check cartridge, empty container, others
Miscellaneous comments: Utilizes a yellow-striped dedicated set to alert the user of epidural infusion

Abbott Laboratories

Address: One Abbott Park Road, Department 993, Building AP30, Abbott Park, IL 60064
Instrument name/model: LifeCare PCA Classic
Instrument cost: $3495 **Set cost:** $4.05
Flow/rate range: 0.1–20 ml
Accuracy: ±5% **Net weight:** a14 lb
Power requirements: AC/DC
System alarms: Check syringe, door open, check settings, lockout, occlusion, low battery, malfunction
Miscellaneous comments: A single-mode PCA infusion device for low-cost PCA procedures

Abbott Laboratories

Address: One Abbott Park Road, Department 993, Building AP30, Abbott Park, IL 60064
Instrument name/model: LifeCare PCA Plus II
Instrument cost: $3495 **Set cost:** $4.05
Flow/rate range: 0.1–200 mg/hr; 10–1000 g/hr
Accuracy: ±5% **Net weight:** 14 lb
Power requirements: AC/DC
System alarms: Check vial, check injection, check syringe, empty syringe, check 4-hr limit, door open, occlusion, reset, low battery
Miscellaneous comments: Device has the ability to dose in μg or mg

Bard Medsystems Division CR Bard, Inc.

Address: 87 Concord Street, North Reading, MA 01864
Instrument name/model: Bard PCA 1 Pump
Instrument cost: $3295 **Set cost:** Not supplied
Flow/rate range: 0–150 ml/hr
Accuracy: ±3% fluid delivery **Net weight:** 4.2 lb, with batteries
Power requirements: 4 "D" cell alkaline batteries
System alarms: 5 ml remaining, end of syringe, occlusion, low battery, others
Miscellaneous comments: Any easy-to-operate syringe pump to meet all I.V. PCA needs

Graseby Medical Ltd.

Address: 8213 Jumpers Hole Road, Millersville, MD 21108
Instrument name/model: Graseby Model "PCAS" Syringe Driver
Instrument cost: Not supplied **Set cost:** Not supplied

Flow/rate range: 01 μg/hr–99.9 mg/hr
Accuracy: ±5%   **Net weight:**   6 lb
Power requirements: AC: 110V or battery
System alarms: 11 alarms
Miscellaneous comments: Uses standard infusion sets and syringes

Ivac Corporation

Address: 10300 Campus Point Drive, San Diego, CA 92121-1519
Instrument name/model: PCAInfuser Model 310
Instrument cost: $3900   **Set cost:**   N/A
Flow/rate range: 0.1–99.9 mg/ml
Net weight: 6 lb
Power requirements: 4 D-cell alkaline batteries
System alarms: Low volume attention, low battery, programming error, syringe not primed, no syringe
Miscellaneous comments: Programmable in mg; accepts wide variety of syringes; PCA mode and continuous rate can be used simultaneously or separately; lightweight; easy to use, intuitive programming

Pharmacia Deltec Inc.

Address: 1265 Grey Fox Road, St. Paul, MN 55112
Instrument name/model: CADD-PCA Ambulatory Infusion Pump, Model 5800
Instrument cost: $3495   **Set cost:** $14.25
Flow/rate range: Continuous: 0–99.5 mg/hr or 0–20 mg/hr; 0–99 mg or 0–6 ml; bolus: 0–99.5 mg or 0.20 ml
Accuracy: ±6%   **Net weight:**   15 oz
Power requirements: 9V alkaline or lithium battery
System alarms: Power-up fault, pump in stop mode, low battery, depleted battery, low reservoir volume, programmed volume depleted, high pressure, system error
Miscellaneous comments: PCA, continuous and/or clinician bolus; programmable in mg or ml; records doses delivered and attempted; model with remote dose card also available

Pumps/Controllers

Abbott Laboratories

Address: One Abbott Park Road, Department 993, Building AP30, Abbott Park, IL 60064
Instrument name/model: LifeCare 5000 Plum
Instrument cost: $3675   **Set cost:** $4.50–$10
Flow/rate range: Macrodrip: 1–999 ml/hr; Microdrip: 0.1–99.9 ml/hr
Accuracy: ±5% total system   **Net weight:**   Approx. 6.0 kg(13 lb) with battery
Power requirements: AC: 115V
System alarms: Full range including distal occlusion, proximal occlusion, air in line, pressure out of range

Miscellaneous comments: Complete drug delivery system that includes programmable operating modes, multiple intermittent piggybacking and syringe capabilities

Baxa Corporation

Address: 13760 E. Arapahoe Road, Englewood, CO 80112-3903
Instrument name/model: MicroMacro 12
Instrument cost: $5,000 to $15,000   **Set cost:** Up to $50
Flow/rate range: Up to 69.4 sec/L
Accuracy: ±0.02 ml   **Net weight:** 16.9 kg
Power requirements: AC: 120V
System alarms: Source container empty, air detection, Mix Check report
Miscellaneous comments: PC-controlled volumetric delivery system with gravimetric check; Micro-Adds from 0.2 ml; up to 12 source solutions

Baxa Corporation

Address: 13760 E. Arapahoe Road, Englewood, CO 80112-3903
Instrument name/model: MicroMacro 23 TPN Compounder
Instrument cost: $20,000 to $30,000   **Set cost:** $50–$90
Flow/rate range: Up to 69.4 sec/L
Accuracy: ±.02 ml   **Net weight:** 19.7 kg
Power requirements: AC: 120V
System alarms: Source container empty, air detection, Mix Check report
Miscellaneous comments: PC-controlled volumetric delivery system with gravimetric check; Micro-Adds from 0.2 ml; up to 23 source solutions

Imed Corporation

Address: 9975 Businesspark Avenue, San Diego, CA 92131-1699
Instrument name/model: PC 1 #1310
Instrument cost: Not supplied   **Set cost:** N/A
Flow/rate range: 0.1–0.999 ml/hr
Accuracy: ±5%   **Net weight:** Not supplied
Power requirements: Not supplied
System alarms: Close door, occluded patient side/fluid side, air in line
Miscellaneous comments: Autotaper; versataper; rapid rate titration; tamperproof; communication through free flow portected administration set

Imed Corporation

Address: 9975 Businesspark Avenue, San Diego, CA 92131-1699
Instrument name/model: PC 2#1320
Instrument cost: Not supplied   **Set cost:** N/A
Flow/rate range: 0.1–0.999 ml/hr
Accuracy: ±5%   **Net weight:** Not supplied
Power requirements: Not supplied
System alarms: Close door
Miscellaneous comments: Free flow protected administration set; rapid rate titration; tamperproof; syringe delivery; communication through an RS-232

Syringe Pumps

Abbott Laboratories

Address: One Abbott Park Road, Department 993, Building AP30, Abbott Park, IL 60064
Instrument name/model: LifeCare Micro Pump System
Instrument cost: $3045 **Set cost:** $5.50–$11
Flow/rate range: 0.1–99.9 ml/hr
Accuracy: ±5% total system   **Net weight:** 13 lb
Power requirements: AC: 117V
System alarms: Infusion complete, air in line, flow error
Miscellaneous comments: Choice of 3 pressure occlusion limits; broad range of special micro pump sets in either 15 or 60 drops/ml

Abbott Laboratories

Address: One Abbott Park Road, Department 993, Building AP30, Abbott Park, IL 60064
Instrument name/model: LifeCare Hyperbaric Pump
Instrument cost: $3360 **Set cost:** $8–$11
Flow/rate range: 10–800 ml/hr
Accuracy: ±10% total system calibrated to ATA   **Net weight:** 14.08 lb
Power requirements: AC: 112V
System alarms: Dose complete, flow occlusion, battery low
Miscellaneous comments: Only device available for volumetric infusion into monoplace hyperbaric chambers

Abbott Laboratories

Address: One Abbott Park Road, Department 993, Building AP30, Abbott Park, IL 60064
Instrument name/model: LifeCare Blues Pump Systems, Models 4, 4H, 4P
Instrument cost: $3045 **Set cost:** $4.50–$10
Flow/rate range: 1–999 ml/hr, in 1-ml increments
Accuracy: ±5% total system **Net weight:** 13 lb
Power requirements: AC: 117V
System alarms: Low battery, occlusion, empty container, malfunction alarm, high/low alarms
Miscellaneous comments: Cannot pump air; choice of pressure limits; titration feature; computer dataway; dual-rate piggybacking

Bard Medsystems Division
C.R. Bard, Inc.

Address: 87 Concord Street, North Reading, MA 01864
Instrument name/model: Bard InfuO.R. Pump
Instrument cost: $1995 **Set cost:** $2.95
Flow/rate range: 0–600 ml/hr
Accuracy: ±3% total system **Net weight:** 2 lb with battery
Power requirements: 4 "C" cell batteries
System alarms: End of syringe, occlusion, low battery

Miscellaneous comments: Offers convenient, single-handed operation; smart labels enable you to select patient weight and bolus doses when applicable

Baxter Healthcare Corporation,
I.V. Systems Division

Address: 1425 Lake Cook Road, Deerfield, IL 60015
Instrument name/model: AS40A Syringe Pump
Instrument cost: List $2395   **Set cost:** N/A
Flow/rate range: .01–360 ml/hr
Accuracy: ±3%   **Net weight:** 1.75 kg (3.85 lb)
Power requirements: AC: 105–125V, 60 Hz
System alarms: Volume limit, dose due, high pressure, idle alert, on charge, low battery, bad battery
Miscellaneous comments: Accepts all syringes 1–60 ml; numerical key pad entry; syringe size recognition; 7 delivery modes; expanded versatility

Baxter Healthcare Corporation,
I.V. Systems Division

Address: 1425 Lake Cook Road, Deerfield, IL 60015
Instrument name/model: AS20S Syringe Pump
Instrument cost: List $1785   **Set cost:** N/A
Flow/rate range: Dependent on syringe selected
Accuracy: ±3% (not including syringe tolerance)   **Net weight:** 24 oz
Power requirements: AC: 105–125V, 60 Hz; DC: internal NiCad rechargeable battery
System alarms: Volume limit, high pressure, on charge, low battery, bad battery
Miscellaneous comments: Infusion modes: continuous, intermittent or standby dosing; single or multiple product delivery

Baxter Healthcare Corporation,
I.V. Systems Division

Address: 1425 Lake Cook Road, Deerfield, IL 60015
Instrument name/model: AS20GH-2 Syringe Pump
Instrument cost: List $2195   **Set cost:** N/A
Flow/rate range: Varies according to programmed information
Accuracy: ±3%   **Net weight:** 127 oz
Power requirements: AC: 105–125V, 60 Hz; DC: internal rechargeable NiCad battery
System alarms: Volume limit, high pressure, on charge, low battery, bad battery
Miscellaneous comments: Infusion modes can be programmed in μg/kg/min, μg/min, or ml/hr automatic rate calculation; programmable bolus

Becton Dickinson Infusion Systems

Address: 2 Bridgewater Lane, Lincoln Park, NJ 07035
Instrument name/model: Rate infuser II/Cat #8994
Instrument cost: $1500   **Set cost:** Not supplied
Flow/rate range: 0.1–99.9 ml/hr

Accuracy: ±3%, ±5% **Net weight:** 2 lb, 10 oz with batteries
Power requirements: 4 "C" alkaline batteries: 240 hr
System alarms: Low battery, wait state, syringe tamper, end of infusion, electronic malfunction, program error
Miscellaneous comments: Easy to use; easily transported; accommodates 1–60 cc syringes; lightweight; large visual display; includes I.V. pole clamp

Becton Dickinson Infusion Systems

Address: 2 Bridgewater Lane, Lincoln Park, NJ 07035
Instrument name/model: 360 infuser/Cat #2800
Instrument cost: $1695 **Set cost:** Not supplied
Flow/rate range: 1.5–360 ml/hr (10–60 min, 2.5 min increments)
Accuracy: ±3% **Net weight:** 2.2 lb with batteries
Power requirements: 4 "C" size alkaline batteries: 400 hr
System alarms: Low battery, infusion rate error, occlusion, syringe tampering, end of infusion, electronic malfunction
Miscellaneous comments: For cost-effective intermittent medication delivery; accommodates 3–60 ml syringes; easy to operate; provides flexibility in delivery for neonatal and pediatric applications

Burron Medical, Inc

Address: 824 12th Avenue, Bethlehem, PA 18018
Instrument name/model: MULTI-AD Pump, MP 3010
Instrument cost: $1540 **Set cost:** $11–$19
Flow/rate range: 1–100 ml in 6 sec
Accuracy: ±1% **Net weight** 12 lb
Power requirements: 12V, normal power grounded
System alarms: NA
Miscellaneous comments: Electronic solid-state system designed for repetitive, volumetric dispensing of diluent or medication, both I.V. and oral, into empty or partial-fill containers and syringes

Graseby Medical Ltd.

Address: 8213 Jumpers Hole Road, Millersville, MD 21108
Instrument name/model: Graseby Models MS16/MS26 Syringe Drivers
Instrument cost: Not supplied **Set cost:** Not supplied
Flow/rate range: 0–60 ml/hr, up to 60 days
Accuracy: ±5% **Net weight:** 6 oz
Power requirements: 9V Mallory battery
System alarms: End of infusion, occlusion, pump failure
Miscellaneous comments: Includes shoulder and belt holsters; uses standard infusion sets and syringes

Ivac Corporation

Address: 10300 Campus Point Drive, San Diego, CA 92121-1519
Instrument name/model: Syringe Pump Model 710
Instrument cost: $1850 **Set cost:** $1.80
Flow/rate range: 0.1–99.9 ml/hr
Net weight: 7 lb

Power requirements: AC: 95–135 V, 50–60 Hz, battery life approximately 8 hr
System alarms: Empty syringe, occlusion, low battery, syringe clamp, zero rate
Miscellaneous comments: Capable of detecting pressure in excess of 6 psi, will alarm, uses 3 manufacturers' syringes

Medfusion Inc.

Address: 3450 River Green Ct., Duluth, GA 30136
Instrument name/model: MedFusion Model 2010 Syringe Pump
Instrument cost: $2445   **Set cost:** $43.75–$123.75/box
Flow/rate range: 0.1–378.0 ml/hr—dependent on syringe size selected
Accuracy: ±3%
Net weight: 2.5 lb
Power requirements: AC adapter; DC internal rechargeable batteries
System alarms: Near-empty, empty, occlusion, system malfunction, low battery, depleted battery, syringe pops out, invalid size, invalid number, check clutch, others
Miscellaneous comments: Delivers in µg/kg/min, µg/kg/hr, mg/kg/min, mg/kg/hr, and ml/hr; automatically senses syringe size

Medfusion Inc.

Address: 3450 River Green Ct., Duluth, GA 30136
Instrument name/model: MedFusion Model 2001 Syringe Pump
Instrument cost: $2195   **Set cost:** $43.75–$123.75/box
Flow/rate range: 0.1–378.0 ml/hr
Accuracy: ±3%
Net weight: 2.5 lb
Power requirements: AC adapter; DC internal rechargeable batteries
System alarms: Near-empty, empty, volume limit, occlusion, system malfunction, low battery, depleted battery, syringe not loaded, keep vein open, others
Miscellaneous comments: Delivers in contuous, volume over time and intermittent modes; automatically senses syringe size

Razel Scientific Instruments, Inc.

Address: 100 Research Drive, Stamford, CT 06906
Instrument name/model: Model A-99, FHM
Instrument cost: $410   **Set cost:**   N/A
Flow/rate range: 0.025–140 ml/hr
Accuracy: ±2%   **Net weight:**   7.5 lb
Power requirements: AC: 115V, 60 Hz
System alarms: End of syringe alarm
Miscellaneous comments: Optional: 12-volt external battery connection; syringe sizes 5–60ml; microsyringe adapter

Razel Scientific Instruments, Inc.

Address: 100 Research Drive, Stamford, CT 06906
Instrument name/model: Model A.EhVY

Instrument cost: $190   **Set cost:** Not supplied
Flow/rate range: 0.1 ml/hr—24 ml/min
Accuracy: ±1%   **Net weight:** 4 lb
Power requirements: AC: 115V, 60 Hz
System alarms: Optional
Miscellaneous comments: Syringe pump shuts off at end of syringe

Pumps

Abbott Laboratories

Address: One Abbott Park Road, Department 993, Building AP30, Abbott
Park, IL 60064
Instrument name/model: LifeCare Provider 5500
Instrument cost: $3495   **Set cost:** $12
Flow/rate range: 0.1–999 ml/hr
Accuracy: ±5%   **Net weight:** 14 oz
Power requirements: 2 9V alkaline batteries
System alarms: Occlusion, air in line (optional), low reservoir, low battery,
system defect
Miscellaneous comments: Continuous, continuous with bolus, bolus only, in-
termittent delivery; no captive reservoir; optional lock box

Abbott Laboratories

Address: One Abbott Park Road, Department 993, Building AP30, Abbott
Park, IL 60064
Instrument name/model: Provider 6000 Dual Channel
Instrument cost: $5195   **Set cost:** $22.92
Flow/rate range: 0.1–250 ml/hr per channel
Accuracy: ±5%   **Net weight:** 31 oz
Power requirements: 2 9V alkaline batteries
System alarms: Occlusion, cartridge improperly inserted, air in line, dose
limit exceeded, low battery, empty container, end of infusion, call-back alert,
system error
Miscellaneous comments: Designed to run 2 independent programs, contin-
uous delivery, continuous with PCA, PCA only and intermittent

Abbott Laboratories

Address: One Abbott Park Road, Department 993, Building AP30, Abbott
Park, IL 60064
Instrument name/model: LifeCare Omni-Flow 4000
Instrument cost: $5665   **Set cost:** N/A
Flow/rate range: 1.4–800 ml/hr
Accuracy: ±4% total system   **Net weight:** 13.25 lb
Power requirements: AC: 120V
System alarms: Cassette unlocked, possible faulty cassette, air in line, oc-
clusion in patient line, empty container, low battery
Miscellaneous comments: 4 medications simultaneously and/or intermit-
tently at different rates and volumes from bags, bottles, syringes; auto dilu-
tion; auto air in line elimination; real-time clock allows preprogramming for
up to 24 hr for continuous or intermittent delivery; needleless connections

Abbott Laboratories

Address: 200 Bullfinch Drive, Andover, MA 01810
Instrument name/model: Omni-Flow Therapist I.V. Medication Management System
Instrument cost: $7995 **Set cost:** N/A
Flow/rate range: 1–700 ml/hr programmable in 9 units of measure
Accuracy: ±4% volume delivered **Net weight:** 15 lb
Power requirements: AC: 120V
System alarms: Cassette unlocked, possible faulty cassette, occlusions in line, full collection bag, air in line, empty container
Miscellaneous comments: Programmable with bar code labels generated by pharmacy; 4 medications simultaneously and/or intermittently from bags, bottles or syringes

Abbott Laboratories

Address: One Abbott Park Road, Department 993, Building AP30, Abbott Park, IL 60064
Instrument name/model: Omni-Flow 4000 Plus
Instrument cost: $6354 **Set cost:** N/A
Flow/rate range: 1–700 ml/hr
Accuracy: ±4% **Net weight:** 13.12 lb
Power requirements: AC: 120V
System alarms: Cassette unlocked, possible faulty cassette, air in line, occlusion in patient line, empty container, low battery
Miscellaneous comments: Same features as Omni-Flow 4000 as well as µg/kg/min dosing; dataway; I.V. history printout capability

Acacia Inc.

Address: P.O. Box 1799, Ojai, CA 93024
Instrument name/model: Pharm Puymp
Instrument cost: $1695 **Set cost:** $375 per 50/case
Flow/rate range: 15 ml/sec
Accuracy: ±1% **Net weight:** 7 lb
Power requirements: AC: 110V, 60 MHz
System alarms: Illogical entry, incorrect entry
Miscellaneous comments: User friendly; can fill PCA syringes and ambulatory medical devices

Applied Science, Inc.

Address: 1300 E. Main Street, Suite 313, Grass Valley, CA 95945
Instrument name/model: UniMed Dispensing Pump
Instrument cost: $1425 **Set cost:** $5.90–$8.25
Flow/rate range: Avg., 10 ml/sec
Accuracy: *Varies with volume* **Net weight:** 8 lb
Power requirements: Wall-mounted, 24V, UL approved AC transformer
System alarms: Audio and visual
Miscellaneous comments: Functions microprocessor controlled; LCD display; lightweight; compact design for all types of admixture procedures; syringe-filling module available

Applied Science, Inc.

Address: 1300 E. Main Street, Suite 313, Grass Valley, CA 95945
Instrument name/model: Gravity-Comp TPN Gravimetric Scale
Instrument cost: $1325 **Set cost:** $5.85–$7.95
Flow/rate range: Approximately 90 sec/L
Accuracy: ±3% or 3 ml, whichever is greater **Net weight:** 4 lb
Power requirements: Wall-mounted, 24 V, UL approved AC transformer
System alarms: Audio and visual
Miscellaneous comments: Functions microprocessor controlled; LCD display; extremely lightweight; compact design; mix 6 solutions; optional printer; RS232 port

Armstrong Medical Industries, Inc.

Address: 575 Knightsbridge Parkway, P.O. Box 700, Lincolnshire, IL 60069
Instrument name/model: AE-1405 MTP Miniature Transport Infusion Pump
Instrument cost: $1975 **Set cost:** Extension Pump Set: $108.75 box of 25
Flow/rate range: 1–499.9 ml/hr, in 1-ml increments
Accuracy: Accurate to ±2% **Net weight:** 4 lb
Power requirements: Hospital grade AC plug and cord; gell cell battery: 8 hr continuous use
System alarms: Tamper alarm; start/stop switch allows halt-resume infusion without loss of microcomputer memory
Miscellaneous comments: Reliable, accurate, user-friendly; adjustable for neonates to adults; accuracy unafffected by position, motion or altitude changes; ideal for transport

Bards Medsystems

Address: 87 Concord Street, North Reading, MA 01864
Instrument name/model: Bard Ambulatory PCA Pump
Instrument cost: $3095 **Set cost:** $8.50
Flow/rate range: 0–20 ml/hr
Accuracy: ±10% **Net weight:** 11 oz
Power requirements: 9V battery
System alarms: Tubing cover open, reservoir cover unlocked, unauthorized entry, occlusion, one-hour limit, system error, end of bag, low battery

Baxa Corporation

Address: 13760 E. Arapahoe Road, Englewood, CO 80112
Instrument name/model: Repeater pump product #095
Instrument cost: $1695 **Set cost:** Varies
Flow/rate range: 13.5 ml/sec (water with a 16-gauge needle)
Accuracy: ±10% at 0.2 ml, ±5% at 0.4 ml, ±2% at 1 ml, ±1% above 2 ml
Net weight: 27.75 lb
Power requirements: AC: 120V, 50–60 Hz, 200 VA
System alarms: Source container empty
Miscellaneous comments: Rapidly pumps any solution and viscosity with accuracy; repeatable precision over prolonged filling operations

Baxter Healthcare Corporation,
I.V. Systems Division

Address: 1425 Lake Cook Road, Deerfield, IL 60015
Instrument name/model: Flo-Gard 8200 Volumetric InfusionPump
Instrument cost: List $3195   **Set cost:** $9.96–$12.80
Flow/rate range: 1–999 ml/hr
Accuracy: ±4%   **Net weight:** 5.5 kg (12.1 lb)
Power requirements: AC: 115V, 60 Hz; DC: Internal lead acid battery
System alarms: Low battery, high and low flow, occlusion, cradle down, no cassette, snooze, malfunctions
Miscellaneous comments: All rate pump with adult and micro modes; flow-check displays, computer-controlled; auto piggyback

Baxter Healthcare Corporation,
I.V. Systems Division

Address: 1425 Lake Cook Road, Deerfield, IL 60015
Instrument name/model: Flo-Gard 6300 Dual-Channel Volmetric Infusion Pump
Instrument cost: List $6694   **Set cost:** Uses standard sets
Flow/rate range: 0.1–1999 ml/hr, in 1-ml increments
Accuracy: ±5%   **Net weight:** 17.5 lb (6.7 kg)
Power requirements: AC: 115V, 60 Hz, 50 W; battery life: 6 hr with one channel operating, 4 hr with two channels operating.
System alarms: Downstream and upstream occlusion, air in line, alarm log, door open, low battery
Miscellaneous comments: Dual rate automatic piggybacking; panel lockout; auto restart; flow check volume; time programming

Baxter Healthcare Corporation,
I.V. Systems Division

Address: 1425 Lake Cook Road, Deerfield, IL 60015
Instrument name/model: Flo-Gard 6200 Dual-Channel Volmetric Infusion Pump
Instrument cost: List $3719   **Set cost:** Uses standard sets
Flow/rate range: 0.1–999 ml/hr, in 1-ml increments
Accuracy: ±5%   **Net weight:** 14 lb (6.7 kg)
Power requirements: AC: 115V, 60 Hz, 10 W; battery life: 6 hr at 125 ml/hr
System alarms: Downstream and upstream occlusion, air in line, door open, low battery
Miscellaneous comments: Dual rate automatic piggybacking; panel lockout

Excelsior Medical Corporation

Address: P.O. Box 1353, Asbury Park, NJ 07712
Instrument name/model: PharmAssist Peristaltic Dispensing Pump
Instrument cost: $1995   **Set cost:** $7.95
Flow/rate range: Up to 14.4 ml/sec
Accuracy: ±1%   **Net weight:** 15 lb
Power requirements: 115V nominal
System alarms: Incorrect entry, end of cycle

Miscellaneous comments: Increase accuracy and speed in many applications; for more information, call (800) 4U-PHARM or (800) 427-4276

Ivac Corporation

Address: 10300 Campus Point Drive, San Diego, CA 92121-1519
Instrument name/model: Variable Pressure Volumetric Pump, Model 570
Instrument cost: $3750   **Set cost:** $4.85
Flow/rate range: 1–999 ml/hr, in 1 ml/hr increments (standard), 0.1–999.9 ml/hr (all-rate range)
Net weight: 14.25 lb
Power requirements: AC: 100–120V, 50–60 Hz, 0.50 A, three-wire grounded, battery approximately 5 hr at 125 ml/hr
System alarms: Occlusion, low battery, open door, air in line, infusion complete, malfunction
Miscellaneous comments: True variable pressure, all-rate range, computer interfaces, optional flow sensor, adjustable air in line setting (50–150 ml)

Ivac Corporation

Address: 10300 Campus Point Drive, San Diego, CA 92121-1519
Instrument name/model: Space Saver Pump, Model 599
Instrument cost: $2400   **Set cost:** $3.10
Flow/rate range: 1–999 ml/hr
Net weight: 6 lb
Power requirements: AC: 90–126V, 50–60 Hz
System alarms: Occlusion, low battery, open door, air in line, set out, discharge battery, malfunction
Miscellaneous comments: Small, lightweight, easy to use, dual rate

Ivion Corporation

Address: 2400 Industrial Lane, Broomfield, CO 80020
Instrument name/model: Ivion KKIDS Large Volume Pump
Instrument cost: $2695   **Set cost:** $150–$280/box
Flow/rate range: 0.1–999.9 ml/hr, in 0.1 ml/hr increments
Accuracy: Not supplied   **Net weight:**   11 lb
Power requirements: AC: 117V nominal, 0.30 A, 60 Hz, internal rechargeable batteries
System alarms: Pump not infusing, cassette/door open, patient occlusion, bottle occlusion, air in cassette, system check, KVO ≤ ml/hr, low battery
Miscellaneous comments: Delivery of maintenance fluids, TPN, blood products and vasopressors; air trapping cassette; patient occlusion monitor

Ivion Corporation

Address: 2400 Industrial Lane, Broomfield, CO 80020
Instrument name/model: Ivion EZ-1 Large Volume Pump
Instrument cost: $2695   **Set cost:** $150–$280/box
Flow/rate range: 0.1–999.9 ml/hr, in 0.1 ml/hr increments
Accuracy: Not supplied   **Net weight:**   11 lb
Power requirements: AC: 117-V nominal, 0.30 A, 60 Hz, internal rechargeable batteries

System alarms: Pump not infusing, cassette/door open, patient occlusion, bottle occlusion, air in cassette, system check, KVO ≤ ml/hr, low battery
Miscellaneous comments: Delivery of maintenance fluids, TPN, blood products and vasopressors; air trapping cassette; patient occlusion monitor

McGaw, Inc.

Address: 2525 McGaw Avenue, Irvine, CA 92713
Instrument name/model: Model 521C MicroRate Plus Intelligent Pump
Instrument cost: $3800   **Set cost:** $4.50–$12
Flow/rate range: 0.1–99.9 ml/hr
Accuracy: ±2%   **Net weight:** 12 lb
Power requirements: AC: 120V
System alarms: Full range including occlusion, air in line, empty container, door open, others
Miscellaneous comments: Micro operation; variable pressure; operations log

McGaw, Inc.

Address: 2525 McGaw Avenue, Irvine, CA 92713
Instrument name/model: Model 521 Plus Intelligent Pump
Instrument cost: $3800   **Set cost:** $4.50–$12
Flow/rate range: 0.1–99.9 ml/hr
Accuracy: ±2%   **Net weight:** 12 lb
Power requirements: AC: 120V
System alarms: Full range including occlusion, air in line, empty container, door open, others
Miscellaneous comments: Automatic TPN ramping; variable pressure; operations log; programmable infusion

McGaw, Inc.

Address: 2525 McGaw Avenue, Irvine, CA 92713
Instrument name/model: Model 522 Intelligent Pump
Instrument cost: $3800   **Set cost:** $4.50–$12
Flow/rate range: 0.1–99.9 ml/hr
Accuracy: ±2%   **Net weight:** 12 lb
Power requirements: AC: 120V
System alarms: Full range including occlusion, air in line, empty container, door open, others
Miscellaneous comments: Variable pressure; automatic piggybacking; titration mode; operations log; panel lockout

McGaw, Inc.

Address: 2525 McGaw Avenue, Irvine, CA 92713
Instrument name/model: Horizon Modular Infusion System
Instrument cost: $4200   **Set cost:** $4.50–$12
Flow/rate range: 0.1–999.9 ml/hr
Accuracy: Not supplied   **Net weight:** 11.9 lb
Power requirements: AC: 90–125V or 180–264V
System alarms: Full range including occlusion, air in line, empty container, door open, others

Miscellaneous comments: Dose rate calculation; stackable; variable pressure; micro/macro rate changes; free-flow protection; computer interface; daisy-chained power cords

Medical Technology Products, Inc.

Address: 107 Woodbury Road, Huntington, NY 11743
Instrument name/model: MVP-1 1000, 1000A
Instrument cost: $1975 **Set cost:** $4.35 each
Flow/rate range: Model 1000: 1–499.9 ml/hr (Volume 1–999 ml); Model 1000A: 0.11–499 ml/hr (volume 1–9999 ml)
Accuracy: ±2% **Net weight:** 4.5 lb
Power requirements: AC: 110–115V available; DC: 12 V adapter, battery life: 6 hr
System alarms: Air occlusion, no flow (empty container), low battery infusion complete (KVO) tamper
Miscellaneous comments: Alarm message displayed on bright LED display; gravity prime set; impact-resistant case; nitro tubing available

3M Infusion Therapy

Address: 3M Center, Bldg. 275-5W-05, St. Paul, MN 55144-1000
Instrument name/model: AVI 480 Infusion Pump
Instrument cost: $2800 **Set cost:** Standard set #201: $5.44
Flow/rate range: 1–999 ml/hr
Accuracy: ±2% **Net weight:** 9.5 lb
Power requirements: AC: 120V
System alarms: Full range of visual and audio alarms
Miscellaneous comments: Continuous, nonpulsatile delivery; needleless upstream air removal; free-flow prevention in set

3M Infusion Therapy

Address: 3M Center, Bldg. 275-5W-05, St. Paul, MN 55144-1000
Instrument name/model: AVI 285 Micro Infusion Pump
Instrument cost: $2900 **Set cost:** Standard set #201: $5.44
Flow/rate range: 1–9.99 ml/hr
Accuracy: ±2% **Net weight:** 9.5 lb
Power requirements: AC: 120V
System alarms: Full range of visual and audio alarms
Miscellaneous comments: Continuous, nonpulsatile delivery; needleless upstream air removal; free-flow prevention in set

3M Infusion Therapy

Address: 3M Center, Bldg. 275-5W-05, St. Paul, MN 55144-1000
Instrument name/model: AVI 880 Dual Channel Infusion Pump
Instrument cost: $5335 **Set cost:** Standard set #201: $5.44
Flow/rate range: 1–999 ml/hr, each channel
Accuracy: ±2% **Net weight:** 16.5 lb
Power requirements: AC: 120V
System alarms: Full range of visual and audio alarms

Miscellaneous comments: Two channels with separate control; continuous nonpulsatile delivery, needleless upstream air removal; free-flow prevention in set

3M Infusion Therapy

Address: 3M Center, Bldg. 275-5W-05, St. Paul, MN 55144-1000
Instrument name/model: AVI 885 Micro Dual Channel Infusion Pump
Instrument cost: $5560 **Set cost:** Standard set #201: $5.44
Flow/rate range: 0.1–99.9 ml/hr
Accuracy: ±2% **Net weight:** 16.5 lb
Power requirements: AC: 120V
System alarms: Full range of visual and audio alarms
Miscellaneous comments: Two channels with separate controls; continuous nonpulsatile delivery, needleless upstream air removal; free-flow prevention in set

Controllers

Abbott Laboratories

Address: One Abbott Park Road, Department 993, Building AP30, Abbott Park, IL 60064
Instrument name/model: Breeze Model 75 Volumetric Controller
Instrument cost: List $1835 **Set cost:** $1.75–$3.50
Flow/rate range: Microdrip 5–250 ml/hr; macrodrip 20–400 ml/hr
Accuracy: ±10% total system **Net weight:** 8 lb
Power requirements: AC: 117V, 60 Hz and 16 V (nominal)
System alarms: Dose end, flow, no flow, low battery, malfunction
Miscellaneous comments: Simple to set up and use; incorporates graphics on screen; uses standard ABBOTT sets

Ivac Corporation

Address: 10300 Campus Point Drive, San Diego, CA 92121-1519
Instrument name/model: Volumetric Controller, Model 262+
Instrument cost: $1800 **Set cost:** $2.50
Flow/rate range: 5–299 ml/hr
Net weight: 13 lb
Power requirements: AC: 115V; 60 Hz; battery life 6 hr (fully charged)
System alarms: Empty fluid container, closed clamp, low battery, occlusion, unattainable rate (under current conditions), mispositioned flow sensor, opened latch
Miscellaneous comments: Flow status indicator, monitoring system capable of detecting most infiltrations, volumetric rate entry, LED display panel, set-up prompts

McGaw, Inc.

Address: 2525 McGaw Avenue, Irvine, CA 92713
Instrument name/model: Model 2001 Intelligent Infusor
Instrument cost: $3800 **Set cost:** $4.50–$12
Flow/rate range: 2–399 ml/hr

Accuracy: ±2%   **Net weight:** 11.5 lb
Power requirements: AC: 90–125 V
System alarms: Full range including low flow, air, door open, low battery
Miscellaneous comments: Volumetric, automatic piggybacking

I.V. Devices

I.V. Flow Regulators

Abbott Laboratories

Address: 1 Abbott Park Road, Abbott Park, IL 60064
Product type: I.V. flow regulators
Product name/model: Plum LifeCare 5000 Enteral Pump Set w/Integral Container #6492
Product cost: Not supplied   **Set cost:** Not supplied
Product specifications: Integral enteral container, 1000 ml volume, top feeding, and special enteral catheter adapter; 105 inches long

Abbott Laboratories

Address: 1 Abbott Park Road, Abbott Park, IL 60064
Product type: I.V. flow regulators
Product name/model: Micro Pump Microdrip Set-SL #9289
Product cost: Not supplied   **Set cost:** Not supplied
Product specifications: Micro pump cassette with Secure Lock may be utilized with LifeCare Micro Pump for delivery of epidural administration

Abbott Laboratories

Address: 1 Abbott Park Road, Abbott Park, IL 60064
Product type: I.V. flow regulators
Product name/model: Venoset Primary Piggyback Set w/IVEX HP-NV, #1792
Product cost: Not supplied   **Set cost:** Not supplied
Product specifications: Automatic primary piggybacking set to be utilized with LifeCare series Macro pumps, model numbers III, IV, IV-P; sterilizing grade high pressure .22 micron filter and Secure Lock male adapter; facilitates use with Model IV-P

Abbott Laboratories

Address: 1 Abbott Park Road, Abbott Park, IL 60064
Product type: I.V. flow regulators
Product name/model: Plum LifeCare 5000 Primary Set w/Capped Secondary Port #11419
Product cost: Not supplied   **Set cost:** Not supplied
Product specifications: 104″ primary vented Plumset with capped secondary port and prepierced reseal; to be utilized in LifeShield needle-less secondary administration; set also contains Secure Lock at male adapter

Abbott Laboratories

Address: 1 Abbott Park Road, Abbott Park, IL 60064
Product type: I.V. flow regulators

Product name/model: 11140, 11137, 11141, and 2422—Miscellaneous sets
Product cost: Not supplied **Set cost:** Not supplied
Product specifications: The pediatric dual-capped port, primary Plumset #2422 may be utilized for various drug delivery applications. Accessories shown facilitate flexibility of delivery therapy in the pediatric neonatology area; able to deliver dual-syringe capability

Baxter Healthcare Corporation

Address: Route 102 & Wilson Road, Round Lake, IL 60073
Product type: I.V. flow regulators
Product name/model: Control-A-Flow Regulator
Product cost: Not supplied **Set cost:** Not supplied
Product specifications: I.V. flow regulator with oscillating membrane technology; keeps flow rates within ±10% despite changes in head height between 30 and 60 inches; reduces risk of "runaway" I.V.s; easy-to-read flow rate dial
Miscellaneous comments: Compatible with any I.V. tubing; extension and in-line sets available

3M Infusion Therapy

Address: 3M Center, Bldg 2754-5W-05, St. Paul, MN 55144-1000
Product type: I.V. flow regulators
Product name/model: 3M IV Flow Regulator, Model 27000
Product cost: $6.72 (list) **Set cost:** Not supplied
Product specifications: Features a unique, patented pressure-sensitive membrane that responds to fluctuations in pressure and automatically compensates to maintain the setflow rate within ±10% accuracy. Clinically tested. Used with central or peripheral lines; any size catheter

Nonelectronic Pump Devices

Healthtek, Inc.

Address: 870 Gold Flat Road, Nevada City, CA 95959
Product type: Nonelectronic pump devices
Product name/model: ADFuse—#AF0630, #AF0650, #AF0690
Product cost: Not supplied **Set cost:** $12.50 each
Product specifications: ADFuse is a user-friendly, compact, completely disposable system used for controlled infusion of small-volume parenteral medications. Up to 60 ml of solution is administered in preset times of 30, 50 or 90 minutes
Miscellaneous comments: Inert materials are compatible with virtually all drugs; can be frozen

Prime Medical Products, Inc.

Address: 2 E. Lakeshore Drive, Round Lake Park, IL 60073
Product type: Nonelectronic pump devices
Product name/model: CADI-120-2, CADI-120-5
Product cost: 120-2, $45.00/120-5, $24.00 **Set cost:** Included
Product specifications: The disposable Continuous-Ambulatory-Drug-Infuser features proven drug-stable 120 ml graduated polypropylene reservoir. De-

tachable fixed rate FlowSet and constant vacuum pressure delivers ±10% accuracy for chemotherapy, antibiotic and pain medications without bursts
Miscellaneous comments: Non-pyrogenic easy-fill syringe-style reservoir exceeds USP Class VI. Call toll-free: 800-488-CADI

3M Infusion Therapy

Address: 3M Center, Bldg. 275-5W-05, St. Paul, MN 55144-1000
Product type: Nonelectronic pump devices
Product name/model: Medifuse small volume infuser
Product cost: $210 (list) **Set cost:** Not supplied
Product specifications: Uses 10 ml to 35 ml Monoject or B-D syringes; infusion rate regulated by Medifuse set; for antibiotic delivery; two sets provide infusion times up to 30 and 60 minutes; no programming; easy to use; no gravity
Miscellaneous comments: For continuous infusions; Medifuse infuser also offers sets that regulate rates as low as 1 ml/hr

Elastomeric Balloon Devices

Baxter Healthcare Corporation,
I.V. System Division

Address: 1425 Lake Cook Road, Deerfield, IL 60015
Product type: Elastomeric balloon devices
Product name/model: Intermate 50 (44050), Intermate 100 (44120), Intermate LV50 (49050), Intermate LV250 (49250), Intermate HPC100 (47100), Intermate 200 (44220)
Product cost: Not supplied **Set cost:** Not supplied
Product specifications: Provides flow rates for: 1/2-, 1-, 2- and 5-hr infusions; offers home infusion patients increased freedom with a portable, safe, effective and discrete system; maximum capacity: 105 ml and 255 ml
Miscellaneous comments: Positive pressure elastomeric technology eliminates gravity flow problems and programming errors

Baxter Health Care Corporation,
I.V. System Division

Address: 1425 Lake Cook Road, Deerfield, IL 60015
Product type: Elastomeric balloon devices
Product name/model: Intermate LV System—100 ml/hr (49100)
Product cost: Not supplied **Set cost:** Not supplied
Product specifications: Delivers 250 ml volume in 2 1/2 hrs. at 100 ml/hr. Ideal for infusing larger volume drugs such as vancomycin and foscarnet. Joins a system for delivery of I.V. antibiotics and drugs often associated with AIDS treatment, such as amphotericin B, ganciclovir and foscarnet
Miscellaneous comments: Offers home infusion patients increased freedom with a portable, safe, effective and discrete elastomeric delivery system

Baxter Healthcare Corporation,
I.V. System Division

Address: 1425 Lake Cook Road, Deerfield, IL 60015
Product type: Elastomeric balloon devices

Product name/model: Multiday Infusor (2C1080), Singleday Infusor (2C1071), Halfday Infusor (2C1073), Sevenday Infusor (2C1082).
Product cost: Not supplied **Set cost:** Not supplied
Product specifications: Provides flow rates for 12-hour, 24-hour, 5-day and 7-day infusion; offers oncology patients the opportunity to continue their daily activities with a portable, safe, effective and discrete elastomeric delivery system
Miscellaneous comments: System provides dependable flow-rate accuracy and wide choice of infusion times

Baxter Healthcare Corporation,
I.V. System Division—Pain Therapy

Address: 1425 Lake Cook Road, Deerfield, IL 60015
Product type: Elastomeric balloon devices
Product name/model: PCA Infusors (Code 2C1073, 2C1955, 2C1954), PCA Module (2C10790)
Product cost: Not supplied **Set cost:** Not supplied
Product specifications: Lightweight, disposable device that dispenses medication at a continuous rate of 0.5 ml/hr (depending on code used), and when used with PCA Module will deliver a bolus dose of 0.5 ml on patient demand every 6, 15, or 60 minutes
Miscellaneous comments: Ideally suited for infusion of analgesics for pain management

Block Medical, Inc.

Address: 5957 Landau Court, Carlsbad, CA 92008
Product type: Elastomeric balloon devices
Product name/model: Elastomeric infusion system Homepump—H101000, H201750, H100020, H102000, H050500, H100050
Product cost: Not supplied **Set cost:** Not required
Product specifications: Volume capacity: 60 ml to 205 ml; preset flow rates ranging from 2 ml/h to 175 ml/h; positive pressure 10 psi. Weight: 4 to 8 oz when filled; in-line air eliminating filter; portable; color-coded flow rate labels
Miscellaneous comments: Self-contained, disposable system for use in antibiotic and chemotherapy delivery; highly drug-compatible elastomeric membrane

Secure Medical/MacLean-Fogg Company

Address: 1000 Allanson Road, Mundelein, IL 60060
Product type: Elastomeric balloon devices
Product name/model: Medflo Ambulatory Infusion Device
Product cost: Not supplied **Set cost:** Not supplied
Product specifications: The new Medflo Ambulatory Infusion Device highlights an easily fillable balloon and unique ergonomic shape with integral stand. Initial introduction includes 100 ml and 200 ml sizes with 50 ml/hr, 100 ml/hr, and 175 ml/hr flow rates
Miscellaneous comments: Drug compatibility data is available for most commonly prescribed antibiotics.

Fluid-Dispensing Systems

Acacia Incorporated

Address: 1482 S. Gage Street, San Bernardino, CA 92408
Product type: Fluid-dispensing systems
Product name/model: 17789, LY100NV, M-1, 1Pharm-6 (single-lead sets)
Product cost: Not supplied   **Set cost:** Up to $7.95/set
Product specifications: New bar connector for easy and consistent insertion into many pumps (Mach One, Mach Two, ADS100, Wheaton, Pharm-Assist and others); sets available in dual and triple leads with the option of finger grips
Miscellaneous comments: Acacia specializes in many pumping chamber assemblies. If you have special needs, please call

Acacia Incorporated

Address: 1482 S. Gage Street, San Bernardino, CA 92408
Product type: Fluid-dispensing systems
Product name/model: Universal Sterile Syringe Tip Adaptor Model #18888
Product cost: $0.65 each, 250/case
Product specifications: Used with a peristaltic pump for syringe batching procedures; can also be used for syringe-to-syringe transfers

Burron Medical, Inc.

Address: 824 12th Avenue, Bethlehem, PA 18018
Product type: Fluid-dispensing systems
Product name/model: Micro-Comp Admixture Compounding System
Product cost: Micro-Comp Stand: $70 each   **Set cost:** 5-unit Micro-Comp Unit: $19.95 each (hospital list)
Product specifications: Designed to meet the individual needs of a pharmacy, Micro-Comp is a compact, self-contained system to access multi-dose additive vials with standard Luer-lock syringes when dispensing micro-nutrients into a TPN bag
Miscellaneous comments: Burron's complete Multi-Ad System is compatible with Micro-Comp

Burron Medical, Inc.

Address: 824 12th Avenue, Bethlehem, PA 18018
Product type: Fluid-dispensing systems
Product name/model: Multi-Ad Syringes—MA-3000, MA-1000, MACC-1000, MAC-1001
Product cost: Range: $9–$12 each   **Set cost:** Not supplied
Product specifications: 10 ml or 30 ml automatic, repetitive dosing system; a choice of either straight or contoured handle on the 10 ml model

Burron Medical, Inc.

Address: 824 12th Avenue, Bethlehem, PA 18018
Product type: Fluid-dispensing systems
Product name/model: Multi-Ad Transfer Set—MAT-4100
Product cost: $4.50 each (hospital list)   **Set cost:** Not supplied

Product specifications: Vented, universal spike and 40″ transfer set connected to automatic two-way valve for closed system approach to multi-dose fluid transfer

Clintec Nutrition Company

Address: 3 Parkway North, Suite 500, Deerfield, IL 60015
Product type: Fluid-dispensing systems
Product name/model: Micromix Compounder
Product cost: Not supplied **Set cost:** Not supplied
Product specifications: Micromix is an automated 10-station gravimetric compounding pump for efficient, accurate "hands-free" transfer of TPN micronutrients or other small-volume I.V. additives. The system maximizes control and efficiency, and reduces potential for touch contamination. The compounder can be interfaced with Clintec's Multitask Operating System (MOS) Software

Clintec Nutrition Company

Address: 3 Parkway North, Suite 500, Deerfield, IL 60015
Product type: Fluid-dispensing systems
Product name/model: Automix 3 + 3 Compounder
Product cost: Not supplied **Set cost:** Not supplied
Product specifications: Automix 3 + 3 is a six-station gravimetric compounding pump for efficient and accurate transfer of TPN base solutions or other large-volume IV fluids. The compounder can optionally be interfaced with Clintec's Multitask Operating System (MOS) software

Clintec Nutrition Company

Address: 3 Parkway North, Suite 500, Deerfield, IL 60015
Product type: Fluid-dispensing systems
Product name/model: Automix Plus Compounder
Product cost: Not supplied **Set cost:** Not supplied
Product specifications: Automix Plus is a three-station gravimetric compounding pump for efficient and accurate transfer of TPN base solutions or other large-volume I.V. fluids. The compounder can optionally be interfaced with Clintec's Multitask Operating System (MOS) software

Healthtek, Inc.

Address: 870 Gold Flat Road, Nevada City, CA 95959
Product type: Fluid-dispensing systems
Product name/model: Filtrare 25-mm Syringe Filters
Product cost: $1.12–$1.31 **Set cost:** Not supplied
Product specifications: Filtrare syringe filters are used for a wide variety of filtering and venting applications. Porosities range from 0.22 to 5.0 microns: color-coded for ease of use
Miscellaneous comments: Low protein binding: no surfactants to wash off

Surgin Inc.

Address: 1030 Richfield Road, Placentia, CA 92670
Product type: Fluid-dispensing systems

Product name/model: ABSOLUTE 0.22 Bacterial Filter
Product cost: $26.75   **Set cost:**   Not supplied
Product specifications: The ABSOLUTE 0.22 micron filter is a high-flow bactrerial filter designed for high-volume retention. The ABSOLUTE filter is bacterial-retentive for 24 hours and is manufactured with appropriate connectors for multiple use
Miscellaneous comments: Cost-effective for high-volume filtration

Surgin Inc.

Address: 1030 Richfield Road, Placentia, CA 92670
Product type: Fluid-dispensing systems
Product name/model: Multi-Spike
Product cost: 5700—$19.00; 5702—$15.00   **Set cost:**   Not supplied
Product specifications: Multi-Spike is a multiple-use fluid dispensing system. It will allow, with standard aseptic technique, the use of a single-dose container for up to three applications
Miscellaneous comments: Safe and effective sterile dispensing system

I.V. Protective Devices

Baxter Healthcare Corporation

Address: Route 120 and Wilson Road RLT-02, Round Lake, IL 60073
Product type: I.V. protective devices
Product name/model: InterLink IV Access System
Product cost: Not supplied   **Set cost:**   Not supplied
Product specifications: Comprehensive needleless system for I.V. administration, blood sampling, heparin lock therapy and drug vial access. Blunt cannula replaces sharp steel needles. Companion injection cap, tubing, vial adapter and prefilled syringes create a versatile system
Miscellaneous comments: Can eliminate up to 80% of needles used in hospitals

Baxter Healthcare Corporation

Address: Route 120 and Wilson Road RLT-02, Round Lake, IL 60073
Product type: I.V. protective devices
Product name/model: Needle*Lock
Product cost: Not supplied   **Set cost:**   Not supplied
Product specifications: Easy-to-use protected needle device helps prevent needlesticks; available with 18- or 20-gauge needles; sold alone or with administration sets; Luer-locks to all Luer connectors; locks to injection sites for secure piggyback connections

Becton Dickinson Division

Address: 1 Stanley Street, Rutherford, NJ 07070
Product type: I.V. protective devices
Product name/model: InterLink I.V. Access System
Product cost: $0.22–$2.00   **Set cost:**   Not supplied
Product specifications: InterLink I.V. Access products reduce needlesticks by eliminating steel hypodermic needles. Blunt plastic cannulas penetrate a

special septum on the InterLink injection site used for intermittent or pig-gyback doses. InterLink system sold jointly by Baxter I.V. and BD
Miscellaneous comments: InterLink products include engineering controls required by OSHA's worker protection regulations

Becton Dickinson Division

Address: 1 Stanley Street, Rutherford, NJ 07070
Product type: I.V. protective devices
Product name/model: Safety-Gard I.V. Needle
Product cost: $0.365/each **Set cost:** Not supplied
Product specifications: Provides passive needlestick protection by eliminating exposed needles for I.V. therapy procedures. Fits most standard heparin locks and Y-sites. Easy to use. Requires no additional parts or changes in systems
Miscellaneous comments: Works particularly well for heparin lock therapy

Critikon, Inc.

Address: P.O. Box 31800, Tampa, FL
Product type: I.V. protective devices
Product name/model: Protectiv I.V. Catheter
Product cost: $2.50 **Set cost:** Not supplied
Product specifications: As the catheter is slid off the introducer needle, a protective guard slides into place over the needle and locks into place permanently before the needle is removed from the catheter hub

McGaw, Inc

Address: 2525 McGaw Ave., Irvin, CA 92713-9791
Product type: I.V. protective devices
Product name/model: Protected Needle N2300, V1921-23, V1922-23, V6312-23
Product cost: $1.82 (list) **Set cost:** Not supplied
Product specifications: Lock onto syringe for I.V. push; protects against accidental needlesticks; snap and lock into place over McGaw Y-site

Medi-Dose, Inc./E.P.S., Inc

Address: 1671 Loretta Avenue, Feasterville, PA 19053-9393
Product type: I.V. protective devices
Product name: ESP Nultraviolet Bag
Product model: PC190, 8" × 14"; PC191, 5" × 7.5"; PC 192, 2.5" × 8.5"; PC193, 2" × 2.5"; PC195, 11" × 18"; RB541220, 12" × 20"
Product cost: PC190, $70/M, $38.50/500; PC191, $30.50/M, $16.75/500; PC192, $18/M; PC193, $10/M; PC195, $125/M; RB541220, $315/M
Product specifications: 96.7% effective against the U/V spectral range. Place over I.V. bottles, bags, or syringe for protection against harmful effects of U/V light
Miscellaneous comments: Toll-free phone: (800) 523-8966, toll-free fax: (800) 323-8966

Medipak, Inc.

Address: P.O. Box 3248, Winchester, VA 22601
Product type: I.V. protective devices
Product name/model: UVLI Bag
Product cost: $38.50/1000 to $165/1000, depending on size and quantity
Product specifications: Clear amber film protects light-sensitive I.V.s. Regularly tested to meet USP standards for light-protective containers. Six sizes for I.V.s, from piggybacks to 4-liter, plus convenient slit-top bags. Also available: six other sizes plus special order sizes
Miscellaneous comments: Telephone (800) 336-9848 for price list and samples

Sanofi Winthrop Pharmaceuticals

Address: 90 Park Avenue, New York, NY 10016
Product type: I.V. protective devices
Product name/model: Carpuject sterile cartridge-needle unit: The Safety System
Product cost: Not supplied **Set cost:** Not supplied
Production specifications: Carpuject Safety System's special safety holder helps protect health care workers from needlesticks by avoiding the necessity of recapping needles. The Carpuject line has heparin, Demerol morphine, Talwin and other injectables
Miscellaneous comments: Clear holder provides 100% visibility for accurate reading of dosage and collaborations and is compatible with all products in Carpuject's line; twist/lock holder makes loading faster and easier with 2-step activation; lightweight, durable holder provides secure, stable injections

Dispensing Pins/Venting Systems

Acacia Inc.

Address: P.O. Box 1799, Ojai, CA 93024
Product type: Dispensing pins/venting systems
Product name/model: Mini Transfer Pin 19999MTP
Product cost: 100/case, $85/case **Set cost:** Not supplied
Product specifications: Acacia's 19999MTP is made of two FDA-approved plastics, giving the product a longer life. Its point remains very sharp after continued use

Acacia Inc.

Address: P.O. Box 1799, Ojai, CA 93024
Product type: Dispensing pins/venting systems
Product name/model: Flow-eze Vented Needle #19999MTP
Product cost: 500/case, $110/case **Set cost:** Not supplied
Product specifications: The Flow-eze Vented Needle has increased the diluent and exhaust ports to aid in ease of delivery of diluent during reconstitution of antibiotic vials

Acacia Inc.

Address: P.O. Box 1799, Ojai, CA 93024
Product type: Dispensing pins/venting systems

Product name/model: Chemo Transfer Pin #19999ChTP
Product cost: 100/case, $165/case **Set cost:** Not supplied
Product specifications: 19999ChTP is made of two FDA-approved plastics giving the product a longer life. Its point remains very sharp after continued use

Becton Dickinson Division

Address: 1 Stanley Street, Rutherford, NJ 07070
Product type: Dispensing pins/venting systems
Product name/model: Sure-Med Dispensing Pin (5230) Safety-Med Dispensing Pin (5231)
Product cost: 5230—$1.25 ea. 5231—$2.35 ea. **Set cost:** Not supplied
Product specifications: Unique pin design allows maximum withdrawal of medication from vial, eliminating need to reposition pin to withdraw remaining residual medication. The Sure-Med includes a 0.45 micron filter; the Safety Med includes a 0.20 micron filter

Burron Medical, Inc.

Address: 824 12th Avenue, Bethlehem, PA 18018
Product type: Dispensing pins/venting systems
Product name/model: Dispensing pins with automatic valve—DP-2500, DP-1500
Product cost: $2.29 each (hospital list) **Set cost:** Not supplied
Product specifications: Standard and mini-spike non-coring dispensing pins allow you to invert any size bag or bottle for easy aspiration and injection without leakage; ideal for large-volume antibiotic reconstitution and compounding
Miscellaneous comments: Shrouds, flanges, and covers minimize the risk of touch contamination

Burron Medical, Inc.

Address: 824 12th Avenue, Bethlehem, PA 18018
Product type: Dispensing pins/venting systems
Product name/model: Chemo Dispensing Pin #CDP-2000
Product cost: $2.45 each (hospital list) **Set cost:** Not supplied
Product specifications: The compact Chemo-Dispensing Pin provides fast venting of powered vials during the reconstitution process with the large-surface 0.2-micron hydrophobic filter
Miscellaneous comments: Used in pharmacies and physicians' offices for more than 10 years

Medi-Dose, Inc./E.P.S., Inc

Address: 1671 Loretta Avenue, Feasterville, PA 19053-9393
Product type: Dispensing pins/venting systems
Product name: Chemo-Spike Reconstitution Device #IV5000
Product model: 50/case: 1–4 cases, $114/case; 5–9 cases, $112/case; 10–24 cases, $111/case; 25–49 cases, $109/case
Product specifications: Angle-mounted 0.22-micron sterilizing filter traps aerosoled meds; streamlining creates short venting pathways and doesn't impede

insertion or aspiration; hinged cap affords additional sterile protection before use, insures security during reconstitution process, provides closed system for disposal; wide finger flange prevents "touch contamination"
Miscellaneous comments: Toll-free phone: (800) 523-8966; toll-free fax: (800) 323-8966

Medi-Dose, Inc./E.P.S., Inc

Address: 1671 Loretta Avenue, Feasterville, PA 19053-9393
Product type: Dispensing pins/venting systems
Product name: I.V. Dispensing-Spike #IV2050
Product model: 50/case: 1–4 cases, $58/case; 5–9 cases, $54/case; 10–24 cases, $52/case; 25–49 cases, $50/case
Product specifications: I.V. Dispensing-Spike for repetitive aspirations from a multiple-dose vial. Natural-color hinged cap on filter opening offers the option of venting or not. The 0.45-micron hydrophobic filter provides proper air displacement. Equipped with a hinged center-port cover-cap, giving additional sterile protection prior to use and ensuring a completely closed system for disposal. Spike design minimizes coring
Miscellaneous comments: Toll-free phone: (800) 523-8966; toll-free fax: (800) 323-8966.

Others

Acacia Inc.

Address: P.O. Box 1799, Ojai, CA 93024
Product type: Filters
Product name/model: FL-1000
Product cost: 100/case, $225/case   **Set cost:** Not supplied
Product specifications: Acacia's FL-1000 has a large 0.22-micron filter area. It is easy to prime and has a longer lifetime of use than the standard round filters sold in hospitals

Bard Access Systems

Address: 5425 West Amelia Earhart Drive, Salt Lake City, UT 84116
Product type: Dual Lumen PICC
Product name/model: Groshong Dual Lumen PICC #7725500
Product cost: 100 tray, $85/case   **Set cost:** Not supplied
Product specifications: The Groshong dual lumen peripherally inserted central catheter is a 5 French catheter with 19 and 20 gauge lumens. The radiopaque silicone catheter incorporates Groshong valves to reduce the possibility of air embolus and blood reflux
Miscellaneous comments: Available in full procedural tray, including repair kit. Bard Access Systems was formerly known as Davol Specialty Access

Baxa Corporation

Address: 13760 E. Arapahoe Road, Englewood, CO 80112
Product type: Luer slip tip caps
Product name/model: Colored Luer Slip Tip Caps Discpac 25 66025 and Discpac 100 66100

Product cost: Not supplied **Set cost:** Not supplied
Product specifications: Sterile self-righting tip caps to fit any Luer syringe. Disk may be reclosed for later use. Will prevent syringe tip breakage and withstand freezing and thawing—25 per Discpac—100 per Discpac
Miscellaneous comments: Available in a wide variety of colors for color coding

Baxa Corporation

Address: 13760 E. Arapahoe Road, Englewood, CO 80112
Product type: Sterile oral dispensers
Product name/model: Sterile Exacta-Med Oral Dispensers Bulk Pack
Product cost: Not supplied **Set cost:** Not supplied
Product specifications: Used for batch filling of sterile or non-sterile respiratory or oral drugs in a sterile environment. Available in a 3 ml, 5 ml or 10 ml oral syringe. Comes with a reclosable disk of sterile oral tip caps

Baxa Corporation

Address: 13760 E. Arapahoe Road, Englewood, CO 80112
Product type: Syringe tip connectors
Product name/model: 13701-Blue, 13901-Pink, 13801 Green, 12701-Clear
Product cost: Not supplied **Set cost:** Not supplied
Product specifications: Blue-sterile Luer-to-Luer connector; pink-sterile Luer-lock-to-Luer-lock connector; green-sterile Luer-lock-to-bag-port connector; clear-Luer to oral connector, sterile or non-sterile
Miscellaneous comments: Luer-to-Luer connector and Luer-lock to Luer-lock connector; available with or without cap

Becton Dickinson Division

Address: 1 Stanley Street, Rutherford, NJ 07070
Product type: Syringes
Product name/model: 10 cc Cornwall Fluid Dispensing Syringe #5224
Product cost: $92.35/case; 10 units **Set cost:** Not supplied
Product specifications: Designed to help overcome fatigue associated with repeated fluid dispensing operations. Equally efficient when used either right- or left-handed. The leaf spring permits faster emptying

Becton Dickinson Division

Address: 1 Stanley Street, Rutherford, NJ 07070
Product type: Needles
Product name/model: No-Kor Filter Needle #5201, Filter Needle 5200
Product cost: Not supplied **Set cost:** Not supplied
Product specifications: No-Kor needle design features eliminate coring and enhance fluid flow. Helps avoid the patient complications and costs that may result from infusion of core-contaminated medication. Unique molded-in membrane filter eliminates possibility of filter disassembly

Becton Dickinson Division

Address: 1 Stanley Street, Rutherford, NJ 07070
Product type: Needles

Product name/model: No-Kor Vented Needle #5213, 5214
Product cost: Not supplied   **Set cost:**   Not supplied
Product specifications: Eliminates the medication waste and patient risk associated with coring. No-Kor needle design features enhanced fluid flow. Speeds medication reconstitution by significantly lowering stopper penetration force

Becton Dickinson Division

Address: 1 Stanley Street, Rutherford, NJ 07070
Product type: Oral medication container
Product name/model: Tamper-Tuf #5203, #5204, #5205, #5206
Product cost: 250/case; $36.00–$46.50/case   **Set cost:**   Not supplied
Product specifications: Provides convenience in a completely self-contained design; no need to purchase and stock vials and caps separately. Eliminates metal cap crumpling and sharp edges

Becton Dickinson Division

Address: 1 Stanley Street, Rutherford, NJ 07070
Product type: Tip Caps
Product name/model: Tip Cap Trays, Catalog #8341
Product cost: 2000/case; $131.20/case   **Set cost:**   Not supplied
Product specifications: Preserves tip cap sterility and enhances syringe filling productivity. Upright positioning allows rapid capping and minimizes contamination

Burron Medical, Inc.

Address: 824 12th Avenue, Bethlehem, PA 18018
Product type: Needle-free system
Product name/model: SAFSITE Needle-free System
Product cost: $1.40 each (hospital list)   **Set cost:**   Not supplied
Product specifications: The SAFSITE System eliminates needles and needle access. The two-way SAFSITE valve attaches to I.V. tubing and opens with standard Luer taper from syringe or IV set. It closes automatically when taper is removed to prevent reflux. When not in use, the SAFSITE valve is capped with a dead-end red cap
Miscellaneous comments: Available with and without extension sets

Burron Medical, Inc.

Address: 824 12th Avenue, Bethlehem, PA 18018
Product type: Syringe caps
Product name/model: Syringe caps—SC-2000, SC-3000
Product cost: $18 each (hospital list)   **Set cost:**   Not supplied
Product specifications: Fully threaded Luer-lock syringe caps available in either red or blue; unique 10-pack blister tray protects sterility of unopened caps and aids in capping
Miscellaneous comments: 500 per case

Chartermed

Address: 170 Oberlin Ave., North Lakewood, NJ 08701
Product type: TPN containers

Product name/model: MixMe
Product cost: Not supplied **Set cost:** Not supplied
Product specifications: New line of automatic and gravity TPN containers; compatible with most automatic compounding systems; quick disconnect feature, eliminates the cut-and crimp process; made of non-DEHP vinyl; 100% leak-tested; available in all sizes

The Clinipad Corporation

Address: 66 High Street, Guilford, CT 06437
Product type: Standard I.V. start kits
Product name/model: I.V. Start Kit #5556
Product cost: $86.25 (case); $1.73 (kit) **Set cost:** Not supplied
Product specifications: Sterile, single-use kit containing the necessary components for I.V. site preparation and dressing change. The featured dressing is Bioclusive. Components include tourniquet, latex gloves, antiseptics, gauze, tape and dressing change label
Miscellaneous comments: Clinipad also has custom kit-manufacturing capabilities

The Clinipad Corporation

Address: 66 High Street, Guilford, CT 06437
Product type: Standard I.V. start kits
Product name/model: IV Start Kit #5550
Product cost: $86.25 (case); $1.73 (kit) **Set cost:** Not supplied
Product specifications: Sterile, single-use kit containing the necessary components for I.V. site preparation and dressing change. The featured dressing is Tegaderm. Components include tourniquet, latex gloves, antiseptics, gauze, tape and dressing change label
Miscellaneous comments: Clinipad also has custom kit-manufacturing capabilities

Conmed Corporation

Address: 310 Broad St., Utica, NY 13501
Product type: I.V. dressing
Product name/model: Veni-Gard
Product cost: $0.35 each **Set cost:** Not supplied
Product specifications: Veni-Gard is a unique I.V. dressing that maximizes stabilization of catheters for all applications, including peripheral, central, PICC, and arterial lines. Veni-Gard helps to minimize restarts, infiltraions, and clinical complications. Veni-Gard offers cost-effective I.V. care
Miscellaneous comments: Five models are available for all I.V. applications

HDC Corporation

Address: 2109 O'Toole Avenue, San Jose, CA 95131
Product type: Catheters
Product name/model: V-Cath #350 Series (2.0 FR), #360 Series (4.0 FR)
Product cost: $25–$51 (small and complete trays) **Set cost:** Not supplied
Product specifications: V-Cath is a radiopaque, silicone catheter (2, 3 and 4 FR) that is inserted into a peripheral vein via a breakaway introducer needle with tip placement in a central or peripheral vein

Miscellaneous comments: For more information, call HDC toll-free: 800-227-8162. In California, call toll-free: 800-752-3999

HDC Corporation

Address: 2109 O'Toole Avenue, San Jose, CA 95131
Product type: Implantable port
Product name/model: Chemo-Port implantable port
Product cost: List prices: $300–350 **Set cost:** Not supplied
Product specifications: Fluid delivery system provides longterm venous access for obtaining blood samples and administering drugs, blood products and TPN; available in regular or low profile size, in titanium and plastic. Available in 4, 7, and 9.6 FR
Miscellaneous comments: For more information, call HDC toll-free: 800-227-8162. In California, call toll-free: 800-752-3999

Healthtek, Inc.

Address: 870 Gold Flat Road, Nevada City, CA 95959
Product type: QC tester
Product name/model: QC tester, QC0102
Product cost: Not supplied **Set cost:** $8.30 each
Product specifications: A complete, convenient and cost-effective method for accurately checking for bacterial contamination of solutions

Ivac Corporation

Address: 10300 Campus Drive, San Diego, CA 92121
Product type: Infusion systems
Product name/model: CRIS System-Controlled Release Infusion System
Product cost: Not supplied **Set cost:** Not supplied
Product specifications: The CRIS adapter is a non-dedicated disposable device designed to facilitate delivery of secondary medications directly from a reconstituted drug manufacturer's 5- to 20-ml vial, eliminating the need for minibags and secondary sets
Miscellaneous comments: The CRIS adapter remains as part of the primary administration set, so it is replaced only as frequently as the set is changed

Medfusion Inc.

Address: 3450 River Green Court, Duluth, GA 30136
Product type: Administration sets
Product name/model: Multiple Administration Sets and Filter Sets
Product cost: Not supplied **Set cost:** Not supplied
Product specifications: Medfusion manufactures needleless mini and low-volume multiple administration sets, such as the Bifuse and Trifuse and mini bifuse and trifuse with lower priming volumes. Filter sets feature low priming volumes and 0.22 micron air venting filters
Miscellaneous comments: Medfusion products are now represented by Medex Inc. Hospital Infusion Systems

Medi-Dose, Inc./E.P.S., Inc.

Address: 1671 Loretta Avenue, Feasterville, PA 19053-7393
Product type: Filter needles

Product name/model: E.P.S. Filter Needle 18 gauge, IV1518; 20 gauge, IV1520
Product cost: Both styles, 50/case; 1–4 cases, $31.00/case; 5–9 cases, $30.00/case; 10–24 cases, $29.00/case; 25–49 cases $27.00/case
Product specifications: Filter needle for medication filtration from rubber-stoppered vials; designed with specially constructed stainless steel, non-shedding, sintered depth filter; equipped with an anti-coring needle point; needles are 18- or 20-gauge lumen, 1 1/2" length
Miscellaneous comments: Toll-free: 800-523-8966; toll free fax: 800-323-8966

Medi-Dose, Inc./E.P.S., Inc.

Address: 1671 Loretta Avenue, Feasterville, PA 19053-7393
Product type: Filter aspirator
Product name/model: E.P.S. Filter Aspirator, Catalog IV1530
Product cost: 50/case; 1–4 cases, $35.00/case; 5–9 cases, $34.00/case; 10–24 cases, $33.00/case; 25–49 cases $31.00/case
Product specifications: E.P.S. Filter Aspirator for medication filtration from ampules. Filter Aspirator designed with specially constructed, stainless steel, cup-shaped, non-shedding sintered depth filter. Aspirator is equipped with an 18-gauge, 3-inch blunt needle
Miscellaneous comments: Toll-free: 800-523-8966; toll free fax: 800-323-8966

Medi-Dose, Inc./E.P.S., Inc.

Address: 1671 Loretta Avenue, Feasterville, PA 19053-7393
Product type: Bag rings
Product name/model: Multi-Dose I.V. Bag Rings, Model #PC2116
Product cost: 500/box; 1–4 boxes, $26/box; 5–9 boxes, $24.75/box; 10–24 boxes, $23.75/box; 25–49 boxes, $23/box
Product specifications: Used to safely and economically identify groupings of I.V. bags by patient, department, time, floor—whatever a facility requires. Rings do not dry out, snap, or fade with use
Miscellaneous comments: Toll-free: 800-523-8966; toll free fax: 800-323-8966

Medi-Dose, Inc./E.P.S., Inc.

Address: 1671 Loretta Avenue, Feasterville, PA 19053-7393
Product type: Luer-lock closures
Product name/model: Combi-Cap Male/Female Luer-Lock Closure, IV2100
Product cost: 100/case; 1–4 cases, $23.00/case; 5–9 cases, $21.00/case; 10–24 cases, $20.00/case; 25–49 cases $19.00/case
Product specifications: Multi-function male/female Luer-lock closure. It is secure and versatile, ideal for capping I.V. syringes, catheters and hypodermic products. Distinctive colors aid in flagging and recognizing medication requiring special handling. Innovative flat base design allows prefilled syringes to stand upright, saving space and guarding against "touch contamination"
Miscellaneous comments: Toll-free: 800-523-8966; toll free fax: 800-323-8966

Medi-Dose, Inc./E.P.S., Inc.

Address: 1671 Loretta Avenue, Feasterville, PA 19053-7393
Product type: Transfer spike

Product name/model: Double-Ended, Medication Transfer Spike, Model TS1800
Product cost: 100/box; $58/box; 360 Bulk Pack, $185/case
Product specifications: For bottle-to-bottle transfer of I.V. fluids, amino acids, etc. Special venting design simultaneously permits air displacement and the transfer of medication, eliminating the use of extra needles. Rigid bell cover protects spike prior to use and minimizes "touch contamination." Wide stopper/flange facilitates aseptic technique. Double spike construction utilizes existing vacuum of IV glass containers
Miscellaneous comments: Toll-free: 800-523-8966; toll free fax: 800-323-8966

Medi-Dose, Inc./E.P.S., Inc.

Address: 1671 Loretta Avenue, Feasterville, PA 19053-7393
Product type: Injection ports
Product name/model: Injection-Port Device, Model #IV2003
Product cost: 100/case; 1–4 cases, $58.00/case; 5–9 cases, $54.00/case; 10–24 cases, $52.00/case; 25–49 cases $50.00/case
Product specifications: The large non-removable, recessed port offers sizable area for injection and protects against "touch contamination." The injection site is made from durable, compressed latex and will reseal after repetitive punctures; clear design shows blood flashback
Miscellaneous comments: Toll-free: 800-523-8966; toll free fax: 800-323-8966

Medi-Dose, Inc./E.P.S., Inc.

Address: 1671 Loretta Avenue, Feasterville, PA 19053-7393
Product type: Filter
Product name/model: 0.45 micron Disposable Disc Filter, Model #IV4500
Product cost: 50/case; 1–4 cases, $58.00/case; 5–9 cases, $55.00/case; 10–24 cases, $52.50/case; 25–49 cases $49.00/case
Product specifications: Sterile, nontoxic, nonpyrogenic 0.45-micron filter for filtration and particulate matter retention; equipped with male and female Luer-locks; filter removes stopper coring ampule fragments and other particulates during admixture procedures
Miscellaneous comments: Toll-free: 800-523-8966; toll free fax: 800-323-8966

Medi-Dose, Inc./E.P.S., Inc.

Address: 1671 Loretta Avenue, Feasterville, PA 19053-7393
Product type: Filters
Product name/model: 0.2 micron Disposable Disc Filter, Model #IV2500
Product cost: 50/case; 1–4 cases, $65.00/case; 5–9 cases, $63.00/case; 10–24 cases, $60.00/case; 25–49 cases $58.00/case
Product specifications: Sterile, nontoxic, nonpyrogenic 0.22 micron sterilizing filter; indicated for sterilization and bacteria-retentive applications; equipped with male and female Luer-locks; prevents spraying, splashing or breaks in sterility; removes stopper coring and other particulates during admixture; design offers minimal internal fluid loss; can be used for both aspiration and injection, withstanding up to 75 psi
Miscellaneous comments: toll-free: 800-523-8966; toll free fax: 800-323-8966

Menlo Care, Inc.

Address: 1350 Willow Road, Menlo Park, CA 94025
Product type: I.V. catheters
Product name/model: Streamline peripheral venous access device
Product cost: Not supplied **Set cost:** Not supplied
Product specifications: Streamline is the only peripheral catheter that expands two gauge sizes and softens in the vessel. Initially rigid, Streamline becomes flexible like silicone after insertion to reduce complications for longer dwell, resulting in fewer restarts (Published references available)
Miscellaneous comments: Cannulas made of Aquavene, a proprietary biomaterial. Gauge sizes 18–26 (16–24 in situ)

Menlo Care, Inc.

Address: 1350 Willow Road, Menlo Park, CA 94025
Product type: I.V. catheters
Product name/model: Landmark Midline Catheter
Product cost: Not supplied **Set cost:** Not supplied
Product specifications: Landmark, which is designed for intermediate-term therapies, allows simple-over-the-needle insertion without guidewires or introducers. Landmark becomes soft and flexible for reduced complications and improved dwell and its needle safety tube prevents accidental needlesticks and blood exposure
Miscellaneous comments: Cannulas made of Aquavene, a new biomaterial. Lengths: 6" and 3". Gauge sizes: 17, 20, 22, 24 (15–22 in situ)

Millipore Corp.

Address: 80 Ashby Road, E8C Bedford, MA 01730
Product type: Syringe filters, transfer sets with filters, QC testing systems, neonatal I.V. filters
Product name/model: Millex Syringe Filters, Millifil Filter Transfer Set, Addichek and Steritest Admixture QC Systems, Cathevex-2 Neonatal I.V. filter set
Product cost: Not supplied **Set cost:** Not supplied
Product specifications: Millipore membrane filtration products help to protect patients from microorganism and particulate contamination. Millex syringe filters are offered in a variety of volume and pore sizes. The AddiChek and Steritest systems meet USP guidelines for sterile product testing

Pall Biomedical Products Corp.

Address: 77 Crescent Beach Road, Glen Cove, New York 11542
Product type: I.V. filter
Product name/model: ELD-96 Set Saver Filter
Product cost: Not supplied **Set cost:** Not supplied
Product specifications: The ELD-96 Set Saver Filter has been approved for up to 96-hr use in the administration of I.V. fluids. It protects patients against inadvertent particulate matter, entrained air, microbial contaminants and any inadvertent endotoxins present in I.V. solutions
Miscellaneous comments: The ELD-96 Set Saver filter is available from Pall Biomedical Products Corporation; phone: 516-759-1900

Pharmacia Deltec

Address: 1265 Grey Fox Road, St. Paul, MN 55112
Product type: Peripheral venous access system
Product name/model: P.A.S. PORT Fluoro-Free Peripheral Venous Access System, Model #21-4501
Product cost: $575 (list) **Set cost:** Not supplied
Product specifications: Peripherally placed ultra-low profile portal system for venous delivery of medications, fluids and nutritional solutions, and for venous blood sampling; eliminates need for fluoroscopy during catheter placement when used with Cath-Finder Catheter Tracking system
Miscellaneous comments: P.A.S. PORT expands options for central venous access; for more information, call toll-free: 800-426-2448

Pharmacia Deltec

Address: 1265 Grey Fox Road, St. Paul, MN 55112
Product type: Implantable epidural access system
Product name/model: PORT-A-PORT Epidural Access System, model #21-0501
Product cost: $695 (list) **Set cost:** Not supplied
Product specifications: Allows long-term, repeated access to the epidural space for the delivery of preservative-free morphine sulfate to relieve intractable pain in cancer patients
Miscellaneous comments: For more information, call toll-free: 800-426-2448

Pharmacia Deltec

Address: 1265 Grey Fox Road, St. Paul, MN 55112
Product type: Implantable venous access system
Product name/model: PORT-A-CATH Venous Access System, Model #21-4000, #21-4010
Product cost: $415 (list) **Set cost:** Not supplied
Product specifications: For parenteral delivery of medications, fluids, and nutritional solutions, and for sampling of venous blood; titanium for lighter weight and ease of imaging; high-density SECUR SITE septum
Miscellaneous comments: Implant tray available; low profile model (unassembled) also available; for more information, call toll-free: 800-426-2448

QI Medical, Inc.

Address: 349 Brock Road, P.O. Box 1329, Nevada City, CA 95959
Product type: Bacterial contamination testers
Product name/model: QuickTest Systems, #QT1000 and QT2000
Product cost: $11.75–$12.75 each **Set cost:** Included
Product specifications: QuickTest provides quick and convenient full filtration testing for bacterial contamination of regular and 3-in-1 TPN admixtures. QT1000 attaches in line with many gravity transfer sets and compounders to eliminate wasted bags and vacuum bottles
Miscellaneous comments: Flow rates 4–10 times faster than other testers; 10–100 times more sensitive than aliquots

Quest Medical, Inc.

Address: 4103 Billy Mitchell Dr., Dallas, TX 75244
Product type: Extension, I.V. sets
Product name/model: No Needles Extension Sets and I.V. sets
Product cost: $2.95–$5.95 **Set cost:** Not supplied
Product specifications: Various designs of No Needles I.V. delivery sets and extension sets, which allow on-handed injection, prevent unwanted retrograding, have no handles to turn, and require no needles
Miscellaneous comments: Available through Quest Medical, 800-627-0226

Quinton Instrument Company

Address: 2121 Terry Avenue, Seattle, WA 98121
Product type: Peritoneal catheters
Product name/model: Peritoneal Catheters
Product cost: Not supplied **Set cost:** Not supplied
Product specifications: Curl Cath and Tenckhoff peritoneal catheters provide reliable access for peritoneal dialysis and intra-peritoneal chemotherapy; assorted lengths and cuff styles, all packaged with Beta-Cap adapter, cap and clamp. Quinton Peritoneal Catheter Kits feature a Pull-Apart Introducer, an alternative to placement by laparotomy

Quinton Instrument Company

Address: 2121 Terry Avenue, Seattle, WA 98121
Product type: Dialysis and apheresis
Product name/model: Mahurkar Dual Lumen Catheters
Product cost: Not supplied **Set cost:** Not supplied
Product specifications: Mahurkar Dual Lumen Catheters are ideal for quick, efficient vaascular access for dialysis and apheresis. Optional curved extensions facilitate dressing and patient comfort. VitaCuff infection control device reduces bacteria fourfold
Miscellaneous comments: Catheters are available in a variety of lengths and convenient kits and trays

Solopak

Address: 1845 Tonne Road, Elk Grove Village, IL 60007
Product type: Syringes
Product name/model: SoloPak Hy-Pod Syringes
Product cost: $0.90–$1.20/prefilled syringe **Set cost:** Not supplied
Product specifications: Disposable prefilled syringes to maintain catheter patency. Available in a range of fill volumes, concentrations and package styles, covering many catheter care protocols and procedures. Can be used with a standard needle, specialty needle, or with needleless systems
Miscellaneous comments: System promotes aseptic technique and reduces patient teaching time

Terumo Medical Corporation

Address: 2100 Cottontail Lane, Somerset, NJ 08873
Product type I.V. catheters

Product name/model: Surflo I.V. Catheters and Surflo I.V. Catheters with wings
Product cost: $97/box; $99.50/box (winged)   **Set cost:**   Not supplied
Product specifications: Over-the-needle I.V. catheters and over-the-needle I.V. catheters with wings for infusion therapy.

Top Corporation c/o Wulf Enterprises

Address: P.O. Box 398, Pleasanton, CA 94566
Product type: Stop cocks
Product name/model: Top Stop Cock
Product cost: $0.45–$0.55   **Set cost:**   Not supplied
Product specifications: Rugged construction with smooth turning design, incorporating additional insert pin to provide added leak-proof feature
Miscellaneous comments: Product in blister/tyvek package with or without Luer-lock and cap

Top Corporation c/o Wulf Enterprises

Address: P.O. Box 398, Pleasanton, CA 94566
Product type: Infusion sets
Product name/model: Top Infusion Sets
Product cost: Not supplied   **Set cost:** $0.60–$0.70
Product specifications: Top infusion sets are designed with highly elastic PVC tubing, which inhibits the formation of kinks. The unique needle point with flexible wings allow for easy anchoring and maximum patient comfort
Miscellaneous comments: Packaged in individual blister/tyvek container in sizes 18 G through 27 G

Wyeth-Ayerst Laboratories

Address: 555 East Lancaster Ave., St. David's, PA 19034
Product type: Injectables
Product name/model: Tubex Injector
Product cost: Free to Tubex users   **Set cost:**   Not supplied
Product specifications: The design of the Tubex injector reduces the risk of accidental needlesticks. It offers a simple twist-and-drop disposal procedure, keeping your hand farther from the point of danger

Index

Page numbers in *italic* indicate figures; numbers followed by "t" indicate tables.